Advances in Healthcare Technology

Philips Research

VOLUME 6

Editor-in-Chief
Dr. Frank Toolenaar
Philips Research Laboratories, Eindhoven, The Netherlands

SCOPE TO THE *'PHILIPS RESEARCH BOOK SERIES'*

As one of the largest private sector research establishments in the world, Philips Research is shaping the future with technology inventions that meet peoples' needs and desires in the digital age. While the ultimate user benefits of these inventions end up on the high-street shelves, the often pioneering scientific and technological basis usually remains less visible.

This 'Philips Research Book Series' has been set up as a way for Philips researchers to contribute to the scientific community by publishing their comprehensive results and theories in book form.

Dr. Rick Harwig

Advances in Healthcare Technology

Shaping the Future of Medical Care

Edited by

Gerhard Spekowius

Philips Research Europe, Aachen, Germany

and

Thomas Wendler

Philips Research Europe, Hamburg, Germany

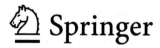 Springer

A C.I.P. Catalogue record for this book is available from the Library of Congress.

ISBN-10 1-4020-4383-X (HB)
ISBN-13 978-1-4020-4383-3 (HB)
ISBN-10 1-4020-4384-8 (e-book)
ISBN-13 978-1-4020-4384-0 (e-book)

Published by Springer,
P.O. Box 17, 3300 AA Dordrecht, The Netherlands.

www.springer.com

Printed on acid-free paper

TABLE OF CONTENTS

PART I: TRENDS IN HEALTHCARE

Chapter 1
Robert Gossink, Jacques Souquet

PART II: DIAGNOSTIC IMAGING

Chapter 2
Falko Busse

Chapter 3
Roland Proksa

Chapter 4
Michael Overdick

Chapter 5
Volker Rasche, Michael Grass, Robert Manzke

Chapter 6
Peter Bornert, Kay Nehrke, Dye Jensen

Chapter 7
Christopher S. Hall

Chapter 8

**PART III: INTEGRATION OF DIAGNOSTIC IMAGING
            AND THERAPY**

Chapter 9

Chapter 10

Chapter 11

Chapter 12

Chapter 13

Chapter 14

PART IV: MOLECULAR MEDICINE

Chapter 15

CONTRIBUTING AUTHORS

Xavier-Louis Aubert PhD
Senior Scientist, Medical Signal Processing, Philips Research Europe - Aachen, Germany

Golo von Basum PhD
Senior Scientist, Care and Health Applications, Philips Research Europe - Eindhoven, The Netherlands

Christopher Bauer
Mechanical Design Engineer, CT Clinical Science Department, Philips Medical Systems, Cleveland, OH, USA

Florian Beyer MD
Radiologist, Institute for Radiology, University Hospital, Münster, Germany

Thomas Blaffert PhD
Senior Scientist, Digital Imaging, Philips Research Europe - Hamburg, Germany

Peter Börnert PhD
Principal Scientist, Tomographic Imaging Systems, Philips Research Europe - Hamburg, Germany

Jörn Borgert PhD
Senior Scientist, Tomographic Imaging Systems, Philips Research Europe - Hamburg, Germany

Andreas Brauers PhD
Research Scientist, Medical Signal Processing, Philips Research Europe - Aachen, Germany

Thomas Bülow PhD
Research Scientist, Digital Imaging, Philips Research Europe - Hamburg, Germany

Falko Busse PhD
Vice President Philips Research, Director Medical Imaging Systems, Philips Research Europe - Hamburg, Germany

Ingwer C. Carlsen PhD
Principal Scientist, Digital Imaging, Philips Research Europe - Hamburg,
Germany

Shelton D. Caruthers PhD
Senior Clinical Scientist, Philips Medical Systems, and
Associate Director, Cardiovascular MR Laboratories, Washington University
School of Medicine, St. Louis, MO, USA

Nicolas W. Chbat PhD
Senior Member of the Research Staff, Healthcare Systems and IT Department,
Philips Research North America - Briarcliff Manor, NY, USA

Eric Cohen-Solal PhD
Senior Member Research Staff, Healthcare Systems and IT, Philips Research
North America - Briarcliff Manor, NY, USA

Ekta Dharaiya
Staff Scientist, CT Clinical Science, Philips Medical Systems, Cleveland, OH,
USA

Nevenka Dimitrova PhD
Research Fellow, Healthcare Systems and IT, Philips Research North America -
Briarcliff Manor, NY, USA

Rufus Driessen
Principal Scientist, Care and Health Applications, Philips Research Europe -
Eindhoven, The Netherlands

Tadashi Egami
Product Manager Motiva, New Ventures, Philips Medical Systems, Milpitas CA,
USA

Matthias Egger PhD
Sales and Marketing Manager PET Europe, Philips Medical Systems, Gland,
Switzerland

Ahmet Ekin PhD
Senior Scientist, Video Processing, Philips Research Europe - Eindhoven, The
Netherlands

Martin Elixmann PhD
Department Head, Connectivity Systems, Philips Research Europe - Aachen, Germany

Thomas Falck
Senior Scientist, Connectivity Systems, Philips Research Europe - Aachen, Germany

Klaus Fiedler PhD
Senior Scientist, Molecular Imaging Systems, Philips Research Europe - Aachen, Germany

Raoul Florent
Principal Scientist, Philips Medical Systems Research, Paris, France

Robert G. Gossink PhD
formerly Managing Director Philips Research Germany and Program Manager Healthcare Systems, presently advisor to Philips Research, Philips Research Europe - Aachen, Germany

Michael Grass PhD
Senior Scientist, Tomographic Imaging Systems, Philips Research Europe - Hamburg, Germany

Holger Grüll PhD
Senior Scientist, Biomolecular Engineering, Philips Research Europe - Eindhoven, The Netherlands

York Hämisch PhD
Product Manager Pre-Clinical Imaging Systems, Molecular Imaging Division, Philips Medical Systems, Böblingen, Germany

Christopher S. Hall PhD
Principal Member Research Staff, Healthcare Systems and IT, Philips Research North America - Briarcliff Manor, NY, USA

Ori Hay
Staff Scientist, CT Clinical Applications, Philips Medical Systems, Haifa, Israel

Eike Hein MD
Radiologist, Institute for Radiology, Charité Hospital, Humboldt University, Berlin, Germany

Horace Hines PhD
Chief Technical Officer, Nuclear Medicine, Philips Medical Systems, Milpitas, CA, USA

Ralf Hoffmann PhD
Principal Scientist, Biomolecular Engineering, Philips Research Europe - Eindhoven, The Netherlands

Hans Hofstraat PhD
Vice President Philips Research, Director Molecular Medicine, Philips Research Europe - Eindhoven, The Netherlands

Leonard Hofstra MD PhD
Associate Professor of Cardiology, Department of Cardiology, Cardiovascular Research Institute Maastricht, University Maastricht, The Netherlands

Claudia Hannelore Igney PhD
Research Scientist, Medical Signal Processing, Philips Research Europe - Aachen, Germany

Dye Jensen PhD
Department Head, Tomographic Imaging Systems, Philips Research Europe - Hamburg, Germany

Wendy B. Katzman
Principal, Decision Point Consulting, Seattle, WA, USA

Michael R. Kaus PhD
Senior Scientist, Digital Imaging, Philips Research Europe - Hamburg, Germany

Kenneth A. Krohn PhD
Professor of Radiology and Radiation Oncology, Adjunct Professor of Chemistry, University of Washington, Seattle, WA, USA

Jochen Krücker PhD
Senior Member Research Staff, Clinical Sites Research, Philips Research North America - Briarcliff Manor, NY, USA

Sascha Krüger PhD
Research Scientist, Tomographic Imaging Systems, Philips Research Europe - Hamburg, Germany

Michael Kuhn PhD
Vice President Technology Strategy, Philips Medical Systems, Hamburg,
Germany

Charles Lagor MD PhD
Senior Member Research Staff, Healthcare Systems and IT, Philips Research
North America - Briarcliff Manor, NY, USA

Gregory M. Lanza MD PhD
Associate Professor of Medicine and Bioengineering, Cardiovascular Division,
Washington University Medical School, St. Louis, MO USA

Chuck Little
General Manager, Philips AED Business, Cardiac Solutions, Philips Medical
Systems, Seattle, WA, USA

Cor Loef
Program Manager Interoperability, Business Group Healthcare IT, Philips
Medical Systems, Best, The Netherlands

William P. Lord
Principal Member Research Staff, Healthcare Systems and IT, Philips Research
North America - Briarcliff Manor, NY, USA

Todd R. McNutt PhD
Assistant Professor, Department of Radiation Oncology, Johns Hopkins School
of Medicine, Baltimore, MD, USA

Sherif Makram-Ebeid PhD
Research Fellow, Philips Medical Systems Research, Paris, France

Robert Manzke PhD
Senior Member Research Staff, Clinical Sites Research, Philips Research North
America - Briarcliff Manor, NY, USA

Chrit T.W. Moonen PhD
Research Director, Laboratory for Molecular and Functional Imaging, Centre
Nationale de la Recherche Scientifique, University 'Victor Segalen Bordeaux 2',
Bordeaux, France

Francisco Morales PhD
Department Head, Care and Health Applications, Philips Research Europe -
Eindhoven, The Netherlands

Charles Mougenot
PhD student, Laboratory for Molecular and Functional Imaging, Centre
Nationale de la Recherche Scientifique, University 'Victor Segalen Bordeaux 2',
Bordeaux, France

Babak Movassaghi PhD
Senior Member Research Staff, Clinical Sites Research, Philips Research North
America - Briarcliff Manor, NY, USA

Jens Mühlsteff PhD
Research Scientist, Medical Signal Processing, Philips Research Europe -
Aachen, Germany

Kay Nehrke PhD
Senior Scientist, Tomographic Imaging Systems, Philips Research Europe -
Hamburg, Germany

Roland Opfer PhD
Research Scientist, Digital Imaging, Philips Research Europe - Hamburg,
Germany

Begonya Otal
Research Scientist, Medical Signal Processing, Philips Research Europe -
Aachen, Germany

Michael Overdick PhD
Department Head, X-ray Imaging Systems, Philips Research Europe - Aachen,
Germany

Jeff Perry
Program Director Motiva, New Ventures, Philips Medical Systems, Milpitas,
CA, USA

Joost Peters PhD
Staff Scientist, Advanced Development, Medical IT, Philips Medical Systems,
Best, The Netherlands

John Petruzzello PhD
Senior Member Research Staff, Healthcare Systems and IT, Philips Research
North America - Briarcliff Manor, USA

Robert Pinter PhD
Research Scientist, Medical Signal Processing, Philips Research Europe - Aachen, Germany

Roland Proksa
Research Fellow, Tomographic Imaging Systems, Philips Research Europe - Hamburg, Germany

Balasundar Raju PhD
Senior Member Research Staff, Healthcare Systems and IT, Philips Research North America - Briarcliff Manor, USA

Volker Rasche PhD
Professor of Cardiovascular Magnetic Resonance Imaging, University of Ulm, Ulm, Germany

Harald Reiter
Senior Scientist, Medical Signal Processing, Philips Research Europe - Aachen, Germany

Chris Reutelingsperger PhD
Associate Professor of Biochemistry, Department of Biochemistry, Cardiovascular Research Institute Maastricht, University Maastricht, The Netherlands

Steffen Renisch PhD
Senior Scientist, Digital Imaging, Philips Research Europe - Hamburg, Germany

Marc S. Robillard PhD
Senior Scientist, Molecular and Biomolecular Engineering, Philips Research Europe - Eindhoven, The Netherlands

Patrik Rogalla MD
Senior Radiologist, Institute for Radiology, Charité Hospital, Humboldt University, Berlin, Germany

Valentina Romano MD
Radiologist, Institute for Radiology, Charité Hospital, Humboldt University, Berlin, Germany

Helen Routh PhD
Research Department Head, Healthcare Systems and IT, Philips Research North
America - Briarcliff Manor, NY, USA

Jörg Sabczynski PhD
Senior Scientist, Digital Imaging Department, Philips Research Europe -
Hamburg, Germany

J. David Schaffer PhD
Research Fellow, Healthcare Systems and IT, Philips Research North America -
Briarcliff Manor, NY, USA

Tobias Schaeffter PhD
Principal Scientist, Tomographic Imaging Systems, Philips Research Europe -
Hamburg, Germany

Kristiane Schmidt PhD
Senior Scientist, Care and Health Applications, Philips Research Europe -
Eindhoven, The Netherlands

David P.L. Simons PhD
Senior Architect, Software Architectures, Philips Research Europe - Eindhoven,
The Netherlands

Kees Smedema
Senior Director Business Development, Business Group Healthcare IT, Philips
Medical Systems, Best, The Netherlands

Jacques Souquet PhD
President, SuperSonic Imagine, SA, Aix-en-Provence Cedex, France

Gerhard Spekowius PhD
Business Development Manager, Philips Research Europe - Aachen, Germany

Lothar Spies PhD
Department Head, Digital Imaging, Philips Research Europe - Hamburg,
Germany

Olaf Such PhD
Senior Scientist, Medical Signal Processing, Philips Research Europe - Aachen,
Germany

Eric Thelen
Department Head, Medical Signal Processing, Philips Research Europe - Aachen, Germany

Jeroen A.J. Thijs
Research Scientist, Medical Signal Processing, Philips Research Europe - Aachen, Germany

Holger Timinger PhD
Research Scientist, Tomographic Imaging Systems, Philips Research Europe - Hamburg, Germany

Roel Truyen
Senior Scientist, Advanced Development, Medical IT, Philips Medical System, Best, The Netherlands

Bert Verdonck
Marketing Director Radiology IT, Business Group Healthcare IT, Philips Medical System, Best, The Netherlands

Thomas Wendler PhD
Research Fellow, Philips Research Europe - Hamburg, Germany

Gordon R. Whiteley PhD
Director, Clinical Proteomics Reference Lab, SAIC-Frederick, Inc., NCI Frederick, Gaithersburg, MD, USA

Samuel A. Wickline MD
Professor of Medicine, Biomedical Engineering, Physics, and Cellular Physiology, Washington University School of Medicine, St. Louis, MO, USA

Rafael Wiemker PhD
Senior Scientist, Digital Imaging, Philips Research Europe - Hamburg, Germany

Dale C. Wiggins
Senior Architect, Patient Monitoring, Philips Medical Systems, Andover, MA, USA

Dag Wormanns MD
Staff Radiologist, Department of Clinical Radiology, University Hospital, Münster, Germany

Jeffrey Yanof PhD
Senior Staff Scientist and Manager Image-Guided Therapy, Clinical Science
Department, Philips Medical Systems, Cleveland, OH, USA

Thomas Zaengel PhD
Vice President Philips Research, Director Monitoring and Treatment, Philips
Research Europe - Aachen, Germany

Michael Q. Zhang PhD
Professor, Computational Biology and Bioinformatics Lab, Cold Spring Harbour
Laboratory, Cold Spring Harbour, NY, USA

PREFACE

Staying healthy and getting appropriate healthcare is certainly one of the most important issues in our society. In a continuous effort, huge investments are made to improve the value of the healthcare system. Among the many ways to optimize medical care, technology plays a predominant role. It not only helps to increase the quality, effectiveness and efficiency of health related procedures, it often stimulates and enables new ways to practise medicine. Apparently, the success of western medicine is to a large extent based on technology driven innovation. In the last century we have increasingly seen breakthrough improvements in medicine that were induced or supported by new technologies, and that were unthinkable without them, leading to better and often revolutionary new ways to detect or solve health problems. Advances in imaging technology, for instance, with the invention of computed tomography (CT) or magnetic resonance imaging (MRI) about thirty years ago, have certainly marked disruptive change for many procedures in diagnosis and therapy.

At the beginning of the new millennium, it is reasonable to expect that the role of technology in the medical innovation process will increase in proportion to the enormous amount of R&D efforts worldwide. The potential impact of research to the medical field is illustrated by the fact that 90% of all researchers - since the beginnings of mankind - live today. The amount of research results that will directly or indirectly influence medicine may easily increase by an order of magnitude over the coming decades.

Medical technology innovation is a complex process, in which industry, academia, clinical institutions and regulatory bodies act closely together. This book has been edited from the perspective of industrial research, and emphasizes the fact that R&D in industry is significantly contributing to many health related innovations and breakthroughs. The material presented here is published as part of a Philips Research book series. Philips, as one of the major players in the field, has a continuous, strong and successful healthcare and wellness oriented research program. This program is addressing very essential topics that will help shape the future of medical care. It is linked to many academic research activities, and to clinical research and validation performed at world-renowned hospital sites.

It is the general intention of this book to present a collection of innovative and valuable contributions to healthcare technology. The chapters were selected to cover different application areas ranging from hospital to home, and to create different views on how technology influences critical aspects of patient care. The aim was to gather a set of high quality contributions, each addressing different aspects of technology and application, resulting in a mix of state-of-the-art overviews, projections to the future, discussion of trends, and - as for most chapters - the presentation of research results for selected areas. Paradigm-changing developments expected for the coming decades are indicated.

In particular, the book is intended to give an overview of recent research results of the Philips healthcare and wellness research program, complemented by contributions from Philips Medical Systems, and chapters provided by distinguished clinical sites or universities. Improvement of medical care is shown as the result of collaboration between industry, academia and clinics. The content spans a combination of long-standing industrial research areas (such as imaging technology), new and rapidly evolving fields (like molecular medicine), important enabling technologies (like medical information technology) and innovations that open up novel ways to look at health care in a changing world (such as personal healthcare home care, and healthcare consumer oriented aspects). Overwiew chapters give general insight for the addressed research fields and also discuss trends that will influence and shape healthcare technology in the future.

How is the book organized? We have prepared the material along a number of specific healthcare related topics, reflected by the 6 independent parts of the book:

The opening **Healthcare trends** part sets the stage for all the following, describing some drivers for recent and future changes in healthcare. These cannot be understood without the socio-economic developments in society, particularly the aging society and the related growth of chronic disease, and the healthcare politics that these developments induce. For advances in technology, some major trends are singled out, such as the impact of Moore's Law on medical imaging, the revolutionary changes anticipated through molecular medicine, and expected new and growing sectors such as e-health and personal healthcare.

Diagnostic imaging is a long-standing and very successful area of innovation and certainly a mainstay for improving diagnosis and therapy, extending far into the future as more specific techniques such as molecular imaging evolve. The past decades have seen an unmatched progress in the optimization of imaging modalities towards better performance in speed and resolution, and for new applications, enabled by computing power, new imaging principles and agents. The attempt to complement anatomical with functional information has seen developments combining the strength of individual modalities. The imaging chapters in the second part give an overview of state-of-the-art and address recent achievements of imaging modalities. For CT, enabling technologies such as detectors and reconstruction techniques are discussed. For X-ray based volume techniques, principles and clinical applications of 3D-rotational X-ray imaging on conventional C-arm systems are presented. Representative for the many advances in MRI, recent problems and methodological solutions are described for coronary magnetic resonance angiography (CMRA). Improvements in ultrasound include four-dimensional ultrasound imaging, which impressively shows real-time rendering of moving anatomy with new applications in interventional cardiology and radiology. In the last 10 years, hybrid imaging systems such as PET/CT and SPECT/CT have become a rapid scientific and commercial success, as they meet strong clinical demands for matching anatomical and functional information. Continuous research is ongoing to improve and optimize the imaging methods as well as techniques for image fusion and co-registration.

The combination of diagnostic imaging with therapy is a significant trend and is paving the road to treatment centres of the future. In image-guided therapy (IGT), imaging is used to plan, implement and follow-up treatment, and to improve treatment accuracy through better planning and precise targeting. Recent trends and innovations in the field are reviewed in part 3. Multi-modality-guided percutaneous ablation based on CT data and a CT-integrated robot system are discussed. Successful techniques are described for catheter-based cardiac interventions that have recently been introduced into clinical practice. The field of high intensity focused ultrasound (HIFU) is presented, a technology to generate therapeutic local hyperthermia inside the body, using MRI guidance of the procedure to allow optimized in situ target definition and the identification of nearby tissue to be spared. Another application shown is image-guidance in adaptive radiation therapy through monitoring the course of treatment. Finally, an example for molecular imaging guided radiation therapy is presented in which the assessment of tumor markers is investigated with the perspective to optimize future radiation therapy.

Molecular medicine is expected to become the big game changer in medical care. Understanding disease phenomena on the molecular level and deriving according methods for diagnosis and therapy will truly be a paradigm shifting change in medicine. Application wise, it has the potential to take the step from a symptom-based diagnosis and treatment to a medicine of the future focussing on prediction, prevention, understanding of disease processes, highly individualized treatment and cure of diseases. Technology-wise, it is marking a shift from traditional research disciplines such as mechanics, electronics, and physics to molecular biology and genetics. The main technologies that enable the field are the *in vivo* identification of disease location through highly specific targeted agents (molecular imaging), and the *in vitro* detection of biomarkers (molecular diagnostics). In part 4, a comprehensive review of molecular imaging systems and their relevant properties (e.g. their sensitivity) is presented, followed by various chapters on biomarkers and agents for diagnosis and therapy including their clinical applications

Medical information technology appears as an important factor for improving the quality and efficiency of patient care, for significantly reducing cost, and as enabler for new methods and applications. IT support has become essential for modern medicine. This part of the book starts with a global view on the IT research field, focussing on technology for physicians, patients and researchers. Challenges in the creation of electronic medical records (EMR), departmental IT systems, and workflow solutions are addressed. A growing field of medical IT research is its application in computer-aided detection (CAD) and computer-aided diagnosis (CADx), for which successful examples in lung nodule detection are presented. Another vital field is covered through research on medical decision support systems (DSS). Bioinformatics research shows that some areas in biology and medicine are strongly based on IT and generate excitement about new potential clinical applications such as clinical genotyping, early diagnosis, prognostic disease models, personalized medicine and wellness monitoring.

Last but not least, the field of **personal healthcare** indicates important changes in the healthcare system, induced by changes in the society such as the aging population, the pressure to rethink healthcare financing, and changing demands of health care consumers. New and rapidly emerging sectors of care move away from the traditional cycle of hospital-based diagnosis, therapy and follow-up: Self care, home care, remote monitoring devices and services hold promises to individualize care while reducing cost. Wellness programs and prevention measures become increasingly attractive that support health and well being preceding the traditional hospital care, and call for novel devices and services. Technology wise, new sensors, easy to use devices for diagnosis, treatment and monitoring, electronics for home and ubiquitous use mark the way to the aspects of personal healthcare as presented in the final part of the book.

Gerhard Spekowius and Thomas Wendler, September 2005

ACKNOWLEDGMENTS

As editors, we thank all authors for their excellent and exciting chapters. Particularly, we appreciate the distinguished contributions provided by academic and clinical researchers. Furthermore, we acknowledge the valuable input of our Philips Medical Systems colleagues

The creation of this book was supported by an editorial board with key members of the Philips Research organization. We like to thank all board members for their assistance in setting up and improving the individual parts:

Helen Routh for the Medical Informatics part,

Falko Busse for the Diagnostic Imaging and Therapy part,

Hans Hofstraat for the Molecular Medicine part, and

Thomas Zaengel for the Personal Healthcare part.

In addition, we like to thank **Rob Gossink** for the initial ideas to create the book, and for taking the responsibility for the Trends in Healthcare part.

ABBREVIATIONS

3D	Three-dimensional
4D	Four-dimensional
AD	Alzheimer's disease
ADC	Analog-to-digital converter
ADT	Admission discharge and transfer
AED	Automated external defibrillator
AES	Advanced event surveillance
AF	Atrial fibrillation
AFA	Atrial fibrillation ablation
ART	Algebraic reconstruction technique
ART	Adaptive radiation therapy
BP	Blood pressure
BTV	Biological target volume
CA	Contrast agent
CAD	Computer aided detection
CADx	Computer aided diagnosis
CDSS	Clinical decision support systems
CHF	Congestive heart failure
CMRA	Coronary magnetic resonance angiography
CNR	Contrast to noise ratio
CPOE	Computerized physician order entry
CRP	Cardiopulmonary resucitation
CRT	Cardiac resynchronization therapy
CSA	Charge sensitive amplifier
CT	Computed tomography
CTA	Computed tomography angiography
CTF	CT fluoroscopy
CVD	Cardiovascular diseases
CZT	Cadmium zinc telluride
DICOM	Standard for digital imaging and communications in medicine
DM	Disease management
DSP	Digital signal processor
DWI	Diffusion-weighted MR imaging
EHR	Electronic health record
ELISA	Enzyme linked immunosorbent assay
EMR	Electronic medical record
EMT	Electromagnetic tracking
EP	Electrophysiology

EPR	Electronic patient record
FDA	Food and Drug Administration
FDG	Fluor-deoxyglykose (^{18}F-fluoro-2-deoxy-D-glucose)
FLT	Fluorothymidine (^{18}F-fluoro-3'deoxy-3'-L-fluorothymidine)
FMISO	^{18}F-Fluoromisonidazole
GPS	Global positioning system
HIFU	High intensity focused ultrasound
HIM	Health information management
HIS	Hospital information systems
HIT	Healthcare IT
HR	Heart rate
HU	Hounsfield unit
ICD	Implantable cardioverter defibrillator
IGRT	Image-guided radiation therapy
IGT	Image-guided therapy
IGT	Impaired glucose tolerance
II-TV	Image intensifier television system
IMRT	Intensity modulated radiation therapy
IR	Infrared
IT	Information technology
IVUS	Intra-vascular ultrasound
KDD	Knowledge discovery from data
LAN	Local area network
LED	Light emitting diode
LOR	Line of response
MAG	Motion adapted gating
MALDI	Matrix enhanced surface desorption ionization
MCI	Mild cognitive impairment
MDx	Molecular diagnostics
MI	Molecular imaging
MIP	Maximum intensity projection
ML	Maximum likelihood
MLC	Multi-leaf collimator
MPI	Magnetic particle imaging
MPR	Multi-planar reconstruction
MR	Magnetic resonance
MRI	Magnetic resonance imaging
MRS	Magnetic resonance spectroscopy
MRT	Magnetic resonance tomography
MTF	Modulation transfer function

NCE	New chemical entities
NCHS	National Center for Health Statistics
NCI	National Cancer Institute
NEC	Noise equivalent count rate
NIH	National Institute of Health
NIR	Near infrared
NLOS	Non-line of sight
NLP	Natural language processing
NM	Nuclear medicine
OPMS	Optical position measurement system
PACS	Picture archiving and communication systems
PCD	Programmed cell death
PET	Positron emission tomography
PFC	Perfluorocarbon
PHC	Personal healthcare
PHR	Personal health record
PMS	Philips Medical Systems
PMT	Photo multiplier tube
PSA	Prostate specific antigen
PTCA	Percutaneous transluminal coronary angiography
PTV	Planned target volume
RA	Rotational angiography
RF	Radio frequency
RFA	Radio frequency ablation
RIS	Radiology information systems
RSNA	Radiological Society of North America
RT	Radiation therapy
RTP	Radiation therapy treatment planning
SCA	Sudden cardiac arrest
SELDI	Surface enhanced laser desorption ionization
SENSE	Sensitivity encoding
SMASH	Simultaneous acquisition of spatial harmonics
SNP	Single nucleotide polymorphism
SNR	Signal to noise ratio
SPECT	Single photon emission computed tomography
TEE	Trans-esophageal echocardiography
TFT	Thin film transistor
TOF	Time of flight
US	Ultrasound
XDS	Cross enterprise document sharing

PART I: TRENDS IN HEALTHCARE

Chapter 1

ADVANCES AND TRENDS IN HEALTHCARE TECHNOLOGY
Stopping Diseases Before They Start

Robert Gossink[1], Jacques Souquet[2]
[1]*Philips Research, Aachen, Germany;* [2]*SuperSonic Imagine SA, Aix-en-Provence Cedex, France*

Abstract: This introductory chapter describes the drivers for recent and future changes in healthcare: (1) socio-economic developments in society (in particular the aging society and the growth of chronic disease), (2) the healthcare politics that these developments induce, and (3) advances in healthcare technology. Three major trends in healthcare technology are singled out: The impact of Moore's Law on medical imaging, molecular medicine, E-health and personal healthcare.

Keywords: Socio-economic developments, the aging society, chronic disease, healthcare politics, medical technology, advances in medical imaging, molecular medicine, E-health, personal healthcare

1.   INTRODUCTION

Society today is in overdrive with no sign of braking or even slowing down. Time and speed are the key parameters guiding our path. From the era of the microsecond, we moved into the world of the nanosecond where everything goes so fast that its representation is frozen, it cannot be captured by the human eye. The Czech novelist, Milan Kundera, wrote: "Speed is the new ecstasy that technology has bestowed on man". By ecstasy, he meant a simultaneous state of both imprisonment and freedom. Man is caught in a fragment of time, totally disconnected from his past and his future. Nowadays there is often reference made to 'real time'. Does it mean that time was 'non-real'? The concept of real time first appeared in the mid 1950s, when mention was made of computers. But computers never dealt with real time, they dealt with simulated time in simulated realities. Only

1

G. Spekowius and T. Wendler (Eds.), Advances in Healthcare Technology, 1-14.
© 2006 *Springer. Printed in the Netherlands.*

recently with the fast increase of compute power, can we think of real time compute applications.

In this fast moving world, also healthcare is changing at rapid speed, influenced both by demographics and by advances in technology, mainly in electronics and in molecular biology.

In this introductory chapter we will consider the main socio-economic, political and technological factors influencing healthcare. After this, we will describe three fields of technology that we see as the major ones in healthcare.

2.   DRIVERS IMPACTING THE GROWTH OF MEDICAL TECHNOLOGIES

2.1   Socio-economics

The number of people of 65 or over is expected to grow in the USA from 35 million in 2000 to 70 million in 2030 (Figure 1-1). By that time one out of five Americans will be 65 or older[1]. The gap between the average age reached by male and by female is closing. Once 65, the remaining life expectancy for male in the USA in 2000 was 16.3 years, whilst that for female was 19.2 years.

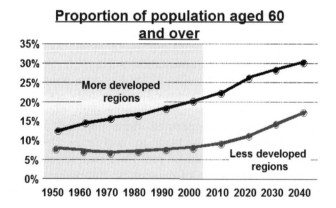

Figure 1-1. Proportion of population aged 60 and over in more and in less developed regions (Source: WHO).

This trend to longer life is mainly due to declines in heart disease and stroke mortality. These have to do with improved medical technology as well as with a healthier life style. Chronic diseases, such a diabetes and high blood pressure, however, are becoming more prevalent among older adults. Also, a considerable proportion of older Americans (about 20%) experience mental disorders. For all developed countries similar trends can be observed[2,3].

The increasing ratio of elderly, often retired, people versus younger people, usually having a job – caused by a combination of longer life and a lower childbirth in the population – puts a great pressure on society. According to a recent study, 60% of healthcare costs are incurred by people of 65 years or older[3]. These developments put pressure on income taxation and other social costs, they put pressure on the level and onset of retirement schemes and – relevant for the present chapter – it puts pressure on the healthcare costs in society.

Healthcare costs show a general increasing trend (in the USA now more than 1.7 trillion dollar/year or more than 15% of GDP, Figure 1-2). Since the mid-1990s healthcare costs in the USA have grown on average by 9%/year[4], the drivers being the above-mentioned aging society with the related phenomenon of long-living individuals with non-lethal chronic diseases, as well as the continuing advances in diagnosis and treatment methods. According to projections by David Cutler[3], healthcare costs will further increase by another 6% of GDP in the coming 30 years, about equally caused by the effects of the aging society and by the introduction of new medical technology.

2.2   Healthcare politics

Although increasing healthcare spending can also be seen as an opportunity for economic growth (more employment in the healthcare system and new opportunities for companies in healthcare technology and services[5]), governments often see it as a threat. This leads to measures to stimulate the efficiency and effectiveness of the healthcare system, whilst (in most countries) trying to preserve the entrance to the healthcare system for all members of the population. It also leads in the healthcare system itself to growing attention for efficiency and effectiveness, leading to concepts like managed care in order to control costs. Also, the tendency to form larger conglomerates of healthcare providers as well as the trend to focus on the core function of the care center (diagnosis and treatment) and to outsource other functions (like the restaurant and hotel function), stem from the drive to more efficiency. This leads to fewer hospital beds, fewer hospitals, conglomerates of hospitals, and transfer of hospitals to for-profit organisations[6].

Another, sometimes opposing trend is that of the self-confident and often well-informed patient. Patients belonging to the more affluent part of the society (including many elderly), when placed in a situation where the government wants to limit access to certain diagnosis or treatment methods, are prepared to use their private resources. In countries like China, this is in many cases anyhow needed to get access to advanced healthcare.

It reminds of the story of the robber directing a pistol at his victim's chest and asking: "your money or your life?" Usually, the choice is easily made. It explains phenomena like 'health tourism' and 'the CT in the shopping mall'. It stimulates the tendency towards privatizations in the healthcare market.

Information on health and disease is abundantly available, in particular through the Internet. Patients thus have the opportunity to better inform themselves, and many do. They may come to their doctor with own ideas and demands on the diagnosis and treatment of their problems.

Governments as well as individuals take prevention more seriously and try to stimulate a healthier life, developing more physical activity for greater fitness and suppressing unhealthy habits like smoking and obesity.

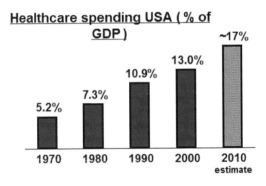

Figure 1-2. Healthcare spending in the USA as a percentage of GDP.

Advances in medicine and medical technology play a dual role in increasing or reducing healthcare costs: They permit better diagnosis and treatment, thus leading to a longer life expectancy and allowing an acceptable quality of life, even for people having one or more chronic diseases. An example is diabetes, where self-analysis and treatment make a long life possible for patients who in earlier times in history or in less developed countries would have died at an early age.

These advances, as we will see later, also help early detection or even prevention of diseases and thus help avoid costs for expensive treatment.

They may also allow more efficient procedures, such as minimal invasive treatment (also reducing the length of hospital stay), faster and more reliable diagnosis by computer-aided detection, and may also enable patients to be monitored at home instead of in the clinic (as in the example of diabetes patients; in the future this will also apply to cardiac patients being able to be monitored at home or underway, whilst nevertheless being in contact with their physician).

Also, modern IT and communication technology has enhanced and will further enhance the efficiency of the healthcare system. It enables much more efficient administrative procedures in the hospital and in the healthcare system at large, it allows much faster access to and interpretation of medical data, and it helps to avoid medical errors. In Germany, in the coming years, a smart card will be introduced for all patients to be used in hospitals, with general practitioners and with pharmacies all over the country, leading to a better integration of and workflow in the healthcare system.

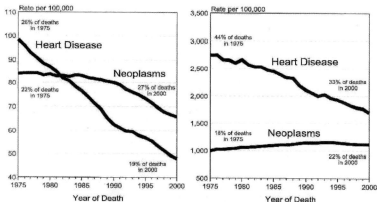

Figure 1-3. Development of death rates in the US over the period 1975-2000 (Source: NCHS public data).

There is a lack of quantitative studies on the net effect of new medical technology on healthcare costs. The fact that the initial effect is spending more money, may lead to sub-optimizations, e.g., by governments limiting investments in advanced diagnostic equipment, thus causing other costs and inconvenience, connected with waiting times for patients, lost economic activity and costs by medical complications due to non-optimal or late diagnosis. It is estimated that in German hospitals alone, there is an 'investment queue' for imaging equipment of 15 million Euros. If factors like gaining working hours by longer life and the value of increased life expectancy are taken into account, the effect of the introduction of new medical technology is clearly positive, as Cutler and McClellan[7] have calculated for a number of disease categories like cardiac disease: "around 70% of the survival improvement in heart attack mortality is a result of changes in technology". History has demonstrated that advances that really help to improve the health of people can never be stopped, only delayed.

2.3   Healthcare technology

In the following sections we will summarize some of the main trends in healthcare technology. There are two key technological drivers for these trends: Ubiquitous electronics and Genomics/Proteomics.

Ubiquitous electronics: mainly enabled by the development in semiconductor technology as described by Moore's Law, we have seen rapid progress over many years in the miniaturization and digitization of electronics, in low-power electronics, in faster computing with ever smaller computers, in data storage (hard-disk drives, optical storage and semi-conductor memories), in larger and flatter displays, in wireless technologies like mobile telephony and wireless LAN, in sensor technology and in rechargeable batteries. This progress is continuing at unchanged speed. These developments in electronics have enabled progress in medical technologies over a wide field, including real-time 3D imaging with ever higher resolution, image processing and computer-aided detection of clinically relevant data, implantable devices, sensor systems in and on the body, and many more.

Genomics and proteomics: the last decade has seen an explosion of the knowledge on the structure and the functioning of the human body at the cellular and molecular level. A major achievement was the unraveling of the human genome. Our knowledge about the relationship how DNA structures translate into proteins and the action of these proteins in the body is growing daily. How this translation process is related to development and treatment of diseases is extremely complex, and most of understanding this still lies ahead of us. Nevertheless, first successes in using targeted contrast media to image diseases at an early stage, have been achieved ('molecular medicine', promise to individualize the detection and treatment of disease.

They may permit measuring predisposition for certain diseases, detection of disease at a very early stage and individual therapy much more effectively than in the generalized approach used today. And even more, molecular medicine may help to develop new pharmaceuticals in a much more efficient way.

2.4 Healthcare in the future

How will medical care look like in a few decades from now? The physician and the hospital concentrate much more on prevention and aftercare, instead of having their focus on the acute phase of medical care ('disease management').

The risk profile of the patient for acute or chronic diseases is assessed on the basis of life style, family history and genetic predisposition; all these data are stored in the electronic patient record (which is accessible to the patient through the internet); the patient carries the essentials of this record with him/her in a smart card with a large memory.

The patient, depending on his/her risk profile, is regularly screened for the possible onset of acute disease or to follow the course of a chronic disease. The patient at home can do part of this screening, if relevant in wireless contact with the physician through a safe and privacy-protected data link.

If the onset of a disease has been detected by molecular diagnosis, the extent and the location of the disease is assessed by molecular imaging using a contrast agent specifically targeted to the disease.

If surgical intervention is needed, this is done using an image-guided minimal-invasive procedure.

Pharmaceutical treatment is individually adapted to the patient in terms of the pharmaceutical and dose chosen, taking into account his/her individual sensitivity to the drug. The dose in which the drug is delivered depends on a feedback system based on continuous measurement of the drug concentration at the targeted site in the body and the effect it has there. If relevant, the drug is only delivered at the site where it is needed ('local drug delivery'), e.g. by focused ultrasound.

If relevant, the patient gets a device implanted that takes over part or whole of the damaged body function. These devices are miniaturized and smart with – helped by their low power consumption – almost infinite battery life. Next to the presently existing smart cardiac pacemakers and defibrillators, there are implantable pumps supporting the heart function, as well as the first generation of complete artificial organs like pancreas, liver and even heart. Neurological diseases, like Alzheimer and Parkinson are kept under control using stable electrodes at the right position, provided with smart electronic signals.

Regenerative medicine and cell therapy have progressed so that parts of the heart that are damaged by heart infarction can be revived.

Personal healthcare systems allow elderly people with chronic disease to stay at home instead of regularly visiting or staying at a care center. Their physician can continuously monitor their health condition and help can be sent immediately when an emergency situation occurs. Similar systems can be employed to measure and improve the fitness of people, young and old, to help preserve their health.

Many examples of the new trends in healthcare technology will be described in subsequent chapters of this book. We would like, however, to set the stage with the three technologies that we consider to be the major ones supporting the drivers mentioned above.

3.   IMPACT OF MOORE'S LAW ON MEDICAL IMAGING

"Doubling the compute power of microprocessors every 18 months" as Gordon Moore stated in the early 1970's has a profound impact on every electronic equipment development, and medical imaging systems are no exception. Besides more processing power in integrated circuits, there is availability of higher bandwidth in networks, ever increasing (almost unlimited) storage at lower cost, development of smarter algorithms leveraging the speed increase to provide better and easier understanding of clinical information. The goal of this new technology is to improve the quality of life of the individuals. We need to not only save lives, but at the same time reduce patient discomfort and minimize the number of avoidable medical errors. A study by the Institute of Medicine estimates the number of deaths in the USA due to avoidable medical errors at about 100,000 persons per year.

Improvement in prevention and early diagnosis will have a dramatic impact on cost reduction and number of lives saved. New technologies leveraging Moore's law with the availability of increased compute power will play an important role. Technologies like real time 3D imaging allow for easier and better understanding of anatomical details. As an example, in Figure 1-4, real time 3D ultrasound allows for early detection of heart anomalies, making this affordable technology available to a greater number of users.

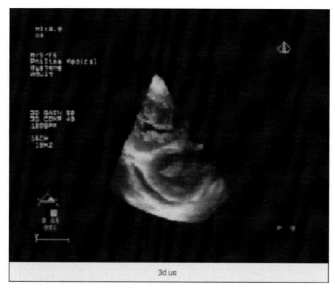

Figure 1-4. Real-time 3D ultrasound image of the heart (Philips Medical Systems).

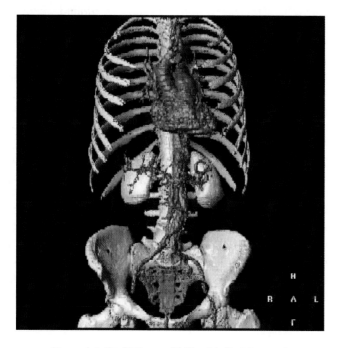

Figure 1-5. 3D CT image (Philips Medical Systems).

Similarly, the on-going revolution in X-ray computed tomography (CT) with faster data acquisition and more detector rows (64 slices) will allow for fast diagnosis where the entire abdomen can be scanned in less that half a minute. One of the major consequences impacting the physician directly related to the acquisition and processing speed, is the overwhelming increase in the amount of data/information he/she has to deal with. Within less than 20 seconds, a complete lung exam takes place with a top of the line CT system. In that time frame more than 2000 images are acquired, images the physician has to analyze. This represents a factor of 10 increase in data volume compared to just a few years ago. The physician is therefore confronted with a new paradigm: the patient spends less and less time for data acquisition and the physician has to spend more and more time in front of an increased volume of data to provide an accurate diagnosis.

This again is where Moore's law finds its way. With increased compute power available, a new generation of support systems is provided to the physician through Computer Aided Detection (CAD) and/or Computer Decision Support Systems (CDSS). These new tools help the user navigate in the huge data set and provide automatic clues for the physician to focus on. Revolutionary 3D visualization techniques allow for virtual inspection of organs like in Figure 1-5.

New techniques like virtual endoscopy greatly improve patient comfort and reduce the threshold for colon cancer.

With faster compute capabilities, medical imaging systems can provide in real time improved spatial and contrast resolution by leveraging signal and image processing techniques. Automatic detection of key features in an image is now becoming a reality. Fusion of data coming from different sources of acquisition plays a role in improving the diagnostic efficacy of the physician.

Another consequence of Moore's law is related to the miniaturization of the equipment. Whilst keeping the level of performance constant, one can today 'shrink' the volume of electronic hardware significantly. There are today in the world about 2 billion cell phones each having the processing power of a mid 1990 personal computer with 100 times less power consumption. Similarly one sees today hand-carried ultrasound imaging systems that have the   processing power of a mid 1990 high-end ultrasound system. This opens a new market for imaging systems, increasing the ubiquitous use of them in the clinical environment, creating new applications and opening new markets. This can be viewed as a disruptive technology as it enforces the following paradigm shifts:

- **Price-performance paradigm:** A high-end, high performance system is not necessarily best suited for all types of exams.

- **Application paradigm:** Ubiquitous usage of imaging systems in the clinical environment.
- **User's paradigm:** Less skilled professionals have access to this new tool.

4. MOLECULAR MEDICINE

The deciphering of the human genome and the arrival on the market of new generations of intelligent contrast agents and markers has been the trigger point for the new field of molecular medicine. This new field includes three linked sub-specialties:

- **Molecular imaging:** Leveraging the use of specific contrast agents designed to target expressed biomarkers to disclose the location and extent of the disease at its onset as well as its fate after and during therapy.
- **Molecular diagnostics:** In vitro test of biomarkers (e.g. proteins) that are expressed in body fluid or tissue to be used to diagnose disease even before clinical symptoms of the disease become evident.
- **Molecular therapy:** Gene-based therapies including targeted drug delivery and targeted cancer drugs.

Already today, cancer drugs (drugs that correct the specific genetic flaws that are the biological causes of cancer) have been approved for sale and are available on the market. The patient lobby being very strong, the cost and sometimes lack of efficacy of the treatment have not prevented the FDA from approving the drugs.

The NIH position statement when analyzing the impact of Molecular Medicine has been: Improving the Health of the Nation. This will be achieved in the following manner:

- **Early diagnosis and prevention:** Especially for cardiovascular diseases, cancer and stroke.
- **Better understanding of disease mechanisms:** For example islet beta cell mass in diabetes, detection of inhaled pulmonary pathogens, neuro-psychiatric disorders…
- **Impacting new therapies** like site targeted drug/gene therapy, stem cell imaging and therapy, organ/tissue transplantation.

The challenges to reach the target are multiple. The first one is to speed up the translation process between what has been achieved on animals to the human. This is a specific goal set up by the National Cancer Institute (NCI) in domains as varied as angiogenesis, anti-angiogenesis, apoptosis, atherosclerosis, and stem cell applications. The second challenge is to recognize that such an effort mandates partnership with partners in complementary arenas of expertise: contrast agents, pharmaceuticals, drug delivery, etc. Such partners can be academic medical centers and/or other industrial partners.

Molecular medicine moves us in the direction of predictive medicine. In the future one should be able to assess the genetic predisposition of individuals for a specific disease. Prediction will replace prevention. Furthermore, during treatment, molecular diagnostics should be able to assess very quickly the efficacy of the therapy. Today the availability of targeted contrast agents has been achieved. Such agents have been designed to target fibrin (for example) responsible for the creation of thrombus in vessels, enhancing the imaging contrast and facilitating the visualization of the location and extent of the thrombus.

Such targeted agents can be designed to be the carrier for a drug, delivering therefore the drug in situ. It thus becomes a targeted drug delivery system. Today experiments are conducted on animal models to validate the technique. The dream of the 'silver bullet' is not too far away.

5. E-HEALTH AND PERSONAL HEALTHCARE

Conventional interactions with patients in the healthcare domain require them to be present in the hospital or clinic. However, leveraging strength in semiconductor and consumer electronic domains, it is entirely conceivable to bring monitoring and treatment technologies to the home. As a matter of fact, the miniaturization of electronics we described earlier is key to this approach: the technology moves where the patient is located and not the patient where the technology is located.

Various initiatives have already started in this domain. A key one is the monitoring of CHF (congestive heart failure) patients at home. Simple and easy to use monitoring equipment is placed at the patient's home. The equipment is connected via an available network (a phone line) to a central server in the hospital. The server is monitored by medical professionals (specially trained nurses or paramedics) who react to the data received by either doing nothing, or calling the patient to modify his/her medication regimen, or having a doctor contact the patient or in the worst case sending an ambulance to bring the patient to the hospital. It has been demonstrated by analyzing reports from various implementations of such systems that, in doing so:

- The quality of care is not diminished.
- The patient feels more responsible for his/her own health.
- The cost compared to the traditional visit of the patient to his/her physician is significantly decreased.

In order for such a system to be successful, it requires complete cooperation across the whole healthcare value chain: insurers, hospitals, physicians, and emergency services.

An extension of this approach is to continuously monitor patients at risk through non-invasive sensing and, why not, implantable sensors. In the case of non-invasive sensing, a conceptual approach is to design intelligent clothing/underwear that carries sensors measuring body activity and embedding simple wireless electronic computing the outcome of the measurement and communicating it to the outside world. An example of such clothing is seen in Figure 1-6.

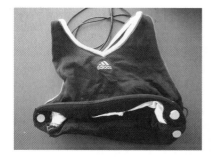 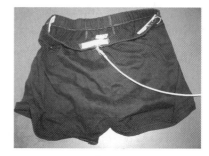

Figure 1-6. Underwear provided with sensors (Philips Research).

An obvious application for such a technology is the monitoring of patients at risk for sudden cardiac arrest. The miniaturized wireless electronics can also incorporate a GPS to help in locating the patient as well as an alarm system triggering the dispatching of an ambulance.

In the future, one can envision implanted sensors in the body, monitoring all kinds of events. Sensors could transmit the outcome of their measurement to each other as well as to some miniaturized central unit located outside the body. A real body LAN is then created.

Besides home blood pressure monitors, the first real therapeutic medical device reaching home in the USA is the Automated External Defibrillator (AED).

Approval for such devices that are crucial to resuscitate patients who have suffered a sudden cardiac arrest event has been granted in the USA in

2005. It is expected to see in the future more and more devices that once were solely used in the hospital environment move into the home.

6.   CONCLUSIONS

We have just touched up on some important new trends in healthcare technology. More examples will be highlighted in the rest of the book like minimally invasive procedures, organ replacement, tissue engineering, regenerative medicine, therapy planning, etc. Each of these new technologies is developed to bring more comfort to the patient and improve the efficacy and cost of diagnostics and treatment. Imaging has made a big impact on healthcare over the last decades and will continue to do so. It is important to promote continuous technology development for better and faster diagnosis whilst lowering cost. The future is bright as true molecular medicine is coming in sight.

Reflecting on the introductory comments on time and speed, it is fair to say that for some time is money; however for us in the health domain, time means life.

REFERENCES

1.   The State of Aging and Health in America, Merck Institute of Aging & Health and The Gerontological Society of America, (2005); www.agingsociety.org.
2.   G. Steingart, *Deutschland, der Abstieg eines Superstars*, (Piper, 2004).
3.   B. Alemayehu and K. E.Warner, The Lifetime Distribution of Health Care Costs, *Health Services Review* (2004).
4.   D. M. Cutler, An International Look at the Medical Care Financing Problem, Harvard University, (July 2003); http://post.economics.harvard.edu/faculty/dcutler/papers/, Cutler Japan paper 7-03.
5.   Medtronic, www.medtronic.com
6.   Studie zur Situation der Medizintechnik in Deutschland im internationalern Vergleich, *Bundesministerium für Bildung und Forschung*, Berlin, (2005).
7.   R. Mullner and K. Chung, Major Trends in Chicago Hospitals 1980-2004, Conference on Chicago Research and Public Policy "The Changing Face of Metropolitan Chicago", (2004); www.about.chapinhall.org/uuc/presentations/MullnerChungPaper.
8.   D. M. Cutler and M. McClellan, Is technological change in medicine worth it? *Health Affairs* **10**, (Sept./Oct. 2001).
9.   W. A. Herman, D. E. Marlowe and H. Rudolph, Future Trends in Medical Device Technology: Results of an Expert Survey, (1998); www.fda.gov/cdrh/ost/trends/toc.html.

PART II: DIAGNOSTIC IMAGING

Chapter 2

DIAGNOSTIC IMAGING
State-of-the-art and Recent Advances

Falko Busse
Philips Research, Hamburg, Germany

Abstract: Medical imaging is the heart of many diagnostic and therapeutic procedures. Starting from the discovery of X-rays in 1895, a number of imaging modalities were invented and later established in clinical practice. Initially these imaging modalities (except PET and SPECT, which target metabolic processes) were aimed to visualize non-invasively anatomical details from within the body. With the improvement of imaging agents, computing power and imaging technology increasingly information about organ function and even metabolism can be measured and used in the clinical decision process. However, all established imaging modalities have strengths and weaknesses. Therefore, a strong trend exists to combine complementary information from different imaging modalities, either through system integration or software fusion. PET-CT is an impressive manifestation of this trend. In addition, work continues to explore novel imaging techniques with the aim to develop new modalities. These would help to close remaining clinical gaps with imaging as the enabler.

Keywords: Imaging modalities, hybrid imaging, functional imaging, molecular imaging, X-ray, CT, PET, SPECT, MR, ultrasound, optical imaging, photoacoustic tomography, magnetic particle imaging

1.   INTRODUCTION

Radiology began as a medical sub-specialty in the first decade of the 1900's after the discovery of X-rays. The development of radiology grew at a moderate pace until World War II. Extensive use of X-ray imaging during the second world war, and the advent of the digital computer and new imaging modalities like ultrasound, computed tomography, magnetic resonance imaging and nuclear imaging have combined to create an

15

G. Spekowius and T. Wendler (Eds.), Advances in Healthcare Technology, 15-34.
© 2006 *Springer. Printed in the Netherlands.*

explosion of diagnostic imaging techniques in the past 25 years. Some of the major milestones in the development of medical imaging technology are summarized in Table 2-1.

Table 2-1. Milestones in medical diagnostic imaging.

Date	Innovation
1895	Wilhelm Conrad Roentgen discovers X-rays. He also produces the first X-ray image of the human body (his wife's hand).
1953	First real-time Ultrasound device built by John Julian Wild and John Reid[1].
1963	Tomographic SPECT reconstruction by David Kuhl and Roy Edwards[2].
1972	CT scanning is invented by Sir Godfrey Hounsfield and Allan Cormack[3].
1974	Clinical PET (Positron Emission Tomography) developed at the University of Washington[4].
1980	First MR imaging of the brain on a clinical patient. MR was developed by Paul Lauterbur and Peter Mansfield[5,6].

Today, imaging systems reveal every organ and lay bare every pathology. They show us three-dimensional, full-color pictures of the beating heart and cross-sectional slices of the abdomen. We can see blood flowing through our arteries, water traveling along nerve fibers, cells dying in a tumor, antibodies battling infection, and, strangest of all, emotions such as fear and love arising in the brain. These devices even analyze the images they produce; they identify malignancies, count plaque deposits in arteries, measure bone loss, and calculate the heart's pumping capacity. They also assist surgeons, tracking the positions of their instruments in real time and letting them know what their scalpels are about to cut into.

The increasing importance of medical imaging in diagnosis and treatment planning is demonstrated by the fact that, in addition to X-ray (W. C. Roentgen), two imaging technologies have been awarded with the Nobel Prize. Allan M. Cormack and Godfrey N. Hounsfield received the prize "for the development of computer assisted tomography" in 1979, and Paul C. Lauterbur and Peter Mansfield "for their discoveries concerning magnetic resonance imaging" in 2003.

2.   TECHNOLOGY TRENDS

The field of medical imaging developed along a few major trends, especially since the mid 1970's. These high level trends can be summarized in a short bullet list:

- Towards fully integrated solid state detectors.
- Towards 3D image matrix.

- Speed-up of acquisition towards 4D (3D+T) images.
- From anatomical to functional to molecular imaging.

The main driver behind this development (or better called enabler) is the exponential growth in performance of silicon devices, both in the area of digital logic as well as processing units. This growth can well observed in e.g. Moore's law[7], which is depicted in Figure 2-1.

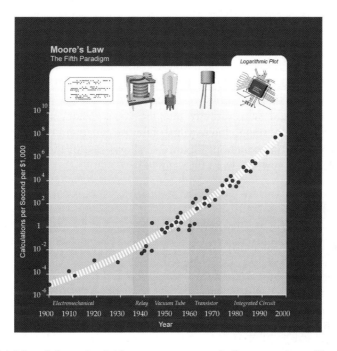

Figure 2-1. Moore's law using Intel processors as example (image courtesy of Intel Corp.).

The general trends in imaging technology, as described above, drive the development of the established imaging modalities. Although the onset and the speed of these developments vary between imaging technologies, the trends can be observed generally throughout the modalities. In the following sections the impact of the trends on improvements in technology will be discussed.

2.1 X-ray

The use of X-rays for diagnostic imaging started shortly after Wilhelm Konrad Roentgen's discovery in 1895. Since X-rays penetrate solid objects, but are slightly attenuated by them, the picture resulting from the exposure reveals the internal structure of the human body. X-ray imaging was and is still used in two applications fields: Radiography and fluoroscopy.

Imaging technology for radiography evolved from plain X-ray film and screen-film combinations to cassette-based computed radiography, introduced 1983 by Fuji[8]. This technology enabled the step of X-ray imaging into the digital domain. However, the conversion from X-rays into digital signals is not performed directly, but requires an intermediate (analog) storage step in photostimulable phosphors[9]. Only recently, a new technology based on large area amorphous silicon plates has been introduced to the market, which converts the incoming X-rays either via a photoconductor layer[10,11] or via a scintillator/photodiode combination[12,13] directly into digital signals. This technology is explained in detail in Chapter 4.

Fluoroscopic imaging initially relied on fluorescent screens. But since doctors then would stare directly into the X-ray beam, such screens were quickly replaced by image intensifiers / television camera combinations after 1954, the year of introduction. Figure 2-2 shows one of the first commercial image intensifier systems from the year 1954.

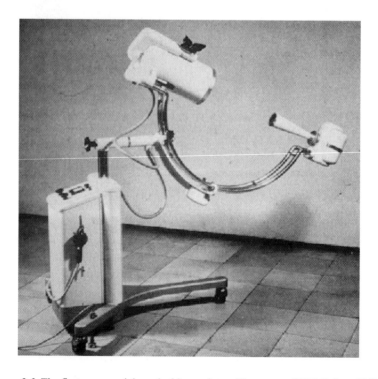

Figure 2-2. The first commercial surgical image intensifier system (BV 20) from Philips.

After the introduction of radiographic detectors based on amorphous silicon technology end of the 1990s, it was only a question of time when the more challenging implementation of fluoroscopic detectors on the same technology would be introduced[14,15]. Due to the advantages of a much more compact design and distortion free images at higher contrast resolution, these detectors have become the mainstream imaging technology in X-ray.

The next technology change already appears at the horizon. Detectors based on large area CMOS technology are available in the early prototype stage for proof-of-concept[16]. The anticipated advantages will be higher spatial resolution, higher readout speed for functional and 3D imaging at potentially lower cost of goods.

The application range of X-ray fluoroscopy spans from classical radiology, interventional radiology, surgery to cardiovascular interventions. As a very successful procedure 3-dimensional rotational X-ray imaging has been introduced in the 1990s[17], expanding the application space into volumetric anatomy and function (compare Chapter 5). There is significant research effort spent to replace the diagnostic interventional procedures performed with X-rays by MR and CT, because of their non-invasive nature.

However, with respect to clinical outcome X-ray is still the gold standard. At the same time, X-ray leverages its real-time capabilities and its high spatial resolution to expand into new and more complex therapeutic applications like integrated navigation (more details in Chapter 11) and cancer treatment (see Chapter 10).

2.2 Computed tomography (CT)

Computed tomography acquires a large number of projection X-ray images from a patient from various angles, usually by rotating X-ray source and detector around the patient. The collection of projection images is then translated into a 3-dimensional volume of linear attenuation coefficients (usually displayed relative to water). Using the first commercial CT systems, scanning just one slice of a human brain took nine hours, with subsequent reconstruction of 2.5 hours. The resulting slice image had a matrix of 80^2 pixels and a contrast resolution of 8 Bit. A picture of one of these first CT systems is shown in Figure 2-3.

Modern CT systems acquire and reconstruct image matrices up to 1024^2 pixels, at a rate of 40 slices per second (for a 512^2 matrix). The contrast resolution of these images is 18 Bit. Reconstruction can be synchronized to breathing and/or cardiac motion, in order to compensate for motion artifacts.

This enormous gain in acquisition speed has been achieved by faster rotation of the gantry (currently at 0.4 seconds per rotation) and by adding more and more detector lines for parallel image acquisition. Current state-of the-art are systems use 64 of such detector lines. In order to avoid that the costs of such systems explode, new paradigms in detector technology have to be pursued, as described in Chapter 4.

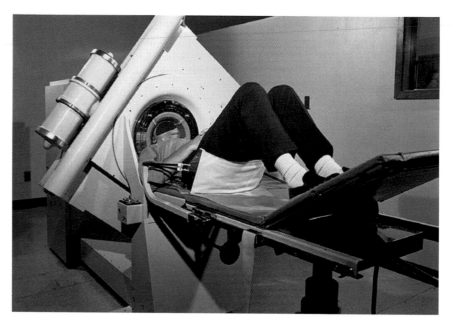

Figure 2-3. Original head CT scanner from EMI (installed at Mayo Clinic, Rochester, Minn.). Image courtesy of the RSNA.

Increasing the detection area generates also challenges to the technology in all other aspects of the system. The bandwidth of the slip ring, through which the data has to be transmitted from the rotating detector to the static part of the gantry, has to multiply in correspondence with the number of detector lines. The reconstruction problem changes drastically, from a fan beam geometry to a cone beam geometry, for which only recently a mathematical approach for an exact solution has been found[18]. A detailed discussion of the state-of-the-art in reconstruction technology is given in Chapter 3.

2.3   Positron emission tomography (PET)

PET images the 3-dimensional distribution of a tracer, which has been injected into the human (or animal) body. The tracer is labeled with a positron-emitting radioisotope. Once emitted, the positrons travel a short distance (0.2 mm for ^{18}F, 0.3 mm for ^{11}C, 0.4 mm for ^{15}O, 0.8 mm for ^{82}Rb, all FWHM), before they annihilate with an electron into two photons of 511 keV that are emitted almost exactly in opposite directions. These two photons are then detected in coincidence.

The fundamental building blocks of PET imaging has not changed over the first 30 years after introduction of the technology. PET detectors consist of a ring shaped layer of scintillation crystals, which are glued to a light guide, and a layer of photomultiplier tubes attached to the outside of the light guide. The scintillator absorbs the incoming γ-rays of 511keV energy and converts them into optical signals. The light guide then spreads the optical photons on several photomultiplier tubes, which allows for an exact reconstruction of the crystal (pixel) which was hit. A more detailed description of PET technology is given in Chapter 8.

Nevertheless, there was significant performance improvement of PET systems over time. This is due to improvements in key components like the scintillation material. The characteristics of the scintillator determine critically the PET imaging performance. Important parameters are especially the detection efficiency, energy resolution, time resolution, emission wavelength, mechanical and hydroscopic properties. Table 2-2 gives an overview of scintillator materials commonly used for PET (adapted from [19]).

Table 2-2. Physical properties of scintillator material commonly used for PET.

Scintillator material	Attenuation length [mm]	Light outout [ph/MeV]	Decay time [ns]	Emission wavelength [nm]	Hydroscopic
BGO	10.4	9000	300	480	No
LSO	11.4	30000	40	420	No
NaI:Tl	29.1	41000	230	410	Yes
CsI:Tl	22.9	66000	900	550	Slightly
GSO	14.1	8000	60	440	No
LuAP	10.5	12000	18	365	No
LaBr3	21.3	61000	35	358	No
LYSO	11.2	32000	48	420	No
LuAG	13.4	5606		510	No

For high intrinsic efficiency, scintillator materials should have both a high effective atomic number Z_{eff} and a high density. The energy (and spatial) resolution is associated with the light yield from the scintillator, since the magnitude of the fluorescent light yield will reduce the statistical spread in accordance with $(n_{ph})^{-1/2}$.

Whereas early PET scanners relied on NaI:Tl and Cesium Fluoride scintillators[20-22], modern PET systems are based on BGO[23], GSO[24] and LSO[25] crystals. Actual developments in the field of new detection technologies are directed towards the use of new cerium doped crystals, the use of layered crystals and other schemes for depth-of-interaction (DOI) determination, and a renewed interest in old technologies such as time-of-flight (TOF) PET[26], taking advantage of excellent timing resolution of new scintillators, along[27]. It appears that cerium doped lutetium orthosilicate (LSO:Ce), lutetium yttrium orthosilicate (LYSO:Ce) and cerium doped lanthanum bromide (LaBr₃:Ce), are the most promising candidates[28].

Recent developments in photodetectors for medical applications should enable efficient collection of the light emanating from the scintillation crystals[29,30]. The design of high resolution imaging devices imposes some additional constraints with respect to the necessity for compact arrays of photodetectors; in turn, this has stimulated the development and use of multichannel position-sensitive photomultiplier tubes (PS-PMT's), Silicon p-i-n photodiodes (PDs) and avalanche photodiodes (APDs)[31,32]. Solid-state photodiodes exhibit many advantages compared to conventional PMT's. They are relatively small, operate at much smaller voltage, and more importantly, and exhibit higher quantum efficiencies. Furthermore, photo-diodes are insensitive to axial and transversal strong magnetic fields and therefore, have the potential to be operated within MRI systems. By using this technology, the sensitive area of the detector could be read out more efficiently.

2.4   Single photon emission tomography (SPECT)

Similar to PET, SPECT images a radioactively labeled tracer. However, the labels in SPECT are γ-emitters, which emit in an energy range between 69 keV (^{201}Tl), and 365 keV (^{131}I), Most commonly used is ^{99m}Tc due to its moderate emission energy of 140 keV, its convenient decay time (6 hours) and its availability in generators.

Shortly after Hal Anger[33] developed the concept of a detector based on a single NaI crystal and an array of photomultiplier tubes, first tomographic images were produced[2]. The detection concept, which includes also a collimator in front of the scintillation crystal for selecting the projection, is still widely used in today's commercial systems.

The main innovations in SPECT therefore occurred in the areas of data acquisition, reconstruction[34] and image analysis.

Nevertheless, there are still attempts to overcome the drawbacks of the Anger camera, namely the reduced sensitivity and spatial resolution due to the collimator, by the means of new imaging technology. A technology that is potentially close to market introduction is the solid-state detector based on the direct conversion material CZT (see Chapter 4 for further information). Solid-state detectors should have intrinsically a better energy resolution, which would lead to lower scatter background. As a consequence, simultaneous dual isotope imaging might be achievable, which would drastically improve workflow of some clinical procedure like stress/rest imaging for cardiac perfusion measurement.

SPECT cameras based on CZT would probably exhibit an improved spatial resolution, but would not solve the intrinsic problem of the reduced sensitivity. One approach to eliminate the collimation at least in one dimension is based on slat detectors with a Slit collimator[35]. The detector together with the collimator would then rotate to achieve some collimation in the second dimension. Such systems exist is a prototype stage, but are not yet commercially available.

Already 1977 the concept of the Compton camera was proposed[36], which tries to replace the mechanical collimation by an electronic one, and thus boost the sensitivity of the detector. This concept has, however, still some significant technical challenges to solve, e.g. to achieve the required detector specifications at reasonable costs and to solve the reconstruction problem.

2.5 Magnetic resonance imaging (MR)

MRI is well recognized as a commonly used medical imaging modality. In spite of its significant growth over the last two decades, technical and application development continues.

Historic developments in image acquisition approaches are summarized in Table 2-3, where the periods of evolution are apportioned into approximately five- to ten-year-long intervals.

Table 2-3. Evolution of MR image acquisition approaches.

Time	Acquisition strategy
Mid 1980s	Identical magnetization level for all phase encodings.
	Identical pulse sequence used for all phase encodings (e.g. FLASH).
Late 1980s	Efficient use of decaying transverse magnetization (e.g. RARE, FSE, TSE).
	Allowance for different magnetization levels for different phase encodings.
	Non-rectilinear k-space trajectories.
Late 1990	Allowance for different pulse sequences for different phase encodings.
	Synthesis of required encodings from sparsely sampled measured set (e.g. SENSE, SMASH).

Two techniques have been developed for the synthesis of data at 'missing' values: Sensitivity encoding (SENSE[37]) and simultaneous acquisition of spatial harmonics (SMASH[38]). Both methods are similar in that an array of receiver coils is used, rather than a single coil. Further, both techniques use the differential response of individual coil elements across the field of view as the basis for generating the missing phase encodings. It has also recently been shown that the SENSE concept can be adapted for the parallel transmission of multi-dimensional RF pulses[39].

One of the driving forces behind MR developments is the need to accommodate increasing image reconstruction demands. A second driver is the emergence of specific research-based methods developed several years ago and the desire to make them more practical. One example of this is functional (f) neuro MRI. With this method a sequence of images of the brain is rapidly acquired over 1 to 2 min while the subject is performing some physical or mental task. A third driving factor is the identification of specific applications in which interactive MR imaging with real-time control is essential. One example of this is the use of real-time navigator echoes to guide the acquisition of data that can be subject to motion degradation (e.g. respiratory motion during a cardiac scan). Another example for which interactive imaging is essential is tracking of catheters and guidewires during interventions.

An example of a procedure that found its way from a research tool into clinical application is diffusion-weighted MR imaging. Perhaps the first clinical application of DWI was reported 1996, showing diffusion deficit in the presence of a stroke[40]. Applications of DWI have developed also into MR tractography, which connects pixels in relation to the anisotropy of the diffusion tensor. The technique can possibly be used to assess white matter tracts as part of neurosurgical planning.

3.   HYBRID IMAGING MODALITIES

Historically, in each major disease category one medical imaging modality of choice has been established as gold standard. Driven by the growing acceptance (reimbursement) of functional and metabolic imaging modalities like PET, this paradigm has changed towards the improvement of sensitivity and specificity of diagnostic imaging also by means of combining information from two (or more) modalities.

Hybrid systems can be realized with different degrees of integration. The architecture of such systems may range from an integrated backend only (with high-speed data exchange and image fusion functionality), over in-line systems that share mechanical components like the patient table, to fully integrated combinations. The choice of the architecture is mainly determined by the clinical value that is provided by the hybrid system, and technical boundary conditions.

Generally speaking, higher degrees of integration will reduce registration errors and will improve workflow for specific applications. In addition, it will allow for the simultaneous imaging with both modalities, which is an enabler for certain diagnostic applications. On the other hand, higher degrees of integration may lead to a reduced flexibility and patient scheduling.

Making an attempt to categorize the field of hybrid imaging modalities, the main driver behind hybrid systems for *diagnostic imaging* purposes has been the improved diagnostic power from combining functional / metabolic and anatomical information. Imaging in the context of molecular therapeutics will also give rise to a large demand for hybrid systems in the area of *therapy response assessment*. Applications of hybrid imaging systems in *image-guided treatment* have been in clinical trials much longer than those for diagnostic imaging. Examples are the integration of X-Ray C-arm systems (also in hybrid combination with CT or MR) with intra-vascular treatment devices, and of MR with high-intensity focused ultrasound (HIFU), and the increasing integration of real-time 3D Ultrasound in interventional treatment.

3.1   Hybrid diagnostic imaging

For PET, with its high sensitivity but low spatial resolution, it was obvious that an anatomical reference image would greatly enhance its value for diagnosis and therapy planning in oncology applications. After some initial debate about whether the images from two separate modalities could simply be fused by suitable image processing algorithms, the market simply decided for *integrated* PET-CT combinations. First systems were introduced in 2001, and today the market for standalone PET systems has virtually disappeared. And even though the CT part of the hybrid combination is running idle ca. 90% of the time during a hybrid exam, the market keeps replacing CT scanners with PET-CT hybrid systems.

Although today still 90% of all PET examinations are performed with ^{18}F-FDG, there is a large research effort spent both in academia as well as in industry to develop and commercialize new imaging agents for PET (compare Chapter 18). These agents will potentially be targeted to metabolic processes or receptors that are very specific to certain diseases. As a consequence, the level of anatomical information in PET images will tend to decrease further, which increases the need for an anatomical reference by a second modality.

With respect to agents, clinical SPECT is further advanced. A number of agents are approved, both for oncology and cardiology applications, and many more are in clinical trials. Some of these agents are targeting specific metabolic processes, and can therefore be called molecular agents already. Therefore, it was a natural step that SPECT-CT was introduced 2004 as the second hybrid modality into the market. Clinical applications for these systems will be both in cardiology (diagnosis and risk stratification of coronary artery disease) and in oncology (diagnosis, staging and follow-up).

As a potential future opportunity for hybrid diagnostic modalities, combinations of MR with either PET or SPECT are considered. These combinations are currently in the research phase, with respect to technology as well as to clinical applications. The main technical challenge for an integrated system is the sensitivity of the photo-multiplier tube, which is a critical component in today's PET and SPECT detectors, to the magnetic field of the MR. Recent successes in replacing the PMTs by Avalanche photodiodes may open a route for a technical realization. Nevertheless, experience from the PET-CT development tells that both modalities in hybrid systems need to have state-of-the-art performance. Such performance still needs to be demonstrated in the case of Avalanche photodiodes, especially if the PET technology moves towards time-of-flight.

3.2   Hybrid imaging in image-guided treatment

Applications of hybrid imaging systems in image-guided treatment have been addressed in clinical trials much earlier than those for diagnostic imaging. However, they have largely remained in the experimental stage and aimed at very specific treatment procedures. They are also less standardized, and have thus not led to spectacular market successes so far. Examples are combinations of X-Ray C-Arm systems with CT and MR (see Chapters 9 and 10), or combinations of optical (microscopic and endoscopic) imaging with MR and Ultrasound. In Cardiology, the increasing attention to detecting vulnerable plaque in coronary arteries and to the treatment of cardiac arrhythmia in the Electrophysiology Lab has stimulated a renewed discussion about the combination of intra-vascular (mainly Ultrasound and Optical) imaging with fluoroscopic modalities like X-Ray (see Chapter 11). Increasingly, also CT and MR are considered for EP guidance, as the 4D fluoroscopic capabilities of these modalities improve. A significant role might evolve for real-time 3D Ultrasound, as the fastest and cheapest '4D-imaging' modality, which is increasingly considered for interventional guidance in a number of application areas (see Chapter 7 for further reading).

3.3   Hybrid imaging to assess therapy response

Apart from the areas mentioned above, there are increasing clinical research efforts in hybrid systems for planning and delivery of non-invasive therapy, in order to provide closed loop solutions in which imaging derived information about the therapeutic procedure is used to control the delivery devices. One example is radiation therapy of tumors using linear accelerators, which are equipped with X-Ray imaging systems for organ motion tracking and corresponding collimation control (see details in Chapter 13). Another oncology procedure is based on non-invasive High-Intensity Focused Ultrasound (HIFU) ablation devices, which are integrated into MR systems. In this combination, the MR system is used for targeting control of the ultrasound focus volume and for monitoring of the resulting 3D temperature distribution. A detailed overview on this technique is given in Chapter 12.

4. NOVEL IMAGING TECHNOLOGIES

Besides the imaging modalities that are already established in clinical practice, there are a number of imaging principles currently in the research phase with the aim to develop them into clinically useful tools for imaging in humans.

Since more than ten years, considerable interest is devoted to optical imaging. Optical imaging is today routinely used only in pre-clinical imaging of small animals. Advancing optical techniques to humans promises high sensitivity without the use of ionizing radiation. However, significant technical challenges have to be overcome, since optical photons are strongly scattered and absorbed by human tissue.

The technical challenges of optical imaging can be somewhat reduced through a technique called photoacoustic tomography. In this concept the optical photons are used only to deposit energy at the location of the imaging agent, and then the resulting temperature increase is imaged with Ultrasound.

Finally, another method to detect small concentrations of an imaging agent is the utilization of the magnetic properties of the imaging agent. Such a technique, called Magnetic Particle Imaging, has recently been proposed.

4.1 Optical imaging

Visual light and near-infrared light offer the opportunity to image biological tissue, even though the predominant interaction processes are scattering and absorption. In the near-infrared window of low water absorption, tomographic optical imaging might be possible. However, due to the strong scattering and absorption of photons, there seems to be a limit for the size of body parts at approximately 10 cm in diameter.

Recently, the emphasis of research in medical imaging with diffuse light has moved away from the pursuit of high spatial resolution and towards functional imaging. It is widely appreciated that diffuse optical imaging can never compete in terms of spatial resolution with anatomical imaging techniques, but offers several distinct advantages in terms of sensitivity to functional changes, safety, cost and use at the bedside.

Three different technology approaches for diffuse optical tomography can be identified: Continuous wave, time domain and frequency domain. Philips Research pioneered the continuous wave approach through the development of a breast imaging system[41] (the prototype is shown in Figure 2-4). A comprehensive comparison of the different approaches as well as a description of the state-of-art of the technology and the clinical applications has been published by Gibson, Hebden and Arrige[42].

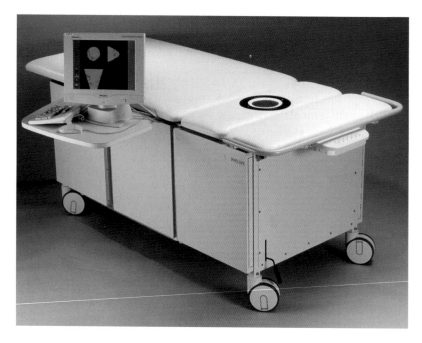

Figure 2-4. Prototype of a diffuse optical tomography system for breast imaging: The Philips 'Mammoscope'.

4.2 Photoacoustic tomography

Biomedical photoacoustic imaging is an imaging technique that is based on the generation of acoustic waves by pulsed light[43,44]. When a short laser pulse heats absorbers inside the tissue (like a specially designed agent), a temperature rise occurs, which is proportional to the deposited energy. As a result, a thermoelastic pressure transient is generated, whose amplitude depends on the amount of absorbed light, being determined by the local energy fluence, and the optical absorption coefficient of the target. From the time this pressure wave needs to reach the tissue surface (detector position), the position of the photoacoustic source can be calculated when the speed of sound in tissue is known.

Photoacoustic tomography overcomes the resolution disadvantages of pure optical imaging, and the contrast and speckle disadvantages of pure Ultrasound imaging. As imaging agents, indocyanine dyes, with strong absorption in the near infrared spectra, are especially useful because of the relatively low absorption of NIR light in human tissue. For example, indocyanine green (ICG), which has been approved by the Food and Drug Administration, in combination with NIR techniques, is employed widely in clinical applications such as cardiac output monitoring, hepatic function study, and angiography in ophthalmology and tumor detection.

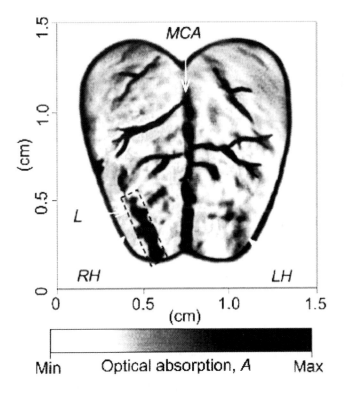

Figure 2-5. Non-invasive photoacoustic tomography image of a superficial lesion (size 1mm x 4mm) on a rat's cerebra, acquired with the skin and skull intact (taken from Wang et al.[45], image courtesy of Nature Publishing Group).

Current research on this technique focuses on animal experiments. Published results indicate that photoacoustic tomography is a noninvasive means for localizing and quantifying regional brain hemodynamic responses to neural activities through the skin and skull with high optical contrast and high ultrasonic resolution in vivo[45] (see also Figure 2-5 for an example). Using multiple wavelengths, photoacoustic tomography should be able to visualize brain neoplasias and brain metastases from distant organs. Imaging of the human brain, although much more difficult, might be feasible.

4.3   Magnetic particle imaging

The use of magnetic particles like SPIOs (super-paramagnetic iron-oxide particles) for MR imaging is already well established in clinical practice. These particles modify the T1 and T2 relaxation times. However, the measurement of the concentration of the imaging agent is limited in sensitivity, since only changes in relaxation times are detected in the presence of a high background signal.

Magnetic Particle Imaging[46] follows a completely different approach. This technique takes advantage of the non-linear magnetization curve of the magnetic particles, and of the fact that the magnetization curve saturates at certain magnetic field strength. Figure 2-6 demonstrates the principle how to translate that into an imaging principle.

If an oscillating magnetic field is applied to a collection of magnetic particles, it will modulate the magnetization M of the magnetic material. The modulation of the magnetization will not only contain the drive frequency, but also a number of higher harmonics, which can easily be separated from the drive frequency.

The effect described above is most pronounced in the absence of any other field except the modulation field. However, if the magnetic particles are exposed to a time constant magnetic field with a sufficiently large magnitude (as shown in part b of Figure 2-6), they saturate and the generation of harmonics is suppressed.

The suppression of harmonics can now be used to perform a spatial encoding, which is a prerequisite for an imaging system. In addition to the modulation field, a time-independent field is superimposed, which vanishes in one point of the imaging device. If there is any magnetic material in the location of the field-free point, it will produce a signal containing higher harmonics. All other material outside the field-free point will remain in saturation. By steering the field-free point through the volume of interest, a tomographic image can be generated.

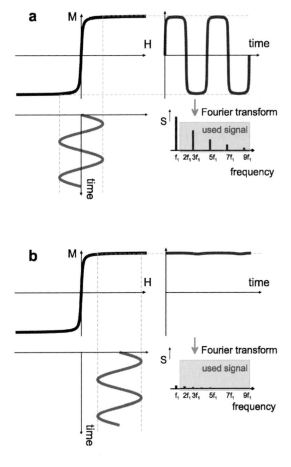

Figure 2-6. Response of magnetic particles to an external magnetic field. a) An oscillating magnetic field is applied to the magnetic material. As the magnetization curve (thick black curve) is nonlinear, the resulting time-dependent magnetization exhibits higher harmonics. b) A time-independent magnetic field is added to the modulation field. The oscillating field does not significantly change the magnetization of the material, as it is always in saturation (pictures courtesy of Nature Publishing Group).

REFERENCES

1. J.J. Wild, J.M. Reid, Echographic visualization of lesions of the living intact human breast, *Cancer Res* **14**, 277-283 (1954).
2. D.E. Kuhl, R.Q. Edwards, Image separation radioisotope scanning, *Radiology* **80**, 653-662 (1963).

3. G.N. Hounsfield, Computerized transverse axial scanning (tomography). Part I: Description of system, *Br J Radiol* **46**, 1016-1022 (1974).

4. M.M. Ter-Pogossian, M.E. Phelps, E.J. Hoffman, N.A. Mullani, A positron-emission transaxial tomograph for nuclear imaging, *Radiology* **114**, 89-98 (1975).

5. P.C. Lauterbur, Image formation by induced local interactions: Examples employing nuclear magnetic resonance, *Nature* **242**, 190-191 (1973).

6. A.N. Garroway, P.K. Grannell, P. Mansfield, Image formation in NMR by a selective irradiative process, *J Phys, C: Solid State Phys* **7**, 457-462 (1974).

7. G.E. Moore, Cramming more components onto integrated circuits, *Electronics* **38**, 114-117 (1965).

8. M. Sonoda, M. Takano, J. Miyahara, H. Kato, Computed radiography utilizing scanning laser stimulated luminescence, *Radiology* **148**, 833-838 (1983).

9. J.A. Rowlands, The physics of computed radiography, *Phys Med Biol* **47**, R123-R166 (2002).

10. W. Zhao, I. Blevis, S. Germann, J.A. Rowlands, D. Waechter, Z. Huang, A flat panel detector for digital radiuology using active matrix readout of amorphous selenium, *The Physics of Medical Imaging, Proc SPIE* **2708**, 523-531 (1996).

11. A. Brauers, N. Conrads, G. Frings, U. Schiebel, M.J. Powell, C. Glasse, X-ray sensing properties of a lead oxide photoconductor combined with an amorphous silicon TFT array, *Mat Res Soc Symp Proc* **507**, 321-326 (1998).

12. L. E. Antonuk, J. Yorkston, W. Huang, J. Boudry, E. J. Morton, R. A. Street, Large area, flat-panel aSi:H arrays for x-ray imaging, *The Physics of Medical Imaging, Proc SPIE* **1896**, 18-29 (1993).

13. U. Schiebel, N. Conrads, N. Jung, M. Weibrecht, H. Wieczorek, T. Zaengel, M.J. Powell, I.D. French, C. Glasse, Fluoroscopic x-ray imaging with amorphous silicon thin-flim arrays, *The Physics of Medical Imaging, Proc. SPIE* **2163**, 129-140 (1994).

14. P.R. Granfors, D. Albagli, J.E. Tkaczyk, R. Aufrichtig, H. Netel, G. Brunst, J.M. Boudry, D. Luo, Performance of a flat-panel cardiac detector, *The Physics of Medical Imaging, Proc. SPIE* **4320**, 77-86 (2001).

15. F. Busse, W. Ruetten, B. Sandkamp, P.L. Alving, R.J. Bastiaens, T. Ducourant, Design and performance of a high-quality cardiac flat detector, *The Physics of Medical Imaging, Proc SPIE* **4682**, 819-827 (2002).

16. T. Graeve, G.P. Weckler, High-resolution CMOS imaging detector, *The Physics of Medical Imaging, Proc SPIE* **4320**, 68-76 (2001).

17. M. Schumacher, K. Kutluk, D. Ott, Digital rotational radiography in neuroradiology, *AJNR Am J Neuroradiol* **10**(3), 644-649 (1989).

18. A. Katsevich, A general scheme for constructing inversion algorithms for cone beam CT, *Int J Math Sci* **21**, 1305-1321 (2003).

19. H. Zaidi, M.-L. Montandon, The new challenges of brain PET imaging technology, *Curr Med Imag Rev* **2**, Bentham Science Publishers, in press (2006).

20. E.J. Hoffman, M.E. Phelps, N. Mullani, C.S. Higgins, B.E. Sobel, M.M. Ter-Pogossian, Design and performance characteristics of a whole-body transaxial tomograph, *J Nucl Med* **17**, 493-502 (1976).

21. C.J. Thompson, Y.L. Yamamoto, E. Meyer, Positome II: A high efficiency positron imaging device for dynamic brain studies, *IEEE Trans Nucl Sci* **26**, 583-589 (1979).

22. M.M. Ter-Pogossian, D.C. Ficke, J.T. Hood, M. Yamamoto, N.A. Mullani, PETT VI: A positron emission tomograph utilizing cesium fluoride scintillation detectors, *J Comput Assist Tomogr* **6**, 125-133 (1982).

23. T.R. deGrado, T.G. Turkington, J.J. Williams, C.W. Stearns, J.M. Hoffman, R.E. Coleman, Performance characteristics of a whole body PET scanner, *J Nucl Med* **35**, 1398-1406 (1994).

24. G. Muehllehner, J.S. Karp, S. Surti, Design considerations for PET scanners, *J Nucl Med* **46**, 16-23 (2002).

25. C.L. Melcher, Scintillation crystals for PET, *J Nucl Med* **41**, 1051-1055 (2000).

26. M.M. Ter-Pogossian, N.A. Mullani, D.C: Ficke, J. Markham, D.L. Snyder, Photon time-of-flight-assisted positron emission tomography, *J Comput Assist Tomogr* **5**, 227-239 (1981).

27. S. Surti, J.S. Karp, G. Muehllehner, Image quality assessment of LaBr3-based wholebody 3D PET scanners: A Monte Carlo evaluation, *Phys Med Biol* **49**, 4593-4610 (2004).

28. P. Dorenbos, Light output and energy resolution of Ce3+-doped scintillators, *Nucl Instr Meth A* **486**, 208-213 (2002).

29. A. Del Guerra, M.G. Bisogni, C. Damiani, G. Di Domenico, R. Marchesini, G. Zavattini, New developments in photodetection for medicine, *Nucl Instr Meth A* **442**, 18-25 (2000).

30. J.L. Humm, A. Rosenfeld, A. Del Guerra, From PET detectors to PET scanners, *Eur J Nucl Med* **30**, 1574-1597 (2003).

31. D. Renker, Properties of avalanche photodiodes for applications in high energy physics, astrophysics and medical imaging, *Nucl Instr Meth A* **486**, 164-169 (2002).

32. Y. Shao, R.W. Silverman, R. Farrell, I Cirignano, R. Grazioso, K.S. Shah, G. Visser, M. Clajus, T.O. Turner, S.R. Cherry, Design studies of a high resolution PET detector using APD arrays, *IEEE Trans Nucl Sci* **47**, 1051-1057 (2000).

33. H.O. Anger, A new instrument for mapping gamma-ray emitters, *Biology and Medicine Quarterly Report UCRL* **3653**, 38 (1957).

34. H.M. Hudson, R.S. Larkin, Accelerated image reconstruction unsing ordered subsets of projection data, *IEEE Trans Med Imag* **13**, 601-609 (1994).

35. G.L. Zeng, D. Gagnon, CdZnTe strip detector SPECT imaging with a slit collimator, *Phys Med Biol* **49**, 2257-2271 (2004).

36. D.B. Everett, J.S. Fleming, R.W. Todd, J.M. Nightingale, Gamma-radiation imaging system based on the Compton effect, *Proc Inst Electr Eng.* **124**, 995-1000 (1977).

37. K.P. Pruessmann, M. Weiger, M.B. Scheidegger, P. Boesiger, SENSE: Sensitivity encoding for fast MRI, *Magn Reson Med* **42**, 952-962 (1999).

38. D.K. Sodickson, W.J. Manning, Simultaneous acquisition of spatial harmonics (SMASH): Fast imaging with radiofrequency coil arrays, *Magn Reson Med* **38**, 591-603 (1998).

39. U. Katscher, P. Boernert, C. Leussler, J.S. van den Brink, Transmit SENSE, *Magn Reson Med* **49**, 144-150 (2003).

40. A.G. Sorenson, F.S. Buonanno, R.G. Gonzalez, L.H. Schwamm, M.H. Lev, Hyperactue stroke: Evaluation with combined multisection diffusion-weighted and hemodynamically weighted echo-planar MR imaging, *Radiology* **199**, 391-401 (1996).

41. S.B. Colak, M.B. van der Mark, G.W. tHooft, J.H. Hoogenraad, E.S. van der Linden, F.A. Kuijpers, Clinical optical tomography and NIR spectroscopy for breast cancer detection, *IEEE J Quantum Electron* **5**, 1143-1158 (1999).

42. A.P. Gibson, J.C. Hebden, S.R. Arridge, Recent advances in diffuse optical imaging, *Phys Med Biol* **50**, R1-R43 (2005).

43. C.G.A. Hoelen, F.F.M. de Mul, R. Pongers, A. Dekker, Three-dimensional photoacoustic imaging of blood vessels in tissue, *Opt Lett* **23**, 648-650 (1998).

44. K.P. Kostli, D. Frauchiger, J.J. Niederhauser, G. Paltauf, H.P. Weber, M. Frenz, Optoacoustic imaging using a three-dimensional reconstruction algorithm, *IEEE J Sel Top Quant* **7**, 918-923 (2001).

45. X. Wang, Y. Pang, G. Ku, X. Xie, G. Stoica, L.V. Wang, Noninvasive laser-induced photoacoustic tomography for structural and functional in vivo imaging of the brain, *Nat Biotechnol* **21**, 803-806 (2003).

46. B. Gleich, J. Weizenecker, Tomographic imaging using nonlinear response of magnetic particles, *Nature* **435**, 1214-1217 (2005).

Chapter 3

RECONSTRUCTION TECHNOLOGIES FOR MEDICAL IMAGING SYSTEMS
Advances in Algorithms and Hardware for CT

Roland Proksa
Philips Research, Hamburg, Germany

Abstract: Medical imaging made immense advances in the last years. Beside new modalities the traditional imaging techniques and systems made rapid improvements. A good example is the improvements of Computerized Tomography (CT) with the introduction of large detector arrays. One of the important technological challenges of most medical imager is the reconstruction technology, which has to deal with complex imaging techniques and steadily increasing requirements. This chapter provides a brief insight into this field and discusses some technological aspects of reconstruction for CT.

Keywords: Reconstruction, CT, hardware acceleration

1.   INTRODUCTION

Most medical imaging devices use physical interactions to generate spatially resolved maps of static properties or functional information. Sensors are used to measure an impact of these physical interactions. Only in few cases the detected signals represent the final images directly (e.g. X-Ray radiography). In most imaging devices, the detected data itself are not useful for medical diagnosis and are usually converted back to the spatially resolved physical effect in the object that causes the acquired signals. The functional chain from the physical interaction up to the detected signal is called the forward problem and is usually well understood. However, the forward problem can become very complex and can include a number of disturbing effects such as scatter radiation, noise, or imperfections of the medical imaging device. Reconstruction is the inversion of the forward

35

G. Spekowius and T. Wendler (Eds.), Advances in Healthcare Technology, 35-47.
© 2006 *Springer. Printed in the Netherlands.*

problem. It estimates the physical interaction from the acquired data given a forward model of the measurement.

Most medical imaging devices have sensors outside the patient and detect data that do not only belong to a single point in the object but to larger areas. An example is a X-Ray beam that undergoes absorption on its way through the patient. The related mathematically forward models usually include integration in the object domain. This integral is usually the key problem of the reconstruction and requires integral transformation techniques. This can be demonstrated with simplified system models of some imaging modalities.

Computerized Tomography generate images of the X-ray absorption coefficient $\mu(x)$ at position x using measurements of the remaining X-ray intensities I of a beam with a primary intensity of I_0 along a line S. The forward problem becomes:

$$I = I_0 e^{-\int_S ds\mu(s)}$$

A simple 2D Magnetic Resonance Tomography generates images of the electromagnetic response m, which is phase encoded with a gradient g_p in y direction applied for time T and frequency encoded with a readout gradient g_r in x direction. With γ being the gyro-magnetic constant, the acquired signal $s(t)$ is described in the forward model by:

$$s(t) = \int \int m(x, y)\, e^{-i\gamma(Tg_p y + t g_r x)}\, dxdy$$

A detector in nuclear medicine (NM) measures the integrated radiation of a line through the object that is caused by a local decay of radioisotopes. Neglecting the absorption and other effects we get:

$$d = \int a(s)ds$$

This chapter gives a brief inside into reconstruction technologies for Computerized Tomography.

2.   CONE-BEAM RECONSTRUCTION IN CT

In recent years, CT scanners were subject to tremendous technological innovations. The most important improvement was the stepwise replacement of the one dimensional detection system with multi-line detectors up to two dimensional, large area detectors. These systems combine ultra-fast acquisition with high spatial resolution. The enhanced clinical value of CT created a push of CT as an important imaging modality. New important clinical application, such as perfusion studies or cardiac imaging came into reach of CT.

From a reconstruction point of view, these systems are Cone-Beam systems. The name reflects the geometrical shape of the x-ray beam, which is a serious challenge for reconstruction technologies. The related problems are twofold. One problem was the development of reconstruction methods and algorithms that produce good images, free of so-called cone-beam artifacts. The other challenge is the enormous amount of processing that came along with the complex reconstruction methods. This very practical problem is a severe burden for the industries, because the clinical workflow of CT imaging should not suffer from long reconstruction times. The use of non off-the-shelf super computer is considered as too expensive.

3.   FROM 2D RECONSTRUCTION TO 3D CONE-BEAM RECONSTRUCTION

The reconstruction of CT images from a 2D scan is a well-defined mathematical problem. After some preparations of the measured data, the problem can be simplified to reconstruct a 2D function from line integrals of this function. The problem can be investigated as a mathematical problem of continuous functions, ignoring the discrete nature of quantities in a real CT scanner such as discrete detector samples or image pixel. The most often used solution is the so-called filtered back-projection, which reads

$$f(x,y) = \int_{0}^{2\pi} \int_{-\infty}^{\infty} p(\phi, u) h(y \cos\phi - x \sin\phi - u) du d\phi$$

with $p()$ being parallel projections and with the distribution

$$h(u) = \frac{1}{2} \int_{-\infty}^{\infty} |p| e^{j2\pi pu} dp$$

which is often called ramp-filter. The inner integral is a convolution of the measured data with the ramp filter. The outer integral is called back-projection because it projects the filtered data back to the image domain.

The 2D filtered back-projection formula is an exact solution to the continuous inverse problem and can be mathematically proven. The general structure of the algorithm, filtering of the projection data and back-projection into the image domain, can also be found for similar reconstruction problems such as cone-beam reconstruction.

Similar to other analytical reconstruction methods that solve the reconstruction problem by means of an analytical reconstruction formula, this solution has to be discretized to finite sets of discrete projection angles, detector samples and image points. For the discrete representation of the data and the reconstruction, care must be taken to use proper sampling patterns and to limit the frequency band of the continuous functions.

The 2D reconstruction formula above assumes parallel ray geometry. Today's CT scanners are usually so-called third-generation scanners with an imaging system that rotates around the patient. A point-like focal spot emits an x-ray beam with a fan or cone shape, which is detected in a 1D or 2D detector array on the opposite side. The problem of the different ray geometry (divergent versus parallel) can be solved with a reformulated version of the reconstruction algorithm or by means of a so-called rebinning step that transform the fan beam data into parallel beam data.

The reconstruction of 3D cone-beam projections has a number of similarities to the 2D problem and again there exists a simple exact reconstruction formula. Unfortunately this formula requires parallel beams similar to the 2D version. Other than in the 2D case, there is no simple way to either reformulate the algorithm or to rebin the data. This was a serious challenge and it took quit some time until proper reconstruction methods became available.

Radon[20] derived a good theoretical framework of the inversion of integral transformations. This framework can directly be used for 2D reconstruction, because *Radon* described the *Radon transform,* which is equivalent to the forward problem and the *inverse Radon transform,* which is a reconstruction. The measured data i.e. the line integrals form the so-called *Radon domain.* The framework can also be applied to 3D functions. The *Radon domain* of a 3D function describes plane integrals of the function. One basic problem of the application of this framework to cone-beam reconstruction is the fact that a cone-beam scanner measures sets of line integrals and not plane integrals. However the framework of *Radon* can be used to consider some theoretical properties of reconstruction methods and it was the base of a class of exact reconstruction methods for cone-beam reconstruction.

3.1 Approximate reconstruction techniques

The absence of proper reconstruction techniques and later the high technological burden to use 3D cone-beam reconstruction techniques lead to a class of reconstruction techniques that performed some transformation or approximation of the acquired cone-beam data in such a way that the final reconstruction could be done with a traditional 2D technique. These simple solutions work fine if the number of detector rows and the related cone angle are small. For large detector arrays and large cone angles, the resulting image quality suffers from the approximation to 2D and shows so-called cone-beam artifacts. One example is the 'nutating slice algorithm'[17] or derivates[10]. This algorithm fits 2D planes to the helical trajectory. The projection data that are closest to this plane are extracted from the cone-beam data and are reconstructed with a 2D technique. Since the orientation of the 2D slices is coupled to the helix of the source trajectory, they are nutated relative to each other.

Another class of approximate algorithms generalizes the basic 2D methods into 3D. Good examples are [4,28,19]. These methods are of the type filtered back-projection. The rules for filtering in these methods are based on heuristics and geometrical considerations. However, there is no proof for exactness. The back-projection is a true 3D back-projection. A key feature of these algorithms is the utilization of the measured data. The framework of *Radon* allows the inspection of the used data in terms of completeness and redundancies, even if the inversion techniques of Radon are not applicable. For limited cone angles, these algorithms perform well and are in use in some clinical scanners. Especially the Wedge algorithm combines little cone-beam artifacts with good dose utilization and insensitivity against motion artifacts. The dose utilization measures, how good the x-ray exposure of the patient is utilized to provide images with good signal to noise ratio. Motion artifacts are image degradations from inconsistent projection data caused by patient motion during the data acquisition.

With the growing detector size in medical CT scanners, the need of helical acquisition techniques becomes less important. For some applications, the cone-beam covers the entire region of interest (40mm with state-of-the-art scanners). This could enable to use a single axial turn of the CT scanner to measure the entire region of interest. Unfortunately this attractive scan protocol has severe shortcomings. Up to now, there is only one basic reconstruction method available for this acquisition[9]. This method and its derivates generate severe artifacts, which can hardly be accepted especially in low contrast applications. Even worse, there is hardly any hope that this problem can be overcome with improved reconstruction techniques. The axial scan trajectory suffers form a so-called missing data problem. It can be shown using the framework of *Radon* or other sufficiency conditions[27,24] that not all data have been measured that are required for an exact reconstruction. It is assumed that this fundamental problem can only be overcome with other scanning trajectories that acquire all or at least more data for accurate reconstruction.

3.2   Exact reconstruction techniques

The first algorithms for exact cone-beam reconstruction[27,8,5,16] required non-truncated projection data and were not applicable for axial truncated data of helical cone-beam CT. Non-truncation in the above sense means that the entire object must be in the cone-beam. This problem was solved with the *Tam-Danielsson* window[25,3]. This window defines a detector shape with some unique features. The most important feature becomes visible if one takes an arbitrary cross section through the scanned object. Inspecting the cross sectional plane of all cones which have the focal spot in this plane, one can see that the plane is segmented into triangles that cover the entire plane completely and without any redundancy. The cross sections can be related to *Radon* planes. Each *Radon* plane is covered by a set of triangles, which are part of the measure cone-beams. Together with an important relation of plane integrals and divergent line integrals[8], it was possible to calculate the derivative of *Radon* planes from cone-beam projections. In the first algorithms based on these results, a limitation of the object support in axial direction by the entire helical scan was still required. This so-called long object problem was later solved[21,22,26]. One shortcoming for clinical applications was the restriction to a fixed pitch, defined as table feed per gantry rotation with a given detector size. This problem has been solved[19] with the *nPI* method that allows a set of discrete pitches.

A breakthrough was achieved with the work of Katsevich[11,12,13]. The basic achievements of Katsevich were later generalized and applied to other reconstruction problems, such as the 3PI acquisition[1,14], or the general nPI acquisition[2]. These methods are filtered back-projection methods, were the filtering direction has to be chosen such, that the *Radon* domain is captured completely and without any redundancy. The framework is very general and can be applied to reconstruction problems, if a proper set of filter directions can be found.

Sidky[23] recently achieved another important exact reconstruction technique with the exchange of the integration order. This novel reconstruction technique performs the back-projection prior to the filtering, which takes now place in the image domain. An important feature was added by Pack[18] and allows the utilization of arbitrary amount of redundant data.

Exact reconstruction methods are currently not used in commercial medical CT scanner although cone-beam artifacts become more important for large detector arrays. A basic shortcoming of these methods is the problem to handle redundant data properly. Redundant data are acquired if the physical detector is larger than required by the Tam-Danielsson window or by consideration to fill the *Radon* domain completely. These redundant data should properly be used to achieve a high x-ray dose utility. Even more important, this data are essential for the reduction of motion artifacts. Recent results[15] that aim to overcome this limitation and combine the absence of cone-beam artifacts from the exact methods with the relative insensitivity to motion artifacts of approximate methods look promising. However, exact reconstruction methods have to demonstrate robustness and practicality.

3.3 Iterative reconstruction techniques

A very different class of reconstruction techniques is called iterative reconstruction. Instead of searching for an analytical solution of a continuous problem, the basic approach of these techniques is to model the imaging process with a discrete system model. A discrete set of image points μ and measurements p are linked with a system matrix A to a simple linear model:

$$p = A\mu$$

The system Matrix A basically describes the system geometry and models how much an image point influences a measurement sample. It can become more complex and take other system aspects of the forward problem into account. Within this model, the reconstruction problem becomes to estimate μ from a measurement p. Several numerical methods exist to solve this problem, typically with an iterative algorithm. From a mathematical point of view, the equation system is usually over determined and inconsistent, because there are more projection samples than image points and the data are inconsistent due to noise.

A powerful method to solve such a problem is ART[7]. ART takes an intermediate image μ^n and applies the forward system matrix to obtain a part of the projection data p^n. A proper part could be a set of parallel rays through the image. These calculated projections are compared to the measured projections p and the difference is used to update the intermediate image. A simplified version of ART is:

$$p^n = A\mu^n$$
$$\mu^{n+1} = \mu^n + \lambda A^T (p - p^n)$$

This process is repeated e.g. with other projection parts, until a stopping criteria is meet. The parameter λ is to control the convergence speed.

Even more powerful techniques take the noise in the measured data into account. A very popular method is the Maximum Likelihood (ML) method. Each projection value is modeled, as a random variable were the measured value is the expected value and the probability distribution is known. A simple noise model is to assume Poisson statistics of the measured data. Given an intermediate image μ, we can calculate the projections p of it. Knowing the probability distribution of each projection value, we can calculate the likelihood of the intermediate image for one projection value or the total likelihood as the product of the individual likelihoods. In other words we can calculate the likelihood $L(\mu)$ of an image, given a set of projections and a noise model. With some iterative numerical methods, we can search for an image that has the highest likelihood. Statistical reconstruction is a science for itself and far beyond the scope of this book. However the simple introduction can help to better understand the features of this reconstruction technique.

ML reconstruction methods have a significantly better signal to noise ratio (SNR) than analytical methods. This is due to the incorporation of a proper noise model. ML reconstruction techniques are widely used in nuclear medicine (NM), were the count rates are typically low and the SNR advantage of ML is essential. Fessler[6] showed that the advantage can also be realized in transmission scans such as CT. SNR improvements between 1.4 and 2 have been reported[29]. This advantage could be used to reduce the x-ray dose by a factor of 2 to 4 and still provide the same SNR as conventional reconstruction methods. Studies with clinical data demonstrated that the image quality is better or equal to standard reconstruction methods. Although the advantages are known, iterative reconstruction methods are not applied in commercial CT scanner due to the enormous amount of processing power required for the reconstruction. The processing time of statistical reconstruction methods is acceptable for NM due to two reasons:

- The processing time depend on the number of image points and the number of detector channel. These numbers are typically low compared to CT (typical number of image points per plane NM 64x64 versus CT 512x512).
- One acquisition in NM lasts typically 15 to 30 min. If a reconstruction takes about as long as the acquisition, the workflow does not suffer to much.

This situation is very different for CT. Unfortunately the number of image points has to be increased compared to an analytical reconstruction technique. To achieve the good results, the entire imaging area has to be reconstructed on a fine grid. This is because the discretization in the image domain goes already into the system model and influences the behavior of the algorithm. The resulting processing time for typical parameter settings and off-the-shelf computer hardware varies between hours and weeks and is not acceptable for clinical use.

However it is expected, that the constantly increasing performance of computer hardware and especially some dedicated computer systems will sooner or later overcome this restriction, and will make the potential dose saving and the other advantages of statistical reconstruction methods available for the clinical use.

As mentioned earlier, iterative techniques allow to integrate more imaging system aspects as just the basic geometry and physics.

4.   HARDWARE ACCELERATION

The reconstruction process of a typical CT system consists of four major parts:

- Raw data correction.
- Data rebinning.
- Filtering.
- Back-projection.

The raw data correction is required to compensate for a number of effects on the measured data. The correction algorithms are usually not very computational intensive and can be realized with off-the-shelf computer systems.

The filtering and the final back-projection are sometimes done in a geometry that differs from the geometry of the CT system itself. This transformation is often called rebinning. One example is the transformation of fan beam data to a parallel geometry. The processing consists of some interpolation steps without high demands on the processing power.

Step number three, the filtering is usually be done in the *Fourier* domain. The processing includes a (Fast) Fourier transform, a multiplication with the filter and an inverse (Fast) Fourier transform. The analysis of the computational effort shows that the required processing power is equivalent to about one state-of-the-art personal computer. The main processing load comes from the Fourier transforms. For costs reasons, a more efficient implementation using off-the-shelf Digital Signal Processor (DSP) accelerator or FGPA based sub-systems can be considered.

The back-projection is much more demanding than the previous processing steps and requires special attention. In the following, an estimate of the computational effort is provided. The estimations are not very precise, because they depend on a number of details. The speed of different implementation can easily vary by a factor of two or more. However they can be used to get an impression of the order of magnitude of the problem.

Back-projection is a simple operation that has to be performed very often. The basic operation is to take one image point, calculate the projection of this point onto one projection, perform an interpolation of the projection and add the result to the image point. In a simple 2D case, this operation requires roughly 20 instructions of a standard processor. The operation has to be repeated 2.5×10^8 times for a 512x512 image slice back projected from 1024 projections. Today's (2005) standard processor can perform this operation with a rate of about 2 images per second. In the 90's, this was a real challenge for the first spiral CT scanners that were able to scan about 1 slice per second. The *easily* available processing power was a few hundred times less. At that time, Philips Medical Systems (PMS) managed this problem with a dedicated processor, which was highly optimized for this operation. Two main architectural choices made it possible to achieve a performance level of about 400 times the performance of off-the-shelf workstation computer systems. The first was to parallelize the operations. Instead of performing the 20 instructions in sequence, a dedicated computational pipeline was able to perform one complete back-projection operation in a single cycle. The second choice was to use multiple units and build a multi-processor system with 14 units. The high specialization of the processor made it possible to increase the operation frequency. All measures together, enabled PMS to build a cost effective accelerator board that reaches real time performance, with a system that could reconstruct two images per second. The price of this attractive reconstruction unit was an investment in processor architecture and design.

The next challenge came with the introduction of cone-beam CT systems. In the beginning of the millennium, the CT systems required:

- Cone-beam reconstruction algorithm without cone-beam artifacts.
- Detector arrays with 16 rows.
- Faster rotation time (0.5 sec).

The effective acquisition speed has increased by a factor of about 30. This was already a serious challenge and some CT manufacturer decided to stay with 2D reconstruction techniques. The 3D cone-beam reconstruction algorithm required about 20 to 30 times more processing power for a basic back-projection operation than the 2D equivalent. An additional problem was that the traditional 2D hardware acceleration systems were not able to perform these more complex 3D operations. Again PMS took the challenge and designed a dedicated 3D cone-beam processor with the latest available semiconductor technology. The result was about the same. It was possible to improve the processing speed by a factor of a few hundred to thousand with dedicated hardware compared to multi-purpose computer systems.

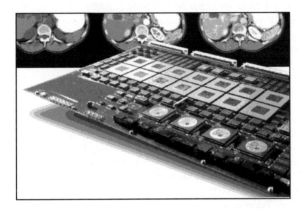

Figure 3-1. The 2D CT Reconstruction accelerator

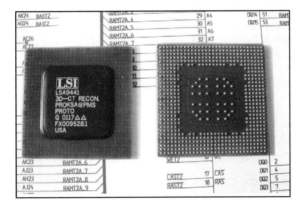

Figure 3-2. The 2nd Generation 3D Cone-Beam Processor

The actual challenges for CT reconstruction are still growing with technological improvements of the CT scanners. They are driven by faster gantry rotation, larger detector arrays (64 rows and more?), the need to use exact reconstruction algorithm or the *wish* to make use of statistical reconstruction methods.

REFERENCES

1. C. Bontus, T. Köhler, R. Proksa, A quasiexact Reconst6ruction Algorithm for helical CT using a 3π Acquisition, *Med Phys* **30**, 2492-2502 (2003).
2. C. Bontus, T. Köhler, R. Proksa, EnPiT, A Reconstruction Algorithm for helical CT, *IEEE Trans Medical Imaging* **8**, 977-986 (2005).
3. P.E. Danielsson, P. Edholm, J. Eriksson, M. Magnusson-Seger, Towards exact 3D-Reconstruction for helical Cone-Beam scanning of long Objects, *Proc 3D'97 Conference, Nemacolin, Pennsylvania, USA*, 141-144 (1997).
4. P.E. Danielsson, P. Edholm, J. Eriksson, M. Magnusson-Seger, H. Turbell, The original PI-method for helical Cone-Beam CT, *Proc 3D'99 Conference, Egmond aan Zee, The Netherlands*, 3-6 (1999).
5. M. Defrise, R. Clack, A Cone-Beam Reconstruction Algorithm using shift-variant Filtering and Cone-Beam Back-Projection, *IEEE Trans Med Imag* **13**, 186-195 (1994).
6. J.A. Fessler, Statistical Image Reconstruction Methods for Transmission Tomography, *Handbook of Medical Imaging*, M. Sonka, J. M. Fitzpatrick (eds.), Vol. 3, 1-70 (SPIE Press, Bellingham,WA 2000).
7. R. Gordon, A Tutorial on ART (Algebraic Reconstruction Techniques), *IEEE Trans Nucl Sci* **21**, 1-23 (1970).
8. P. Grangeat, Mathematical Framework of Cone-Beam 3D Reconstruction via the First Derivative of the Radon Transformation, *Mathematical Methods in Tomography*, 66-97, (Springer, Berlin 1991).
9. L.A. Feldkamp, L.C. Davis, J. W. Kress, Practical Cone-Beam Algorithm, *J Opt Soc Am*, A 1, 612-619 (1984).
10. M. Kachelrieß, S. Schaller, W.A. Kalender, 2000, Advanced Single-Slice Rebinning in Cone-Beam Spiral CT, *Med Phys* **27**, 754-772 (2000).
11. A. Katsevich, Theoretically exact FBP-type inversion Algorithm for Spiral CT, *Proc 3D'2001 Conference, Asilomar, USA*, 6-9 (2001).
12. A. Katsevich, Analysis of an Exact Inversion Algorithm for Spiral Cone-Beam CT, *Phys Med Biol* **47**, 2583-2597 (2002).
13. A. Katsevich, Theoretically exact FBP-type inversion Algorithm for Spiral CT, *SIAM J Appl Math* **62**, 2012-2026 (2002).
14. A. Katsevich, On two Versions of a 3π Algorithm for Spiral CT, *Phys Med Biol* **49**, 2129-2143 (2004).
15. T. Köhler, C. Bontus, P. Koken, A new Approach to handle redundant Data in helical Cone-Beam CT, *Proc 3D'2005 Conference*, Salt Lake City, Utah, 19-22 (2005).
16. H. Kudo, T. Saito, Derivation and Implementation of a Cone-Beam Reconstruction Algorithm for non-planar Orbits, *IEEE Trans Med Imag* **13**, 196-211 (1994).
17. G. Larson, C.C. Ruth, C.R. Crawford, Nutating Slice CT Image Reconstruction Apparatus Method, *US Patent 5,802,134* (1998).
18. J.D. Pack, F. Noo, R. Clackdoyle, Cone-Beam Reconstruction using the Backprojection of locally Filtered Projections, *IEEE Trans Med Imag* **24**, 70-85 (2005).
19. R. Proksa, T. Köhler, M. Grass, J. Timmer, The n-PI-method for helical Cone-Beam CT, *IEEE Trans Med Imag* **19**, 848-863 (2000).

20. J. Radon J., Über die Bestimmung von Funktionen durch ihre Integralwerte längs gewisser Mannigfaltigkeiten, Berichte Sächsische Akademie der Wissenschaft, *Math Phys* **69**, 262-267 (1917).
21. F. Sauer, S. Samarasekera, K.C. Tam, Practical Cone-Beam Image Reconstruction using local Region-of-Interest, *US Patent 6009142* (1999).
22. S. Schaller, F. Noo F. Sauer K.C. Tam, G. Lauritsch, T. Flohr, Exact Radon Rebinning Algorithm for the long Object Problem in Helical Cone-Beam CT, *IEEE Trans Med Imag* **19**, 361-375 (2000).
23. E.Y. Sidky, Y. Zou, X. Pan, Minimum Data Image Reconstruction Algorithms with shift-invariant Filtering for helical, Cone-Beam CT, *Phys Biol* **50**, 1643-1657 (2005).
24. D. Smith, Cone-beam convolution formula, *Comput Bio Med* **13**, 81-87 (1983).
25. K.C. Tam, Three-dimensional Computerized Tomography Scanning Method and System for large Objects with smaller Area Detectors, *US Patent 5,390,112* (1995).
26. K.C. Tam, Exact local Region-of-interest Reconstruction in Spiral Cone-Beam filtered Backprojection CT: Theory, *Proc SPIE Medical Imaging,* SPIE **3959**, 606-519 (2000).
27. H.K. Tuy, An inversion formula for cone-beam reconstruction, *SIAM J Appl Math* **43**, 546-552 (1983).
28. H.K. Tuy, 3D Image Reconstruction for helical partial Cone Beam Scanners, *Proc 3D'99 Conference*, Egmond aan Zee, The Netherlands, 7-10 (1999)
29. A. Ziegler, D. Heuscher, T. Köhler, T. Nielsen, R. Proksa, Systematic Investigation of the Reconstruction of Images from Transmission Tomography using a Filtered Back-Projection and an iterative OSML Reconstruction Algorithm, *Proc IEEE Medical Imaging Conference, Rome*, on CD, M02-181 (2004).

Chapter 4

DETECTORS FOR X-RAY IMAGING AND COMPUTED TOMOGRAPHY
Advances and Key Technologies

Michael Overdick

Philips Research, Aachen, Germany

Abstract: Medical X-ray imaging and Computed Tomography (CT) rely heavily on the performance of the imaging detectors used in these modalities. This article gives an overview over the key technologies involved in the construction of such imaging detectors. Apart from the conversion of the X-rays also photodiodes and the associated electronics constitute important technology fields. For both X-ray and CT the development of the technologies over the last decade is reviewed, the state of the art is described and some current and envisaged developments are emphasized.

Keywords: X-ray, CT, detector, scintillator, direct conversion, photodiode, pixel electronics, integrating, counting

1.   INTRODUCTION

Signal detectors are a central element in any medical imaging system. In the imaging modalities X-ray, CT, SPECT and PET the information is carried by ionizing radiation, more precisely X-rays or γ-quanta. The imaging detectors consist of a multitude of detector channels, for modern X-ray detectors up to several million picture elements (pixels). In this article, the main emphasis will be on detectors for X-ray and CT. SPECT and PET will be briefly touched upon in the outlook section at the end of the article.

In general, detectors for X-ray and CT imaging comprise a conversion stage for converting the X-ray quanta ultimately into electrical signals. The conversion stage is followed by pixel electronics, i.e. the electronic circuitry belonging exclusively to one detector channel. The pixel electronics are then

G. Spekowius and T. Wendler (Eds.), Advances in Healthcare Technology, 49-64.

usually connected to further circuitry, which is shared by many or all detector channels. The general scheme is shown in Figure 4-1a.

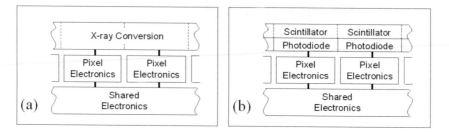

Figure 4-1. a) General representation of an X-ray or CT detector, b) with indirect conversion.

In the majority of today's detectors for dynamic X-ray imaging and CT imaging, the conversion is indirect (Figure 4-1b), i.e. the X-rays are first converted into visible light, which is converted further into an electrical signal by a photosensitive device, usually a photodiode in the case of X-ray and CT. Although the photodiodes are a part of the overall conversion stage, they will be discussed in a separate section of this chapter.

There are many design and performance parameters related to imaging detectors. Detection efficiency, spatial resolution, signal-to-noise ratio, dynamic range and temporal resolution are most important[1]. This article cannot cover all these parameters for all key technologies in depths, so only some main relations will be mentioned.

2. CONVERSION MATERIALS

Conversion materials should efficiently detect (i.e. absorb) the incoming X-ray quanta and convert them into light (for scintillating materials) or directly into electrical signals (for direct conversion materials). The extremely strong influence of the conversion stage on the overall imaging performance makes both scintillator and direct conversion materials key technology items for imaging detectors. Main characteristics of conversion materials are:

- Detection efficiency.
- 'Sensitivity', i.e. the light yield for scintillators or the charge yield for direct conversion materials.
- Spatial resolution, often expressed as the Modulation Transfer Function (MTF).
- Temporal resolution.

It is very important to note the difference between detection efficiency and sensitivity. As X-ray and CT imaging are governed by the noise of the X-ray quantum flux, the detection efficiency should be as high as possible, e.g. 80% or more of the incoming quanta should be detected. Too low a detection efficiency cannot be recovered by increasing the sensitivity of the detector.

2.1   Scintillators

There are many materials emitting visible light when energy is deposited in the material, e.g. by X-rays or energetic charged particles. Such materials are known as scintillators. For the efficient detection of X-rays usually inorganic compounds containing some heavy element are used. Sodium iodide (NaI) or cadmium tungstate (CdWO$_4$) are well known examples. Extensive overviews have been given by van Eijk[2]. To achieve the high detection efficiency at quantum energies of 60 keV or higher, the typical thickness of a scintillator can range from 0.3 to 2.5 mm for X-ray and CT imaging.

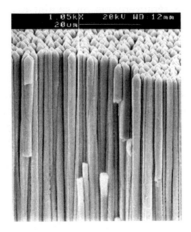

Figure 4-2. Columnar structure of a CsI:Tl scintillator.

X-ray imaging requires a fine spatial resolution of the order of 100 µm at the detector. Cesium iodide (CsI) is often used for this application, as it can be grown with a columnar structure as shown in Figure 4-2. This structure limits the lateral spread of the scintillation light, thus helping significantly in achieving an acceptable spatial resolution. For the use with amorphous silicon photodiodes (see section 3.1), the CsI is doped with traces of thallium which works as an activator shifting the maximum of the light emission spectrum into the green region[3]. The light yield of CsI:Tl is about 60 photons per keV of deposited energy[1,2]. CsI:Tl exhibits a significant afterglow of about 1% after 10 ms[2,4]. However, for X-ray imaging this is an acceptable value. After strong X-ray illumination the light yield of the CsI:Tl increases slightly, the effect being known as 'bright burn'[4].

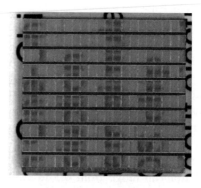

Figure 4-3. Array of CdWO$_4$ crystals for CT imaging.

For CT imaging the requirements on spatial resolution are only of the order of 1 mm at the detector, while the fast gantry rotation and the large number of projections demand signal integration times as low as 100 µs and therefore a very good temporal behaviour of the scintillator. Frequently cadmium tungstate (CdWO$_4$) or gadolinium oxysulfide (GOS, Gd$_2$O$_2$S) are chosen[5]. CdWO$_4$ has a light yield of 20 photons per keV, whereas GOS, depending on the doping, reaches 35-60 photons per keV [2]. The scintillator crystals are machined into small pieces of about 2-5 mm^3, which are then mounted next to each other with reflective material between them to avoid lateral cross-talk of the scintillation light between the individual crystals (Figure 4-3).

2.2   Direct conversion materials

Direct conversion materials generate measurable charge signals when absorbing X-ray quanta. Usually these materials have a high resistivity (10^{10} to 10^{16} Ωcm) and are operated with relatively strong electric fields (between 0.1 and 20 V/µm). For applications in X-ray imaging, several classical photoconducting materials have been studied,[6] such as amorphous selenium[7-9] (a-Se) and the polycrystalline materials lead iodide[10,11] (PbI$_2$), lead oxide[12-14] (PbO) and mercury iodide[11,15,16] (HgI$_2$). Some properties of these materials are listed in Table 4-1. The main advantage of direct conversion materials is their inherently excellent spatial resolution. Even for finely spaced pixel electrodes (e.g. 100 μm pitch or below) the charge signal usually remains within the pixel area in which the X-ray quantum was absorbed. This is due to the relatively high and well-defined electric fields in the materials and due to a rather small lateral diffusion of the charge carriers. Figure 4-4 shows an X-ray image obtained with a PbO detection layer[13]. Until now, only amorphous selenium is used in commercial X-ray detectors[7, 9], the other materials still being in their research phases.

Table 4-1. Selected properties of some direct conversion materials.

	a-Se	PbO	HgI$_2$	cryst. CZT
Typ. el. field	10-20 V/μm	5 V/μm	1-2 V/μm	0.1 V/μm
Resistivity	10^{14}-10^{16} Ωcm	10^{12}-10^{13} Ωcm	10^{12}-10^{13} Ωcm	$3\cdot10^{10}$ Ωcm
Charge yield	20-30 e$^-$/keV	60 e$^-$/keV	100 e$^-$/keV	200 e$^-$/keV

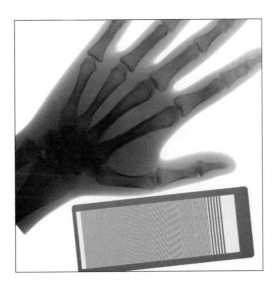

Figure 4-4. X-ray image acquired with a PbO detection layer.

A common problem of the amorphous or polycrystalline direct conversion materials is their temporal behavior. Some materials show strong residual signals, i.e. a decaying surplus dark current after X-ray illumination, which can be in the range of several percent still 1 s after switching off the X-rays. Amorphous selenium exhibits a reduced sensitivity (reduced charge yield) after X-ray illumination. This so-called ghosting effect[8] decays even slower, it can be present for minutes. The mechanism of charge trapping cannot account for all of the observed temporal effects in direct converters. Also charge injection invoked by charge accumulation layers may often play a role[14].

There are also crystalline direct conversion materials. Classical examples are silicon and germanium, but both are not very heavy materials and germanium detectors usually have to be cooled during operation. A room-temperature detector material receiving much research attention is cadmium zinc telluride (CZT, roughly $Cd_{0.9}Zn_{0.1}Te$)[17]. Some of its properties are also stated in Table 4-1. CZT has a high charge yield of about 200 e⁻ per keV deposited energy, and its temporal behavior is much better than that of amorphous or polycrystalline materials. The use of CZT detector crystals is considered for X-ray, CT and also for SPECT. However, the material is still somewhat expensive and cannot be produced in arbitrary sizes. CZT can also be operated in counting mode allowing the detection of individual X-ray or γ-quanta, as will be discussed in the outlook in section 4.

3.   PHOTODIODES AND PIXEL ELECTRONICS

3.1   Flat X-ray detectors based on amorphous silicon

3.1.1   State of the art

The field of dynamic X-ray imaging detectors has gone through significant technologies change over the last five years. From the 1970's the standard technology were image intensifier systems (II-TV) based on sizeable vacuum tubes incorporating electron optics, phosphor screens and optical cameras. Roughly from the year 2000 onwards, flat dynamic X-ray detectors[18-21] utilizing amorphous silicon technology have been introduced for cardiology, neurology, vascular imaging and other applications. Also for static X-ray imaging, e.g. in general radiography, the amorphous silicon technology is now frequently employed in new systems.

The majority of the flat X-ray detectors are based on indirect conversion using CsI:Tl as the scintillation material, as discussed in section 2.1. The optical light is detected by amorphous silicon photodiodes in the large area electronics panel[22-24]. The a-Si photodiodes exhibit only small leakage currents and have their maximal sensitivity in the green where the CsI:Tl shows its highest light emission. The circuit diagram for an indirect conversion flat detector pixel is shown in Figure 4-5a. Each pixel has an a-Si thin film transistor (TFT) as the switching element, allowing a row-wise read-out of the pixel array. The pixel diode and its associated capacitance are discharged by the light from the scintillator during X-ray illumination. During read-out an external charge sensitive amplifier (CSA) connected to the read-out column re-charges the pixel diode to a fixed reverse bias voltage, typically 5 to 10 V. In this charge read-out configuration, the dominant noise sources are the reset noise of the diode (also referred to as kTC-noise as it is given by kTC_{pix}, where C_{pix} is the pixel capacitance) and the noise of the charge sensitive amplifier. The shot noise of the diode's leakage current is among the smaller noise contributions.

In addition to the temporal effects in the scintillator, the amorphous silicon photodiode and the TFT in the pixel also show temporal effects[25-28], namely residual signals, photodiode gain effect (similar to ghosting) and incomplete read-out. The first two effects are attributed to trapping states in the a-Si. Both can be reduced by illuminating the a-Si photodiodes with additional light (refresh light)[28].

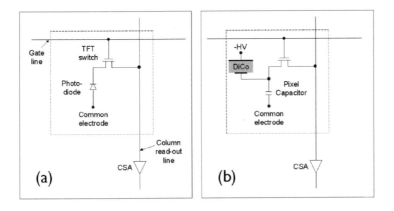

Figure 4-5. a-Si pixel circuits for (a) indirect and (b) direct conversion.

The introduction of flat X-ray detectors based on a-Si technology on the medical market is very successful. Compared to the previous II-TV systems, the flat detectors are less bulky, have a distortion-free imaging geometry and almost completely suppress a long-range blurring effect known as low-frequency drop. For many applications this opens up a larger usable dynamic range.

The flat detectors based on direct conversion materials (see section 2.2) also utilize a-Si technology for the large area substrates[9,13]. The pixel circuit is very similar, as shown in Figure 4-5b. A collection electrode and a capacitor on which the charge signals are integrated during X-ray illumination replace the a-Si photodiode. The read-out operates in a similar way as described for the indirect conversion circuit.

3.1.2   Advanced amorphous silicon flat detectors

After the radical technology switch from image intensifiers to flat X-ray detectors, research and development in this field are currently concentrating on improving the a-Si based X-ray detectors. Improvement topics are the signal-to-noise ratio at low X-ray doses, dynamic range and spatial resolution. Also reducing the production costs and implementing additional functionality within the a-Si technology are natural directions.

One way of improving the signal-to-noise ratio is to enhance the fill factor of the pixel, i.e. the fraction of the pixel area that is sensitive to light. To this end, several methods to increase the size of the photodiode in the pixel have been developed, including diode-on-top technologies[29, 31] and infinite photodiode layers[30]. An increased fill factor also allows to construct detector arrays with smaller pixels and therefore enhanced spatial resolution.

Another way to achieve a higher signal-to-noise ratio would be to amplify the signal already in the pixel. Several circuits for in-pixel amplifiers have been proposed[32-34]. Many suffer from some poor electrical properties of the amorphous silicon TFTs, especially their low charge carrier mobility and the drift of the threshold voltage over time. In more complex circuits also additional noise sources have to be taken into account. An example of a pixel circuit with signal amplification is drawn in Figure 4-6.

Other advanced pixel circuit concepts include the integration of sample-and-hold stages or the suppression of the pixel's reset noise by means of correlated double sampling. Additional functionality can also come in the form of integrated dose sensing allowing the control of the X-ray generation equipment during the X-ray pulse. One concept for integrated dose sensing[35] avoiding any additional active elements in the pixel is shown in Figure 4-7. The dose sensing information is sensed non-destructively through tiny capacitors C_{tap} attached to each pixel node. Using appropriate external electronics this yields coarsely resolved images at a very high rate (e.g. 10 kHz) from which the information relevant for the dose control can be derived.

Apart from pure a-Si technology, also advanced technology versions or other large area electronics technologies are investigated. Examples are poly-silicon electronics[34], or flexible electronics produced by inexpensive roll-to-roll processes, including ink jet printing methods and polymer-based electronics[36]. Also CMOS array detectors have been proposed which can offer excellent performance[37]. However, achieving very large area detectors with sufficient yield may be an issue with this technology.

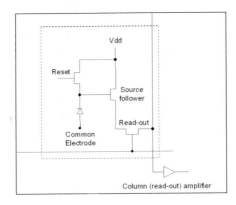

Figure 4-6. Pixel circuit with signal amplification (source follower).

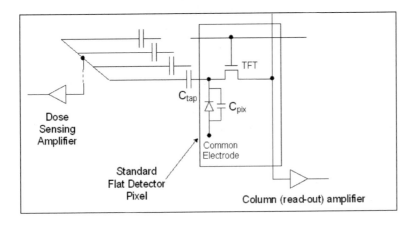

Figure 4-7. Diagram illustrating integrated dose sensing.

3.2 Detectors for multi-slice CT

3.2.1 State of the art

In Computed Tomography (CT) the last decade has been dominated by two trends, faster gantry rotation and more detection slices in the axial direction of the patient (multi-slice CT)[38]. Both trends led to a dramatic reduction of the scanning times, shortening a whole body scan, for example, from about 20 minutes to about half a minute. At the same time, the spatial resolution was improved, leading to even finer resolved volume images of the human body and all organs of interest.

The basic construction scheme of a CT detector has stayed roughly the same. The detector elements are arranged on a ca. 1 m long arc of a circle, sometimes called the 'detector banana'. Each detector pixel consists of a scintillator crystal and a corresponding photodiode. The photodiode is then connected to the electronics channel, typically comprising an amplifier and an analog-to-digital converter (ADC) optimized for the CT detector operation.

The photodiodes have evolved from individual diodes or linear arrangements into two-dimensional arrays of photodiodes. All of these photodiodes are made from crystalline silicon, which has an excellent linearity and temporal behavior. The illumination is from the front of the photodiode, and the pixel contacts are routed on that same side to one or two edges of the photodiode array. With the number of axial slices in the CT exceeding 32, the routing of the many pixel connections to the edges became more and more difficult. This problem is now addressed using back-illuminated photodiodes, where the routing of the pixel contacts is no longer needed[39,40]. The connection from the pixel is made directly to a substrate using modern interconnect technology.

For the electronics, the increasing number of detector slices led to a strong trend to shrink and integrate the channel electronics, also in order to decrease cost and power consumption and to minimize the noise by keeping the distances between the photodiodes and the electronics short. In current CT detectors, the electronics channels of e.g. 32 pixels fit into an integrated circuit that outputs the digitized data. Also in this context, high density interconnect technologies such as bump bonding are getting more and more important in the field of large area radiation detectors.

3.2.2 Advanced technology for CT

Although today's CT detectors show an excellent performance, some technologies are being investigated for future CT detectors. One concept brings the integration of the detector one step further by combining the photodiodes and the channel amplifier in a common CMOS chip[41,42]. To achieve the necessary dynamic range of about 17 bit, the amplifier is constructed as an integrator with an automatic gain switch selecting one of two sensitivities. The pixel electronics is located in areas which are in the shadow of the anti-scatter grid of the detector. In this way, the electronics are not wasting valuable fill-factor and are shielded from too much radiation, so that the CMOS pixel electronics is not harmed by the X-rays. Figure 4-8 shows a detector module with 20 by 20 pixels and a zoom into the pixel area.

Other investigations analyze the use of direct conversion materials also for CT. Due to the required excellent temporal behaviour (see section 2.1), the known amorphous and polycrystalline direct conversion materials cannot be used in CT. Only crystalline direct conversion materials are fast enough. Consequently, materials such as cadmium zinc telluride (CZT, see section 2.2) are regarded as possible candidates for use in CT detectors. However, some studies analyzing the behaviour of CZT under high X-ray fluxes indicate some issues with the material[43, 44].

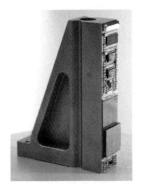 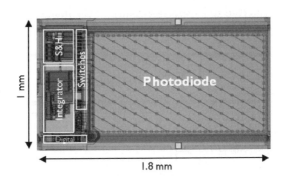

Figure 4-8. CT Detector module based on integrated CMOS photodiodes and pixel electronics. On the module, only one of two scintillator arrays is mounted.

4.   OUTLOOK

The trends towards higher performance and at the same time cost reduction will continue for detectors in X-ray and CT imaging. In the long run, direct conversion and a further integration of the electronics are probable directions. Apart from this, also qualitative changes in the functionality of the detectors are expected, for example moving from integration mode to counting mode detectors. Until now, both X-ray and CT detectors operate in integration mode, i.e. they sum up the 'intensity' of the measured X-ray flux during the signal integration time. An alternative approach is to detect and count the X-ray quanta individually, a mode known as counting operation. Due to the high fluxes that can occur in both X-ray and CT imaging (of the order of 10^9 quanta per second per mm² at the detector), counting has so far been considered unfeasible. However, advances in pixelled counting detectors[45, 46] may trigger investigations in this direction.

It is also possible to combine counting and integrating operation, as sketched in Figure 4-9. This would yield additional information as the counting channel records the number of the detected quanta, whereas the integrating channel sums up the energies of the detected quanta. Thus the mean energy of the X-ray quanta can be calculated per detector pixel by simply dividing the integrated signal by the counted signal. The mean energy is a measure for the beam hardening in the patient and can give some information about the material composition along the X-ray beam in the patient. With even more complex electronics it may also become feasible to measure the spectrum of the detected radiation in each pixel[47]. This concept is referred to as spectral X-ray or CT imaging.

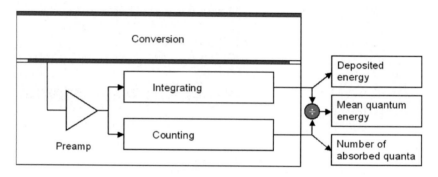

Figure 4-9. Combined counting and integrating detector pixel.

At this point it is interesting to compare the detector technology in X-ray and CT imaging with the methods used in nuclear medicine, i.e. SPECT and PET imaging. In SPECT and PET it is mandatory to measure the energy of the individual γ-quanta to suppress scatter events, so spectral imaging is already a standard in nuclear medicine. However, the fluxes are much lower (1-100 quanta / s mm² for SPECT and about 100 quanta / s mm² for typical PET applications) which eases the design of the spectrally resolving detector. The architecture still most commonly used in nuclear medicine comprises scintillator crystals optically connected to arrays of photo-multipliers. The energy of a detected quantum is calculated by summing up the signals from several adjacent photomultipliers, while the spatial information is retrieved using a centroid calculation. This is the so-called Anger method already in use since the 1960s for two-dimensional scintigraphy. For nuclear medicine a technology change towards solid-state detection with indirect conversion or direct conversion is being contemplated, but most commercial systems still rely on the photomultiplier technology and discrete electronics. More information about the imaging modalities of nuclear medicine can be found in Chapter 8 of this volume.

5.   CONCLUSIONS

For medical X-ray and CT imaging, the detectors play a significant role for the overall system design and performance. The key technologies comprise:

- X-ray conversion (using scintillators or direct conversion materials).
- Photodiodes (in connection with scintillators).
- Pixel electronics.
- Interconnect technology.

Both X-ray and CT detectors have seen tremendous advances in these key technologies over the last decade. In X-ray imaging the last years brought a rapid technology change from image intensifiers towards flat X-ray detectors based on a-Si large area electronics. This technology is being improved to achieve further enhancements in the detector performance and reductions of the production costs.

For CT detectors, the number of axial slices has increased dramatically and the faster gantry rotation requires shorter and shorter signal integration times. Technically, these challenges have been met by going to back-illuminated photodiodes and highly integrated electronics chips. Also cheap and reliable interconnect technology plays an increasingly important role.

As long-term trends the use of direct conversion materials and even more highly integrated electronics have been identified for both modalities. The future may even bring a qualitative change from integrating detectors to counting detectors also in the field of X-ray and CT imaging.

ACKNOWLEDGEMENTS

The overview presented here is partly based on the detector related activities at Philips Research Laboratories Aachen, Germany, Philips Research Laboratories Redhill, United Kingdom, Philips Medical Systems X-ray, Best, The Netherlands and Philips Medical Systems CT, Cleveland, Ohio, USA and Haifa, Israel.

The author would like to thank all colleagues from these groups for their contributions and the good long-standing collaboration.

REFERENCES

1. J. Beutel, H.L. Kundel, R.L. van Metter (eds.), *Handbook of Medical Imaging, Vol. 1*, (SPIE, Bellingham, 2000).
2. C.W.E. van Eijk, Inorganic scintillators in medical imaging, *Phys Med Biol* **47**, R85-R106 (2002).
3. H. Wieczorek et al., CsI:Tl for solid state X-ray detectors, *Proc Int Conf. on Inorganic Scintillators and their Applications (Delft University of Technology)*, 547-554 (1996).
4. H. Wieczorek and M. Overdick, Afterglow and hysteresis in CsI:Tl, *Proc. 5th Int Conf on Inorganic Scintillators and their Applications*, M.L. Lomonosov Moscow State University, 385-390 (2000).
5. B.C. Grabmeier, Luminescent materials for medical applications, *J Luminescence* **60&61**, 967-970 (1994).
6. S.O. Kasap and J.A. Rowlands, Direct-conversion flat-panel X-ray image sensors for digital radiography, *Proc IEEE* **90**(4), 591-604 (2002).
7. O. Tousignant et al., Spatial and temporal characteristics of a real-time large area a-Se X-ray detector, *Phys of Med Imaging, Proc SPIE* **5745**, 207-215 (2005).
8. W. Zhao, G. DeCrescenzo, S.O. Kasap, and J.A. Rowlands, Ghosting caused by bulk charge trapping in direct conversion flat-panel detectors using amorphous selenium, *Med Phys* **32**(2), 488-500 (2005).
9. D.C. Hunt, O. Tousignant, J.A. Rowlands, Evaluation of the imaging properties of an a-Se-based flat panel detector for digital fluoroscopy, *Med Phys* **31**(5), 1166-1175 (2004).
10. G. Zentai et al., Improved properties of PbI$_2$ X-ray imagers with tighter process control and using positive bias voltage, *Phys of Med Imaging, Proc SPIE* **5368**, 668-676 (2004).
11. R.A. Street et al., Comparative study of PbI$_2$ and HgI$_2$ for direct detection active matrix X-ray image sensors, *J Appl Phys* **91**(5), 3345-3355 (2002).
12. A. Brauers et al., X-ray sensing properties for a lead oxide photoconductor combined with an amorphous silicon TFT array, *Mat Res Soc Proc* **507**, 321 (1998).
13. M. Simon et al., PbO as direct conversion X-ray detector material, *Phys of Med Imaging, Proc. SPIE* **5368**, 188-199 (2004).
14. M. Simon et al., Analysis of lead oxide (PbO) layers for direct conversion X-ray detectors, accepted for *IEEE Trans Nucl Sc* **52**(5), 2035-2040 (2005).
15. G. Zentai et al., Mercuric iodide medical imagers for low exposure radiography and fluoroscopy, *Phys of Med Imaging, Proc SPIE* **5368**, 200-210 (2004).
16. L.E. Antonuk et al., Systematic development of input-quantum-limited fluoroscopic imagers based on active matrix flat-panel technology, *Phys of Med Imaging, Proc SPIE* **5368**, 127-138 (2004).
17. C. Scheiber and G.C. Giakos, Medical applications of CdTe and CdZnTe detectors, *Nucl Instr Meth A* **458**, 12-25 (2001).
18. N. Jung et al., Dynamic X-ray imaging based on an amorphous silicon thin-film array, *Phys of Med Imaging, Proc SPIE* **3336**, 396-407 (1998).
19. P. R. Granfors, Performance characteristics of an amorphous silicon flat panel X-ray imaging detector, *Phys of Med Imaging, Proc SPIE* **3659**, 480-490 (1999).
20. T. Ducourant et al., Optimization of key building blocks for a large area radiographic and fluoroscopic dynamic digital X-ray detector based on a-Si:H/CsI:Tl flat panel technology, *Phys of Med Imaging, Proc SPIE* **3977**, 14-25 (2000).
21. F. Busse et al., Design and performance of a high-quality cardiac flat detector, *Phys of Med Imaging, Proc SPIE* **4682**, 819-827 (2002).
22. M.J. Powell et al., Amorphous silicon image sensor arrays, *Mat. Res. Soc. Symp. Proc.* **258**, 1127-1137 (1992).

23. R.A. Street et al., Large area 2-dimensional a-Si:H imaging arrays, *Mat Res Soc Symp Proc* **258**, 1145-1150 (1992).
24. L.E. Antonuk et al., Large area, flat-panel a-Si:H arrays for X-ray imaging, *Phys of Med Imaging, Proc SPIE* **1896**, 18-29 (1993).
25. H. Wieczorek, Effects of trapping in a-Si:H diodes, *Solid State Phen* **44-46**, 957-972 (1995).
26. J.H. Siewerdsen and D.A. Jaffray, A ghost story: Spatio-temporal response characteristics of an indirect-detection flat-panel imager, *Med Phys* **26**, 1624-1641 (1999).
27. S. Pourjavid and P.R. Granfors, Compensation for image retention in an amorphous silicon detector, *Phys of Med Imaging, Proc SPIE* **3659**, 501-509 (1999).
28. M. Overdick, T. Solf, H.-A. Wischmann, Temporal artefacts in flat dynamic X-ray detectors, *Phys of Med Imaging, Proc SPIE* **4320**, 47-58 (2001).
29. M.J. Powell et al., Amorphous silicon photodiode thin-film transistor technology with diode on top structure, *Mat Res Soc Symp Proc* **467**, 863-868 (1997).
30. J.T. Rahn et al., High-resolution high fill factor a-Si:H sensor arrays for medical imaging, *Phys of Med Imaging, Proc SPIE* **3659**, 510-517 (1999).
31. R.L. Weisfield et al., Performance analysis of a 127-micron pixel large-area TFT/photodiode array with boosted fill factor, *Phys of Med Imaging, Proc SPIE* **5368**, 338-348 (2004).
32. N. Matsuura, W. Zhao, Z. Huang, J.A. Rowlands, Digital radiology using active matrix readout: Amplified pixel array for fluoroscopy, *Med Phys* **26**(5), 672-681 (1999).
33. K.S. Karim, S. Yin, A. Nathan, J.A. Rowlands, High dynamic range architectures for diagnostic medical imaging, *Phys of Med Imaging, Proc SPIE* **5368**, 657-667 (2004).
34. L.E. Antonuk et al., Investigation of strategies to achieve optimal DQE performance from indirect detection, active matrix flat-panel imagers (AMFPIs) through novel pixel amplification architectures, *Phys of Med Imaging, Proc SPIE* **5745**, 18-31 (2005).
35. M. Overdick et al., Flat detector with integrated dose sensing, *Phys of Med Imaging, Proc SPIE* **5030**, 246-255 (2003).
36. R.A. Street et al., Printed active-matrix TFT arrays for X-ray imaging, *Phys of Med Imaging, Proc SPIE* **5745**, 7-17 (2005).
37. T. Graeve and G.P. Weckler, High-resolution CMOS imaging detector, *Phys of Med Imaging, Proc SPIE* **4320**, 68-76 (2001).
38. J. Hsieh, *Computed Tomography: Principles, Design, Artifacts and Recent Advances*, (SPIE, Bellingham, 2003).
39. R. Luhta et al., Back illuminated photodiodes for multislice CT, *Phys of Med Imaging, Proc SPIE* **5030**, 235-245 (2003).
40. A. Ikhlef et al., Volume CT (VCT) enabled by a novel diode technology, *Phys of Med Imaging, Proc SPIE* **5745**, 1161-1169 (2005).
41. L. Spies et al., Performance of prototype modules of a novel multislice CT detector based on CMOS photosensors, *Phys of Med Imaging, Proc SPIE* **5030**, 490-503 (2003).
42. R. Steadman et al., A CMOS photodiode array with in-pixel data acquisition system for computed tomography, *IEEE J Solid-State Circ* **39**(7), 1034-1043 (2004).
43. A. Jahnke and R. Matz, Signal formation and decay in CdTe X-ray detectors under intense irradiation, *Med Phys* **26**(1), 38-48 (1999).
44. Y. Du et al., Temporal response of CZT detectors under intense irradiation, *IEEE Trans Nucl Sc* **50**(4), 1031-1035 (2003).
45. P. Fischer et al., A counting CdTe pixel detector for hard X-ray and γ-ray imaging, *IEEE Trans Nucl Sc* **48**(6), 2401-2404 (2001).

46. X. Llopart and M. Campbell, First test measurements of a 64k pixel readout chip working in single photon counting mode, *Nucl Inst Meth A* **509**, 157-163 (2003).

47. M. Lindner et al., Medical X-ray imaging with energy windowing, *Nucl Instr Meth A* **465**, 229-234 (2001).

Chapter 5

3D-ROTATIONAL X-RAY IMAGING
Advances in Interventional Volume Imaging

Volker Rasche[1], Michael Grass[2], Robert Manzke[3]
[1]University Hospital Ulm, Ulm, Germany; [2]Philips Research, Hamburg, Germany; [3]Philips Research, Briarcliff Manor, NY, USA

Abstract: 3D-rotational X-ray imaging is a rather new volume imaging technique on conventional C-arm X-ray systems. This contribution covers the basics of the underlying mathematics of three-dimensional X-ray imaging, the data acquisition protocols, and calibration and reconstruction techniques. Furthermore, an overview of the current clinical application of 3D-rotational X-ray imaging is presented.

Keywords: 3D-rotational angiography, C-arm calibration, cone beam reconstruction

1. INTRODUCTION

Three-dimensional rotational X-ray imaging (3D-RX) is a rather new imaging method based on the rotational angiography (RA) technique, which was introduced in the early 90s. RA is an extension of the conventional angiography technique, in which the gantry of an X-ray system is rotated around the patient while acquiring X-ray projections during continuous contrast agent (CA) injection. Initially, the main application of RA was in the field of interventional neuroradiology[1,2]. Compared to conventional angiography the improved visualization of vascular anatomy by the multiple angles of view available from the rotational acquisition results in superior information on complex 3D vascular structures. This additional anatomic information significantly improved e.g. the angiographic assessment of aneurysms making it an excellent adjunct in e.g. the investigation of subarachnoid hemorrhage. In the following years RA has been introduced to various other fields including assessment of the renal arteries[3,4] and

G. Spekowius and T. Wendler (Eds.), Advances in Healthcare Technology, 65-80.

visualization of the coronary artery tree, in which a significant reduction of overall X-ray and contrast agent dose could be realized[5].

Based on the RA protocols, the projection data acquired during a RA run have been utilized for volume reconstruction, resulting in the so-called 3D rotational angiography (3D-RA) technique. Since then, the application of volume reconstruction has become more and more standard in interventional neuroradiology e.g. for improved assessment of the shape and size of aneurysms[6], the planning of radiation treatment of arterialvenous malformations (AVM)[7], or just to get more insights in the vascular structure[8]. With increasing availability, other applications such as the renal arteries[9] and peripheral angiography[10] have been added.

Up to now, the application of 3D-RA has been limited to high-contrast objects such as selectively enhanced vascular trees. With the advent of new X-ray systems providing significantly improved characteristics for volume reconstruction, the application of 3D-RA to more general volume X-ray imaging (3D-RX) is on its verge.

This contribution covers the basic mathematics of three-dimensional X-ray imaging, the basics of acquisition, calibration and reconstruction on current X-ray systems and gives an overview on clinical application of 3D-RX.

1.1   Mathematical description of the 3D reconstruction from X-ray projections

1.1.1   The Radon transformation

The Radon transformation R of a three-dimensional object function $f(x,y,z) = f(\vec{x})$ is defined as the complete set of integrals over planes E through the object. With

$$E : \vec{x} \cdot \vec{\xi} = \rho \qquad \vec{x} = \begin{pmatrix} x \\ y \\ z \end{pmatrix} \qquad \vec{\xi} = \begin{pmatrix} \sin\theta\cos\lambda \\ \sin\theta\sin\lambda \\ \cos\theta \end{pmatrix}$$

the Radon transform $Rf(\rho, \lambda, \theta) = Rf(\rho\vec{\xi})$ at a specific distance ρ to the origin with orientation $\vec{\xi}$ (Figure 5-1) can be calculated according to

$$Rf(\rho\vec{\xi}) = \int_{-\infty}^{+\infty}\int_{-\infty}^{+\infty}\int_{-\infty}^{+\infty} f(\vec{x})\delta(\vec{x}\cdot\vec{\xi} - \rho)d\vec{x}, \qquad\qquad [1]$$

which can be reformulated as

$$Rf(\rho\vec{\xi}) = \int\limits_{-\infty}^{+\infty}\int\limits_{-\infty}^{+\infty} f(\rho\vec{\xi},s,t)\,ds\,dt,$$ [2]

with $\rho\vec{\xi}$ defining the orientation and position of the plane and s and t being two variables running along two orthogonal axes in the plane.

A complete Radon transformation of an object function $f(\vec{x})$ requires the calculation of all Radon values $Rf(\rho\vec{\xi})$ with $\rho\in$ [-∞,∞], $\lambda\in$ [-π/2,π/2) and $\theta\in$ [0,2π).

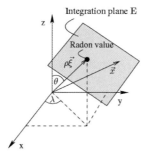

Figure 5-1. A single Radon value is obtained by integration of the object function over a specific plane, defined according to its location and orientation in space.

1.1.2   The X-ray projection

In the ideal basic X-ray imaging experiment (Figure 5-2), the subject of investigation $f(x,y,z)$ is irradiated by an X-ray beam along a line L, along which an intensity I_0 is emitted from the X-ray tube towards the detector element. While the X-ray beam is passing through the subject, its intensity is attenuated according to the tissue-specific attenuation factor $f(x,y,z)$. Finally, the intensity I_{out} of the attenuated X-ray beam is measured by means of an X-ray detector. For simplicity, in the following description of the mathematics, the attenuation coefficients are assumed to be independent on the energy of the X-ray photons and no non-ideal effects such as scatter are considered.

According to the law of Lambert-Beer, the attenuated intensity of the X-ray beam I_{out} can be calculated as

$$I_{out} = I_0 e^{-\int\limits_L f(x,y,z)\,dl}.$$ [3]

Equation [3] can be easily reformulated to the so-called line integral value p, the value of which is independent on the initial intensity I_0 and hence only depending on the tissue attenuation properties

$$p = \ln \frac{I_{out}}{I_0} = -\int_L f(x,y,z)dl .$$ [4]

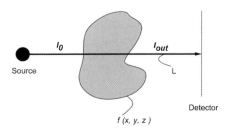

Figure 5-2. The basic X-ray imaging experiment.

As shown in Figure 5-3, with $\vec{T}$ being the position of the focal spot, each line on the detector belongs to a certain plane $E(\rho\vec{\xi})$ through the object and the projection value $p(\vec{T},s,t)$ can be rewritten as $Xf(\rho\vec{\xi}, \kappa)$ with κ being the angle between the central beam and the specific X-ray beam along the s-direction. With r being the distance along the ray, $Xf(\rho\vec{\xi}, \kappa)$ can be calculated according to

$$Xf(\rho\vec{\xi},\kappa) = \int_{-\infty}^{+\infty} f(\rho\vec{\xi},r,\kappa)dr$$ [5]

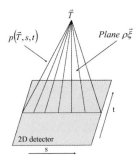

Figure 5-3. Relation between a single projection value and the corresponding Radon plane.

1.1.3 Relation between the X-ray projection and the Radon transformation

The calculation of the integral of a certain plane $E(\rho\vec{\xi})$ involves the integration of $Xf(\rho\vec{\xi},\kappa)$ along the line on the detector, which results to

$$\int_{-\frac{\pi}{2}}^{+\frac{\pi}{2}} Xf(\rho\vec{\xi},\kappa)d\kappa = \int_{-\frac{\pi}{2}}^{+\frac{\pi}{2}}\int_{-\infty}^{+\infty} f(\rho\vec{\xi},r,\kappa)drd\kappa. \qquad [6]$$

Transformation of equation [2] into the X-ray coordinate systems yields

$$Rf(\rho\vec{\xi}) = \int_{-\frac{\pi}{2}}^{+\frac{\pi}{2}}\int_{-\infty}^{+\infty} f(\rho\vec{\xi},r,\kappa)rdrd\kappa, \qquad [7]$$

which differs from equation [6] by the proportional factor r and hence the Radon transform values can not directly be obtained by integration along lines on the detector. In 1991 Grangeat[11] presented a mathematical framework, which relates the X-ray values to the 1st derivative of the Radon transform

$$\frac{\partial}{\partial\rho} Rf\left(\rho\vec{\xi}\right) = \frac{1}{\cos^2\beta}\frac{\partial}{\partial s}\int_{-\infty}^{+\infty}\frac{\overline{SO}}{\overline{SA}} Xf\left(s\left(\rho\vec{\xi}\right),t\right)dt. \qquad [8]$$

Here, SO defines the source detector distance, SA the distance between the source and the respective detector element (s,t) and β defines the angle between the central beam and the detector t-value. This mathematical framework enables the calculation of Radon transform values from X-ray projection data.

1.1.4 Radon inversion formula

An inversion formula to reconstruct an object function from its Radon transform data was introduced by Natterer[12] in 1986

$$f(\vec{x}) = -\frac{1}{8\pi^2} \int_{-\frac{\pi}{2}}^{+\frac{\pi}{2}} \int_{0}^{2\pi} \frac{\partial^2}{\partial \rho^2} Rf\left((\rho\vec{\xi})\cdot\vec{\xi}\right)\sin\theta d\lambda d\theta. \qquad [9]$$

This formula represents the basis for all exact reconstruction algorithms based on Radon inversion.

1.1.5   Data sufficiency criteria

During a real imaging experiment, data are acquired while moving the X-ray tube and detector around the patient. To ensure complete filling of Radon space, for each plane with normal $\rho\vec{\xi}$ at least one source point position, which belongs to that plane, must be available. Tuy[13] and Smith[14] formulated the so-called sufficiency condition as:

If on every plane that intersects the object, there exists at least one cone beam source point, then one can reconstruct the object.

1.2   3D-RX

The 3D-RX imaging method is directly based on the 3D Rotational Angiography (3D-RA) data acquisition protocol[14]. The underlying projection data is acquired on conventional C-arm systems. During continuous projection data acquisition, the C-arm gantry is rotated around the object under investigation by at least 180°. To get to the final volume information, the projection data has to be calibrated and reconstructed.

The different steps involved are elucidated in the following subsections.

1.2.1   Data acquisition

A schematic view of the projection data acquisition procedure is presented in Figure 5-4 for the example of an Angiography acquisition. Projection data are normally acquired along a planar trajectory by rotating the C-arm gantry around the patient either in head or lateral position. Depending on the anatomy, a caudal or cranial tilt of the gantry of up to 30° is used during data acquisition. The target area is positioned in the center-of-rotation (iso-center). Depending on the application, projection images are taken at a frame rate between 12.5 and 60 fr/s and the rotation speed of the system may be up to 55°/s. Valid combinations of frame rate and rotation speed are defined by the number of projections required for a certain application and a clinically acceptable maximal acquisition time. For high-contrast applications such as conventional three-dimensional rotational angiography applications, in which a reconstruction of a contrast-agent enhanced vascular tree is obtained, typically 100 projections are taken within 4s over an angular range of 220°. In case of more soft-tissue contrast applications such as brain imaging to check for intracerebral bleedings, up to 750 projections are being used acquired within 25s.

1.2.2 Calibration

Due to the open design of conventional X-ray C-arm systems, during rotation of the gantry, the relative position of the tube to the detector is changing due to slight bending and vibration of the gantry and, in case of image intensifier based systems, distortions to the projections are introduced by earth magnetic field interactions and vignetting. For 3D reconstruction, however, the knowledge of the accurate position of the tube and the detector and distortion-free projections are mandatory to avoid image quality degradation. The measurement of the real projection geometry and the projection image distortions is one of the most important steps in 3D-RX.

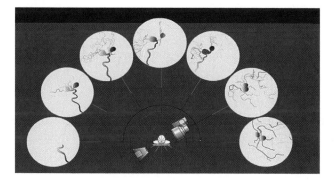

Figure 5-4. Example of a 3D-RX data acquisition for 3D rotational angiography.

A variety of calibration approaches have been introduced[16-19]. Among these, the utilization of dedicated geometrical phantoms with known markers represents a very stable approach to achieve calibration results of high accuracy. For each trajectory used, the calibration and projection parameters are measured once during the installation of the system and normally remain constant over months due to the excellent reproducibility of the systems.

The calibration procedure is separated into the acquisition of projection data of two phantoms, used for the measurement of the image distortions and focal spot position, and the projection geometry.

The first phantom consists of two parallel grid plates (Figure 5-5) manufactured in glass fiber. Grid 1 for the II-distortion measurement consists of equally spaced grid-points (e.g. 1.5 mm bronze beads; grid-distance equal to15 mm). Grid 2 for the focal spot measurements consists of grid-points (e.g. 2 mm bronze beads) arranged on a circle equally spaced at 7.5°. Both test grids are coupled by rods and mounted in front of the detector housing.

The second phantom (Figure 5-5) used for measurement of the projection direction consists of 20 beads, positioned in the corners of a regular polyeder (dodecaeder). Three additional markers are placed on the z-axis of the geometry phantom.

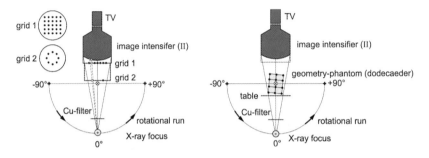

Figure 5-5. Principle of the two-step calibration approach.

1.2.2.1   Measurement of the image distortion

The projected beads of the grid are automatically determined in each projection image and the functional relation between the imaged grid points and the real grid points is determined by modeling the distortions along the x-axis and the y-axis by bivariate polynoms[20] independently for each projection view. Once the distortion coefficients are known, each projection image is warped by means of bilinear interpolation before reconstruction.

1.2.2.2   Focal spot determination

The automatically recognized points of grid 2 are matched to a circle in a least-square-fit. From the diameter of the determined circle and its location relative to the detector, the position of the focus spot is estimated independently for each view. A typical measurement of the focal spot position is shown in Figure 5-6 for a half circular trajectory. The average error in the determined focal spot position is in the order of 0.1mm.

1.2.2.3   Geometrical projection parameter determination

After automatic extraction of the projected beads, a comparison between the forward projected position of the known phantom beads with known projection orientation and the real projection of the phantom is used for determination of the projection direction. For performing a sufficient least squares error fit, all 23 beads of the object are considered during the optimization. A typical outcome of the measurement of the projection geometry is shown in Figure 5-6.

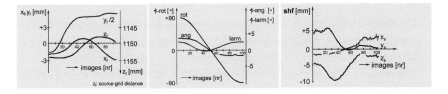

Figure 5-6. Typical values for the tube position (left), projection orientation (middle) and the iso-center measurement (right) for a 180° trajectory.

1.2.3   Reconstruction

After distortion correction, the knowledge of the accurate projection geometry is used to apply a 3D cone-beam reconstruction from the projection data. It can be shown that the inverse Radon transformation results into a simple three-dimensional convolution back projection in case the projection data are acquired on a circular trajectory. This so-called Feldkamp reconstruction technique was introduced in 1984 by Feldkamp, Davis, and Kress[21]. The original Feldkamp algorithm is described by:

$$f(x, y, z) = \frac{1}{2} \int_0^{2\pi} \left(\frac{D}{d}\right)^2 [(p(s,t,\phi)\cos\gamma) * h(s)] d\phi.$$ [10]

Here, (s,t,ϕ) describes the detector element at (s,t) acquired with angle ϕ of the circular trajectory, γ is the angle between the vector from the source to the center of the detector and the vector from the source to the detector element (s,t), $h(s)$ describes the convolution kernel, D is the distance from the origin to the position of the source and d is the length of the vector from the source to the voxel under consideration projected onto the central ray. $h(s)$ is chosen as a pure band-limited ramp filter tangential to the ideal source-detector trajectory as

$$h(s) = \frac{1}{2}\sin c(s) - \frac{1}{4}\sin c^2\left(\frac{s}{2}\right).$$

[11]

In equation [10] a perfectly circular trajectory with equiangular spacing of the source position along the trajectory is assumed. These conditions are not met for a typical 3D-RX acquisition. In order to compensate for the deviations from the ideal trajectory, three modifications to the original Feldkamp algorithm must be applied[22]:

- Consideration of the true detector and source position as measured during the calibration process. Since the deviations from a planar circular trajectory are usually small, a modification of the filter direction is not required. It is kept parallel to the projection of the source trajectory onto the detector.
- Compensation for an uneven sampling density along the circular trajectory, caused by the acceleration and the deceleration of the gantry during the rotational acquisition. This is achieved by calculating the sample distance of projection measurements along the source trajectory. Each projection measurement represents a certain part of the acquisition path and its relation to the complete path length yields the corresponding weight.
- Finally, for acquisition paths, which represent a circular arc with more than a half circle plus the fan angle, a Parker weighting is applied in order to compensate for rays measured redundantly[23].

1.2.4   System performance

Due to certain system limitations such as the improperly filled Radon space caused by the circular trajectory, the limited dynamic range, spatial extent and speed of the current detectors, and limited suppression of scatter, the volume imaging performance in 3D-RX does not yet meet the standards of CT. However, analysis of the imaging performance reveals[24,25] that the small pixel size of the X-ray detectors down to $165^2 um^2$ enables volume imaging at unique isotropic spatial resolution of up to 30lp/cm in all spatial directions. Furthermore, utilizing the high dynamic range of up to 14Bit in case of the recent flat panel detectors enables significantly improved contrast resolution below 30 Hounsfield units[25] (Figure 5-7).

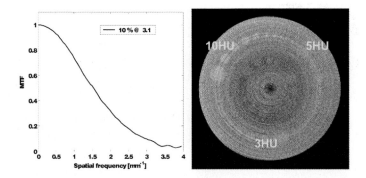

Figure 5-7. Modulation transfer function (left) and contrast-resolution (right) of 3D-RX performed on a Philips Allura FD10 X-ray system. The curve on the left shows the average MTF of all spatial dimensions. The image on the right shows an image of the soft-tissue section (CTP515 of the Catphan 500, The Phantom Laboratory, Cambridge, USA). Data courtesy of Dr. Georg Rose, Philips Research Aachen.

1.3   Future directions

Future directions in 3D-RX are aiming for providing CT-like image quality on interventional C-arm systems. Major targets are the improved compensation for projection truncations[26] and the complete filling of Radon space by using dedicated trajectories, which perform rotations around more than a single axis[27]. Further work focuses on the reduction of the impact of scatter[28].

Furthermore, so-called hybrid systems combining some CT components such as closed gantry concepts with X-ray components such as real two-dimensional detectors are currently entering clinical evaluation[29].

2.   CLIINICAL EXAMPLES

In the following, some examples of the use of 3D-RX in the current clinical environment are given. The current application can roughly be categorized into high-contrast applications, in which the contrast between the object and the background is typically in the order of several hundred HU, and medium- to soft-tissue contrast applications, in which the contrast difference may go down close to 20 HU. For all applications, currently circular trajectories covering an angular range of about 220° are utilized. Major differences results from the number of projections utilized for the projections and the exposure settings. For high contrast objects, typically less projections and higher kV settings are used.

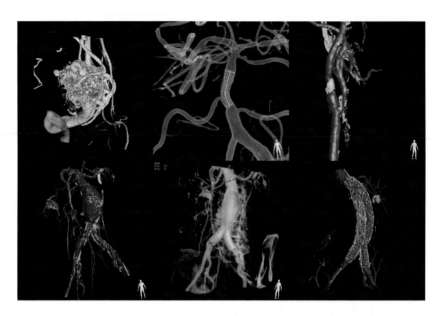

Figure 5-8. Examples of typical vascular application of 3D-RX. Examples show reconstruction of an AVM (upper left), stent planning for intracerebral stenting (upper middle), carotid stenosis with calcified plaque (upper right), abdominal aortic aneurysm (AAA) with calcified plaque (lower left), stent planning for AAA (lower middle) and stent visualization after deployment (lower right).

2.1   High contrast applications

The use of 3D-RX for providing high-quality three-dimensional angiograms is still the paramount clinical application. Here, a typical high-contrast protocol is applied since the vascular structures are selectively enhanced by direct injection of the contrast media into the vascular structure under investigation. Most applications are in the field of interventional neuroradiology for improved assessment of three-dimensional vessel structures and quantitative assessment of vascular and aneurysm properties. Furthermore, due to the intrinsic high contrast of calcium, the angiographic information can be augmented by superposition of the calcified structures. With deeper clinical penetration of the techniques, application in the fields of abdominal aortic aneurysm as well as for other abdominal and peripheral arterial structures have become more common. Some typical examples of the usage of 3D-RX in the vascular field are shown in Figure 5-8.

Besides the angiographic application, the application of 3D-RX for bone imaging in the field of surgery and orthopedics is getting more and more attention. Here the projection data is normally obtained on mobile surgery

C-arm systems[30,31] with motorized propeller rotation. Main anatomical targets are the head, spine, joints and extremities. Figure 5-9 and 5-10 show the application of 3D-RX on a surgical system for providing anatomic information prior to ear-nose-throat (ENT) surgery and for guiding a cochlea implant implantation procedure.

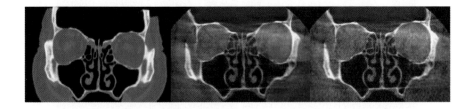

Figure 5-9. Comparing of conventional CT to of an intact post mortem head to 3D-RX on a mobile surgery X-ray system (upper row). From left to right a CT, 3D-RX high quality (375 projections) and a 3D-RX normal quality (151 projections). Data courtesy of Prof. Dr. med. et Dr. med. dent. Beat Hammer, Cranio-Faciales-Centrum, Hirslanden Clinic, Aarau, Switzerland.

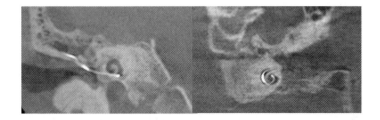

Figure 5-10. Example of the intra-surgical use of 3D-RX during the implantation of a cochlea implant. (Data courtesy of Dr. B. Carelsen, AMC, Amsterdam, The Netherlands).

2.2   Medium- to soft-tissue contrast applications

With the introduction of the new flat panel detectors providing up to 14 bits of dynamic range, the application of 3D-RX in the field of medium- to soft-tissue contrast resolution is approached. Recent studies proved the applicability of 3D-RX for the assessment of e.g. fresh intra-cerebral bleedings as depicted in Figure 5-11.

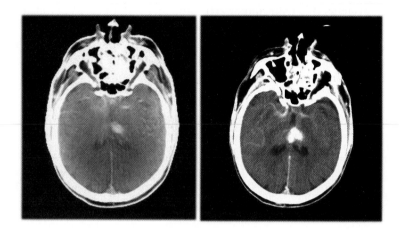

Figure 5-11. Comparison 3D-RX (left) with CT (right) for imaging of fresh intra-cerebral bleeding. (Data courtesy of Prof. Moret, Foundation Ophthalmologique de Rothshild, Paris, France).

3.   DISCUSSION

In conclusion, three-dimensional imaging on X-ray systems (3D-RX) has dramatically progressed over the last years. The application of 3D-RX in the field of interventional neuroradiology has entered clinical routine. New application of 3D-RX, especially in the field of surgery and orthopedics, are on the horizon and initial clinical evaluations show promising results. The extension of 3D-RX to other fields demanding medium- to soft-tissue contrast is a continuous process, which will likely be accelerated by the introduction of new X-ray systems.

From the current perspective, 3D-RX will remain in the realm of interventional imaging providing three-dimensional information during interventional procedures without the need for additional imaging equipment such as MRI or CT.

The major advantage of 3D-RX results from the huge two-dimensional detectors, which enable full organ coverage during a single rotation at very high spatial resolution. Whether that will motivate its application to diagnostic imaging may be questioned, especially since the ever increasing number of detector elements in CT systems will get close to the X-ray detectors.

REFERENCES

1. M. Schumacher, K. Kutluk, D. Ott, Digital rotational radiography in neuroradiology, *AJNR Am J Neuroradiol* **10**(3), 644-649 (1989).
2. D.J. Hoff, M.C. Wallace, K.G. ter Brugge, F. Gentili, Rotational angiography assessment of cerebral aneurysms, *AJNR Am J Neuroradiol* **15**(10), 1945-1948 (1994).
3. H.M. Klein, D. Vorwerk, J. Neuerburg, R.W. Gunther, Rotational angiography of the renal arteries, *Rofo* **162**(3), 249-251(1995).
4. H.R. Seymour, M.B. Matson, A.M. Belli, R. Morgan, J. Kyriou, U. Patel, Rotational digital subtraction angiography of the renal arteries: technique and evaluation in the study of native and transplant renal arteries, *Br J Radiol* **74**(878), 134-141 (2001).
5. J.T. Maddux, O. Wink, J.C. Messenger, B.M. Groves, R. Liao, J. Strzelczyk, S.Y. Chen, J.D. Carroll., Randomized study of the safety and clinical utility of rotational angiography versus standard angiography in the diagnosis of coronary artery disease, *Catheter Cardiovasc Interv* **62**(2), 167-174 (2004).
6. T. Hirai, Y. Korogi, K. Suginohara, K. Ono, T. Nishi, S. Uemura, M. Yamura, Y. Yamashita, Clinical usefulness of unsubtracted 3D digital angiography compared with rotational digital angiography in the pretreatment evaluation of intracranial aneurysms, *AJNR Am J Neuroradiol* **24**(6), 1067-1074 (2003).
7. F. Colombo, C. Cavedon, P. Francescon, L. Casentini, U. Fornezza, L. Castellan, F. Causin, S. Perini. Three-dimensional angiography for radiosurgical treatment planning for arteriovenous malformations, *J Neurosurg* **98**(3), 536-543 (2003).
8. R. Anxionnat, S. Bracard, J. Macho, E. Da Costa, R. Vaillant, L. Launay, Y. Trousset, R. Romeas, L. Picard, 3D angiography. Clinical interest. First applications in interventional neuroradiology, *J Neuroradiol* **25**(4), 251-262 (1998).
9. G. Hagen, J. Wadstrom, L.G. Eriksson, P. Magnusson, M. Magnusson, A. Magnusson, 3D rotational angiography of transplanted renal arteries: influence of an extended angle of rotation on beam-hardening artifacts, *Acta Radiol* **46**(2), 170-176 (2005).
10. J.C. van den Berg, F.L. Moll, Three-dimensional rotational angiography in peripheral endovascular interventions, *J Endovasc Ther* **10**(3), 595-600 (2003).
11. P. Grangeat, Mathematical framework of cone–beam 3D reconstruction via the first derivative of the radon transform In: G.T. Herman, A.K. Louis, F. Natterer (eds.), *Mathematical Methods in Tomography, Lecture Notes in Mathematics*, 66-97 (Springer, Berlin, 1991).
12. F. Natterer, *The Mathematics of Computerized Tomography*, ISBN 0-471-90959-9 (John Wiley and Sons, New York 1986).
13. H.K. Tuy, An Inversion Formula for Cone-Beam Reconstruction, *SIAM J Appl Math* **43**(3), 546-552 (1983).
14. B.D. Smith, Image reconstruction from cone-beam projections. *IEEE Trans Med Img* **4**(1), 14–25 (1985).
15. R. Kemkers, J. Op de Beek, H. Aerts, R. Koppe, E. Klotz, M. Grass, J. Moret, 3D Rotational Angiography: First Clinical application with use of a standard Philips C-arm system, *Proc Computer Assisted Radiology, 13th International Congress and Exhibition, Tokyo, 182-187 (1998)*.
16. A. Rougee, C. Picard, C. Ponchut, Y. Trousset, Geometrical calibration for 3D X-ray imaging, *Proc SPIE Medical Imaging, Image Capture, Formatting, and Display* Vol.**1897**, 161-169 (1993).
17. R. Koppe, E. Klotz, J. Op de Beek, H. Aerts, 3D vessel reconstruction based on Rotational Angiography, *Proc Computer Assisted Radiology, 9th International Congress and Exhibition, Berlin, 101-107 (1995)*.

18. R. Koppe, E. Klotz, J. Op de Beek, H. Aerts, Digital stereotaxy/stereotactic procedures with C-arm based Rotation-Angiography, *Proc Computer Assisted Radiology, 10th International Congress and Exhibition, Paris, 17-22 (1996)*.

19. R. Fahrig, M. Moreau, D.W. Holdsworth, Three-dimensional computed tomography reconstruction using a C-arm mounted XRII: Correction of image intensifier distortion, *Med Phys* **24**(7), 1097-1106 (1997).

20. P. Haaker, E. Klotz, R. Koppe, R. Linde, Real-time distortion correction of digital X-ray II/TV-systems, *Int Journal of Card Imaging* **6**, 39-45 (1990/91).

21. L.A. Feldkamp, L.C. Davis, J.W. Kress, Practical Cone-Beam Algorithms, *J Opt Soc Am* **6**, 612-619 (1984).

22. M. Grass, R. Koppe, E. Klotz, R. Proksa, M.H. Kuhn, H. Aerts, J. Op de Beek, R. Kemkers, Three-dimensional reconstruction of high contrast objects using C-arm image intensifier projection data, *Comp Med Imag Graph* **23**, 311-321 (1999).

23. D.L. Parker, Optimal short scan convolution reconstruction for fanbeam CT, *Medical Physics* **9**(2), 254 – 257 (1982).

24. V. Rasche, C. Graeff, M. Grass, T. Istel, E. Klotz, R. Koppe, G. Rose, H. Schomberg, B. Schreiber, Performance of image intensifier equipped X-Ray systems in three dimensional imaging, *Proc Computer Assisted Radiology, 10th International Congress and Exhibition, London, 187-192 (2003)*.

25. V. Rasche, B. Schreiber, J.N. Noordhoek, P. van de Haar, D. Schaefer, J. Wiegert, Comparison of Flat Panel Detectors and Image Intensifiers for Volume Imaging on Interventional C-Arc Systems, *RSNA, 83rd Scientific Session* (2003).

26. H. Schomberg, Image Reconstruction from Truncated Cone-Beam Projections, *Proc 2004 IEEE International Symposium on Biomedical Imaging: From Macro to Nano*, 575-578 (2004).

27. H. Schomberg, Complete Source Trajectories for C-Arm Systems and a Method for Coping with Truncated Cone-Beam Projections, *Proc 6th International Meeting on Fully 3D Image Reconstruction in Radiology and Nuclear Medicine*, 221-224 (2001).

28. J. Wiegert, M. Bertram, D. Schaefer, N. Conrads, J. Timmer, T. Aach, G. Rose, Performance of standard fluoroscopy antiscatter grids in flat-detector-based cone-beam CT, *Proc SPIE Medical Imaging, Physics of Medical Imaging*, Vol. **5368**, 67-78 (2004).

29. J. Lisauskas, M. Ferencik, F. Moselewski, S. Houser, R. Gupta, R. Chan, Morphologic Measurements of ex-Vivo Coronary Arteries from High-Resolution Volume CT, *RSNA* (2004).

30. T. van Walsum, E.B. van de Kraats , B. Carelsen, S.N. Boon, N.J. Noordhoek, W.J. Niessen, Accuracy of Navigation on 3DRX Data Acquired with a Mobile Propeller C-Arm, *Proc 4th Annual Meeting of Computer Assisted Orthopedic Surgery, 22-23 (2004)*.

31. B. Carelsen, N.H. Bakker, S.N. Boon, W.J. Fokkens, N.J.M. Freeling, N.J. Noordhoek, Mobile 3D rotational X-ray: comparison with CT in sinus surgery, *Medica Mundi* **48**(3), 4-10 (2004).

Chapter 6

CORONARY MAGNETIC RESONANCE ANGIOGRAPHY
Methodological Aspects

Peter Börnert, Kay Nehrke, Dye Jensen
Philips Research, Hamburg, Germany

Abstract: This chapter gives a brief overview over recent methodological advances of Coronary Magnetic Resonance Angiography (CMRA). To cope with the major problem of cardiac and respiratory motion, techniques for motion correction and appropriate data sampling schemes based on advanced hardware technology are discussed, and examples of CMRA data are shown.

Keywords: Magnetic resonance imaging, MRI, coronary artery imaging, navigator, motion, motion correction

1.   INTRODUCTION

According to the WHO, coronary artery disease is the major cause of morbidity in the western civilisation. This is despite the recent improvements in diagnostic technology and the huge efforts spent on prevention. The gold standard for the diagnosis of this disease is x-ray coronary angiography, which involves the catheterisation of the patient and the application of iodinated contrast agent. Each year, up to 1 million X-ray based diagnostic procedures are performed, in Europe and the US, but only a fraction of the examined patients (40%) show significant disease[1]. Due to the risks of the invasive procedure and the high associated costs, alternative diagnostic approaches are desirable, either as a gatekeeper for the cath-lab or as safe follow-up techniques to control appropriate re-vascularisation procedures.

Magnetic Resonance Imaging (MRI) is a well-established diagnostic imaging modality, which exhibits an excellent soft-tissue contrast and which has found important application in cardiovascular diagnostics[2]. MRI has a

81

G. Spekowius and T. Wendler (Eds.), Advances in Healthcare Technology, 81-97.

very high versatility with respect to contrast providing a wealth of information and allows to visualise cardiac morphology, evaluate the cardiac function, the myocardial perfusion, local necrosis and to assess arteriosclerosis[2].

Much effort has been spent on the development of coronary magnetic resonance angiography (CMRA), which represents an essential prerequisite for MRI-based cardiovascular diagnostics[3]. In contrast to x-ray coronary angiography, CMRA does neither expose the patient and the cardiologist to ionising radiation nor involves the use of iodinated contrast agents. However, human CMRA remains technically challenging despite many advances over the past decade. MRI requires long measuring times compared to X-ray, making CMRA vulnerable to all kinds of motion effects. Furthermore, the spatial resolution, which is reaching the sub-millimetre range, is not as high as the one of X-ray.

Thus, a lot of research effort is necessary to overcome the technical shortcomings and to provide high-resolution three-dimensional information of the coronary artery tree.

Motion compensation for respiration and cardiac motion is a core element of CMRA. Therefore, in this chapter, methodological advances will be discussed to cope with the motion problem. EKG triggering and advanced navigator gating allow motion to be largely frozen at the cost of an increased total scanning time. To further increase image quality and/or to shorten the scanning time, prospective motion compensation techniques have been devised based on motion models steered by navigators in real-time.

Also the MR imaging sequence itself bares a significant potential to further reduce motion sensitivity. In particular, certain k-space sampling schemes are suited to provide this feature.

While initially thin slab double-oblique 3D imaging techniques have been used to visualise the proximal to mid portion of the coronary artery tree, whole heart 3D coronary MRA is gaining more and more importance. The associated advantages and disadvantages will be the third topic of this chapter.

2.   MOTION

Coronary MR angiography demands a high spatial and temporal resolution. The limited signal intensity in magnetic resonance requires a trade-off in measurement time, signal-to-noise ratio (SNR) and spatial resolution. Typically, the measurement times exceed several minutes, making the scan vulnerable to all kinds of physiological and bulk patient motion. The adverse consequences of motion on the imaging process are similarly to photography, where serious image blurring occurs, if the object, from which a picture shall be taken, moves during capturing. The same holds for MRI.

The main sources of motion to be considered are the cardiac motion and respiratory motion superimposed. Both represent the major forms of bulk motion coronary MRA has to cope with. In the following sections, appropriate correction- and/or compensation techniques will be discussed.

2.1   Cardiac motion and motion sensors

During the cardiac cycle, the coronaries, which are located on the epicardium, move along with the contracting and relaxing myocardium. Neglecting respiration, this motion component easily exceeds the vessel dimension making synchronization or motion compensation mandatory.

Cardiac MR[4,5,6] and X-ray coronary angiography measurements have been performed to study the motion of the coronary vessels during the cardiac cycle and to identify intervals of minimal motion. The displacements are different for the different coronary arteries, but in general, there are two possible sampling windows: one at mid-systole (during isovolumetric relaxation) and the other one at mid-diastole (during the relaxation period of the heart). The timing of these windows is patient- and heart rate-dependent. Thus, the most appropriate way to determine these quiescent periods is a patient-specific measurement based on a multi-heart phase scan, that can easily be performed in a short single breath-hold[6]. Using image processing, the cardiac motion pattern can be extracted, and the corresponding timing can be obtained automatically[7]. This approach is illustrated in Figure 6-1.

Both of the two possible cardiac acquisition windows, indicated by the maxima in Figure 6-1, can be used for data acquisition in clinical practice, and some authors recommend using both simultaneously[8] to increase the scan efficiency. However, in most of the patient examinations, an acquisition window in diastole is preferred. Nevertheless, in patients with very high heart rates or strong heart rate irregularities, a mid-systolic window can yield better image quality.

It is important to note, that also the duration of the cardiac acquisition window is limited by cardiac motion (see Figure 6-1). It has been found in patients, that a duration of 80-90ms represents an acceptable compromise[9]. Longer windows can result in serious image blur.

To synchronize the MR data acquisition with the cardiac motion, EKG triggering is performed, which basically relies on the detection of the QRS-complex. The magneto-hydro-dynamic effect and the switching of gradients and RF pulses, involved in MR imaging, corrupt the measured electrical potentials. Thus, an EKG signal sampled in an MR scanner is not of diagnostic value. Simple signal evaluation algorithms used to detect the QRS-complex often fail, which make cardiac triggering difficult. However, due to the introduction of the multi-dimensional vector EKG[10], R-wave detection became very reliable (near 100%) even at very high field strengths.

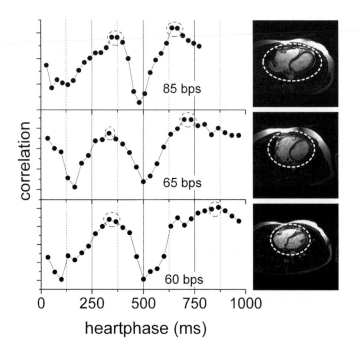

Figure 6-1. Cardiac motion and cardiac sampling window. During the cardiac cycle, the heart is continuously moving. To find the optimal acquisition window automatically, a cross correlation is performed on single-slice cine MR data obtained during a short breath-hold. The maxima in the curves represent periods of little motion, which can be used as cardiac acquisition windows. Data from three different volunteers are shown. Each dot represents an image measured in the cine scan. The automatically found windows correspond with those selected manually (circles) by visual inspection of the cine images.

The detected R-wave is used as a reference point within the current cardiac cycle. Assuming a fixed heart rate, the corresponding cardiac phase is selected by an appropriate delay, and MR data acquisition is permitted (see Figure 6-2). The data acquisition itself usually takes place in mid/end diastole, which is far away from the R-peak. This makes CMRA prone to slight heart rate irregularities, which result in a mixing of different heart phases giving rise to image blur. Advanced arrhythmia rejection algorithms[11] or real-time adjustments would be desirable[12] in that respect.

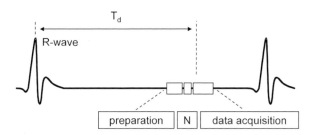

Figure 6-2. Schematic representation of a CMRA imaging sequence. The EKG triggered data acquisition starts after a heart-rate dependent delay T_d. Prior to data acquisition, longitudinal magnetisation is prepared to maximise image contrast. A navigator (N) is applied for respiratory motion sensing and prospective motion correction.

Based on the cardiac synchronisation of the data sampling procedure, the principle building block of a CMRA sequence can be illustrated as shown in Figure 6-2. However, such a sequence is only capable of sampling a sub-set of data necessary to reconstruct a full MR image. Therefore, the sequence has to be repeated several times, making data acquisition potentially prone to respiratory artefacts.

2.2 Respiratory motion and motion sensors

The respiration is a rather complicated process, which involves a large number of different muscle groups[13]. During respiration, the diaphragmatic excursion reaches up to about 30 mm. This motion results in blurring and ghosting artefacts, unless corrected. To cope with this problem, breath-hold techniques have been devised[14]. Their main problem is patient comfort and stability; therefore, free-breathing techniques are preferred, which minimise patient stress and the need for an active co-operation.

To monitor the respiratory motion, pressure belts or pressure pillows have been used earlier, which have typically been replaced by more reliable navigators[15,16], allowing the measurement of the motion of the organ of interest. MR navigators are one-dimensional MR sub-measurements, which are able to sense the position of an arbitrary organ with high spatial resolution[13]. Their basic principle is shown in Figure 6-3.

In most applications, the position of the right hemi-diaphragm at the lung-liver interface is monitored. During scanning, the displacement is determined with respect to a pre-stored reference position. This information can be used to take the accept/reject decision for the acquired data in real-time[17]. Such a gating procedure usually employs an acceptance window of several millimetres. This allows freezing the data acquisition to the end-expiratory state, which is the most frequent and most reproducible respiratory motion state. The navigator sequence, schematically shown in Figure 6-3 has to be applied in close temporal proximity to the MR data acquisition so as to maximise the accuracy of the motion information used for the gating decision[18]. Gating can be performed either retrospectively[19] during image reconstruction or prospectively[20], which allows the correction of the slice position during scanning.

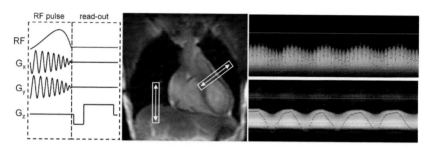

Figure 6-3. Pencil beam navigator and application: Navigator pulse sequence using a spiral-based 2D selective excitation RF pulse to excite magnetisation along a beam shaped volume, which is read out using gradient echo along the direction of the beam. Thus, quasi one-dimensional information is available to monitor tissue interfaces. Navigators were placed on the right hemi-diaphragm and on the heart. The measured navigator profiles are shown as a function of time (right top and bottom). The cardiac navigator (top right trace) clearly shows a superposition of the cardiac and the respiratory motion. The red dots indicate the displacements derived by the evaluation algorithm and used for gating to steer the MR acquisition. G_x, G_y, G_z represent the gradient fields, RF: denotes the excitation radio frequency. Read-out indicates the MR data acquisition.

Besides a simple accept/reject algorithm, a number of more sophisticated prospective gating algorithms have been developed to freeze the respiratory motion in the final data. Among them are the diminishing variance algorithm (DVA)[21], which performs an automatic auto-focusing during a data reacquisition phase, the motion adapted gating approach (MAG)[22], which introduces a k-space-dependent gating function to improve scan efficiency and the phase ordering with adapted window selection algorithm (PAWS)[23], which performs gating with multiple gating windows, while an image is reconstructed from the data of that gating window, for which the total sampling is finished first.

All of these algorithms run automatically and show some potential to cope with the diaphragmatic drift problem[24,25]. This is a serious problem in long-lasting gated scans, where an acceptance window has to be defined at the beginning of the scan, which can be wrong at it's end, resulting in a considerable drop of scan efficiency.

In general, the total scan efficiency depends of the size of the gating window. For usual windows of 3-5mm, the resulting gating efficiency varies between 30-50%[3].

2.2.1 Prospective respiratory motion compensation

However, the described gating techniques leave significant residual motion in the measured data. For instance, for a 5mm gating window, the residual spatial variation is still larger than the diameter of the coronaries. Further measures are necessary to improve and to correct the data. Again, the navigator information can be used for such a motion correction. A simple one-dimensional rigid body motion model can be employed. It assumes a fixed, patient-independent, linear relationship between the feet-head positions of the diaphragm and the heart[26]. This allows for prospective slice tracking, making sure that the same portion of the object is excited and measured in each sub-experiment[27]. Thus, based on such a simple rigid body motion model, it is possible to correct for the through-plane and in-plane components prospectively in real-time[28]. This is schematically shown in Figure 6-4. The corresponding transmit/receive frequencies and phases of the subsequent sequence elements are modified immediately to adapt the data acquisition. This approach is rather hardware demanding, but shows significant advantages over a retrospective motion correction approach.

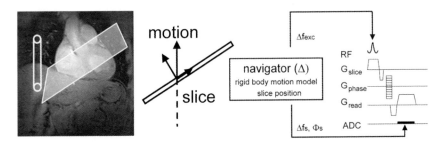

Figure 6-4. Prospective correction of rigid body motion (translation). The diaphragmatic displacement (Δ) measured using the navigator is decomposed into its through-plane and in-plane components. The through-plane component is compensated by an appropriate frequency offset during signal excitation. The in-plane components are compensated during signal reception by changing the demodulation frequency and its phase. The G_i represent the corresponding gradients of the MR imaging sequence.

Major limitations of the slice-tracking approach based on diaphragmatic navigators are the restriction to one-dimensional translation, the limited correlation between the motion of the diaphragm and the motion of the heart, and finally, the non-consideration of the patient specificity. Recently, more sophisticated patient-specific calibrated affine models based on multiple navigators have been introduced for prospective motion correction[29]. The affine motion model takes into account more complex motion such as 3D-translation, rotation, sheering and stretching[30]. To accommodate sufficient degrees of freedom provided by the affine model, a patient-specific calibration is performed[31]. Core of this prospective correction is the motion model, schematically shown in Figure 6-5. It is steered by multiple navigators to allow a fast parameter update for the model. The navigators are placed at different anatomical positions (e.g. diaphragm, chest, abdominal wall, heart) to improve the correlation between the navigator measurements and the actual respiratory motion.

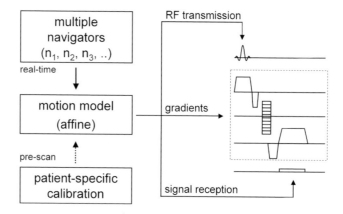

Figure 6-5. Scheme of the patient-specific prospective motion correction approach. Multiple, real-time navigators steer the affine motion model, which has been adapted to the specific patient in a preceding calibration scan. Prospective correction of the object parameters of the MR imaging sequence objects is performed by linear transformation of the gradient coordinate system and the (de-) modulation of the transmitted and received RF signal. This allows the compensation of affine motion including translation, rotation, sheering and stretching in the three-dimensional space.

These improvements allow an extension of the gating window and thus an increase of the scan efficiency while maintaining image quality[32]. Consequently, the total imaging time of such a scan can be reduced to increase patient comfort. Corresponding results are shown in Figure 6-6.

In contrast to prospective motion correction, retrospective techniques[33] are performed after data acquisition[34,35], which significantly limits their use. The main drawback is that slice tracking is not possible. This increases the risk of not exciting the anatomical structures of interest, which can result in serious image artefacts.

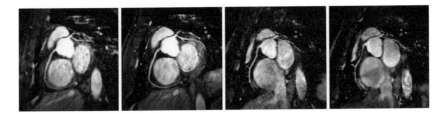

Figure 6-6. Free-breathing coronary angiography. Reformatted images of the right coronary artery (RCA) are shown for 3D Cartesian (first, second from left) and 3D radial imaging sequences (third, fourth) of two different volunteers. Two different motion compensation schemes were used for the two sequences: a 20 mm gating window with prospective correction based on a calibrated affine motion model (first, third) and a 5 mm gating window with slice-tracking (second, fourth). Using the 20 mm affine correction approach, the total scan times were halved to two minutes in total.

3. MR IMAGING SEQUENCE

The MR imaging sequence, which is EKG-triggered and motion corrected, comprises a magnetisation preparation part and a sampling part (see Figure 6-2). The duration of the data sampling is not only limited by the cardiac motion, but also by the live time of the contrast imprinted by the magnetisation preparation.

3.1 Contrast manipulation

Due to the tissue-dependent relaxation times (T_1, T_2), the chemical composition (especially fat) and various other MR-relevant parameters (like proton density, diffusion, flow, etc.), the MR image contrast can be manipulated with a great variability and flexibility for the benefit of the diagnosis. The most common way is the preparation of the longitudinal magnetisation shortly before the signal sampling.

One essential preparation is the fat signal suppression, because the coronary arteries are embedded in epicardial fat[14]. By suppressing the fat signal, the contrast between the coronary blood pool and the surrounding tissue can be enhanced[36,37]. Fat suppression is achieved either by nulling the longitudinal fat magnetisation during the subsequent sampling of the low spatial k-space data in the acquisition block or by applying a spectral spatial RF excitation pulse[38]. The latter solution is, however, limited to selected MR sequences[39].

To enhance the contrast between the myocardium and the arterial blood in the coronary vessels, a T_2-preparation pre-pulse sequence[40,41] is applied.

Due to the T_2 differences, the ratio of the longitudinal magnetisation of arterial blood and the myocardium is changed. This preparation furthermore reduces the signal of the deoxygenated venous blood signal, present in the coronary veins, which eases the vessel identification in the final images.

Regional signal pre-saturation can additionally be performed using slice selective excitation followed by gradient-based signal de-phasing to suppress high signal components from the anterior chest-wall. Thus, residual respiratory motion artefacts originating from the anterior chest wall can be minimised and potential fold-back of unwanted signal from outside the field of view (FoV) can be reduced.

Most of the contrast manipulations previously discussed are dedicated to bright blood CMRA, which has shown great potential for the non-invasive assessment of intra luminal coronary artery disease[42]. However, the majority of acute coronary syndromes occur at sites with non-flow limiting stenoses[43]. Recently, black blood imaging techniques[44] have been elaborated to perform coronary MR vessel wall and plaque imaging[44,45,46]. For this purpose, the magnetisation preparation shown in Figure 6-2 is modified, using global inversion recovery schemes with local re-inversion, to null out the magnetisation of the blood lumen leaving the signal in the coronary wall almost untouched. These preparations in combination with appropriate signal sampling allow a direct assessment of the wall thickness and the visualization of focal atherosclerotic plaque.

In addition, the imaging sequence itself bears high potential to optimise the image contrast and SNR. Among the conventional standard T_2- and T_1-weightings, achieved by Spin-Echo or Gradient-Echo sequences, steady-state sequences received a lot of attention recently[47]. Balanced FFE or true FISP[48] represent the most interesting candidate for CMRA. This very time-efficient sequence generates a T_2/T_1 contrast, which yields a very high SNR for the blood to be imaged in the lumen.

3.2   *k*-Space sampling schemes

The second and very important part of the sequence is the actual sampling period. Besides the different motion compensation measures described above, the MR sampling employed to acquire the actual MR data has an impact on the motion sensitivity and on the image quality. MR data sampling is performed in the so-called *k*-space, and the corresponding trajectory or sampling scheme describes, how this space of measurement data is traversed.

Cartesian scanning schemes are the most common ones in MRI due to their low system and reconstruction requirements. In general, this is a very simple and rather robust scanning scheme. As illustrated in Figure 6-7, *k*-space data sampling is performed in a uniform way, which even holds for a three-dimensional sampling pattern. Image reconstruction from the measured *k*-space data can be done very efficiently.

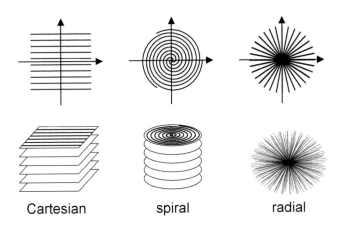

| Cartesian | spiral | radial |

Figure 6-7. Schematic representation of Cartesian, spiral and radial *k*-space sampling schemes. In the upper row, the 2D schemes are shown, whereas in the lower row selected 3D variants are shown (Cartesian, stack of spirals and 3D radial).

In contrast, non-Cartesian *k*-space trajectories offer some advantages due to their specific properties. For example, the spiral sampling scheme samples *k*-space very time-efficiently and is robust against flow/motion effects[49]. It allows very short effective echo times and exhibits a high SNR per unit time[50]. However, the spiral scheme suffers from off-resonance sensitivity, which can be caused by local main field inhomogeneities or chemical shift. To achieve a spatial resolution in three dimensions, the stack-of-spirals approach[51] is preferred, in which conventional phase encoding is used for spatial encoding in the slice selection direction.

Radial imaging is another candidate for signal sampling (Figure 6-7). The technique is known for its low motion sensitivity[52], and thus, is attractive in combination with balanced FFE type sequences. Such modern and robust steady state sequences yield a very high SNR[53]. The radial sampling can be extended to 3D using the same ideas as mentioned for the spiral, i.e. the use of stack-of-stars. However, a real 3D radial sampling as shown in Figure 6-7 easily allows volumetric/whole heart sampling. This scheme has a high robustness against motion, but shows a slight loss of SNR compared with a Cartesian scheme of the same total measuring time[54].

In Figure 6-8, some selected examples for Cartesian and spiral-based CMRA are shown obtained in healthy volunteers.

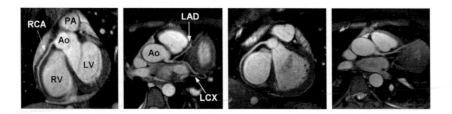

Figure 6-8. Coronary MRA images. Reformatted images are shown (cropped) obtained from different subjects using 3D free breathing techniques. Examples for the mid RCA / proximal RCA and left main (LM) / left anterior descending (LAD) / circumflex (LCX) portions of the vessels are well visualized. Additionally, some anatomical structures are indicated (RV: right ventricle, LV: left ventricle, Ao: aorta, PA: pulmonary artery). The two left images represents data sets obtained using the 3D Cartesian segmented k-space gradient echo scheme. The two right ones show data obtained using the 3D single-interleaf spiral imaging approach.

The Cartesian scanning techniques, which are slightly more motion-sensitive, offer a number of interesting features as well. They can easily be combined with half Fourier[55] and parallel imaging techniques, which allow a considerable reduction of the scan time, without the need for complicated image reconstruction.

3.3   Parallel imaging for scan acceleration

Parallel imaging has received considerable interest during the last few years and will have an important impact on the way of scanning in the future. It is based on the idea that the spatially varying sensitivities of individual coil elements forming a receive coil array can be used to instantaneously encode spatial information during signal reception[56,57]. This inherent signal encoding allows the reduction of the number of necessary phase encoding steps conventionally required for MR imaging. Thus, the acceleration of scanning or the increase of spatial resolution keeping the total scan time constant.

Parallel imaging is based on the phased array coil technology[58], which helps to improve the SNR and has, therefore, been applied to CMRA very early[56]. Multiple independent and decoupled reception coils, each connected to an individual receiver, allow a local signal reception minimizing the noise, dominated by the object itself and restricted by the sensitive volume of the coil. Different algorithms have been elaborated to combine the individual coil data and to compensate for the residual reception inhomogeneities[58].

This basic concept allows further scan acceleration by subsampling the data in *k*-space without compromising the image quality. With the recent hardware advances, massively parallel imaging becomes feasible, which is a very promising technique for future CMRA.

3.4   Whole heart

One of the main advantages of MRI compared to other imaging modalities is its ability to measure single slices (2D) or thin-slab 3D volumes in arbitrarily double-oblique orientations. Most of the recent studies are using volume targeted thin-slab double-oblique 3D imaging techniques[59] to visualize portions of the coronary artery tree.

However, whole-heart coronary MRA techniques have recently been re-introduced, which allow the whole coronary tree to be imaged in a single acquisition[60]. These new approaches provide several advantages compared with conventional volume targeted approaches[59,37]. The volumetric coverage enables the reconstruction of arbitrary views, and the reduced planning effort improves ease-of-use aspects of coronary MRA. On the other hand, the long acquisition time of whole-heart acquisitions[60] (up to 20 min) results in an increased dependence on motion such as heart rate variations or respiratory drifts. However, with the introduction of the new generation of MR scanners supporting many receive channels and a corresponding number of reception coil elements, the SNR can be increased, and a significant acceleration of these protocols becomes feasible. Thus, whole heart coronary MRA might become feasible in a single breath-hold[61]. However, these breath-holds are still rather long, not applicable to the majority of patients, and the spatial resolution is limited.

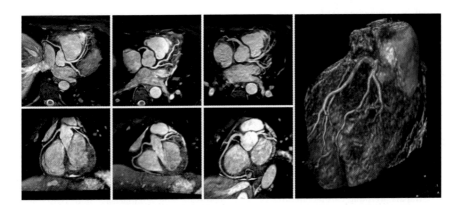

Figure 6-9. Free-breathing, whole heart 3D coronary MR angiograms. Different reformatting (top row left: LM/LAD/LCX, bottom row: RCA/LCX) are shown for three selected volunteers (from left to right). A surface rendered reconstruction of such a data set shows the LM/LAD branch. Measurements were performed using a 32-channel MRI system with a total scan acceleration factor of 6, resulting in a total scan time of four minutes during free breathing.

More robust approaches, which potentially address a larger part of the patient population, employ advanced multi-channel technology for navigator based free-breathing techniques. This allows the whole heart to be imaged with sufficient resolution and SNR in about a few minutes, which is quite acceptable with respect to the clinical workflow and patient comfort (see Figure 6-9).

4.   CONCLUSION

The recent improvements in motion correction and the advances in hardware and scanning methodology enable coronary magnetic resonance angiography in comparably short total measuring times at high patient comfort with high diagnostic value. Further technical and clinical developments can be anticipated strengthening the role of MRI in the cardiac arena.

REFERENCES

1.   M.J. Budoff, D. Georgiou, A. Brody, A.S. Agatston, J. Kennedy, C. Wolfkiel, W. Stanford, P. Shields, R.J. Lewis, W.R. Janowitz, S. Rich, B.H. Brundage, Ultrafast computed tomography as a diagnostic modality in the detection of coronary artery disease: a multicenter study, *Circulation* **93**, 898-904 (1996).
2.   W.J. Manning, D.J. Pennel, *Cardiovascular Magnetic Resonance,* (Churchill Livingstone, New York 2002).
3.   W.Y. Kim, P.G. Danias, M. Stuber, S.D. Flamm, S. Plein, E. Nagel, S.E. Langerak, O.M. Weber, E.M. Pedersen, M. Schmidt, R.M. Botnar, W.J. Manning, Coronary magnetic resonance angiography for the detection of coronary stenoses, *N Engl J Med* **27** (345), 1863-1869 (2001).
4.   D.K. Sodickson, M.L. Chuang, V.C. Khassgiwala,W.J. Manning, In-plane motion of the left and right coronary artery during the cardiac cycle. *Proceedings of the 5th Annual Meeting of ISMRM, Vancouver, Canada,* 910 (1997).
5.   M.B. Hofman, S.A. Wickline, C.H. Lorenz, Quantification of in-plane motion of the coronary arteries during the cardiac cycle: implications for acquisition window duration for MR flow quantification, *J Magn Reson Imaging* **8**, 568-576 (1998).
6.   W.Y. Kim, M. Stuber, K.V. Kissinger, N.T. Andersen, W.J. Manning, R.M. Botnar, Impact of bulk cardiac motion on right coronary MR angiography and vessel wall imaging, *J Magn Reson Imaging* **14**, 383-390 (2001).
7.   C. Jahnke, I. Paetsch, K. Nehrke, B. Schnackenburg, R. Gebker, E. Fleck, E. Nagel, Rapid and complete coronary arterial tree visualization with magnetic resonance imaging: feasibility and diagnostic performance, *Eur Heart J*, (Jun 29, 2005).
8.   D. Manke, P. Börnert, K. Nehrke, E. Nagel, O. Dossel, Accelerated coronary MRA by simultaneous acquisition of multiple 3D stacks, *J Magn Reson Imaging* **14**, 478-483 (2001).

9. R.M. Botnar, M. Stuber , P.G. Danias, K.V. Kissinger, W.J. Manning, Improved coronary artery definition with T2-weighted, free-breathing, three-dimensional coronary MRA, *Circulation* **99**, 3139-3148 (1999).

10. S.E. Fischer, S.A. Wickline, C.H. Lorenz, Novel real-time R-wave detection based on the vectorcardiogram for accurate gated magnetic resonance acquisitions, *Magn Reson Med* **42**, 361-370 (1999).

11. R.M. Botnar, T. Leiner, K.V. Kissinger, G. van Yperen, W.J. Manning, Improved motion compensation in coronary MRA, *Proceedings of the 14th Annual Meeting of ISMRM, Kyoto, Japan,* 2555 (2004).

12. M. Buehrer, S. Kozerke, P. Boesiger, Trigger delay adaptation during coronary MRA by prediction of heart rate variations, in: *Proceedings of the 13th Annual Meeting of ISMRM, Miami, USA,* 2240 (2005).

13. K. Nehrke, D. Manke, P. Börnert, Free-breathing cardiac MR imaging: study of implications of respiratory motion - initial results, *Radiology* **220**, 810-815 (2001).

14. R.R. Edelman, W.J. Manning, D. Burstein, S. Paulin, Coronary arteries: breath-hold MR angiography, *Radiology* **181**, 641-643 (1991).

15. J. Pauly, D. Nishimura, A. Macovski, A k-space analysis of small-tip-angle excitation, *J Magn Reson* **81**, 43–56 (1989).

16. K. Nehrke, P. Börnert, J. Groen, J. Smink, J.C. Bock, On the performance and accuracy of 2D navigator pulses, *Magn Reson Imaging* **17**, 1173-1181 (1999).

17. T.S. Sachs, C.H. Meyer, B.S. Hu, J. Kohli, D.G. Nishimura, A. Macovski, Real-time motion detection in spiral MRI using navigators, *Magn Reson Med* **32**, 639-645 (1994).

18. E. Spuentrup, M. Stuber, R. M. Botnar, W.J. Manning, The impact of navigator timing parameters and navigator spatial resolution on 3D coronary magnetic resonance angiography, *J Mag Reso Imaging* **14**, 311-318 (2001).

19. F.S. Prato, R.L. Nicholson, M. King, R.L. Knill, L. Reese, K. Wilkins, Abolition of respiration movement markedly improved NMR images of the thorax and upper abdomen, *Magn Reson Med* **1**, 227-229 (1984).

20. V.M. Runge, J.A. Clanton, C.L. Partain, A.E. James Jr., Respiratory gating in magnetic resonance imaging at 0.5 Tesla, *Radiology* **15**, 521-523 (1984).

21. T.S. Sachs, C.H. Meyer, P. Irarrazabal, B.S. Hu, D.G. Nishimura, A. Macovski, The diminishing variance algorithm for real-time reduction of motion artifacts in MRI, *Magn Reson Med* **34**, 412-422, (1995).

22. M. Weiger, P. Börnert, R. Proksa, T. Schäffter, A. Haase, Motion-adapted gating based on k-space weighting for reduction of respiratory motion artefacts, *Magn Reson Med* **38**, 322-333 (1997).

23. P. Jhooti, P.D. Gatehouse, J. Keegan, N.H. Bunce, A.M. Taylor, D.N. Firmin, Phase ordering with automatic window selection (PAWS): a novel motion-resistant technique for 3D coronary imaging, *Magn Reson Med* **43**, 470-480 (2000).

24. M. Taylor, P. Jhooti, F. Wiesmann, J. Keegan, D.N. Firmin, D.J. Pennell, MR navigator-echo monitoring of temporal changes in diaphragm position: implications for MR coronary angiography, *J Magn Reson Imaging* **7**, 629-636 (1997).

25. R. Sinkus, P. Börnert, Motion pattern adapted real-time respiratory gating, *Magn Reson Med* **41**,148-155 (1999).

26. Y. Wang, S.J. Riederer, R.L. Ehman, Respiratory motion of the heart: kinematics and the implications for the spatial resolution in coronary imaging, *Magn Reson Med* **33**, 713-719 (1995).

27. M.V. McConnell, V.C. Khasgiwala, B.J. Savord, M.H. Chen, M.L. Chuang, R.R. Edelman, W.J. Manning, Prospective adaptive navigator correction for breath-hold MR coronary angiography, *Magn Reson Med* **37**, 148-152 (1997).

28. Y. Wang, R.C. Grimm, J.P. Felmlee, S.J. Riederer, R.L. Ehman, Algorithms for extracting motion information from navigator echoes, *Magn Reson Med* **36**, 117-123 (1996).

29. D. Manke, K. Nehrke, P. Börnert, Novel prospective respiratory motion correction approach for free-breathing coronary MR angiography using a patient-adapted affine motion model, *Magn Reson Med* **50**, 122-131 (2003).

30. D. Manke, K. Nehrke, P. Börnert, P. Rösch, O. Dössel, Respiratory motion in coronary MR angiography - a comparison of different motion models, *J Magn Reson Imaging* **15**, 661-671 (2002).

31. D. Manke, P. Rösch, K. Nehrke, P. Börnert, O. Dössel, Model evaluation and calibration for prospective motion correction in coronary MR angiography based on 3D image registration, *IEEE Trans Med Imag* **21**, 1132-1141 (2002).

32. C. Jahnke, I. Paetsch, K. Nehrke, B. Schnackenburg, R. Gebker, E. Fleck, E. Nagel, Rapid and complete coronary arterial tree visualization with magnetic resonance imaging: feasibility and diagnostic performance, *Eur Heart J* **26**, 2313-2319 (2005).

33. M. Hedley, H. Yan, Motion artifact suppression: a review of post-processing techniques, *Magn Reson Imaging* **10**, 627-635 (1992).

34. D. Atkinson, D.L. Hill, P.N. Stoyle, P.E. Summers, S.F. Keevil, Automatic correction of motion artifacts in magnetic resonance images using an entropy focus criterion, *IEEE Trans Med Imaging* **16**, 903-910 (1997).

35. A. Manduca, K.P. McGee, E.B. Welch, J.P. Felmlee, R.C. Grimm, R.L. Ehman, Autocorrection in MR imaging: adaptive motion correction without navigator echoes, *Radiology* **215**, 904-909 (2000).

36. D. Li, C.B. Paschal, E.M. Haacke, L.P. Adler, Coronary arteries: three-dimensional MR imaging with fat saturation and magnetization transfer contrast, *Radiology* **187**, 401-406 (1993).

37. M. Stuber, R.M. Botnar, P.G. Danias, D.K. Sodickson, K.V. Kissinger, M. Van Cauteren, J. DeBecker, W.J. Manning, Double-oblique free-breathing high resolution three-dimensional coronary magnetic resonance angiography, *J Am Coll Cardiol* **34**, 524-531 (1999).

38. C.H. Meyer, J.M. Pauly, A. Macovski, D.G. Nishimura, Simultaneous spatial and spectral selective excitation, *Mag Reson Med* **15**, 287-304 (1990).

39. P. Börnert, M. Stuber, R.M. Botnar, K.V. Kissinger, W.J. Manning, Comparison of fat suppression strategies in 3D spiral coronary magnetic resonance angiography, *J Magn Reson Imaging* **15**, 462-466 (2002).

40. J. H. Brittain, B.S. Hu, G.A. Wright, C.H. Meyer, A. Macovski, D.G. Nishimura, Coronary angiography with magnetization-prepared T2 contrast, *Magn Reson Med* **33**, 689-696 (1995).

41. R.M. Botnar, M. Stuber, P.G. Danias, K.V. Kissinger, W.J. Manning, Improved coronary artery definition with T2-weighted, free-breathing, three-dimensional coronary MRA, *Circulation* **99**, 3139-3148 (1999).

42. W.J. Manning, W. Li, R.R. Edelman, A preliminary report comparing magnetic resonance coronary angiography with conventional angiography, *N Engl J Med* **328**, 828-832 (1993).

43. W.C. Little, M. Constantinescu, R.J. Applegate, M.A. Kutcher, M.T. Burrows, F.R. Kahl, W.P. Santamore, Can coronary angiography predict the site of a subsequent myocardial infarction in patients with mild-to-moderate coronary artery disease?, *Circulation* **78**, 1157-1166 (1988).

44. Z.A. Fayad, V. Fuster, J.T. Fallon, T. Jayasundera, S.G. Worthley, G. Helft, J.G. Aguinaldo, J.J. Badimon, S.K. Sharma, Noninvasive in vivo human coronary artery

lumen and wall imaging using black-blood magnetic resonance imaging, *Circulation* **102**, 506-510 (2000).

45. R.M. Botnar, M. Stuber, K.V. Kissinger, W.Y. Kim, E. Spuentrup, W.J. Manning, Noninvasive coronary vessel wall and plaque imaging with magnetic resonance imaging, *Circulation* **102**, 2582-2587 (2000).

46. R.M. Botnar, W.Y. Kim, P. Boernert, M. Stuber, E. Spuentrup, W.J. Manning, 3D coronary vessel wall imaging utilizing a local inversion technique with spiral image acquisition, *Magn Reson Med* **46**, 848-854 (2001).

47. M.T. Vlaardingerbroek, J.A. den Boer, *Magnetic Resonance Imaging theory and practice*, (Springer, Berlin, 1997).

48. A. Oppelt, B. Graumann, H. Barfuss, H. Fischer, W. Hartl, W. Schajor, FISP-a new fast MRI sequence, *Electomedica* **54**, 15-18 (1986).

49. H. Meyer, B.S. Hu, D.G. Nishimura, A. Macovski, Fast spiral coronary artery imaging, *Magn Reson Med* **28**, 202-213 (1992).

50. P. Börnert, M. Stuber, R.M. Botnar, K.V. Kissinger, P. Koken, E. Spuentrup, W.J. Manning, Direct comparison of 3D spiral vs. Cartesian gradient-echo coronary magnetic resonance angiography, *Magn Reson Med* **46**, 789-94 (2001).

51. P. Irarrazabal, D.G. Nishimura, Fast three dimensional magnetic resonance imaging, *Magn Reson Med* **33**, 656-662 (1995).

52. G.H. Glover, J.M. Pauly, Projection reconstruction techniques for reduction of motion effects in MRI, *Magn Reson Med* **28**, 275-289 (1992).

53. C. Larson, O.P. Simonetti, D. Li, Coronary MRA with 3D undersampled projection reconstruction TrueFISP, *Magn Reson Med* **48**, 594-601 (2002).

54. C. Stehning, P. Börnert, K. Nehrke, H. Eggers, O. Doessel, Fast isotropic volumetric coronary MR angiography using free-breathing 3D radial balanced FFE acquisition, *Magn Reson Med* **52**, 197-203 (2004).

55. D.A. Feinberg, J.D. Hale, J.C. Watts, L. Kaufman, A. Mark, Having MR imaging time by conjugation: demonstration at 3.5 kG, *Radiology* **161**, 527-531 (1986).

56. K. Sodickson, W.J. Manning, Simultaneous acquisition of spatial harmonics (SMASH): fast imaging with radiofrequency coil arrays, *Magn Reson Med* **38**, 591-603 (1997).

57. K.P. Pruessmann, M. Weiger, M.B. Scheidegger, P. Boesiger, SENSE: Sensitivity encoding for fast MRI, *Magn Reson Med* **42**, 952-962 (1999).

58. P.B. Roemer, W.A. Edelstein, C.E. Hayes, S.P. Souza, O.M. Mueller, The NMR phased array, *Magn Reson Med* **16**, 192-225 (1990).

59. P. Börnert, D. Jensen, Coronary artery imaging at 0.5 T using segmented 3D echo planar imaging, *Magn Reson Med* **34**, 779-785 (1995).

60. O.M. Weber, A.J. Martin, C.B. Higgins, Whole-heart steady-state free precession coronary artery magnetic resonance angiography, *Magn Reson Med* **50**, 1223-1228 (2003).

61. T. Niendorf, C.J. Hardy, H. Cline, R.O. Giaquinto, A. K. Grant, N.M. Rofsky, D.K. Sodickson, Highly accelerated single breath-hold coronary MRA with whole heart coverage using a cardiac optimized 32-element coil array, *Proceedings of the 13th Annual Meeting of ISMRM, Miami, USA,* 702 (2005).

Chapter 7

4-DIMENSIONAL ULTRASONIC IMAGING
Technology Advances and Medical Applications

Christopher S. Hall
Philips Research, Briarcliff Manor, NY, USA

Abstract: Four-dimensional ultrasound is a relatively newcomer to the diagnostic imaging market. With real-time rendering of moving anatomy, 4-D ultrasonic techniques promise to permit many new applications in the realms of interventional cardiology and radiology, as well as to improve specific existing two-dimensional applications. In this chapter, we will review some of the technical advances that have enabled 4-D ultrasound imaging including hardware and quantification tools, remaining technical challenges, initial clinical applications, and novel areas of medicine to which the technology can be applied.

Keywords: 4-D ultrasound; four-dimensional ultrasound; real-time imaging

1.   INTRODUCTION

In this chapter, we will examine the increasingly important role of four-dimensional ultrasound in specific clinical applications and discuss the key technological advances that have enabled the construction of 4-D ultrasound clinical imaging systems. Four-dimensional (4-D) ultrasound is often used as a key marketing phrase and may have different meanings to each reader. In the context of this chapter, we will refer to 4-D ultrasound as any means of providing time-varying volumetric images. This designation will include both real-time and non-real-time techniques for volume acquisition. Often 4-D ultrasound is referred to as 3D + T or real-time 3-D or RT3D to explicitly break out the time-varying component from the spatial dimensions. The reader may also wish to consult other excellent summaries of the state of the art in 4-D ultrasonic medical imaging[1-3].

G. Spekowius and T. Wendler (Eds.), Advances in Healthcare Technology, 99-116.

Why four dimensions? The history of medical ultrasound has progressed from the early days of A-line or 1-D imaging, to B-mode presentation of multiple A-lines as a two-dimensional imaging technique, to three-dimensional presentation of multiple B-modes as a volume. This progression has been driven in part by 'technology push' as well as 'clinical pull'. 'Technology push' describes the advances in the technical realm that allow the possibility of performing novel forms of imaging in an affordable and repeatable manner. This concept will be discussed in greater depth in the next section, Technological Advances. However, without actual clinical needs ('clinical pull') for technology, there is little impetus for further development. The section, Clinical Applications, describes many of the clinical applications for four-dimensional ultrasound. In all of these cases, the need is for an imaging modality that is capable of capturing three-dimensional volumes that vary rapidly with time. In human physiology, almost all processes change with time, but of course, the concept of clinical imaging is that the change is on a time-scale that is relevant to the health of the patient.

Four-dimensional ultrasound allows for a richer description of pathology that can often be lost with traditional two-dimensional (2D + T) imaging. Full time-varying volume imaging allows for reduced intra- and inter-variations thereby increasing the clinical utility of ultrasonic imaging. Quantification tools both on-line and off-line allow for rapid, repeatable, and robust calculation for empirically determined clinical metrics of health.

2.   TECHNOLOGICAL ADVANCES

The advent of four-dimensional ultrasonic imaging has been made possible by key advances in ultrasonic transducer fabrication including inter-connect and cabling technology, micro-processor miniaturization, real-time beam-forming including micro-beam forming technology, increased processing power of personal computers and graphic processing units, visualization tools for complex data sets, and many other enabling technologies. This section will give an overview of these key areas and discuss some of the remaining challenges.

2.1   Current 4-D imaging methods

The current approaches to four-dimensional medical ultrasonic imaging can be separated into two categories: non-real-time and real-time imaging. Depending on the clinical application, the benefit/cost ratio of each approach dictates the adoption of the specific solution.

Non-real-time four-dimensional imaging is sometimes referred to as 'gated acquisition'. Typically this approaches uses the acquisition of multiple scan planes or volumes either prospectively or retrospectively triggered by a physiologic signal. The signal is often the electrocardiogram or sometimes the breathing motion induced by the expansion of the lungs and movement of the diaphragm. The motion of the volume of interest is assumed to be perfectly periodic with respect to the physiologic signal. This assumption allows for different imaging planes / volumes to be acquired in each period and then a simple geometric- or more complex, image-based fusion of the separate imaging volumes is performed.

The category of non-real-time four-dimensional imaging includes several techniques for acquiring multiple imaging planes/volumes. These techniques include mechanical movement of linear probes constructing two-dimensional (2-D + T) images in rapid succession. This approach has been used in trans-esophageal echocardiography with movement of a sector array in a fan-like motion. Various mechanical scanning approaches are also used for trans-thoracic and for trans-abdominal imaging techniques. Similar techniques using a 'pull-back' approach where the operator moves the 2-D probe in a prescribed motion, usually a linear movement at a constant velocity that allows for stitching of the various imaging planes into a three-dimensional volume. This same technique has been used for intra-vascular applications where the catheter is either advanced or withdrawn at a specified rate so that three-dimensional images can be captured.

Another technique for acquiring 3D volumes that can be off-line reconstructed into four-dimensional imaging through the use of gated acquisition involves the use of positioning systems. These systems allows the identification of the ultrasonic probe in three-dimensional space with respect to the previously captured volume / plane images. The assumption is that the multiple acquisitions are in a constant plane of reference with respect to the patient, i.e. the patient has not moved substantially during the entire imaging sequence. These positioning systems can involve such technologies as a positioning arm, infrared location markers, and RF magnetic tracking systems. With the three-dimensional information for the position of the probe with respect to the patient, it is possible to retrospectively gate the captured imaging volumes and fuse them together to form a complete data set. Such approaches are limited by several important clinical practicalities such as the difficulty maintaining a patient-probe reference frame (no patient motion), and the complexity of conveying to the operator in real-time if sufficient data has been collected to reconstruct a full three-dimensional volume.

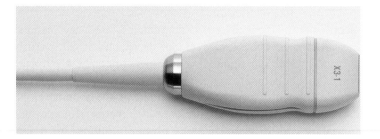

Figure 7-1. A two-dimensional array (X3-1 Philips) for real-time four-dimensional cardiac imaging.

The second category of four-dimensional ultrasound imaging is real-time imaging. Real-time imaging refers to the class of imaging that shows the rendering of the ultrasonic volume in a time frame that can be associated with other clinical monitoring technologies (such as the electrocardiogram). It is often useful to remember that real-time may have different meanings depending on the context of the application. Real-time almost never means at the exact same time as the physiologic change in morphology. In ultrasound, the limitation of speed of sound propagation places a fundamental limit on the time it takes to observe the structure of the body versus the actual motion occurring. In the case of four-dimensional ultrasound, it is helpful to note that real-time refers to rate at which the skilled clinician or sonographer can perceive changes in structure or blood flow as if they were observing with the naked eye. In practice, the concept of real-time coincides with the frame-rate of the presentation of data and is for most purposes identical to the frame-rate necessary for all moving images (TV, motion pictures, etc.) of between 10 to 75 times a second.

The advantages to real-time imaging are manifold but so too are the technical challenges. Real-time imaging obviates the use of retrospective or prospective gating techniques because the entire imaging volume can be captured in a single pass. This implies that the assumption of periodic motion of a structure need no longer be made, and the movement of tissue / blood can be made as it occurs. This property allows the sonographer or clinician a more intuitive interface for capturing four-dimensional images as movement of the probe is directly reflected in the imaging volume acquired. In addition, data can be captured more quickly and with a higher degree of certainty. However, the technical requirements of performing such approaches to imaging are tremendous and necessitate advances in several areas that will be detailed in the sub-section, Enabling technologies.

2.2   Technical challenges

From a technical point of view, the challenges for four-dimensional ultrasonic imaging are manifold. In the next section, we will detail many of the enabling solutions for addressing the technical challenges. In this section, we will attempt to detail the clinical requirements and thereby technical challenges that must be solved.

The basic clinical requirement is to image three-dimensional human anatomy with ultrasound in such a way to make clinical diagnoses reliable, repeatable, and robust. The often unspoken corollary to these requirements is that the imaging modality must be cost-effective per diagnosis.

For real-time versus non-real-time imaging approaches, the technical challenges are slightly different. In either case, roughly 30 volumes per second are required. In the case of real-time imaging, this means that for a transmit line density of 64 lines per scan plane, roughly 64^2 lines must be fired. Each line if propagated to a depth of 20 cm requires a round trip time of (2 x 20 cm / 0.15 cm/μsec) = 266 μsec, and thereby for a full volume 64x64x266 μsec is 1.1 seconds. Obviously this straightforward approach will only allow a single volume per second.

In addition, the signal-processing path must be capable of handling enormous data throughput. A typical received line will be digitized to 12 or 16 bits of accuracy at a rate of approximately 40 Megasamples/second for 30 volumes per second of line densities of 128 per received scan plane. This requires on the order of (266 μsec * 40 Samples / μsec * 2 bytes / sample * 30 volumes / sec * (128 x 128) lines / volume) = 10 GBytes/sec throughput.

These data are then scan converted and presented to the user in various forms (as detailed in the section called Presentation to the clinician). The ability to construct a presentation format that accounts for correct user-to-volume positioning, shading, transparency, and lighting needs to be accomplished at 30 volumes/sec.

2.3   Enabling technologies

In order to make four-dimensional ultrasound imaging a clinical reality, key technological advances have had to occur. In this section, several of the important advances in transducer design, microelectronics, beam forming, and computing power are discussed. The emphasis in this section will be on the real-time implementation of 4-D ultrasonic imaging.

Mechanically scanned probes are limited often by the speed at which they can move for various reasons such as the time to propagate sound to construct a single imaging plane, the vibration of the probe, the time to return the probe to the first imaging plane, the difficulty of having multiple focal zones, and the often necessary continuous movement of the probe. As a result, the desired approach for constructing four-dimensional ultrasound images is through the use of electronically steered arrays (see Figure 7-1). In order to perform this approach, it is necessary to have fully sampled two-dimensional transducer technology. A typical 1-D ultrasound array usually has on order of 128 elements in a single direction. The addition of another dimension in order to construct three-dimensional volumes means that on order of 128^2 elements is needed. Current implementations of matrix arrays usually have on order of 2000 to 3000 elements. The first two-dimensional arrays were constructed by van Ramm and Smith in the late 1980's and early 1990's[4]. Their design was then adopted by the spin-off company Volumetrics Imaging Systems, Inc.

The fabrication of such transducer arrays is challenging for several reasons. The first is the difficulty in construction of a transducer with several thousand individual elements. This can be a challenging manufacturing problem to have high yields and a high degree of reliability. The second challenge is individually connecting each element to a different channel (the 'inter-connect' problem). The third challenge is the approaches necessary to address each transducer element individually in transmit and receive (the 'channel-count' problem) modes.

Interesting solutions have been explored for these challenges. The 'inter-connect' problem can be summarized as how do you connect a limited number of cables/channels to multiple elements in a finite amount of space provided by the transducer surface? Flex-circuit technology can be employed to breakout the connections to a larger connection area to ensure a smaller footprint (necessary for cardiac or pediatric probes). In addition, techniques that use flip-chip technology, circuitry that can be bonded directly to the transducer electrodes allow for handling the vast number of interconnects.

The 'channel-count' problem describes the need to have several thousand independent channels while minimizing the cables from the ultrasound machine to transducer. This problem is driven by the user-experience of the clinician or sonographer to not have a large and heavy cable tied to the transducer. In addition, increasing the channel count can increase the cost of an ultrasonic scanning system considerably. Ideally, four-dimensional imaging should be available for a comparable cost to the traditional two-dimensional (2D + T) imaging techniques. Multiplexing signals is one approach although not a very practical one considering the large element number count. Another approach is to examine micro-beam forming technology.

Micro-beam forming describes an approach that groups elements together with a fixed relative beam forming rule. In typical delay and sum beam-forming, the electrical signal sent to each element is delayed relative to adjacent elements in order to geometrically focus the transmitted or received ultrasonic signal. For several thousand elements, this would entail a corresponding 1:1 element to channel count in order to apply the necessary delays. In the micro-beam forming solution, the elements are grouped together in patches of nearby elements and a pre-calculated constant offset from one of the patches' elements is applied to the other patch elements. This approach allows for only one channel per patch to be needed and therefore reduces the number of channels needed on the system.

2.4   Presentation to the clinician

Four-dimensional ultrasonic images are rich in information, but conveying the relevant information to the physician to enable effective diagnoses can be challenging. Many techniques have been developed to address the problem of displaying complex volumetric data in an intuitive manner. The approach that is taken is often driven by the application for which the image is needed or by the desired clinical workflow. Real-time reading and reaction to the clinical volume images might be necessary to provide immediate feedback to the sonographer as he/she gathers the images or for the interventional radiologist as he/she adapts a procedure in response to image information. In off-line or non-real-time reading, the demands of visualization may require more customizability to allow for quick reading so as to not alter or add to the existing two-dimensional (2-D + T) workflow.

The means of visualization require several steps. The first step involves the scan conversion of the captured ultrasonic information into a three-dimensional volume. Advances in computing power of general CPU's have made this step possible in the controlling computer instead of in dedicated hardware implementations. The second step involves the choice of appropriate display. In practice, there is a choice between three dimensional rendering and 2-D cross-sections (MPR or multi-planar reconstruction, see Figure 7-2 for a compromise approach). The three-dimensional rendering can be direct volume rendering with appropriate light source, viewpoint, and surface reflectivity. It can also be a maximum intensity projection where the maximum pixel brightness along a line of site from the dataset to viewpoint is shown. Other methods include selecting a specific opacity of the overlying tissue to allow for a slightly transparent view into deeper tissues. All of these approaches can be used for trimmed datasets where the extraneous overlying image data are removed to reveal hidden structures.

Often the clinician will utilize multiple two-dimensional views to visualize planes at specific geometrical orientation to each other. In cardiac applications, the physician may for example choose to look at a short-axis, 2-chamber long-axis, and 4-chamber long axis views simultaneously. This approach is very useful as the two-dimensional views are the manner in which many clinicians have been taught to read ultrasonic images and therefore are the most intuitive.

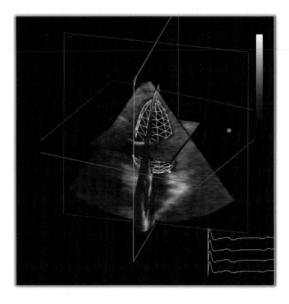

Figure 7-2. A presentation format combining two MPR planes and a wireframe volumetric display.

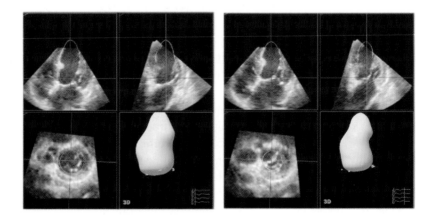

Figure 7-3. Semi-automatic detection of the endocardial borders allows characterization of the left ventricle shape at end systole and end diastole.

2.5   Analysis tools and quantification

One of the key goals of introducing four-dimensional ultrasound is to allow the physician to make more reliable and reproducible diagnoses while at the same time minimally impacting the time per exam. Three-dimensional datasets can often be quite difficult to interpret with a great deal of effort spent orienting the observer in relation to anatomical landmarks. When multiple measurements are necessary as is the case with time-varying volumes, it is often helpful to have semi- or fully- automated means of quantification. These analysis tools are key to the adoption of 4D ultrasound.

The analysis tools can vary from the automatic selection of standard 2-D views of anatomical structures from the 3-D volumes to automate means of volume, area, length, and timing measurements. For the detection of volumes, algorithms to detect the border of the anatomy of interest (endocardial wall, tumor margins, etc.) are necessary (Figure 7-3). Segmentation algorithms from other fields as well as novel approaches can be used to determine the anatomical borders.

In the case of echocardiography, automation of the detection of the endocardial surface allows for calculation of the maximum end systolic, end diastolic volumes, and the ejection fraction. Tracking of mitral valve leaflets can determine if they close fully or if there is an opening for mitral regurgitation. In obstetrics, it is sometimes desirable to obtain the features of the fetus in utero in order to diagnose a cleft palate or other abnormalities. The ability to detect and delineate the fetus' face with respect to other surrounding tissue such as the uterine wall is greatly aided by automated approaches to segmentation. Automatic detection and measurement of the femur length, head size, and other fetal metrics can greatly aid quick and accurate reading.

In the area of analysis tools for four dimensional ultrasound clinical images, there are a few competing products. TomTec Imaging Systems, Inc. offers several products compatible with 4D scanning systems (Volumetrics, Inc. and Philips Sonos 7500, IU22, and IE33 platforms) aimed at the off-line reading of four-dimensional ultrasound clinical images. Philips Medical Systems offers an integrated solution, Qlab®, on the imaging system and also available in off-line mode for analysis of specific metrics to address the needs of each clinical sub-specialty.

2.6   Future technologies

Although the power of 4D ultrasound imaging has been demonstrated in several key clinical applications (see section 3), there are several advances that are necessary unleash its full potential in some outstanding clinical needs. In echocardiography, it would be desirable to 1) image the entire volume of the heart and not just the left ventricle in real-time; 2) capture a large volume while simultaneously detecting Doppler flow; 3) detect motion of the heart wall to measure contractility; 4) tracking myocardial tissue to determine wall motion; 5) perfusion mapping of the myocardium in 4D; and many others.

The underlying technological challenges that need to be met to address these areas include novel transducer design, multi-line transmissions with increased field of view and conserved frame rate, increased channel/element count, new automated analysis techniques, and implementation of contrast-specific settings.

In the realm of novel transducer design, there are several needs driven by traditional and non-traditional markets for ultrasound. In echocardiography, the need for 4D ultrasound in TEE, pediatric, and small-footprint trans-thoracic applications will necessitate new form factor and probe design. In the area of general imaging, a wider field of view will drive transducer design with larger aperture and therefore a corresponding increase in element count. Novel applications, such as the movement of ultrasound into the interventional suites in cardiology and oncology may require transducer design that seamlessly integrates into the already crowded interventional workspace.

Increasing the field of view also drives the need for novel beam forming approaches. As was discussed in earlier sections, the fundamental limitation of the speed of sound within the body can reduce the effective frame rate for a volume with the desired line densities. This limitation becomes even more serious when a larger volume must be captured, not to mention if in conjunction with real-time multi-transmit modalities such as Doppler flow. Similarly, the introduction of contrast settings may also drive a need for clever transmit schemes since most contrast specific modes employ multi-transmit lines (e.g. pulse inversion, power modulation, etc.).

The increased channel count necessary to drive larger aperture probes can place an inordinate requirement on the ultrasound system because of the added cost for each transmit / receive channel. Novel ways of supplying the interconnects for the large number of elements, increased yield for large multi-element transducers, and standardized approaches for connecting the channels to elements to allow for re-use of design templates are all necessary technologies to maintain the cost effectiveness of the technology.

Although, all of the above technologies need to be fully developed in the future to expand the clinical utility of four-dimensional ultrasound, perhaps no where is the need for future technologies more obvious to the physician that through the tools and presentation technologies for the clinical images. Advances in the integration of the analysis toolsets and the corresponding reporting mechanisms will be necessary to ensure that the 4-D ultrasound imaging technology is adopted and positively impacts the clinical workflow. These analysis toolsets will need to automate fully many of the analyses such as volume, length, and timing measurements with minimal and effortless oversight from an expert reader. The results then need to be presented to the physician in such a way as to allow for effective and cost-conscious diagnoses. In this area, the use of parametric representation of specific parameters such as wall motion, contractility timing, contrast agent kinetics and other relevant parameters superimposed over the anatomical volumetric image will be extremely useful.

3.   CLINICAL APPLICATIONS

Commercially available four dimensional ultrasound clinical imaging systems have been available only in the last ten years (1994, Volumetrics, Inc. released its first real-time scanning system, and in 2002, Philips released its first real-time three-dimensional scanning system). Since the inception of these devices, the clinical adoption has in part been driven by the availability of specific settings and devices tailored for a specific clinical sub-specialty. The advent of the X4 matrix array on the Philips Sonos 7500 was released for the cardiac market in 2002 while the C6v2 probe on the Philips IU22 was released in early 2004 for the obstetrics market. The clinical need in these markets was more obvious and therefore the 'clinical pull' allowed the technology to be deployed and evaluated. The following sections will describe work performed in many of the clinical sub-specialties to evaluate the suitability of four-dimensional ultrasound.

3.1   Obstetrics / gynecology

One of the clinical areas that first found use for 3-D ultrasound was the area of obstetrics (Figure 7-4). Initially the use of 3-D was to provide useful information about specific developmental deformities such as facial abnormalities to rule out cleft lip or to detect spinal deformations[5]. The means of acquiring 3-D images was usually through image fusion of several 2-D planes or through the use of a mechanically driven probe. These approaches were limited in scope by the movement of the patient, the fetus, or variations in the pressure applied to the hand-held probe. The advent of real-time 3-D imaging allows for reduction in the effect of motion and thereby expands the utility of ultrasound for clinical diagnosis. The current application for 4-D ultrasound in obstetrics is the monitoring of the fetus' heart in utero. Many developmental diseases are reflected in cardiac abnormalities such as arterial malposition, single ventricle, septal defects, Ebstein's anomaly, and other congenital diseases.

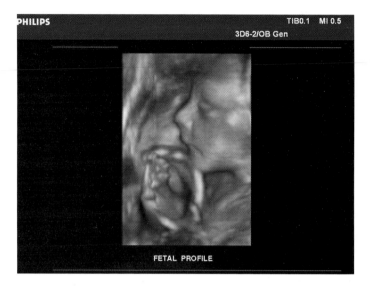

Figure 7-4. Three-dimensional view of a fetus in utero.

3.2   Cardiology

3.2.1   Chamber volume / heart mass

Perhaps one of the most pervasive measurements in cardiology applications of ultrasound is the observation of the change in heart chambers' volumes as a function of the heart cycle. Ejection fraction or the percentage of the heart chamber volume ejected during systole has considerable clinical merit as a surrogate of heart failure. In order for four-dimensional ultrasound to obtain acceptance, it is necessary to show that the method is superior in some ways than the traditional imaging approaches. Initial measurements in vitro with phantoms of human and porcine right ventricles showed accurate quantification of the right ventricle volumes and stroke volumes without the necessary geometric assumptions used in the Simpson's rule for calculating volume from B-scan images[6]. Other studies have shown that real-time three dimensional imaging reduces inter- and intra-observer variability in comparison to traditional two-dimensional approaches when compared to a gold standard, MRI heart volume assessment[7-9].

Of course, in addition to cardiac output, there have been many studies of the benefit and suitability of real-time 3D ultrasonic imaging in cardiology. The motion of the heart walls can reveal underlying pathology of the blood supply to the heart muscle. Kuo et al. showed that left-ventricular akinesia or dyskinesia in a canine model was detectable with wall motion tracking using real-time three-dimensional ultrasound[10]. Tustsui et al. provided a case study of the use of three-dimensional echocardiography in diagnosis of large left circumflex coronary aneurysm[11]. And Cheng et al. used RT3D ultrasound to find that 3D assessment of septal defect diameters correlated much better than two-dimensional assessment when compared to surgical findings in 38 patients[12].

3.2.2   Valvular diseases

Another important area where four-dimensional ultrasound has found an emerging role is in the diagnosis of specific valvular diseases such as mitral stenosis and prolapse and the concomitant regurgitation[13]. As is the case in adoption of cardiac output applications, it is necessary to show that 4-D ultrasound provides an added benefit to the accepted procedures. In patients with mitral valve stenosis, Xie et al. showed that 4-D ultrasound showed good correlation of mitral valve area with 2-D ultrasound approaches, but allowed for faster exam times and choice of the optimal plane of the smallest mitral valve orifice[14]. Other studies showed that 3D echocardiography was superior to multi-plane transesophageal in 75 patients undergoing mitral valve repair for identification of the commissures[15].

3.3   General imaging / oncology

The applications for four-dimensional ultrasound have been not as forthcoming in the field of general imaging. This is due primarily to the lack of a suitable product aimed at this clinical segment. However, there have been several studies looking at the use of real-time 3-D ultrasonic imaging in the breast[16,17] (detailed below in the section, Interventional Radiology and Other Applications), the brain[18], and for parathyroid ablation[19]. Trans-cranial 3-D color Doppler flow scans and perfusion maps of the brain were accomplished with a bolus injection of contrast agent into the internal carotid artery[18]. In another study using contrast agents, Kitaoka showed that the visualization of the 3D vasculature of the large vessels within the brain could be accomplished with ultrasound[19].

3.4   Interventional suite

One of the very promising areas for four-dimensional ultrasound is in the interventional suite. In this medical application, ultrasound is used for several reasons. One is to visualize the soft tissue pathology where it is currently not available, i.e. under rotational x-ray or fluoroscopic illumination. Another compelling reason is to allow for guidance of the interventional tool (biopsy needle, catheter, rf ablation needle, or other device) to the location of the pathology. In the next two sections, two interesting areas will be examined: the electrophysiology interventional suite and the interventional radiology suite.

3.4.1   Interventional cardiology

Two procedures in the electrophysiology suite have been growing in popularity in the past few years: cardio-resynchronization therapy (CRT) and atrial fibrillation ablation (AFA). The goal of CRT is to address the case where a patient's heart is not beating in the most efficient manner. This can be due to hypertrophy altering the conduction pathways and causing segments of the heart to contract at different times. One approach to solving this problem is to place additional electrical sources into the heart to 're-synchronize' the various portions of the heart. Such a procedure is usually performed under fluoroscopic guidance with physician's mental image of the heart anatomy. By introducing four-dimensional ultrasound, it is possible not only to visualize directly the heart tissue within the procedure but also to observe its response to the electrical stimulus (see Figure 7-5).

3.4.2   Interventional radiology and other applications

Clinical applications of 4-D ultrasound occur in interventional radiology for biopsy needle guidance, rf ablation of liver and other tumors, and even in cases of in utero surgery. Nelson's laboratory has pioneered much of the work in the interventional suite. One such study examined the role of 3-D ultrasound images in the interventional laboratory with emphasis on the suitable displays to provide to the intervening physician[20]. The study showed that volume rendered images did not provide as good visualization as multiple MPR views of the same volume.   Such a MPR (and volume rendered) display was used by Won et al. for the guidance of biopsy of hepatic masses in 12 patients and was shown to optimize the needle position in 67% of the patients in the same exam time as using two dimensional ultrasound techniques[21]. A three-dimensional ultrasonic guided breast biopsy device was constructed and tested on phantoms and ex vivo tissue with an accuracy of 0.43 to 1.71 mm[17] and a 94.5% success rate for lesions 3.2 mm in size[16].

3.5   Future applications

Although the list of possible future applications of four-dimensional ultrasound could be quite extensive, this section will concentrate on several areas that hold great clinical promise.

The use of ultrasonic contrast agents has helped to delineate endocardial borders and quantify perfusion in the myocardium and other tissues using two-dimensional ultrasound. The combination of contrast imaging and four-dimensional ultrasound promises to be one that is extremely powerful. In many cases the endocardial border is difficult to detect, and by utilizing contrast agents, the physician can help ensure the accuracy of the assessment of heart wall motion, blood volume, and perfusion. In addition, contrast agents may help visualize structures that before were not apparent on traditional two-dimensional exams. Figure 7-6 shows such a case where the three-dimensional structure of part of the coronary tree is visualized with the combination of real-time 3D imaging and contrast agents.

One of the areas where four-dimensional ultrasound will play an important role is in the assessment of cardiac function after administration of a stress exam. Currently, the stress exam occurs after either physically or pharmaceutically induced stress. The time that the echocardiographic exam takes can often complicate accurate readings since the patient may be in different states of recovery from the stress challenge when the specific two-dimensional views are gathered. In addition, it is often difficult to obtain the exact same views of the heart pre- and post-stress which can obscure the correct reading. As a result, much of the diagnosis is subjective and prone to reader variability. By introducing real-time volumetric acquisition, it is possible to capture all views of the leftventricule within a few heartbeats. This approach can allow for objective and reproducible diagnoses. Initial studies on patients and volunteers showed promise for correctly spatially registering pre- and post-images while preserving stress-induced changes[22].

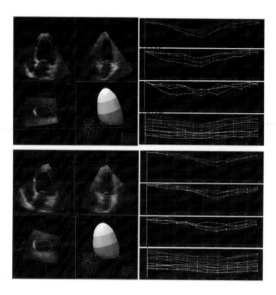

Figure 7-5. The top two panes show the detected endocardial walls and the corresponding motion in each of the 15 segments. The bottom panes show the same wall motion after bi-ventricular pacing has been applied.

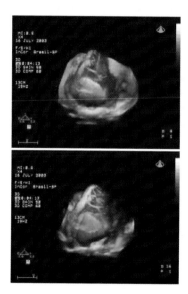

Figure 7-6. Two volume displays at different portions of the heart cycle showing the progressive perfusion of the coronary arteries.

4. CONCLUSION

Although four-dimensional ultrasound has only been available for the last 14 years and only commercially available in two products since 1994 (Volumetrics) and 2002 (Philips), its utility has been shown in clinical applications from echocardiography to obstetrics to the interventional suite. Reduced intra- and inter-user variability promises to increase further the utility of ultrasound as a diagnostic imaging modality. Future improvements in field-of-view, frame-rate, and automated quantification packages guarantee many exciting and clinically beneficial prospects for four-dimensional ultrasound.

5. ACKNOWLEDGMENTS

The author would like to thank Sham Sokka, Ivan Salgo, and Jean Pergrale for their help and contributions to this chapter. In addition, thank you to Brad Robie and Leigh White for providing some of the images.

REFERENCES

1. J.C. Somer, The history of real time ultrasound, *International Congress Series* **1274**, 3-13 (2004).
2. R.C. Houck, J. Cooke, E.A. Gill, Three-Dimensional Echo: Transition from Theory to Real-Time, A Technology Now Ready for Prime Time, *Current Problems in Diagnostic Radiology* 34(3), 85-105 (2005).
3. I.S. Salgo, Three-dimensional echocardiography, *Journal of Cardiothoracic and Vascular Anesthesia* 11(4), 506-516 (1997).
4. S.W. Smith, G.E. Trahey, O.T. von Ramm, Two-dimensional arrays for medical ultrasound, *Proc IEEE Ultrasonics Symposium*, 625-628 (1991).
5. F. Forsberg, Ultrasonic biomedical technology; marketing versus clinical reality, *Ultrasonics* 42(1-9), 17-27 (2004).
6. S.T. Schindera, et al., Accuracy of Real-time Three-dimensional Echocardiography for Quantifying Right Ventricular Volume: Static and Pulsatile Flow Studies in an Anatomic, In Vitro Model, *J Ultrasound Med* 21(10), 1069-1075 (2002).
7. C. Jenkins, Reproducibility and accuracy of echocardiographic measurements of left ventricular parameters using real-time three-dimensional echocardiography, *J Am Coll Cardiol* 44(4), 878-86 (2004).
8. R.S. Von Bardeleben, et al., 914 Contrast enhanced live 3D echo in acute myocardial infarction determines accurate left ventricular wall motion and volumes compared to cardiac MR imaging, *European Journal of Echocardiography* 4(Supplement 1), S119 (2003).
9. H.P. Kuhl, et al., High-resolution transthoracic real-time three-dimensional echocardiography: Quantitation of cardiac volumes and function using semi-automatic

border detection and comparison with cardiac magnetic resonance imaging, *Journal of the American College of Cardiology* **43**(11), 2083-2090 (2004).

10. J. Kuo, et al., Left ventricular wall motion analysis using real-time three-dimensional ultrasound, *Ultrasound in Medicine & Biology* **31**(2), 203-211 (2005).

11. J.M. Tsutsui, et al., Noninvasive evaluation of left circumflex coronary aneurysm by real-time three-dimensional echocardiography, *European Journal of Echocardiography*, in press (2005).

12. T.O. Cheng, et al., Real-time 3-dimensional echocardiography in assessing atrial and ventricular septal defects: An echocardiographic-surgical correlative study, *American Heart Journal* **148**(6), 1091-1095 (2004).

13. G. Valocik, O. Kamp, C.A. Visser, Three-dimensional echocardiography in mitral valve disease, *European Journal of Echocardiography*, in press (2005).

14. M.X. Xie, et al., Comparison of Accuracy of Mitral Valve Area in Mitral Stenosis by Real-Time, Three-Dimensional Echocardiography Versus Two-Dimensional Echocardiography Versus Doppler Pressure Half-Time, *The American Journal of Cardiology* **95**(12), 1496-1499 (2005).

15. A. Macnab, et al., Three-dimensional echocardiography is superior to multiplane transoesophageal echo in the assessment of regurgitant mitral valve morphology, *European Journal of Echocardiography* **5**(3), 212-222 (2004).

16. K.J.M. Surry, et al., The development and evaluation of a three-dimensional ultrasound-guided breast biopsy apparatus, *Medical Image Analysis* **6**(3), 301-312 (2002).

17. W.L. Smith, et al., Three-dimensional ultrasound-guided core needle breast biopsy, *Ultrasound in Medicine & Biology* **27**(8), 1025-1034 (2001).

18. S.W. Smith, et al., Feasibility study: Real-time 3-D ultrasound imaging of the brain, *Ultrasound in Medicine & Biology* **30**(10), 1365-1371 (2004).

19. M. Kitaoka, Clinical application of three-dimensional contrast imaging on parathyroid percutaneous ethanol injection therapy (PEIT), *Ultrasound in Medicine & Biology* **29**(5) Supplement 1, S94 (2003).

20. S.C. Rose, T.R. Nelson, R. Deutsch, Display of 3-Dimensional Ultrasonographic Images for Interventional Procedures: Volume-Rendered Versus Multiplanar Display, *J Ultrasound Med* **23**(11), 1465-1473 (2004).

21. H.J. Won, et al., Value of Four-dimensional Ultrasonography in Ultrasonographically Guided Biopsy of Hepatic Masses, *J Ultrasound Med* **22**(2), 215-220 (2003).

22. R. Shekhar, V. Zagrodsky, V. Walimbe, 3D Stress echocardiography: development of novel visualization, registration and segmentation algorithms, *International Congress Series* **1268**, 1072-1077 (2004).

Chapter 8

CLINICAL HYBRID IMAGING: IMAGE CO-REGISTRATION AND HARDWARE COMBINATION FOR PET/CT AND SPECT/CT

Combining Biochemical and Morphological Information for Better Diagnosis and Treatment

Y.Hämisch[1], M. Egger[1], H. Hines[2], K. Fiedler[3], I. Carlsen[4]

[1]*Philips Medical Systems, Böblingen, Germany;* [2]*Philips Medical Systems, Milpitas, CA, USA;* [3]*Philips Research, Aachen, Germany;* [4]*Philips Research, Hamburg, Germany*

Abstract: Hybrid imaging systems have been conquering medical imaging practice more rapidly and rigorously than any other imaging technology before, meeting strong medical and logistical demands from clinicians and researchers. Despite efforts of combining just images and the higher technical complexity and costs of combined systems the improvements in diagnostic accuracy and ease of patient logistics are too convincing. The rapid development of hybrid devices only occurred in the last 10 years and is still ongoing. Technological advances are made on a yearly pace.

Keywords: Hybrid imaging, SPECT/CT, PET/CT, molecular imaging, FDG, FLT, image registration, rigid transformation, elastic warping, Time-of-flight (TOF)

1.   THE NEED FOR COMBINED IMAGING

Tomographic imaging has become the preferred and widely accepted form of clinical diagnostic imaging since the invention of the first x-ray based tomographic imager by Hounsfield and Cormack in 1973[1,2]. Computer Tomography (CT) and later also Magnetic Resonance Tomography[3] (MRT) scanners are a standard component of most radiological departments in the world.

In parallel, isotope based imaging in nuclear medicine also evolved from planar scintigraphy into a tomographic method, called Single-Photon-

117

G. Spekowius and T. Wendler (Eds.), Advances in Healthcare Technology, 117-138.

Computed-Tomography (SPECT) and has been established in nuclear medicine departments across the world[4]. In the late 80's, after long years in research[5], another isotope based imaging modality, Positron-Emission-Tomography[6] (PET) started to enter medical practice but was only widely accepted clinically in the early 90's because of its complexity, higher costs and more difficult tracer logistics due to the short half life of positron-emitting isotopes[7]. However, those challenges have been overcome in many countries already and today PET, because of its superior sensitivity and diagnostic accuracy, is the driving modality for combined imaging[8,9].

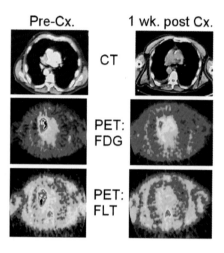

Figure 8-1. Transaxial cross-sections through the chest of a patient with small cell lung cancer prior (left column) and one week after onset (right column) of chemotherapy. Shown are cross-sections from CT (upper row), F-18FDG-PET (middle row) and F-18-FLT-PET (bottom row). (Images courtesy of K. Krohn, Univ. of Washington, Seattle).

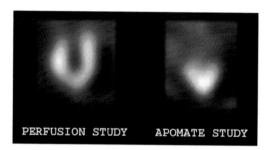

Figure 8-2. Vertical long axis cross-section through the heart of a patient with an acute myocardial infarction: perfusion study (left) and apoptosis study (using Tc-99m labeled Annexin-V 'Apomate') (right). (images courtesy of Heart Medical Center, Eugene, Oregon).

In order to understand the need for combined imaging it is important to recognize that isotope based imaging modalities like SPECT and PET are providing fundamentally different, however, complementary information to morphological imaging methods like CT and MRT. In most cases, SPECT and PET are providing insight into biochemical processes like e.g. metabolism or cell proliferation with a rather poor spatial resolution of 3-10 mm but high sensitivity, whereas CT and MRT are delivering high resolution (sub-mm) images of anatomical structures and physiological function like e.g. blood flow. SPECT and PET are based on a 'tagging' (labeling) of biological molecules with radioactive isotopes that are incorporated and the subsequent observation of their accumulation and distribution in cells, organs and organ systems with a camera or tomograph[10]. The latter are based on the attenuation of x-rays applied from outside in biological tissues (CT)[11] or on the measurement of the magnetic properties of the water content of tissue (MRT)[12].

Figure 8-1 illustrates the different nature of information of the modalities and their impact on treatment decisions in oncology. Shown are transaxial cross-sections through the chest of a patient with small cell lung cancer prior (left column) and one week after onset of chemotherapy (right column). The upper row are cross-sections from x-ray CT, where there is no visible difference in tumor extend between left and right. The middle row shows PET images taken with the tracer F-18-FDG, the most common tracer in oncology diagnosis and treatment monitoring, depicting increased glucose uptake into malignant cells due to higher concentrations of glucose transporters on the membranes of those cells. The labeled F-18-FDG accumulates in the malignant cells and is not metabolized like normal glucose. Here one can easily observe a difference between the image on the left (prior to therapy) and on the right (one week after onset of therapy) by the reduced size and metabolic intensity of the tumor (depicted by the color scale: black & red – very high metabolism, blue – low metabolism). This represents a first indication for the effectiveness of the therapy. An even stronger indication is provided by the PET images with the tracer F-18-FLT. Shields & Griesson first reported the application of F-18-FLT in humans as a tracer to image tumor proliferation and DNA replication in 1998[13]. Here on the right image the tumor seems to have completely disappeared, but in fact, only its proliferating (DNA replicating) activity has been stopped by the therapy. As a control, normal proliferative activity is still seen in the bone marrow of the spine on the right image as well as on the left. It is certainly imaginable what impact the addition of biofunctional information will have on patient management, both in terms of patient outcome and prognosis as well as overall costs of care.

Another strong driver for the increasing use of combined imaging is the development of so-called molecular imaging agents, which are characterized by their very high specificity and almost complete lack of any anatomical background information[14,15]. In PET one could count e.g. the above-mentioned F-18-FLT into that category. An example of a SPECT molecular imaging agent is shown in Figure 8-2, displaying vertical long axis cross-sections through the heart of a patient with an acute myocardial infarction. Shown on the left side is the perfusion study using a common SPECT perfusion tracer labeled with ^{99m}Tc, on the right side the same cross-section, obtained with the new apoptosis marker Annexin-V ('Apomate'), a human protein labeled with [99m]Tc. Apoptosis is the process of 'programmed cell death' and is part of the natural cell turnover (e.g. in skin cells) but also e.g. in infarcted myocardial cells. The apoptotic cells release the phospholipid phospatidylserine (PS) to which the Annexin-V binds and therefore accumulates. This allows to e.g. exactly determine the extent and severity of an infarct as shown in Figure 8-2, but more importantly answer the question about a potential revitalizability of the myocardial tissue[16]. Comparing the two images of Figure 8-2, the reduction in anatomical information is remarkable, going from the flow tracer (left), where at least the left ventricle can still be delineated, to the apoptosis marker (right), where only the apoptotic cells are highlighted. For any kind of further therapeutic decision this information needs to be correlated to anatomical information.

The probably strongest driver for combined imaging currently is its application in the planning and monitoring of oncological treatment, in particular radiation treatment[17-19]. Especially the combination of (FDG-PET) and CT has become a valuable tool to improve the accuracy and effectiveness of radiation treatment by applying the metabolic information from the FDG-PET to refine the treatment plan in IMRT (Intensity Modulated Radiation Treatment)[20-23]. An example of such an application is shown in Figure 8-3.

The above examples demonstrate the medical necessity and benefits of combined imaging. In the case of brain studies this combination might be achieved by software based overlay of the different images from different instruments, due to the skull providing a solid anatomical frame. In other areas of the body this approach is rather challenging (as described in section 2 of this chapter), due to patient positioning differences, organ position differences, bowel filling etc.[9].

Besides the diagnostic benefits there are other strong drivers and motivators for the development of combined imaging instruments, like temporally different patient anatomy (organ positions, bowel filling) and physiology (blood sugar levels, metabolic and heart rates etc.). Aside from those are the patient (one investigation vs. two, one image reading vs. two, one report vs. two or more etc.) and hospital logistics (availability of imaging data, incompatibility of data formats, time consuming manual alignment of different studies, necessary coordination of staff from different departments).

With the appearance of the first combined imaging devices it became clear that in particular those 'non-diagnostic' factors represent a very strong driving force for the installation of a combined system. These logistical benefits have contributed significantly to the extremely rapid acceptance of those devices in the medical community. For PMS alone, the fraction of combined vs. single devices in PET changed from <10% to >95% of all instruments sold within 3 years[24]. Those instruments are also starting to change structures in hospitals and to force collaborations of previously rather separated departments and people[25]. However, with the increasing use and acceptance of those devices it also became clear that some of the above issues persist, due to the non-simultaneity of the studies, providing justification for the ongoing development of sophisticated image co-registration methods as described in the next section[26].

2. IMAGE CO-REGISTRATION TECHNOLOGIES AS A PRE-REQUISITE TO MULTI-MODALITY IMAGING

2.1 The role of image registration in medical imaging

In general, the medical images to be combined in diagnosis or therapy may have been acquired

- with the same or different imaging modalities, e.g. CT, PET, Magnetic Resonance Imaging (MRI), Ultra-Sound (US) etc.,
- simultaneously or at different times,
- from the same or different patients.

Unless acquired simultaneously, however, anatomical structures are likely to have changed their positions between the acquisitions due to patient or organ motion, tumor growth or shrinkage, breathing, heart motion, bladder and rectum filling, etc. Combining these images thus requires their geometric warping so that corresponding image structures correctly align - this is the purpose of *image registration*.

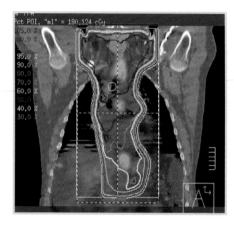

Figure 8-3. Patient with a squamous cell carcinoma of the esophagus. Example of an IMRT treatment plan, based on the information obtained by a combination of PET (thermal scale) and CT (grey scale). The colored lines are dose isocontours determined by the information about malignant foci and the degree of their malignancy from PET. Anatomical corrections and finetuning (e.g. the spare-out of important organs or vessels) is done based on the information from CT. (image courtesy of Mary Bird Perkins Cancer Center and The Lady of the Lake PET Imaging Center, Baton Rouge, LA).

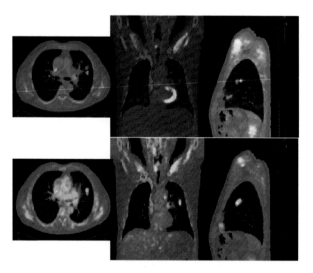

Figure 8-4. Color-coded PET image overlaid to a CT image after rigid (top row) and elastic (bottom row) registration. The images have been acquired independently of each other. Please note the different body and lung outlines in the top images due to the different breathing status of the patient. Elastic registration compensates for the breathing motion and aligns not only the lung volumes, but also a hot spot in the PET image with a lesion in the CT image indicative of a malignant, i.e. cancerous, tumor (images courtesy of K. Hahn, Ludwig Maximilians University, Munich).

Aligning images for combined visual inspection (fusion, Figure 8-4) is, however, only one of many applications of registration in medical imaging. More often and less visibly, registration techniques are deployed for motion compensation during acquisition and reconstruction of medical images as well as segmentation and classification of medical images.

The first step to registration is to compensate for translations and rotations between the input images. This *rigid registration* - rigid because it treats the human as a rigid body - compensates e.g. for different patient positioning. Often this needs to be extended to *affine registration* by including also scaling and skewing along the body axes to align e.g. different sampling and acquisition geometries. Both registrations have become standard techniques provided as an automatic or at least semi-automatic operation by workstations of all major vendors in the medical arena. However, the human body is not rigid and significant deviations remain after affine registration.

To compensate for those, *elastic registration* needs to be applied. Contrary to its rigid/affine counterparts, elastic registration has not yet become a standard technique that is used on a routine basis, the reason being that elastic registration is much more difficult to achieve and, as of yet, no generally accepted solution has made it into clinical practice.

2.2 Why is elastic registration so difficult?

Rigid and affine transformations are easy to be unequivocally formulated in simple mathematical terms and need only very few parameters to be adjusted for registration, namely in 3 (2) dimensions: 3 (2) translations, 3 (1) rotations, 3 (2) scaling factors, and 3 (1) skewing factors.

The situation looks dramatically different as soon as it comes to elastic registration as this involves non-linear transformations for which many possible mathematical formulations exist, e.g. polynomials, rational functions, or one of the many varieties of spline functions some of them explicitly modeling the elastic properties of the tissue imaged. The choice of the correct formulation is crucial for the success of elastic registration and depends on the anatomical region and the clinical target application. For example, the quite regular global motion pattern in the thoracic region due to breathing is very different from the much more irregular motion pattern in the abdominal region due to peristaltic motion. And this in turn looks very different from the local motion pattern in the cardiac region that deviates significantly from the local deformation due to tumor growth or tumor resection. In other words, one choice is unlikely to fit all - it strongly depends on where you are looking for what and for what purpose. Once the choice of the proper class of mathematical transformations has been made, it remains to find the member that optimally aligns the images. This normally demands for the optimization of hundreds or thousands of control parameters, an operation that is not only extremely computationally intensive, but also may not have a unique solution. This requires additional application-specific constraints to be imposed to finish optimization within reasonable time and to make it converge into clinically relevant solution.

In view of these challenges, it is not astonishing that there is currently no generally accepted solution for elastic registration that serves all clinical purposes.

2.3   Configuration of registration algorithms

Two fundamentally different approaches to registration can be taken - feature-based or volume-based registration.

Feature-based registration uses features such as point-like anatomical landmarks, organ surfaces etc. that are extracted interactively or (semi-) automatically from the input images. The geometric transformation that optimally aligns the landmark locations between the input images is determined and subsequently the underlying image is subjected to this transformation. The basic problem with this approach is that it involves a segmentation step for extracting the landmarks from the original image data and a pattern-matching step for identifying corresponding landmarks. Both tasks are difficult and in full generality still unsolved problems unless done under interactive control. Any error occurring during the initial segmentation step is very hard to correct afterwards. However, the great advantage of this approach is, that once the features have been identified, the rest of the registration task is solved fairly quickly as only a small subset of the original data, namely the discrete set of features, has to be manipulated.

Volume-based registration circumvents feature extraction and matching and strives for the direct alignment of the intensity values of the images. This avoids the error-prone segmentation and pattern matching steps at the expense of longer computation times due to the large amount of data involved. However, the resulting methods are often more robust and less application-specific than feature-based registration.

For each of those, several reliable methods exist that serve as a common methodological basis for the configuration of dedicated registration algorithms that address specific requirements of the target application.

2.4 Validation and future directions

Registration algorithms that have been configured for a specific target application also have to be validated in view of the application requirements. Any deficiencies detected lead to re-configuration resulting in a configuration-validation cycle incrementally refining the algorithm until it (hopefully) meets all application requirements.

Validating registration algorithms requires some *ground truth* or *gold standard* from which the quality of a registration result can be inferred. For rigid/affine registration, due to the linear behavior of the affine transformation and the few parameters involved[27,28], such ground truth can be produced using external fiducials serving as landmarks visible in all images to be registered. This approach fails, however, for elastic registration due to the prohibitive number of fiducials required to check the large number of control parameters involved and, more importantly, due to the non-linear behavior over the inter-fiducial space. Phantom images or artificially, but realistically deformed images provide a ground truth for a *technical validation* to estimate robustness, consistency, and accuracy of a registration algorithm and to improve its configuration. However, the resulting algorithm will be more mature in a technical sense only, but will form a better candidate for a subsequent *clinical validation* where its performance will be evaluated on clinical data by clinicians.

Elastic registration will develop in two major directions. First, the distinction between feature- and volume-based registration is going to dissolve into methods integrating segmentation and registration technology. These methods will help with the registration of highly disparate modalities that provide insufficient image structures for either purely feature- or volume-based registration. Second, application-specific a priori information will be explicitly added to each of the major procedural steps to speed-up and disambiguate the search for the optimal image alignment. Anatomical and motion models can give the expected anatomy, its deformation and elastic properties to guide the search for the global optimum, physical/ physiological models can describe the contrast generating mechanisms supporting the segmentation/enhancement of matching features etc.

However, a fundamental limit of software-based registration is reached whenever images do not show any well-defined structures that can be unambiguously matched. This limit will be reached for example when matching Molecular Imaging using highly specific agents. The more specific a tracer the less general tissue uptake it shows that correlates with anatomical morphology. This problem of lost anatomical context can only be handled by dedicated acquisition protocols supporting registration or by combined hardware devices as described in the next section.

3.   TECHNOLOGY OF COMBINED IMAGING DEVICES

3.1   Combined imaging development

Innovation in healthcare technology can be driven in two fundamental ways: medical/diagnostic needs requiring a new technical solution, or new ideas of scientists/engineers are opening up new fields of application and enabling new levels of diagnostic and therapeutic accuracy. In the case of combined morphologic/functional imaging both approaches have been subsequently combined. Considering the benefits of combined imaging one might be surprised that those combination devices like PET/CT and SPECT/CT did not enter mainstream clinical practice earlier than 2000/2001.

There are several reasons that can be speculated about. In the context here focus shall be on the technical aspects. In short, the challenge was to combine a fast, high-resolution modality (CT) with a slow, low-resolution modality (SPECT, PET). To underline the difference, figures of data acquisition times for a 90 cm whole body study may serve as an indicator: In the mid 90's, a PET-study took 60-90 minutes, a CT 1-2 minutes. Today a PET-study takes 12-15 minutes, a CT less than 1 minute. These figures indicate that the technologies have been converging in terms of imaging times, making them better suited for a 'marriage' in one device. And this process is going on, driven by further innovations particularly in PET[25].

Historically, the most widely applied PET tracer F-18-FDG, accumulating in many organs, muscles and structures of the body often providing seemingly sufficient anatomical background for the reader, has been reducing the pressure for the use of a combined device in the past. Also, primarily nuclear medicine physicians only, familiar with reading isotope emission based images, have interpreted PET studies.

With SPECT tracers generally providing even less anatomical background and the even lower spatial resolution of SPECT (compared to PET) it is not surprising that the first combined imaging instrument coming to market was a SPECT/CT[29]. Even that this first generation of combined instruments struggled for clinical acceptance due to implementation issues (e.g. low resolution, non-diagnostic CT) the clinical benefits already started to show[30].

With the increasing clinical use of PET in the late 90's and it's clinical and administrative acceptance in the healthcare system, especially of the US, patient numbers on clinical PET scanners rose significantly. Now two major issues started to surface, preventing further increases of patient throughput, but also impacting diagnostic accuracy and acceptance: i) attenuation correction for PET images, performed with external sources, added up to 50% to the investigation times per study and increased image noise. Therefore many clinical studies were read on images uncorrected for attenuation; and ii) referring physicians increasingly started to base their clinical decisions on the information provided by PET where they faced difficulties in correlating the functional information due the lack of anatomy provided.

The need for additional anatomical information was recognized in oncology[8], but computer algorithms (as described in section 2) did only work well in the brain[31]. Attempts have been made to extend the application of those algorithms to other parts of the body[9], also by the use of external markers and operator intervention during manual alignment. However, the obvious solution to this problem appeared to be the acquisition of both functional (PET) and anatomical (CT) data sequentially with a single scanner without the necessity of moving the patient between those studies.

The first development of a combined PET/CT device was started by Townsend & Beyer in the late 90's and first realized at Pittsburgh University. This device employed a partial ring rotating PET system and a single-slice, spiral CT, again a rather low-end approach[32]. However, first clinical experiences were so convincing[33] that a next generation system was designed immediately[34]. At this point the medical industry picked up the development and all three big players (GE Healthcare, Siemens Medical Solutions, Philips Medical Systems) started to offer combined PET/CT systems. Today, as mentioned before, those systems have almost completely taken over the market from single PET systems and at the same time significantly expanded it[35]. This is a proof of a very rapid clinical acceptance of a new technology and underlines how strong the medical and logistical demand for such devices has been and still is.

The rapid success and acceptance of PET/CT also significantly revitalized the interest in SPECT/CT, with several systems now being on the market. The technology of those systems will be described in more detail in the following sections.

3.2   PET/CT

3.2.1   Introduction to PET technology

Since CT technology is described in detail in chapter 4 of this book this section will focus on describing the elements and key features of a modern PET system.

The scintillating crystal is the first element of the detection chain in a PET system. The light it produces is read out by an arrangement of light sensitive devices. Though photodiodes will likely be used in future designs, all industrial PET tomographs today use photo multiplier tubes, in different shapes and sizes. As a good system energy resolution is key to high quality data acquisition in 3D PET, new detector designs with a highly uniform spatial response were introduced recently to best maintain intrinsic crystal energy resolution through the light collection stage, while supporting high count rates[36]. Philips introduced the Pixelar™ panel technology in its Allegro™ PET system in 2001: small individual GSO crystal elements are coupled to an optically continuous light guide (Figure 8-5). This light guide controls the spread of light, and exhibits identical properties regardless of the position along the circumference or the axis of the cylindrical detector. Round photo multipliers are densely packed in a hexagonal array at the back of the light guide. When trigger channels detect two photon absorptions in coincidence, clusters of seven photo multipliers are dynamically allocated to read out position and energy of each of the two photons. No edges, corners or boundaries between blocks disturb light collection homogeneity.

Signal processing, correction steps and image reconstruction are equally important links in the quest for the best possible image. Faster and smaller electronic components increase the processing bandwidth and support high count rate acquisitions. High statistics transmission images are obtained for measured attenuation correction of the emission data: Karp & Muehllehner introduced a fast single-photon Caesium (^{137}Cs) based transmission method as early as 1995, allowing attenuation correction to become reality in clinical routine[37]. Nowadays, PET/CT scanners use the CT image as a very fast acquired and virtually noiseless transmission image for PET attenuation correction[38].

PET image reconstruction benefited from a number of improvements in recent years. Extended, spherically symmetric basis functions were introduced to replace voxels in the image description[39] and the first industrial implementation in 1999 of a fully three-dimensional, maximum-likelihood based, iterative image reconstruction algorithm eliminated a number of approximations and improved image quality significantly[40]. Recently, reconstruction algorithms have been further enhanced to reflect the acquisition geometry more closely and take into account the irregular sampling of the object by the lines between detector pairs (LOR reconstruction)[41].

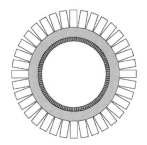 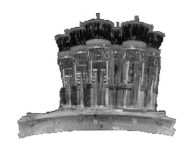

Figure 8-5. Left: cross-sectional schematic view of the Pixelar panel detector, with individual GSO crystals coupled to an optically continuous lightguide (grey) and read out by a densely packed array of photomultipliers; Right: Twenty-eight of these modules are assembled to form the cylindrical detector; optical coupling ensures continuity across mechanical boundaries (pictures: Philips Medical Systems).

3.2.2 Hybrid PET/CT development

Ideally, hybrid PET and CT imaging would make use of a single detector, capable of counting 511 keV photons one by one, and integrating high photon fluxes at X-ray energies. However, as the previous paragraphs have shown, current commercially available PET and CT detectors rely on different technologies: all PET/CT designs today combine two different scanners under a common cover with a common patient pallet, allowing sequential CT and PET imaging without removing or repositioning the patient on the couch.

An outstanding feature of the Philips' PET/CT development is the particular emphasis on patient centred design. An about 30 cm wide gap separates the CT portion from the PET portion of the machine (Figure 8-6): patients experience a feeling of openness and light and feel more at ease than in a long closed tunnel. Communication and visual contact with staff or parents is reassuring, especially for claustrophobic and paediatric patients. Patient comfort has a direct impact on image quality: patient motion due to nervousness is reduced, and so is increased muscle uptake of FDG due to tension. Also, experience has shown that claustrophobic patients tolerate the study well, and prefer undergoing an examination on an open gantry scanner.

The open gantry design of the Gemini™ even goes a step further: the PET portion can be moved back to increase the gap to about one meter, which allows even better access to the patient. This option is regularly used to study patients under anaesthesia, who require direct monitoring by an anaesthetist (figure 8-7). Other applications include interventional work on the CT, direct positioning for brain and cardiac PET, or brain PET examinations that require equipment to be placed within the patient's sight.

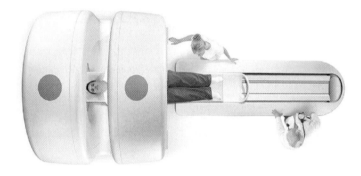

Figure 8-6. The open gantry of Gemini™ PET/CT was designed to maximize patient comfort.

The use of the CT image goes beyond its interpretation as a traditional radiology study. The matching of lesions and the confident localisation of functional abnormalities – shown by PET – backed by the accurate anatomical representation – provided by CT – is the tremendous advantage of a hybrid device. PET attenuation correction is a further direct benefit: a map of attenuation coefficients at 511 keV is required to correct for the attenuation (absorption, scatter) of annihilation photons in the body. Radioisotope based transmission images are used in standalone PET and require acquisition times of several minutes to cover a standard whole-body study. After rescaling CT numbers to linear attenuation coefficients at 511 keV, the CT image provides virtually noiseless PET attenuation maps in a fraction of that time.

Differences exist in the acquisition techniques of PET and CT on standalone machines, which need to be resolved by either adapting acquisition protocols, or developing new technologies.

While PET/CT instrumentation and data processing methods continue to improve, patient throughput rates of 25 per day become common, and the amount of image data produced for each patient increases, the usability and performance of image review tools become a critical factor in the workflow of a PET/CT facility. The reading physicians need to easily navigate through large image volumes, switch between different views, fused or not, extract quantitative information, distribute and store images and reports in electronic form on hospital wide information systems. Most manufacturers chose to integrate PET/CT review and reporting on their radiology reading platforms, as Philips did on its Extended Brilliance Workspace™. This modern, scalable system meets the requirements of the busiest radiology departments and provides an appropriate base to implement future advanced PET/CT applications.

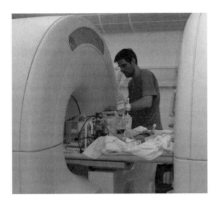

Figure 8-7. A patient under anesthesia is being scanned on Gemini™ PET/CT: the gantry is separated to allow access to the anesthetist and his equipment (Picture courtesy of I. Kastrup, Herlev Hospital, Copenhagen).

3.2.3   Future technologies: Time-of-flight-PET (TOF)

One of the main goals in the design of PET scanners is to maximize the noise equivalent count rate (NEC), which translates into reduced scan times and increased signal-to-noise in the reconstructed image. In today's 3D-PET scanner designs, the NEC is mainly determined by detector parameters like scintillator geometry and stopping power (improve sensitivity), energy resolution (suppresses scattered events) and coincidence timing resolution (reduces random events).

A very promising and effective method of significantly increasing the effective NEC is the incorporation of time-of-flight (TOF) information in the image reconstruction. As shown in Figure 8-8, a PET event consists of a line of response (LOR) between two coincident gamma quanta. Since a single event only indicates a positron annihilation somewhere along this line, the full LOR is back projected into the image matrix (see Figure 8-8a). Given a sufficient coincidence timing resolution dt of the PET detectors, it is however possible to narrow down the position along the LOR by measuring the time difference between the detection of the two gamma quants (see figure 8-8b). The corresponding position uncertainty is given by $dx = dt \cdot c/2$. For a cylindrical phantom of diameter D, the gain in effective NEC can be approximated by D/dx[42].

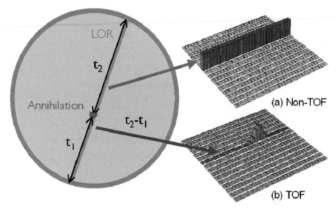

Figure 8-8. Illustration of a line of response (LOR) in a PET scanner (a) without incorporation of time-of-flight information, and (b) with incorporation of time-of-flight information.

For typical patient diameters in full-body PET scanners (> 20 cm), a coincidence timing resolution of <1 ns has to be achieved to realize a significant improvement in scan time and image quality. This imposes additional requirements on both the scintillator properties (light output, rise time, decay time) and the light detection chain (PMT, analog electronics, digitization) of the system[43]. While early implementations of TOF[44] met the timing requirements, the employed scintillators like BaF_2 and CsF did not provide the energy and spatial resolution needed in 3D PET scanners. However, recent advances in the development of inorganic scintillators like LYSO and $LaBr_3$ have opened up the possibility to combine high stopping power with sub-ns time stamps and good energy resolution. Using typical PET scintillator geometries, a coincidence timing resolution of less than 600 ps at $\approx$12% energy resolution can be achieved with LYSO. For $LaBr_3$ crystals, which feature slightly less stopping power, values of less than 300 ps at 4.5% energy resolution, have been measured[44].

The impact of TOF information on the PET image quality is the topic of ongoing research activities[45]. To illustrate the potential reduction in scan time, Figure 8-9 shows a simulation study of a 27 cm cylinder phantom in a 3D PET scanner. Depending on the coincidence timing resolution, a scan time reduction of up to a factor of six can be realized without changing the contrast recovery and the image noise. Likewise, the visual image quality improves significantly with better timing resolution when using a constant number of events (see Figure 8-10; ref[46] contains a quantitative analysis). As expected, the image noise decreases with $\sqrt{dx}/D$ when incorporating TOF information in the image reconstruction.

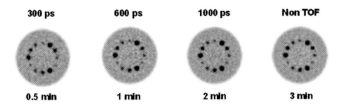

Figure 8-9. Benefit of time-of-flight information for reducing scan time at constant image quality. The images are based on simulation studies with a 27 cm cylinder phantom and an uptake ratio of 4:1 in the hot spheres[46].

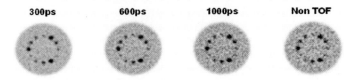

Figure 8-10. Benefit of time-of-flight information for improving image quality at constant scan time (0.5 min). The images are based on simulation studies with a 27 cm cylinder phantom and an uptake ratio of 4:1 in the hot spheres[46].

Based on the current advances in the development of PET scintillators, TOF-PET therefore represents a promising method of further reducing the scan time and improving the image quality in future PET scanners.

3.3   SPECT/CT

As outlined before, a SPECT/CT system combines the detailed anatomical information from CT with the metabolic and molecular imaging capabilities of SPECT. The anatomical background provided by CT allows the physician to access a large number of very specific SPECT tracers that can image physiological processes.

SPECT/CT imaging provides the benefit of improved efficiency for both the patient and the interpreting physician. During the same episode of care, the patient can have both the SPECT and CT data acquired without having to move from the patient bed. Images of both modalities are provided instantly. Registered functional and anatomical images allow more accurate diagnosis and staging by providing more precise localization. Additionally, the presence of anatomical CT information can help the referring physician contextualize the functional SPECT data and gain additional confidence, important for the effectiveness of subsequent therapies.

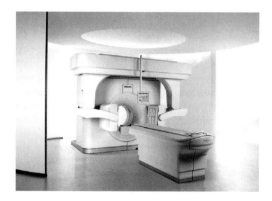

Figure 8-11. Example of a high-end SPECT/CT system (Philips Precedence™). The CT gantry (in the back) holds two flexible arms with SPECT detectors that are closely moving around the patient during the SPECT study. For the subsequent CT study the patient is advanced on the pallet through the CT gantry opening without changing position. (Picture: Philips Medical Systems).

For example, a bone SPECT study is a very sensitive examination but does not allow accurate localization of pathology in the bone. The fused images in Figure 8-12 show that the lesion is not located in the ostigonum as previously suspected.

In Cardiology, SPECT imaging is considered the gold standard for myocardial perfusion imaging[47]. The addition of the CT component can enhance clinical information by improving SPECT image quality or by providing complimentary data. Attenuation artifacts, a significant source of false positive studies in cardiological SPECT, are due to the presence of dense tissue between the heart and the detector as the camera moves from right anterior oblique to left posterior oblique. SPECT/CT performs x-ray based attenuation correction to remove these types of artifacts that are prevalent in women with large breasts or patients with high diaphragms. Additionally, the CT can provide complimentary data to the perfusion information, in the form of calcium scoring. Calcium scoring, combined with patient history, and myocardial perfusion imaging can be a powerful risk stratification tool[48].

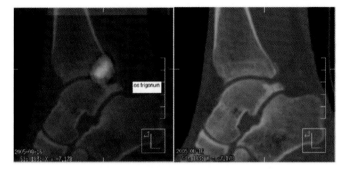

Figure 8-12. Images of a patient with a bone lesion, which was suspected to be in the ostigonum by evaluating SPECT data alone. The combination image with CT (left) shows the correct position in the bone. The lesion is not visualized by CT alone (right).

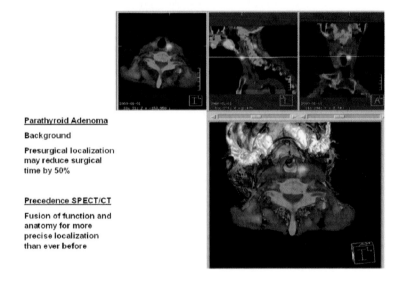

Parathyroid Adenoma

Background

Presurgical localization may reduce surgical time by 50%

Precedence SPECT/CT

Fusion of function and anatomy for more precise localization than ever before

Figure 8-13. The fused SPECT and CT image above shows the location of the parathyroid to the left lateral side of the esophagus. The surgeon can use this information in planning the surgical route that may reduce time in the operating room and trauma to the patient (Images courtesy of S. Scharf, Lenox Hill Hospital, New York).

The combination of SPECT perfusion data with coronary artery CT-angiography (coronary CTA) may provide the cardiologist with data to guide treatment; the SPECT data being used to evaluate the severity of perfusion abnormalities and the coronary CTA data to determine which vessels contain lesions and their severity. These data may provide improved patient management by determining which patients are treated medically or will have a stent or bypass surgery. Furthermore, this data may be useful in planning the therapeutic catheterization procedure.

In oncology, SPECT/CT is an ideal tool to help plan patient treatment. In pre-surgical planning, the SPECT can be used to visualize the tumor and the CT for accurate localization. As shown in Figure 8-13, the parathyroid can be accurately localized and the CT exam be used for surgical planning. In the future, the image quality of the SPECT images may be improved through more accurate reconstruction by incorporating the CT data into the SPECT reconstruction process. One goal is to make the SPECT images quantitative. In order to do this, the reconstruction process must include corrections for scatter, attenuation, collimator resolution effects and partial volume effects. The CT can provide high quality attenuation and scatter maps as well as structure sizes for partial volume corrections. Quantitative SPECT may be useful as a prognostic indicator, in assessing a patient's response to therapy, or following the progression of disease. As SPECT/CT systems become more prevalent, they may promote the validation and acceptance of new molecular imaging radiopharmaceuticals. Since molecular imaging agents are more specific with high lesion uptake and less non-target uptake, they are likely to receive significant benefit from the co-registered anatomical CT images. An example currently in FDA phase II trials is ^{99m}Tc-ethylene-dicystine-glucose[49] that may enable SPECT tumor imaging similar to FDG-PET.

REFERENCES

1. G.N. Hounsfield, Computerized transverse axial scanning (tomography). Part I: Description of system, Part II: Clinical applications, *British Journal of Radiology* **46**, 1016-1022 (1973).
2. A.M. Cormack, Reconstruction of densities from their projections, with applications in radiological physics, *Physics in Medicine and Biology* **18**, 195-207 (1973).
3. P.C. Lauterbur, NMR zeugmatographic imaging in medicine, *J Med Syst* **6**(6), 591-597 (1982).
4. S. Webb, *From the Watching of Shadows,* (Adam Hilger, Bristol and New York 1990).
5. M. Reivic, D. Kuhl, A. Wolf, J. Greenberg, M. Phelp, T. Ido, V. Casella, J. Fowler, E. Hoffmann, A. Alavi, P. Som, and L. Sokoloff, The [18F-FDG] fluorodeoxyglucose method for the measurement of local cerebral glucose utilization in man, *Circular Research* **44**, 127-137 (1979).
6. G.L. Brownel, J.A. Correi, and R.G. Zamenho, Positron Instrumentation, in *Recent Advances in Nuclear Medicine*, J.H. Lawrence, T.F. Budinger (eds.), Grune & Stratton, New York, 1-49 (1978).
7. L.G. Straus, P.S. Cont, The application of PET in clinical oncology, *J Nucl Med* **32**, 623–648 (1991).

8. W.B. Eubank, D.A. Mankof, U.P. Schmied, et al., Imaging of oncologic patients: benefit of combined CT and FDG PET in the diagnosis of malignancy, *AJR* **171**, 1101–1110 (1998).

9. R.L. Wahl, L.E. Quint, R.D. Cieslak, et al., Anatometabolic tumor imaging: fusion of FDG PET with CT or MRI, *J Nucl Med* **34**, 1190 (1993).

10. M.N. Wernic, J.N. Aarsvold, *Emission Tomography: The fundamentals of PET and SPECT*, Academic Press, ISBN-0127444823 (2004).

11. W.R. Webb, W. Brant, N. Major, *Fundamentals of Body CT*, Elsevier/Saunders, ISBN-1416000305 (2005).

12. E.M. Haacke, R. Brown, M.R. Thompson, R. Venkatesan, *Magnetic Resonance Imaging: Physical Principles and Sequence Design*, Wiley-Liss, ISBN-0471351288 (1999).

13. A.F. Shields, J.R. Grierson, B.M. Dohmen et al., Imaging proliferation in vivo with [F-18-FLT] and positron emission tomography, *Nature Medicine* **4**, 1334-1336 (1998).

14. R. Weissleder, Molecular Imaging: Exploring the next frontier, *Radiology* **212**, 609-614 (1999).

15. F. Jaffer, R. Weissleder, Molecular Imaging in the Clinical Arena, *JAMA* **293**(7), 855-862 (2005).

16. F.G. Blankenberg, et. al., Imaging of Apoptosis (Programmed Cell Death) with 99m-TC Annexin V, *J Nuc Med* **40**, 184-191 (1999).

17. I.F. Ciernik, E. Dizendorf, B.G. Baumert, et al., Radiation Treatment Planning with an Integrated Positron Emission and Computer Tomography (PET/CT): a feasibility study, *Int J Radiat Oncol Biol Phys* **57**, 853-863 (2003).

18. J.D. Bradley, C.A. Perez, F. Dehdashti, B.A. Siegel, Implementing biologic target volumes in radiation treatment planning for non-small cell lung cancer, *J Nucl Med* **45** (suppl1), 96S-101S (2004).

19. A.L. Grosu, M. Piert, W.A. Weber, et al., Positron Emission Tomography for Radiation Treatment Planning, *Strahlenther Onkol* **181**(8), 482-499 (2005).

20. A.C. Paulino, M. Koshy, R. Howell, D. Schuster, L.W. Davis, Comparison of CT- and FDG-PET-defined gross tumor volume in intensity-modulated radiation therapy for head-and-neck cancer, *Int J Radiat Oncol Biol Phys* **61**(5), 1385-92 (2005).

21. C.L. Holloway, D. Robinson, B. Murray, et al., Results of a phase I study to dose escalate using intensity modulated radiotherapy guided by combined PET/CT imaging with induction chemotherapy for patients with non-small cell lung cancer, *Radiother Oncol* **73**(3), 285-287 (2004).

22. J. Esthappan, S. Mutic, R.S. Malyapa, et al., Treatment planning guidelines regarding the use of CT/PET-guided IMRT for cervical carcinoma with positive paraaortic lymph nodes, *Int J Radiat Oncol Biol Phys* **58**(4), 1289-97 (2004).

23. J.T. Yap, J.P. Karney, N.C. Hall, D.W. Townsend, Image guided cancer therapy using PET/CT, *Cancer J* **10**(4), 221-233 (2004).

24. Philips Medical Systems, BL Nuclear medicine, Internal Market Data 2001-2004

25. D.W. Townsend, J.P. Karney, J.T. Yap, N.C. Hall, PET/CT today and tomorrow, *J Nucl Med* **45**, 45-145 (2004).

26. P.J. Slomka, Software approach to merging molecular with anatomic information, *J Nucl Med* **45** (suppl.), 36S-45S (2004).

27. J.V. Hajnal, D.L.G. Hill, D.J. Hawkes (eds.), *Medical Image Registration*, (CRC Press, Boca Raton 2001).

28. J. Modersitzky, *Numerical Methods for Image Registration*, (Oxford University Press, 2004).

29. B.H. Hasegawa, H.R. Tang, A.J. Da Silva, K.Iwata, M.C.Wu, K.H. Wong, Implementation and applications of a combined CT/SPECT system, *Conference Record of the 1999 IEEE Nuclear Science Symposium and Medical Imaging Conference, Seattle, WA* (1999).

30. O. Israel, Z. Keidar, G. Iosilevsky et al., The fusion of anatomic and physiologic imaging in the management of patients with cancer, *Semin Nucl Med* **31**(3), 191-205 (2001).

31. R.P. Woods, S.R. Cherry, J.C. Maziotta, Paoid automated algorithm for aligning and reslicing PET images, *J Comput Assist Tomogr* **16**, 620-633 (1992).

32. T. Beyer, D.W. Townsend, T. Brun, P.E. Kinahan, et al., A Combined PET/CT Scanner for Clinical Oncology, *J Nucl Med* **41**, 1369-1379 (2000).

33. M. Charon, T. Beyer, N.M. Bohnen, et al., Image analysis in patients with cancer studied with a combined PET and CT scanner, *Clin Nucl Med* **25**, 905-910 (2000).

34. D.W. Townsend, T. Beyer, A combined PET/CT scanner: The path to true image fusion, *Brit J Radiol* **75** (supplement), 24-30 (2002).

35. T. Beyer, Kombinierte Positronen-Emissions-Tomographie/Computertomographie (PET/CT) für die klinische Onkologie: Technische Grundlagen und Akquisitions-protokolle, *Der Nuklearmediziner* **27**, 236-245 (2004).

36. S. Surti, J.S. Karp, R.Freifelder, F. Liu, Optimizing the performance of a PET detector using discrete GSO crystals on a continuous lightguide, *IEEE Trans Nucl Sci* **47**(3), 1030-1036 (2000).

37. J.S. Karp, G. Muellehner, H. Qu, X.H. Yan, Singles transmission in volume imaging PET with a ^{137}Cs source, *Phys Med Biol* **40**, 929-944 (1995).

38. P.E. Kinahan, D.W. Townsend, T. Beyer, D. Sashin, Attenuation correction for a combined 3D PET/CT scanner, *Med Phys* **25**, 2046-2053 (1998).

39. R.M. Lewitt RMAlternatives to voxels for image representation in iterative reconstruction algorithms, *Phys Med Biol* **37**, 705-716 (1992).

40. M.E. Daube-Witherspoon, S. Matej, J.S. Karp, R.M. Lewitt, Application of the row action maximum likelihood algorithm with spherical basis functions to clinical PET imaging, *IEEE Trans Nucl Sci* **48**(1), 24-30 (2001).

41. D. Kadrmas, LOR-OSEM: statistical PET reconstruction from raw line-of-response histograms, *Phys Med Biol* **49**, 4731-4744 (2004).

42. S. Surti, et al., Investigation of lanthanum scintillators for 3-D PET, *IEEE Trans Nucl Sci* **50**(3), 348-354 (2003).

43. A. Thon, et al., Exact modeling of analog pulses for PET detector modules, *IEEE NSS-MIC Conference Recor* (2003).

44. T.F. Budinger, Time-of-flight positron emission tomography: Status relative to conventional PET, *J Nucl Med* **24**, 73-78 (1983).

45. A. Kuhn, et al., Design of a lanthanum bromide detector for TOF PET, *IEEE Trans Nucl Sci* **51**(5), 2550-2557 (2004).

46. S. Surti, et al., Image quality improvement in TOF-capable fully 3D PET scanners, presented at the *annual meeting of the Society of Nuclear Medicine, Toronto, Canada* (2005).

47. R. Hachamovitch, D.S. Berman, The use of nuclear cardiology in clinical decision making, *Semin Nucl Med* **35**(1), 62-72 (2005).

48. P. Raggi, D.S. Berman, Computed tomography coronary calcium screening and myocardial perfusion imaging, *J Nucl Cardiol* **12**(1), 96-103 (2005).

49. D.J. Yang, C.G. Kim, N.R. Schechter, A. Azhdarinia, et.al., Imaging with 99mTc ECDG targeted at the multifunctional glucose transport system: feasibility study with rodents, *Radiology* **226**(2), 465-473 (2003).

PART III: INTEGRATION OF DIAGNOSTIC IMAGING AND THERAPY

Chapter 9

NEW TECHNOLOGY FOR IMAGE-GUIDED THERAPY
Trends and Innovations

Jeffrey Yanof[1], Michael Kuhn[2]

[1]*Philips Medical Systems, Cleveland, OH, USA;* [2]*Philips Medical Systems, Hamburg, Germany*

Abstract: Image-Guided Therapy (IGT) uses imaging to plan, implement, and follow-up treatment. Typical goals are personalized treatment planning, accurate targeting, therapeutic effectiveness, decreased procedure time, minimal side effects, and responsive follow-up. Many IGT technologies involve pre-, intra-, and post- procedure stages. Intra-procedure processes include targeting, monitoring, and controlling[1]. Trends and innovations are reviewed for multi-modality-guided percutaneous ablation, catheter ablation for cardiac arrhythmias, MR-guided therapeutic ultrasound, and advanced radiation therapy. These technologies have a role in treatment centers of the future, and will ultimately be measured in terms of improved patient outcomes.

Keywords: Medical trends, medical imaging, diagnosis, image-guided therapy, minimally invasive surgery, HIFU, RFA, radiation therapy, molecular imaging

1.   OBJECTIVES OF IMAGE GUIDED THERAPY

The Tricorder, used by Dr. 'Bones' McCoy in the Star Trek Sci-Fi series[2,3], was a hand-held, fully integrated 'Sense-Cure' device. By hovering the device near the afflicted area, it could both *sense and cure* (space-age) ailments in a matter of seconds.

The idealized capabilities of the Tricorder, unfortunately, represent formidable clinical and technical challenges in present day, especially when implying potentially curative outcomes for major chronic diseases such as

139

G. Spekowius and T. Wendler (Eds.), Advances in Healthcare Technology, 139-146.
© 2006 *Springer. Printed in the Netherlands.*

cancer, heart disease, and diabetes; nevertheless, some aspects of the Tricorder are being realized in state-of-the-art technology and their advancements.

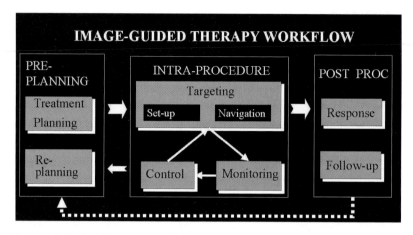

Figure 9-1. Typical 'See-Treat' workflow for many image-guided therapy procedures.

Instead of 'Sense-Cure' capabilities, many state-of-the-art technologies in image-guided therapy seek to facilitate the following objectives (some of which, in an imaginary sense, may be intrinsic to Dr. McCoy's Tricorder):

- Image, accurately detect, and localize the tissue targeted for treatment,
- Quickly develop a patient-specific treatment plan for the target tissue (e.g., in less then two minutes) while minimizing risk to nearby structures and minimizing side effects,
- Quickly and easily implement the plan by accurately targeting the lesion during the procedure with minimal risk, side effects, and ionizing radiation to healthy tissue,
- Directly monitor the treatment's effectiveness in 'real-time' and use this information to adjust targeting and the treatment plan,
- Accurately assess the post-procedure treatment response,
- If the treatment is incomplete or if the original treatment plan for fractionated treatment is no longer valid, then update the plan with re-imaging in some cases.

2.   CLINICAL PROCEDURE STAGES IN IGT

Prototypes, concepts, and investigations to meet these image-guided therapy objectives are discussed in the sections and chapters ahead. Each of them typically involves Pre-, Intra-, and Post-procedure stages (Figure 9-1), and the intra-procedure stage typically includes Targeting, Controlling, and Monitoring processes.

These stages and processes are not always clearly delineated; they can overlap and can be iterative. For example, information obtained while monitoring the treatment can be displayed on images from, and used to update, the pre-procedure plan. Another example is that simultaneous planning and targeting processes can be used when repositioning or refocusing devices based on imaging feedback.

3. TRENDS AND ADVANCES IN IGT

3.1 Less-and-less invasiveness

Rapid advances in medical imaging have enabled these IGT objectives and processe to be performed with less-and-less invasiveness. Laparoscopic procedures, via keyholes, are often replacing open surgical procedures; transcutaneous procedures, via extracorporeal delivery, are replacing percutaneous procedures. Less-invasive and non-invasive procedures inherently need tomographic, projection, or sector imaging to increase visualization of the interventional field and target treatment locations.

Extra-corporal, i.e., transcutaneous, non-invasive procedures such as Radiation Therapy, Therapeutic Ultrasound, and Lithotripsy require imaging for *planning* and, in some cases, for intra-procedurally *monitoring* the treatment. Virtual 'Radiation Therapy' (RT) Simulation is now commonly used with large bore, multi-detector row CT scanners. The 3-D coordinates of a solid tumor can be localized online, with digitally reconstructed radiographs (DRRs), immediately after acquiring a multi-phasic CT data set. These coordinates are sent to CT-integrated lasers, which enable the skin to be marked for subsequent positioning on a LINAC. Methods are under investigation to decrease inaccuracies of the RT due to respiratory motion and organ shift (Chapter 13). A retrospectively gated CT scan can be used to include respiratory motion in the therapy planning stage. Also, improved model-based segmentation algorithms are being investigated to further automate *planning* processes, and help to more accurately predict doses to targets and critical structures.

In MR-Guided Therapeutic Ultrasound, i.e., High-Intensity Focused Ultrasound (HIFU) (Chapter 12), the MR scanner provides both a 3-D anatomical map and 'thermometry' to *monitor* and *control* heat delivery. Treatment of uterine fibroids with MR-guided HIFU has recently been FDA approved. Diagnostic Ultrasound, registered with 3-D CT data, is also being investigated for *targeting* and *monitoring* HIFU therapy (Chapter 10).

3.2   Endoscopy often replaces open surgery

Many image-guided treatments cannot presently be administered extracorporally. Continuous and pulsed HIFU is being investigated for ablation and local drug-delivery within the liver; but, these techniques may not be applicable when high frequency acoustic energy cannot penetrate to the target tissue or when direct manipulation of tissue is needed.

Endoscopic surgery was first used in the late 1970s and a significant amount of training was required for obstetric and gynecology physicians. After being adopted for gall bladder resection in the 1980s, laparoscopic surgery was extended to the appendix, spleen, colon, stomach, kidney, and liver in the 1990s. Robotic assistance for remote endoscope manipulation was introduced at this time, but has been slowly adopted, potentially due to its high cost and marginal value for well-trained surgeons.

Endoscopic examinations of the colon, i.e., colonoscopy, – with on-line polyp resection – is today one of the most successful examples of an integrated, non-invasive approach to screening and diagnosis combined with minimally invasive therapy.

Multi-modality imaging is being investigated to enhance abdominal laparoscopic procedures. A miniature electromagnetic sensor (Chapter 10) is attached to the tip of an ultrasonic laparoscope and registered and tracked in a recently acquired 3-D tomographic data set. Combining real-time imaging, e.g., ultrasound, angiography, MR or CT Fluoroscopy, with the 3-D retrospective data sets is an emerging concept in multi-modality image-guidance (see below and Chapter 10).

Another recent innovation in the area of endoscopy is the integration of imaging and non-invasive therapy using a pill-sized endoscopic capsule, first introduced in 2001. Current models are 1 cm x 2 cm and can wirelessly capture 0.4 megapixel video at up to 30 frames/second. In the future, these capsules could have a remotely controlled camera direction, take tissue samples, and deliver medications – like a telemetric version of Asimov's '3 micra' submarine, Proteus, in the Fantastic Voyage[4].

3.3   New procedures for the cardiac cath lab

Using fluoroscopy during interventions, to track minimally invasive instrument-based intervention, has lead to the growing discipline of Interventional Radiology and the exponential growth of catheter-based procedures, which – together with the availability of ever more complex stents - have since steadily replaced open surgery in the heart, abdomen, and brain, to name the most important areas. The 'Catheter Lab' developed into a truly integrated approach to diagnostic imaging and therapy.

Complex procedures are performed today in the Electrophysiology (EP) laboratory (see Chapter 11) to interrupt arrhythmia-causing nerve conduction with highly accurate catheter-based ablation while *monitoring* ECG signals. The catheter tips carry tiny electromagnetic coils for accurate non-line-of-sight localization. Cone-beam CT data sets are being investigated to assist EP 3-D treatment *planning* and for intra-procedure registration with the real-time Angio imaging, and MR-guided EP procedures are also under investigation.

3.4 Multi-modality guidance and molecular imaging

As with combining real-time imaging with retrospective data sets, there is, more generally, an increasing trend of inter- and intra- modality registration in both diagnostic and therapeutic imaging. As an important example in diagnostic imaging, Positron Emission Tomography (PET) and Single-Photon Emission Computed Tomography (SPECT) are now integrated and share a patient table with CT imagers. Furthermore, CT and MRI anatomical imaging is also being complemented with functional MRI (brain activity, metabolism in MR-spectroscopic images, and diffusion imaging). These and other hybrid imagers enable the registration of 3-D morphological images with functional imaging of molecular processes and pharmakinetic/dynamic properties of new agents. Examples include imaging of metabolism, apoptosis/inflammation, angiogenesis, anti-angiogenisis, and immunological processes. In the new paradigm of Molecular Imaging (MI), these imaging modalities (and also optical and ultrasound imaging) are used in combination with molecular contrast agents[5] which are targeted to disease-specific proteins and receptors, thus providing enhanced image signals from the pathology.

Registration and fusion of multi-modality data sets to plan Radiation Therapy or Surgery is presently available. In oncology, further use of multi-modality imaging could enable: The accurate delineation of heterogenous tumors for image-guided percutaneous ablation (Section 3.5), perfusion visualization for targeted drug delivery with HIFU, or more accurate tumor targeting with image-guided radiotherapy (Chapter 13) or particle beam therapy. Many new approaches combine targeted drugs with contrast agents, such that a real-time 3-D imaging modality can be used to monitor the distribution and localization of a therapeutic agent as it delivers its payload. Multi-modality molecular image approaches are also being investigated for monitoring the response to radiation therapy (Chapter 14).

3.5   Interventional oncology and percutaneous ablation

The first CT guided biopsy was reported by Dr. John Haaga in 1976[6]. Radiologists' have since typically become relatively skilled at placing needles with CT or Ultrasound (US) guidance for percutaneous biopsies and fluid drainages. Some needle-based procedures involving double angles, deep targets, and targets near critical structures or the diaphragm, however, may pose more challenges. These may require more use of real-time imaging and breath-hold reproducibility techniques.

The transition from needles to Radiofrequency electrodes for percutaneous ablation of hepatic tumors was first suggested in 1990[7,8]. Since then, the technique has rapidly expanded to treatments of other areas such as kidney, lung, and bone tumors, and has developed into a new field of 'Interventional Oncology'.

The leading RFA application has been the treatment of solid liver tumors, especially indicated when these are un-resectable. Presently, tumors larger than 3 cm can be difficult to treat, without risking marginal recurrence, due to the potential difficulty of placing multiple electrodes to cover the tumor. Innovations being investigated to meet this challenge include: point-and-click treatment planning and simulation with virtual electrodes, targeting with CT-integrated robots, electromagnetically tracked electrodes, and CT-Ultrasound image registration (Chapter 10). Heat-activated drug delivery during RFA is another recent method being investigated to combat marginal recurrence.

An example of personalized medicine in the post-genomic era aims to use proteomic and genomic analysis of biopsy tissue samples to evaluate drug effect and investigate tumor genetics. This requires a biopsy sample of a heterogeneous tumor at precisely the same location pre- and post therapy. New devices such as a CT-integrated robot with inter- and intra-modality image-based planning, as discussed in Chapter 10, may facilitate more reproducible sequential biopsy sampling. Eventually, molecular imaging may alleviate the need for biopsy in the process of developing personalized medicines.

3.6   Real-time imaging and virtual tracking

In the mid 1990s, 'frameless stereotactic' approaches were developed for the operating room using optical (line-of-sight) navigation systems (Chapter 10). After registering the surgical tool, the operating field, and the image-space coordinates, the optical camera enabled the tracking of a surgical tool within a pre-operative CT or MR data sets.

A prerequisite for sufficient accuracy in these approaches was the proper correction of geometric distortions, which are inherent not only to MRI (dependent on acquisition protocol and anatomical area), but to some extent also in CT image data. Also, navigation in static CT or MR data sets, as a form of virtual reality, did not reflect intra-procedural, morphological changes in tissue. Accordingly, applying frameless stereotactic techniques to the areas such as the lung and abdomen can pose challenges due to respiratory motion and organ shift/deformation. This can be mitigated with the use of real-time imaging in combination virtual tracking of instruments in recently acquired image data sets (Chapter 10).

In view of the X-Ray dose to both patients and clinicians during fluoroscopy, attention is increasingly being paid to alternative fluoroscopic imaging modalities such as 3-D ultrasound and MRI. In this context, recent advances in the real-time localization of MR-microcoils have paved the way for integrating catheter or instrument localization with the MR data acquisition.

Also, new visualization methods and dose mitigation strategies are being investigated for volume CT-fluoroscopy (Chapter 10). CT-integrated robots are being investigated to remotely steer interventional devices during real-time Volume (3-D) CT-fluoroscopy imaging.

4.   SUMMARY

New technologies for image-guided transcutaneous, percutaneous, and endoscopic procedures will be reviewed in the following chapters. In the future, the ideal treatment paradigm would enable the multi-modality (including molecular) image-based treatment planning, guidance, monitoring, and controlling of treatment effectiveness in one seamlessly integrated platform. Imaging, tools, and devices can be easily accessed before and during the procedure to simplify workflow, within and between stages, to achieve the therapeutic objectives.

Trade-offs often exist between approaches, associated tools, and alternatives, and these depend on the application and venue. For example, real-time imaging can increase targeting accuracy and decrease the procedure time; but the use of ionizing radiation may require strategies to decrease x-ray dose to the physician and the patient. Registration and real-time tracking of interventional tools in a static 3-D data set may provide real-time navigational feedback in virtual reality space, but may not always be a sufficient substitute for continuous or intermittent fluoroscopic imaging of the interventional field and surgical devices.

With some image-guided applications, the clinical protocols and technical methods are under varying stages of clinical investigation. There may be multiple approaches to achieve the same therapeutic objectives and they can have complex trade-offs. Clinical protocols and use of technology may vary between, or even within institutions, and always depend on the presentation of each patient. For instance, there are presently at least seven types of chemical and thermal energies used to destroy tumors, e.g., RFA, laser ablation, alcohol installation, cryogenic, etc. These are often used in combination with other treatments and are the subject of many international studies[9].

For a new device, imaging method, or procedure to be accepted or embraced by the clinical community, it must be of significant benefit without adding cost, time, or the need for a non-trivial amount of training. For some procedures, this may first occur in less challenging regions such as those easier to target and monitor. Interdisciplinary teams, e.g., researchers, surgeons, oncologists, interventional radiologists, and cardiologists, must work synergistically to understand and re-visit requirements associated with the new devices.

The Star Trek Tricorder is not light-years away. Ultimately, here on earth, the value of IGT technology will be always measured in terms of a better outcome for the patient.

REFERENCES

1. S.N. Goldberg, et al., Image Guided Tumor Ablation: Standardization of Terminology and Reporting Criteria, *Radiology Online* **10**, 1148 (2005).
2. M. Okuda, D. Okuda, D. Mirek, *Encyclopaedia of Star Trek*, Star Trek, (Updated edition December 1997).
3. I. Bitter, The Star Trek Tricorder for Diagnosis and Treatment, Graphics and Vitual Informatics Lab Workshop, U. Maryland College Park (2003); http://www.cs.umd.edu/gvil/seminar/2003.shtml
4. I. Asimov, *Fantastic Voyage*, (Houghton, Mifflin, 1966).
5. S. Johnston, M.W. Lee, M.F. Hawthorne, Development of cell-surface protein targeted CT and MR contrast agents, *Applied Radiology Online* **32**(6) (June 2003).
6. J. Haaga, R. Afidi, et al., Precise Biospy Localization By Computed Tomography, *Radiology* **118**, 603-607 (March 1976).
7. J.P. McGahan, P.D. Browning, J.M. Brock, H. Teslik, Hepatic ablation using radiofrequency electrocautery, *Invest Radiol* **25**, 267-270 (1990).
8. S. Rossi, F. Fornari, C. Pathies, L. Buscarini, Thermal lesions induced by 480 KHz localized current field in guinea pig and pig liver, *Tumori* **76**, 54-57 (1990).
9. G.D. Dodd, M.C. Soulen, R.A. Kane, T. Livraghi, W. Lees, Y.Yamashita, A.R. Gillams, O.I. Karahan, H. Rhim, Minimally Invasive Treatment of Malignant Hepatic Tumors: At the Threshold of a Major Breakthrough, *Radiographics* **20**, 9-27 (2000).

Chapter 10

IMAGE-GUIDED THERAPY (IGT): NEW CT AND HYBRID IMAGING TECHNOLOGIES
Devices for the Interventional Radiology (IR) Suite and the OR

Jeffrey Yanof[1], Christopher Bauer[1], Steffen Renisch[2], Jochen Krücker[3], Jörg Sabczynski[2]
[1]*Philips Medical Systems, Cleveland, OH, USA;* [2]*Philips Research, Hamburg, Germany;* [3]*Philips Research , Briarcliff Manor, NY, USA.*

Abstract: Integrated multi-modality IGT prototypes are described for IR and OR suites of the future including procedures guided with CT and hybrid imaging devices. Radiofrequency Ablation (RFA) is an exemplary application, and the prototypes can be adapted to other procedures. To investigate pre-planning[1], a software prototype enables virtual electrode placement. Intra-procedurally, a CT-integrated robot aligns its laser to planned trajectories. Interventional tools and mini-imaging devices are registered to imagers and 3-D data sets by attaching them as robot hands, or by tracking them with electromagnetic or optical systems. Tissue response is monitored with new 3-D real-time imaging. The ultimate goal is to simplify treatment and provide benefit to the patient.

Keywords: Percutaneous ablation; image-guided therapy; interventional radiology; surgical navigation; virtual reality; medical robotics; image registration

1.   INTRODUCTION

Prototype modules and devices for percutaneous, extracorporeal, and laparoscopic procedures are described in the pre-, intra-, and post procedure stages primarily for CT, X-ray C-arm based systems, and other imaging devices. These imagers allow the integration of and access to many types of equipment including navigation devices, such as robots and instrument tracking devices, and other imaging equipment such as PET, SPECT, and Ultrasound imagers.

G. Spekowius and T. Wendler (Eds.), Advances in Healthcare Technology, 147-166.

The leading application in the new field of 'Interventional Oncology' has been the treatment of solid tumors with percutaneous Radio-frequency Ablation (RFA). Accordingly, many of the investigative tools in this chapter are illustrated by percutaneous RFA; however, they can be adapted to other research areas such as drug delivery, gene transfection, and biological implantation, etc. Furthermore, there are many techniques used to locally and directly treat tumors such as cryogenic, brachytherapy[2], and microwave, and presently it is not known which may have clear advantages over the other.

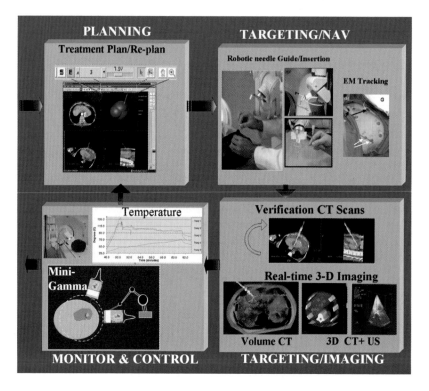

Figure 10-1. Investigative concepts and devices for RFA workflow. Upper Left: Treatment planning display to specify virtual electrodes. Upper Right: The plan is sent to a CT-integrated robot and an electromagnetic tracking system, which are used for targeting in conjunction (lower right) with real-time imaging. Lower Left: Temperature signals[3] and molecular tracers[4] can be used to monitor the target tissue location in shared 3-D coordinates.

The objectives for RFA include the general objectives for image-guided therapy (IGT) discussed in Chapter 9 and the specific objective: To accurately place single or multiple electrodes to cover the entire treatment region without heating critical structures such as the heart.

2. PRE-PROCEDURE PLANNING

For many image-guided procedures such as needle biopsies, disposable positioning grids and estimated angles may be sufficient for planning; however, there are IGT applications where computer-based treatment planning can potentially be useful. Examples include cases involving large tumors (greater than 3cm), tumors near critical structures, multiple targets, and multiple treatments.

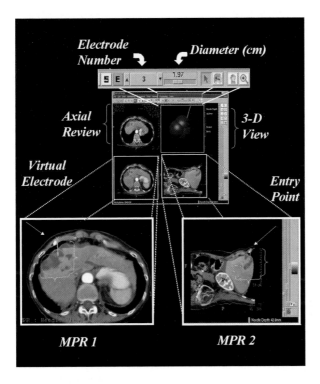

Figure 10-2. On-line RFA pre-planning screen that uses a CT data set to specify the trajectory and placement of virtual electrodes (green) with associated tumor conforming, overlapping isothermal contours (green) and skin entry point (red)[5].

On-line treatment planning is used on the scanner's host computer after the patient is scanned. Reconstructed image data sets can be automatically registered with the interventional field provided that the patient remains immobile and methods are used to manage respiratory motion[6]. If planning requires more than several minutes, however, the image data can be transferred to another computer, as is done with radiation therapy planning.

However, additional registration steps and patient positioning may be needed to implement the plan.

2.1   Treatment planning for RFA with CT data set

A prototype for on-line, point-and-click RFA planning, as shown in Figure 10-2, was developed in collaboration with Bradford Wood, M.D., NIH Clinical Center. After the patient is scanned, the 3-D CT data set is loaded and virtual electrodes are interactively placed on bi-sectional CT multi-planar reformatted (MPR) views. Each electrode contains a graphical skin entry point, a target, and a spherically-shaped ablation zone. The physician can simultaneously adjust MPR views and virtual electrode positions, and the 3-D treatment plan is updated automatically. The set of virtual electrodes form a 3-D ablation plan based on overlapping spheres. Isothermal contours are computed and displayed as overlapping circles resulting from MPR-sphere intersections (outer contours only). A shaded-surface representation of the plan is also displayed in a 3-D view port.

For review and refinement of the treatment plan, the physician can step through virtual electrodes and view the 50°C contours associated with the set. Axial images can be scrolled in a separate view port to verify that the contours cover the imaged tumor with a sufficient margin. Also, the set of virtual electrodes are stored in a patient-specific database for reference to subsequent CT scans.

The planned distance from the skin entry point to the tip of electrode is computed automatically and displayed. Also, the distance from the imaged tumor to nearby, heat sinking blood vessels can be measured.

The spherical geometry was used to model the Rita XLi electrode, but other treatment shapes could be represented in the form of ellipsoid, disc, rice kernel for High-Intensity Focused Ultrasound (HIFU, Section 4.4), and ice-ball shaped regions (cryoablation).

This prototype also provides a framework for investigation of new concepts for RFA planning such as: 1) optimization of electrode placement based on segmentation results, 2) multi-modality image-guided ablative therapies as discussed in the next section, 3) simulation and display of multiple isotherms indicating the treatment and blood flow effects, and 4) an intra-procedural means to merge treatment monitoring with the plan for re-planning.

2.2   Multi-modality planning

Inter- or intra-modality registration can provide synergistic information for both diagnosis and therapy[7] (see Chapter 9). Image-guided pre-planning based on multi-modality data sets is being investigated for RF ablation and biopsy. The point-and-click treatment planning prototype in Figure 10-2 can be extended to use multi-modality data sets. A pre-planning screen based on pre-registered PET-CT data from the Philips Gemini scanner is shown in Figure 10-3[8]. As virtual electrodes are interactively positioned, the dual-modality data set is displayed and updated with fused axial and MPR views.

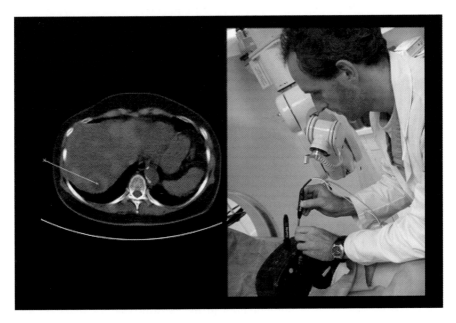

Figure 10-3. Left: $F^{18}DG$ PET-CT data set used with point-and-click GUI to plan trajectories for CT Guided robot. Right: Dr. Wood uses laser guidance to place a Radionics triple-cluster RFA electrode in a CIRS Model 57 (CIRS Norfolk, VA) abdominal phantom.

Robotic or passive tracking systems can be integrated with the planning display and the PET/CT imager to provide intra-operative assistance, as discussed in the next section.

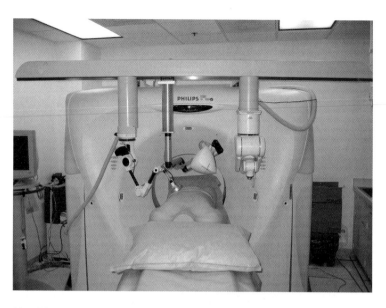

Figure 10-4. Three navigation tools integrated with the Brilliance 16 CT at the NIH Clinical Center. Left: Passive position-sensing arm tracking a US-HIFU assembly. Center): Electromagnetic generator for instrument-tip tracking. Right: Six-axis robot with laser end-effector. The retractable CT gantry frame registers diagnostic and therapeutic devices in multiple (detent) positions and in the CT's coordinate system, and facilitates their easy deployment.

3.   INTRA-PROCEDURE STAGE

The treatment plan is implemented in the intra-procedure stage (Figure 10-1), with assistance from targeting (i.e., navigation) and monitoring devices. Passive navigation is an interactive 3-D search process to align a physical device (e.g., needle or electrode), in some cases to a preplanned trajectory, by tracking a corresponding virtual device within one or more static, registered tomographic data sets. Passive systems can be based on an electromagnetic sensor-generator (section 3.1.2, Figure 10-4 middle), an optical camera with LEDs (section 3.1.3), or a position-sensing articulated arm (Section 4.3, Figure 10-4 left). Each presently has advantages and trade-offs, as mentioned below. Active navigation uses a robot for automatic alignment and targeting, inside or outside the CT's aperture, based on commands received from a planning screen (shown in Figure 10-2) or a remote device (section 3.1.1).

As in the pre-planning stage, multi-modality data sets and imaging can be used in this stage. To assist with the tracking of organ and target motion, for instance, one modality can be real-time (live) and the other can be based on a recently acquired, inter- or intra-modality (e.g., contrast enhanced) image data set. Also, to combine inter-modality information, one data set can be used to plan the acquisition of another.

During the procedure, there may be deviations from the original plan and instances where it needs to be updated. This could be due to variations in electrode placement, organ shift, or patient re-positioning. Another indication for re-planning is when the monitoring process indicates under-treated areas.

3.1.1   CT-integrated robotics

Active navigation, unlike passive navigation, does not involve a manual 3-D search process to align with a pre-planned trajectory[9,10]. Instead, a robot can automatically align its end-effector or hand, such as a guidance laser. The robot, with new end-effectors, can also assist with percutaneous needle insertion and control, inside the CT's aperture, with force feedback during fluoroscopy[11]. The PAKY (Percutaneous Kidney Access) needle driver, supported with a RCM (Rotational Center of Motion) and a manual support arm, was among the first custom prototypes for robot needle insertion to be tested clinically[12].

A CT-integrated robotic system is being investigated with Dr. Wood. A six-axis Kawasaki FS-2 robot (Figure 10-3, right, Kawasaki LTD, Wixom, MI) is rigidly attached at its base to the CT gantry (Philips Brilliance 16) and is pre-registered into the CT's 3-D coordinate system during installation. A tool coordinate is also pre-determined for the end-effectors, e.g., the laser angles. Since the patient remains on the imaging table during the procedure and since the robot software tracks table motion inside or outside the CT aperture, the robot, planning data set, and patient are mathematically co-registered at the completion of each scan without the need for intra-procedure registration steps.

After the on-line pre-planning screen in Figure 10-2 is used to place virtual electrodes, the 3-D coordinates for each electrode, specifically the target and skin entry points, are sent from the CT's host computer to the robot's C70 controller via an RS-232 serial line. The controller then semi-autonomously and automatically moves the robot to align its class II laser with the electrode's planned trajectory to assist with electrode placement. Also, the CT patient support automatically moves the interventional field into the robot's reachable workspace.

For the laser end-effector, the robot and controller are designed with redundant safety mechanisms to maintain a minimum distance of 15 cm from the patient for contact free operation. Another safety feature is that the physician must continuously press a button to enable the robot to move between its home and target-alignment positions.

The physician then aligns the physical RFA electrode with the laser beam and advances the electrode, with verification CT scans, to the pre-measured depth. To compare planned and actual electrode positions, the verification image data set is loaded into the pre-planning software. Each pre-stored virtual electrode can be selected and its position can be compared and aligned with the corresponding imaged electrode, which then updates the ablation plan. The physical electrode or the remaining virtual electrodes in the plan can then be repositioned to decrease the likelihood of under treated tissue.

Miniature (e.g., hand-held) imaging and extracorporeal therapeutic devices can also be attached to the hand of the robot, which automatically registers them into the CT's 3-D coordinate system (see Figure 10-4, left and Figure 10-11 left and right), either inside or outside the CT's aperture.

3.1.2   Electromagnetic tracking

Tracking sensors can be attached to interventional, surgical, or imaging devices to provide real-time 3-D positional information of the device. The position information can be used to display the actual position of the device relative to real-time or pre-acquired images once the transformation between tracking space coordinates and image coordinates has been established. This registration transformation can be determined manually, semi-automatically, or automatically.

Non-line-of-sight systems[13] such as EM tracking only require the tracked device to be anywhere in the operating range of the system, with no requirements for visibility, which opens up the possibility of tracking devices inside the patient during interventional and minimally-invasive procedures.

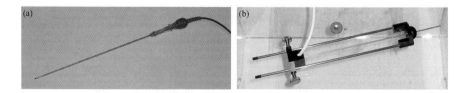

Figure 10-5. (a) Tracked stylet/sheath combination for biopsies, and (b) tracked needle guidance device for radiofrequency ablations (Traxtal Inc.). For biopsies, the tracked stylet is removed from the sheath and replaced by the actual biopsy needle once the device is in place. For radiofrequency ablations, the RFA needle with up to 3 prongs can be inserted through coaxial holes in the guidance device.

The accuracy of EM tracking systems can be compromised by secondary electromagnetic fields, such as those generated by eddy currents in conductive metal plates. The smaller sensor size, however, in combination with the ability to track non-line-of-sight, can outweigh some of the limitations.

For example, when tracking a laparoscope[14], an optical tracking sensor has to be attached near the handle. Any small error in the tracked orientation of the device is amplified to a larger positional error at the tip. With EM tracking, the sensor can be attached very close to the tip, thus providing accurate positional information of the relevant part of the instrument without the need for position extrapolation.

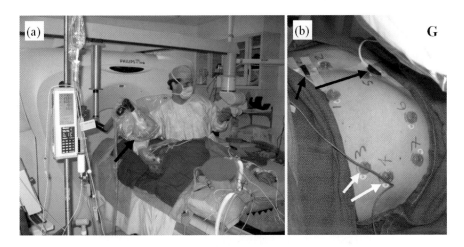

Figure 10-6. (a) The EM field generator (black arrow) is attached to the CT scanner using an articulated arm, and is positioned close to the needle insertion point during the intervention. (b) Close-up of the sterilized area shows the EM generator (G), the fiducial skin markers used for registration (white arrow), and 6 DOF reference trackers used for motion compensation studies (black arrows).

The feasibility of using EM tracking to guide biopsies and RFA procedures in conjunction with pre-operative CT scans is being investigated in collaboration with Dr. Wood. In this study, needles with integrated miniaturized EM sensor coils are used (Figure 10-5). The EM field generator (Northern Digital Imaging, Waterloo, CA) is attached to the CT scanner (Philips Brilliance 16) using an articulated arm, and is manually positioned and locked above the patient near the skin entry point (Figure 10-6). The pre-operative CT scan is obtained after placing six fiducial skin markers in the workspace of the tracking system. The image data is automatically transferred to a workstation, which runs the custom tracking software. To register EM tracking coordinates with image coordinates, the fiducial markers are manually identified in the pre-operative image, and the markers are momentarily contacted with a tracked needle. Once registration is established, a virtual image of the tracked needle is shown relative to MPRs of the CT volume at the needle location. After identification of the target location using a single mouse click in the pre-procedure image, an additional target display shows the location of the target relative to the needle tip. It provides visual feedback about the distance between needle tip and target, and about the angular deviation between the current and targeted needle direction (Figure 10-7). Additional skin trackers are used to monitor respiratory and patient motion.

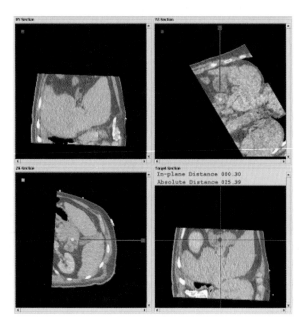

Figure 10-7. The tracked needle is visualized relative to the pre-op CT scan using three orthogonal MPRs at the tip of the needle. The yellow spot indicates the manually selected target position. The target display in the lower right provides visual and numeric information about the current distance from the target and about the alignment of the needle with the target.

3.1.3   Optical tracking in the operating room

Although EM navigation systems can track devices within the body, optical tracking may have advantages over EM tracking (EMT) in the fully equipped OR. The accuracy of EMT in the OR could be susceptible to interference of metal devices such as surgical instrument trays, anesthesia carts, etc. Also, the larger working range of optical systems may be advantageous in the OR.

The Optical Position Measurement System (OPMS), introduced in the early 1990's by several manufacturers and referred to as 'frameless stereotaxy', enables special surgical instruments to be tracked in real-time and displayed in registration with a pre-operative CT or MR data set. These instruments are equipped with infrared emitting diodes (IRED), which can be seen by OPMS cameras to triangulate their position in 3-D space. Registration, as with other tracking devices, is the calculation of the coordinate transformation from the coordinate system of the pre-operative images to the coordinate system of the intra-operative position measurement system. During surgery, the position measurement system continuously measures the position and orientation of surgical instruments (*tracking*) and the position of the instruments is visualized in the pre-operative image, i.e., 'virtual reality'. This allows the surgeon to accurately navigate in the pre-operative images without having direct visual contact to the structures of interest and helps him or her to perform complex manual tasks.

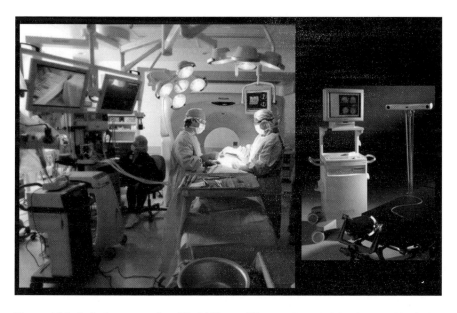

Figure 10-8. Left: Intra-operative CT (Philips Brilliance 16) at Celebration Health Florida Hospital in collaboration with Drs. Gary Onik and Joseph Redan. Right: The Philips EasyGuide, an early surgical navigation system consisting of a computer, a monitor, an optical position measurement device, and special surgical instruments.

Soon after the first optical navigation systems were used clinically, questions arose regarding how accurate these systems were in comparison to free-hand surgery and well-established tools like stereotactic frames. A crucial issue for the clinical acceptance of surgical navigation systems is the overall application error. Application error is the positioning error occurring between target locations in pre-operative images versus the position in intra-operative patient space. Simulations[15] showed that application error strongly depends on the clinical protocol used (especially on the registration method), the position and orientation of the surgical instrument, and the resolution of the images used. However, in a typical clinical setup the accuracy of navigation systems is comparable to the accuracy of stereotactic frame systems[16].

4.   MONITORING AND CONTROLLING

During image-guided procedures in the interventional radiology suite or the operating room, the physician monitors, measures, or visualizes the effect of the treatment. This important feedback is used to make adjustments in treatment delivery to decrease the risk for under-treated tissue. Techniques for image-guided monitoring are expected to grow rapidly as active areas of research. Future intra-procedural monitoring will include targeted contrast agents and many other types of real-time molecular imaging such as tracer-labelled monoclonal antibodies or liposomes with therapeutic payloads.

For the example application of RFA, some early measurements and devices for monitoring include: temperature or current impedance feedback, dynamic visualization of CT contrast enhancement, and live 3-D ultrasound registered with CT.

4.1   Temperature monitoring

In vivo temperature measurement is obviously an important measurement during thermal ablation. The measurement can be derived from the thermocouples embedded in the electrode tine tips (XLi, Rita Medical, Fremont, CA) and is used by RFA generators (Rita Medical) to adjust the power delivered to the electrode.

Temperature measurements can also be superimposed on the original planning images and compared with simulations and resulting isotherms. Image-based temperature monitoring with MR is established and is under feasibility investigation with CT. The image-based feedback can be used by the physician to re-position electrodes, e.g., more heat may be required to heat a tumor near a large blood vessel. Since this electrode re-positioning is a form of targeting and targeting requires some form of planning, it can be seen that the stages of image-guided therapy can overlap.

4.2 Volume CT fluoroscopy

Volume (3-D) CT fluoroscopy could improve feedback during image-guided procedures. Increasing rows of detectors in CT enables CT Fluoroscopy (CTF) to be extended from 2-D to 3-D visualization modes at increasing frame rates. The simulation of 3-D visualization methods, previously restricted to retrospective review on a workstation, are under investigation for 3-D CTF[17]. Volume CTF for the 3-D deployment of RFA tines is shown in Figure 10-9. A sequence of images is presented from axial, coronal, and sagittal viewpoints using an abdominal phantom with simulated respiratory motion. A blood orange was embedded in the phantom to simulate a 5 cm diameter tumor.

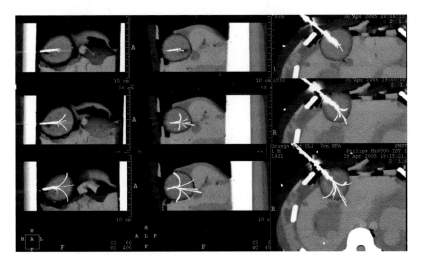

Figure 10-9. Simulated volume CT fluoroscopy (three selected frames) with left (coronal view), middle (sagittal view), and right columns (Axial view). Volume Maximum Intensity Projection is used to visualize the deployment of electrode tines in an abdominal phantom with blood orange representing a tumor.

Volume CTF could also be used for dynamic perfusion imaging[16] of the tumor to monitor the treatment effects like coagulation necrosis. Other applications for 3-D CTF include the insertion of a skinny, bending needle with a double angle trajectory toward a 5 mm target and advancing a catheter in a vascular tree.

Dose mitigation strategies, such as intermittent volume CTF, low tube current, anti-scatter grids, and needle holders, can be deployed.

4.3   Live ultrasound combined with CT data set

An emerging multi-modality technique is to register real-time imaging (projection, tomographic, or sector) with a 3-D retrospective image data set. This can be accomplished with a 3-D tracking system (electromagnetic, optical, or position sensing arm).

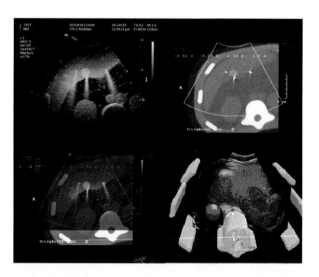

Figure 10-10. An ultrasound transducer is tracked in 3-D CT data. This co-display shows the registration on three markers[18]. (Supported by a Grant from the SIR Foundation-formerly CIRREF-Pilot Research Grant Program). The lower right shows a real-time US image registered with segmented CT[19].

Accordingly, the position and orientation of the US transducer is tracked in the CT's 3-D coordinates and used to automatically select CT MPR planes, which are co-planar and registered with the US images. Ultrasound-CT registration and fusion take advantage of the temporal resolution of US (30 frames per second) and the spatial resolution of CT (21 line-pairs per cm). This technique, which has been extended to 3-D US, may be extremely useful during the targeting process, when shadowing from bone or gas resulting from the burn can obscure visualization of the interventional field. Also, US contrast agents, co-located with CT, could have an important role in the future.

4.4   HIFU guided with CT and diagnostic US

Intra-procedure IGT can be extended to three imaging modalities (e.g., CT, US, NM) and these, along with therapeutic devices, can each be co-registered into a common coordinate system. A tri-axial probe for image-guided High Intensity Focused Ultrasound (HIFU) was fabricated[20] (Focus Surgery, Indianapolis, IN): A diagnostic US transducer was co-axially embedded in a 1 MHz therapeutic US transducer. The dual-US assembly is attached as end-effectors on a position sensing and lockable articulated arm. The arm registers the diagnostic US probe into 3-D CT coordinates to reformat CT images that are co-planar with the live US images.

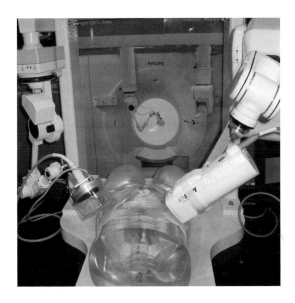

Figure 10-11. Three-modality image-guided therapy: Imaging and therapeutic devices for targeting and monitoring can be attached as hands of navigation devices, thereby registering them into the CT's 3-D coordinate system. A mini-gamma camera is attached to the robotic arm (right) and a dual modality (therapeutic and diagnostic) ultrasound transducer is attached to the position-sensing arm (left). Both can be navigated, aligned, and locked onto the target tissue location (RSNA'04 infoRad Exhibit, Photo by A. Viswanathan, NIH Research Fellow).

4.5 X-ray imaging in the operating room

Using static pre-operative image data can have limitations. In neurosurgery the phenomenon of brain shift was discovered, i.e. after opening the dura for brain tumour resection, the brain deforms and the pre-operative images no longer reflect the intra-operative morphology. This is more significant after the tumour has been resected. A strategy to circumvent these problems of tissue deformation and patient movement is intra-operative imaging. Almost all imaging modalities, which are used for diagnostic purposes, can also be used in the OR. Intra-operative X-ray and ultrasound have been in use for some time, and intra-operative CT (Figure 10-8) and MRI are either in use or are being investigated.

Intra-operative imaging also allows for further automation of the procedure. While non-integrated navigation devices require a manual registration procedure, intra-operative imaging with an integrated navigation device can bypass the registration step. If during imaging, the geometrical imaging properties of the imaging system are known and its position relative to the patient is determined, e.g. with the help of a position measurement system, the registration transformation can be calculated automatically. In order to determine the imaging properties of the imaging system, a *calibration* procedure must be done, either at the installation of the imaging system or pre-operatively. For this purpose, a calibration phantom with known geometry or markers is imaged. The calibration phantom must also be visible to the position measurement system in order to allow registration of the calibration image with the external coordinate system.

C-arm x-ray is used intra-operatively on a routine basis in many surgical disciplines and in Interventional Radiology (IR). Applications range from orthopedics and traumatology to cardiology. Navigation systems using intra-operative X-ray images offer several advantages over conventional methods. Since navigation uses position measurements to generate an overlay of the instrument on the image, radiation dose for both staff and patient can be significantly reduced in comparison to real-time imaging.

4.5.1 Instrument tracking with C-arm fluoroscopy

For navigation using intra-operative X-ray images, a surgical C-arm can be used. As when tracking a US probe or mini-gamma camera in the CT's coordinates, the C-arm can be equipped with a tracker of the position measurement system in order to measure its position and orientation[21,22]. In order to overlay instrument positions onto X-ray images, the imaging properties of the X-ray system must be known. The imaging properties of a surgical C-arm consist of the X-ray generation and detection part, which can be modelled by a simple pinhole camera model, and the image intensifier. Image distortions due to the image intensifier can be described as a pin-cushion distortion due to the curved form of the X-ray entry window, an image shift, an image distortion, and an 'S'-shaped distortion due to an external magnetic field[23,24]. These distortions can be corrected for by a third order polynomial approach with sufficient accuracy[21].

Prior to the first operation a calibration phantom (see Figure 10-11) is attached to the image intensifier, which allows collecting data for image intensifier distortion correction and determination of the position of the focal point of the X-ray tube. The phantom is removed before the operation.

The image intensifier distortion is influenced by external magnetic fields such as the earth's magnetic field. Therefore the model parameters to describe the imaging geometry of the C-arm depend on its position and orientation. The calibration step thus needs to be repeated for typical positions of the C-arm.

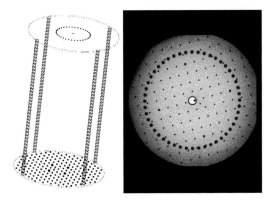

Figure 10-12. Calibration phantom (left) to correct for image intensifier distortion and position of focal spot of the X-ray tube. X-ray image (right) of the calibration phantom. (From[22], Copyright: Robotic Publications Ltd., 2004).

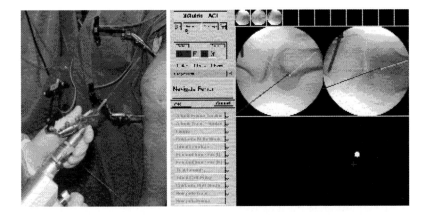

Figure 10-13. Left: Intra-operative situation during drilling of the femoral canal. Note that femur, tibia, and drill guide are equipped with trackers for the position measurement system. Right: Screen shot during drilling of the femoral hole. The red line shows the drill guide in both a-p and lateral C-arm images. The green and blue lines are the planned tibial and femoral canals. In the lower right a targeting tool provides additional geometrical feedback. (From[22], Copyright: Robotic Publications Ltd., 2004).

The surgical navigation system described above has been used in orthopedics for computer-assisted replacement of the Anterior Cruciate Ligament (ACL)[21]. Rupture of the ACL is a common trauma in sports. The common reconstruction is by an autologous tendon, usually the medial third of the patellar tendon or semitendinosus tendon. This procedure is a biomechanically difficult task. The correct placement of the graft, especially the isometry of the tibial and femoral insertion points, is critical to the success of the procedure and the stability of the knee. During conventional arthroscopy the planning of the insertion points and accurate execution of the plan is difficult due to limited overview in the knee.

5.   POST-PROCEDURE TREATMENT RESPONSE

Whether performed in the OR or IR suite, many procedures require imaging as treatment follow-up. Ideally, in some interventional oncology cases, post-procedure imaging would not be needed if sufficient and conclusive intra-procedure feedback was provided as to whether or not the local treatment was complete. This ideal has not yet been realized, but could be with advances in molecular imaging.

After an episode of RFA treatment, imaging is used to determine if a portion of the tumor is untreated; thereby, necessitating re-treatment. For RFA, this is typically a contrast enhanced CT scan between 1-7 days after the procedure.

To check for marginal recurrence, tumor size can be tracked over longer periods with sequential CT scans using established criteria for measuring tumor size, e.g., RESIST or WHO, or a 3-D criteria. More recently, on some protocols, PET-CT, SPECT-CT, or dynamic MR are being used to track the response of the tumor with a potentially higher accuracy than CT. This can help further differentiate a heterogeneous tumor and indicate the need for re-treatment based on functional or molecular information.

6.   SUMMARY

New technologies for IGT were reviewed for the interventional radiology suite and the operating room of the future. This included new methods for multi-modality, point-and-click treatment planning, multi-modality image targeting with active and passive navigation devices, monitoring with real-time 3-D imaging, and post treatment follow-up.

Some of the devices, such as optical, electromagnetic, and articulated arm navigation systems, have advantages and trade-offs. In some cases, more investigation is needed for further automation, verification and validation, and to determine which methods or devices are best for a given application and venue. Some prototypes and projects are in the early exploratory phase, and others are being used in clinical protocols.

Multi-modality treatment planning and real-time targeting and monitoring will eventually become seamlessly integrated, more fully automated, and easier to access and use during the procedure. Many devices and imagers can be integrated, used in combination, and can share common coordinate systems and image data.

Further merging of molecular imaging and image-guided therapy will significantly increase the amount of pre- and intra-procedure visualization. Integrating image-guidance devices with this additional visualization will lead to significant benefits for the patient and will ultimately, at least in some cases, facilitate the need for only one episode of image-guided care.

REFERENCES

1. S.N. Goldberg, et al., Image Guided Tumor Ablation: Standardization of Terminology and Reporting Criteria, *Radiology Online* **10**, 1148 (2005).
2. J.M. Hevezi, M. Blough, D. Hoffmeyer and J.H. Yanof, Brachytherapy using CT PinPoint, *Medica Mundi* **46**(3), 22-27 (2002).
3. B.J. Wood, D. Uecker; J.H. Yanof, P. Klahr, C. Bauer, Integration of Pre-Procedural Treatment Planning and Intra-Procedural Temperature Visualization for CT-guided, Robot-assisted RF Ablation (RFA) of Liver Tumors, *RSNA,* 755 (2003).
4. B.J. Wood, J.H. Yanof, C. Bauer, A.M. Gharib, V. Frenkel, K.C. Li, Molecular Imaging System for Treatment Planning and Robot-assisted Intervention: Utilization of New Nuclear Medicine (NM) Tracers as the Ultimate MS-CT Contrast Agent, *RSNA,* 830 (2004).
5. S. Renisch, J. Yanof, C. Bauer, L. Achint, P. Klahr, B. Wood, CT-integrated treatment planning for robot-assisted thermal ablation and laser guided sphere packing, *Proc Computer Assisted Radiology and Surgery,* 1361 (2004).
6. E.A. Kelley, J.H.Yanof, J.P. Lipuma, CT-Integrated Breath Monitor for Intervention: Evaluation of Pre- and Intra-Operative Breath-Hold Congruency, *Society Interventional Radiology, Supplement to JVIR* **13**, s104 (2002).
7. W.F. Bennett, J.H. Yanof, Image Fusion of Octreotide SPECT and CT, *RSNA,* 478 (1994).
8. B. Wood, J. Yanof, M. McAuliffe, S. Renisch, J. Hvizda, K. Cleary, PET-CT Treatment Planning Interface for Robot-assisted Biopsy and Tumor Ablation, Abstract, *RSNA,* 789 (2003).
9. J.H. Haaga, J.H. Yanof, D. Nakamoto, L. Kelley, D. Kwartowitz, U. Shreter, Computer-radiologist Interface with Tactile Feedback for Robot-assisted CT-guided Interventional Procedures, *RSNA,* 726 (2002).
10. B. Wood, F. Banovac, M. Friedman, Z. Varro, K. Cleary, J. Yanof, et al., CT-Integrated Programmable Robot for Image-Guided Procedures: Comparison of Free-Hand and Robot-Assisted Techniques, *Society Interventional Radiology, Supplement to JVIR* **14**, s62 (2003).

11. J. Yanof, C. Bauer, B. Wood, Tactile feedback and display system to assist CT guided robotic percutaneous procedure, *Proc Computer Assisted Radiology and Surgery,* 521-526 (2004).

12. S. Solomon, B. Patriciu A, Bohlman, M.E. Kavoussi, L. Stoianovici, Robotically Driven Interventions: A Method of Using CT Fluoroscopy without Radiation Exposure to the Physician, *Radiology* **225**, 277-282 (2002).

13. B.J. Wood, H. Zhang, A. Durrani, N. Glossop, S. Ranjan, D. Lindisch, E. Levy, F. Banovac, J. Borgert, S. Krueger, J. Kruecker, A. Viswanathan K. Cleary, Navigation with Electromagnetic Tracking for Interventional Radiology Procedures: A Feasibility Study, *Journal of Vascular and Interventional Radiology* **16**, 493-505 (2005).

14. J. Krücker, A. Viswanathan, J. Borgert, N. Glossop, Y. Yang, B.J. Wood, An electro-magnetically tracked laparoscopic ultrasound for multi-modality minimally invasive surgery, *Proc Computer Assisted Radiology and Surgery,* 746-751 (2005).

15. M. Fuchs, H.-A. Wischmann, A. Neumann, J. Weese, W. Zylka, J. Sabczynski, M.H. Kuhn, Th.M. Buzug, G. Schmitz, P.M.C. Gieles, Accuracy analysis for image-guided neurosurgery using fiducial skin markers, 3D CT imaging, and an optical localizer system, *Proc Computer Assisted Radiology and Surgery,* 770-775 (1996).

16. W. Zylka, J. Sabczynski, G. Schmitz, A Gaussian approach for the calculation of the accuracy of stereotactic frame systems, *Med Phys* **26**(3), 381-391 (1999).

17. J.H. Yanof, K. Read, T.R. Fleiter, A. Viswanathan, J. Locklin, B. Wood, Volume Visualization Methods Using Multidetector CT Volume Fluoroscopy during Image-guided Interventions, accepted *RSNA* (2005).

18. B.J. Wood, J. Hvizda, J. Kruecker, Z. Neeman, J.H. Yanof, Registration and Fusion of Multi-Slice CT (MS-CT) and Real-time 3-D Ultrasound (3D-US) for RF Ablation (RFA) of Liver Tumors, *RSNA,* 789 (2004).

19. J. Berg, J. Kruecker, H. Schulz, K. Meetz, and J.Sabczynski, A hybrid method for registration of interventional CT and ultrasound images, *Proc Computer Assisted Radiology and Surgery,* 492-497 (2004).

20. B.J. Wood, R. Seip, N. Sanghvi, J.H. Yanof, P. Klahr, K.C. Li, Dual-modality Navigation and Display System for Targeting High-intensity Focused Ultrasound (HIFU) Therapy for Drug Delivery or Thermal Ablation: Utilization of Multislice-CT (MS-CT) and Real-Time Ultrasound (US), *RSNA,* 830 (2004).

21. J. Sabczynski, E. Hille, S. Dries, W. Zylka, L. Tafler, P. Haaker, T. Istel, Computer assisted arthroscopic anterior cruciate ligament reconstruction, *Proc Computer Assisted Radiology and Surgery,* 263-268 (2002).

22. J. Sabczynski, S.P.M. Dries, W. Zylka, E. Hille, Image-guided reconstruction of the anterior cruciate ligament, *Int J Medical Robotics and Computer Assisted Surgery* **1**(1), 125-132 (2004).

23. M. Grass, R. Koppe, E. Klotz, R. Proksa, M.H. Kuhn, H. Aerts, J. op de Beek, R. Kemkers, Three-dimensional reconstruction of high contrast objects using C-arm image intensifier projection data, *Comput Med Imaging Graph* **23**(6), 311-321 (1999).

24. R. Koppe, E. Klotz, J. op de Beek, H. Aerts, 3D vessel reconstruction based on rotational angiography, *Proc Computer Assisted Radiology and Surgery,* 101-107 (1995).

Chapter 11

DEVELOPMENTS IN CARDIAC INTERVENTIONS
Image Improvement, Reconstruction, Guidance, and Navigation

Jörn Borgert[1], Raoul Florent[2], Sascha Krueger[1], Sherif Makram-Ebeid[2], Babak Movassaghi[3], Holger Timinger[1] and Volker Rasche[4]

[1]*Philips Research, Hamburg, Germany;* [2]*Philips Medical Systems, Paris, France;* [3]*Philips Research, Briarckiff Manor, NY, USA;* [4]*University Hospital Ulm, Ulm, Germany*

Abstract: Over the last decades, X-ray imaging technology in the catheterization laboratory (cath lab) has dramatically evolved. On latest X-ray equipment, new functionalities such as low-dose imaging, three-dimensional imaging and improved navigation technology aiming for further improvement of existing interventional procedures as well as enabling future procedures are on the verge. This contribution provides a brief overview on some new technologies, which have recently been introduced into clinical practice. Furthermore, some representative examples of ongoing research activities are presented.

Keywords: 3D coronary angiography, stent boosting, noise reduction, motion-compensated navigation

1.   INTRODUCTION

The guidance of cardiac interventional procedures such as PTCA and stent deployment has been the domain of X-ray fluoroscopy for the last decades. The introduction of new technologies has significantly improved the imaging performance of the X-ray imaging equipment. For example, the recent commercial availability of flat detector X-ray imaging systems has dramatically improved image quality while further reducing radiation dose. Recent X-ray system geometries for cardiac catheterization laboratories (cath lab) typically provide multiple degrees of freedom enabling the acquisition of X-ray projections from multiple angulations without moving the patient, while maintaining sufficient patient accessibility (see Figure 11-1).

167

G. Spekowius and T. Wendler (Eds.), Advances in Healthcare Technology, 167-182.
© 2006 Springer. Printed in the Netherlands.

On the other side, almost 50 years after Mason Sones (1919-1985) acquired the first coronary angiogram, the basic principle of selective angiography has not changed with the introduction of modern X-ray systems. Considering the two-dimensional projective nature of conventional angiography, some limitations such as superposition of vascular structures and vessel foreshortening are obvious. Quantitative measurements of the vessels properties such as length, cross-sectional area, and orientation cannot precisely be retrieved from the two-dimensional projections and there is always the risk that the target lesion is visualized foreshortened or superimposed by other structures. Furthermore, new complex procedures such as interventional multi-vessel disease treatment, patent foramen ovalis (PFO) closures[1], transluminal valve repair and replacement[2], and the injection of biological material in the myocardial wall[3] are currently on the verge.

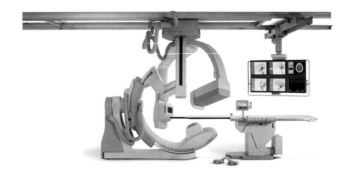

Figure 11-1. Recent bi-plane cardiovascular X-ray system.

Recent technical developments for improving the interventional guidance focus on a further reduction of the X-ray dose, on providing three-dimensional information, and on the integration of advanced navigation technologies.

This contribution will focus on some specific recent developments for dose reduction by means of image processing, three-dimensional reconstruction from projection data, enhancement of stent visualization, and motion-compensated navigation.

2. IMAGE NOISE REDUCTION

Interventional cardiovascular procedures still involve considerable X-ray dose to the patient and staff, for which the accumulated dose received is still a great concern. Increasing workloads and case complexity will likely place further pressure on X-ray dose levels, which makes X-ray dose reduction an important topic in the field of X-ray-guided interventions.

To reduce X-ray dose, different approaches, such as the use of high power X-ray tubes in combination with heavy filtration of the X-ray beam, have been applied. Although these techniques may provide a reduction of the X-ray dose, the possible maximal reduction is still limited by image noise.

Recently, dedicated filters were introduced, which could significantly reduce X-ray image noise while preserving important image characteristics, for example edges. The proposed cardiac enhancement filter (CEF) was initially developed for conventional ultrasound imaging[4,5] and later modified to be used specifically for X-ray projections. As depicted in Figure 11-2, the filter utilizes a multi-resolution Laplacian Pyramid decomposition as defined by Burt and Adelson in their 1983 paper[6].

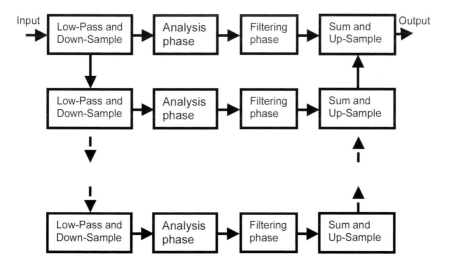

Figure 11-2. Block diagram showing the processing in X-ray noise reduction filtering.

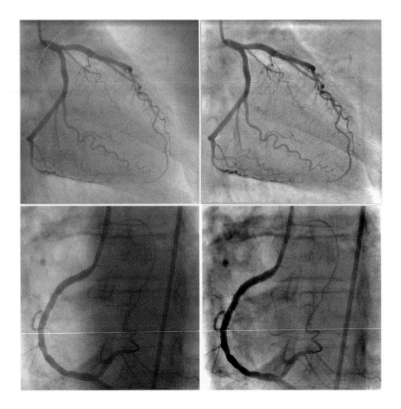

Figure 11-3. Low-dose X-ray projection images before (left) and after (right) filtering by the dedicated cardiac enhancement filter.

Each slice image is decomposed into a succession of sub-bands representing different levels of resolution from coarse to fine. Within each sub-band, pixels are segmented into high contrast regions (edges and ridges) and weakly textured regions. Highly anisotropic filtering is applied to the high contrast regions using adaptive smoothing kernels that are elongated along the ridges and edges and that may optionally provide some enhancement in the direction normal to those ridges and edges. In this way edges and ridges are not blurred and can even be slightly enhanced. In the weakly textured regions, slight isotropic filtering is applied to reduce high frequency random noise without appreciably altering the texture. These operations are applied to each of the individual sub-bands before recomposing the pyramid. As outlined in the figure, the processing at each resolution includes an analysis phase in which each sub-band is segmented into high contrast and weakly textured regions. In the analysis phase, the edge and ridge feature orientations are computed for determining the required filter kernels size and anisotropy. In the subsequent filtering phase, pixel adaptive filtering is implemented.

The described multi-resolution filter technique allows a significant improvement of the signal-to-noise and the contrast-to-noise ratios and enables the application of significantly reduced X-ray doses (see Figure 11-3), while maintaining the clinical value of the images.

3. VOLUME RECONSTRUCTION FROM PROJECTION DATA

Stent deployment is the preferred vascular interventional procedure for coronary stenosis treatment, making coronary angiography and angioplasty two of the most widespread diagnostic and interventional procedures performed worldwide. These procedures are currently carried out based on information provided by two-dimensional (2D) projection angiograms of the coronary arteries. However, the projective nature of the acquisition results in vessel foreshortening and vessel overlap, which still are major obstacles in X-ray guided fluoroscopic procedures. There is a strong demand for adding three-dimensional morphological and functional data for improving the assessment of the degree and relevance of a certain stenosis or even to enable quantitative three-dimensional assessment of vessel properties. Recent X-ray systems offers the ability to acquire data while constantly moving the gantry at high speed around the patient. This so-called Rotational Angiography (RA) functionality is utilized for providing more detailed information on the vascular morphology during the intervention.

3.1 Rotational angiography

In Rotational Angiography, projection data are acquired along a planar trajectory by rotating the C-arm gantry around the patient either in head or lateral position. The target anatomic area is positioned in the center-of-rotation. During the rotation, contrast agent (Iodine, 300mg/ml, 1.5 – 3 ml/s flow rate) is selectively injected into the root of the vascular structure under investigation. In applying RA to the coronary arteries, projections are normally taken from RAO 55° to LAO 55°, providing projective information on the coronary arteries over a huge angular range from a cine data acquisition using a single contrast injection only. Several studies by investigators[7,8] using X-ray systems from multiple vendors have documented the safety and clinical utility of this approach. In fact, some of these studies demonstrated that in clinical practice by utilizing RA, the overall amount of contrast injected and the X-ray dose can be significantly reduced in comparison to the traditional non-rotational technique. Figure 11-4 shows an example of multiple projections obtained from a single rotational acquisition.

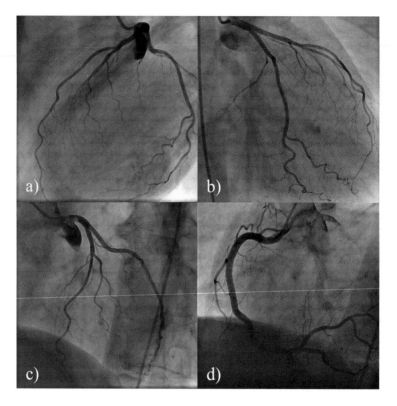

Figure 11-4. Example of coronary rotational angiograms, where a-c) show three different views of the LCA obtained during a single rotational run, and d) shows a single projection of the RCA selected to ensure minimal foreshortening of the medial section.

3.2 Coronary modeling

To further improve the value of X-ray imaging during cardiovascular interventions, in recent years much work has been performed to expand the current 2D imaging modality into 3D, utilizing a number of 2D X-ray projection images obtained during a single rotational angiography data acquisition. Current methods[9-11] generate a three-dimensional representation of the coronary arteries by means of so-called 'coronary modeling techniques'. In 3D modeling, the 2D projected center- and borderline of the vascular tree are extracted in at least two projections. In combination with the accurate knowledge of the projection geometry, the knowledge of the 2D projected center- and borderline can be used for generation of a 3D representation of the vascular tree (see Figure 11-5). The resulting 3D representation of the coronary artery tree enables an accurate assessment of the three-dimensional structure of the anatomy of the coronary tree and can be applied for localization of lesions. Besides volumetric quantitative analysis of the degree of stenosis, the 3D representation enables the automatic generation of optimal view-maps for the extraction of those projection directions providing minimal foreshortening and vessel overlap for a specific segment of the vascular tree (see Figure 11-5).

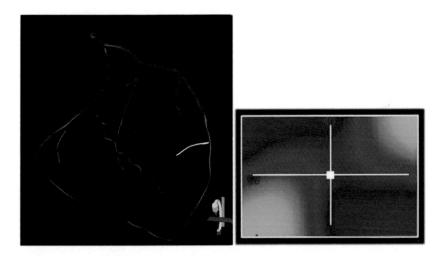

Figure 11-5. 3D model of a left coronary artery tree (left) and the respective optimal view map (right), obtained for the yellow-colored vessel branch. Green indicates little foreshortening and vessel overlap, whereas red indicates severe foreshortening and vessel overlap, depending on the angulation (y-axis) and the rotation (x-axis) of the X-ray gantry.

3.3 Three-dimensional reconstruction

From a user's perspective, a major limitation of 3D modeling is the required user-interaction for guiding the segmentation of the center- and borderlines in the 2D projections. Either a significant reduction in the amount of user interaction or perhaps even a fully automated generation of a three-dimensional coronary reconstruction may be beneficial in expediting the generation of 3D images for diagnostic and therapeutic purposes. In recent years, three-dimensional reconstructions at high spatial resolution have been demonstrated for non-moving vascular structures based on calibrated 2D X-ray projection data acquired during a rotational run. The application of these acquisition and reconstruction methods to the coronary arteries requires additional correction procedures for cardiac and respiratory motion. Initial studies have been performed in which breath-hold data acquisition techniques have been combined with ECG-gated[13] and motion-compensated techniques[14,15].

In ECG-gated techniques, projection data acquired in the same cardiac phase are used for performing a full three-dimensional reconstruction. To obtain sufficient projections from a single rotational data acquisition and to ensure enough angular coverage for the reconstruction, the acquisition protocols have been modified to cover an angular range of about 220° in about 8s. The acquisition protocol was tested in eight pigs. It was well tolerated by all animals and neither a significant venous enhancement nor an obvious hypoxia-induced change in the contraction pattern or heart rate could be observed. After acquisition, the projections were clustered based on delays relative to the R-peaks of the ECG signal. Three-dimensional back-projection was done using a slightly modified Feldkamp algorithm[16] considering the real projection geometry and compensating for the non-equidistant angular sampling. Reconstructions were performed using a spatial resolution between 0.13^3 mm^3 and 0.43^3 mm^3 as shown in Figure 11-6.

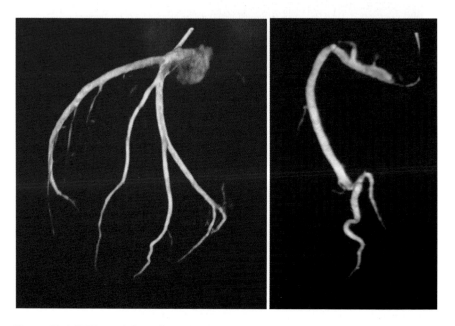

Figure 11-6. ECG-gated three-dimensional reconstruction of a LAD (left) and RCA (right). Data courtesy of Prof. Dr. A. Buecker, RWTH Aachen, Germany.

4. STENT BOOST FLUOROSCOPIC IMAGING

During conventional coronary stenting procedures, the assessment of the stent after deployment is crucial for ensuring optimal outcome. The applicability of conventional X-ray fluoroscopy imaging is limited by the contrast between the stent and the background. Stent boost fluoroscopic imaging (StentBoost) is a new technique, in which a motion-compensated sum over several successive X-ray fluoroscopic projections is formed for improving the visibility of the stent in the final image.

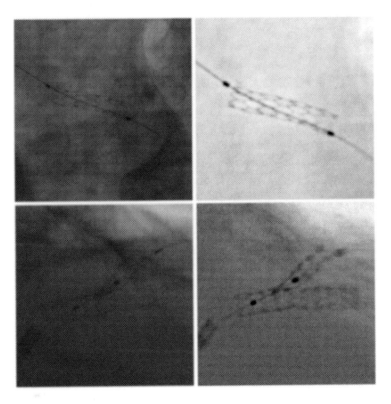

Figure 11-7. Raw X-ray fluoroscopy images (left) and corresponding StentBoost X-ray fluoroscopy images (right).

The motion compensation is based on fully automated tracking of the positions of the markers on the balloon catheter used for deployment of the stent. The tracked positions are utilized for generation of a motion vector field describing the motion of the markers over time. Assuming that the stent moves similar to the balloon markers, the derived motion vector field is used for performing a motion-compensated summation of temporally successive projections. By motion-compensated summation, all structures moving synchronously with the balloon markers are enhanced, while other structures are smeared off, thereby increasing the visibility of the stent (see Figure 11-7). The summation produces a highly augmented image of the deployed stent in coronary arteries – while the catheter is still in place. The StentBoost image helps clinicians to make a thorough check of stent expansion, and see the position of stents in relation to other objects, e.g. other stents, without the use of extra contrast agent or intra-vascular imaging modalities.

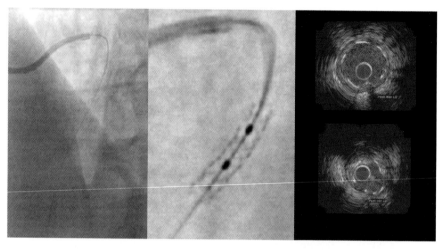

Figure 11-8. Raw X-ray fluoroscopy images (left), corresponding StentBoost X-ray fluoroscopy images (mid) and IVUS image (right). Data courtesy of Prof. AD Michaels, UCSF, California, USA.

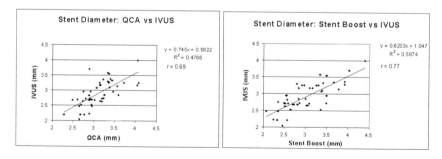

Figure 11-9. Comparison of stent diameter measurements between QCA and IVUS (left) and between StentBoost and IVUS (right).

Comparison of quantitative coronary angiography (QCA), intravascular ultrasound (IVUS) and StentBoost[17] for the determination of adequate stent expansion revealed that in direct comparison Stent Boost provided a significantly better correlation of stent diameter measurements (n = 47; r = 0.77; p < 0.001) than QCA (n = 47; r = 0.69; p < 0.001). Bland-Altman analysis showed a mean difference of -0.09mm (95% CI -0.19 to +0.01mm) for StentBoost where for QCA a mean difference of 0.21mm (95% CI 0.12 to 0.31mm) resulted when compared to IVUS (see Figure 11-8 and 11-9).

5.   MOTION COMPENSATED NAVIGATION FOR CARDIOVASCULAR APPLICATIONS

The general aim of motion compensated navigation using virtual roadmaps and non-line-of-sight (NLOS) localization technology for navigation and guidance in interventional procedures is to reduce contrast agent and dose burden to both patient and physician while at the same time conserving or improving the accuracy of the guidance. Tracking systems used for the NLOS localization task perform spatial measurements of position and orientation. However, for the correlation of the position and orientation information to *static* virtual roadmaps, the measurements have to be compensated for internal organ motion due to heartbeat and respiration. NLOS localization is normally done by means of magnetic tracking systems (MTS), which is a technology allowing for real-time position measurements of medical devices without line-of-sight restrictions. It has therefore been used to track interventional devices like catheters, needles or endoscopes inside the human[18-23].

One of the most prominent challenges of applying MTS for the tracking of medical devices is the presence of large amounts of conductive or ferromagnetic materials, which cause a distortion of the magnetic field. In cases where the magnetic environment remains constant, registration between the imaging modality and the NLOS system can be established. Focusing on the conventional interventional equipment including an X-ray system, a registration will only be valid for one given orientation of the gantry. Whenever the gantry rotates or the detector is shifted, this registration will become inaccurate due to changes in the magnetic environment. To avoid magnetic field variation due to movement of the gantry, the MTS can be attached to the gantry[21] to ensure a static situation between MTS and gantry.

The problem of organ motion has widely been investigated in the field of motion-compensated image reconstruction. Such motion compensation strategies include, among others, gated acquisition protocols or the use of parameterized motion models, which are driven by the ECG or a respiratory sensor signal, inspired by motion compensated MR image acquisition, where rigid or affine parameterized motion models are commonly used[24,25]. Here, the parameterization is accomplished by means of a respiratory sensor signal, which is derived from diaphragm tracking using 1D-pencil beams acquired by the MR scanner. A similar idea was used for tracking the diaphragm for motion compensation in 2D X-ray projection images[26]. These techniques can also be applied to motion compensated interventional navigation.

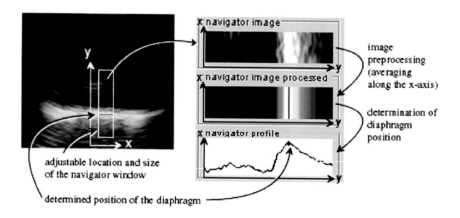

Figure 11-10. Example of sensing the respiratory position by monitoring the position of the diaphragm in an U/S image. The image on the left depicts a typical U/S image with superimposed navigator box applied for the diaphragm position extraction. The image on the right shows the involved steps for deriving the diaphragm position from the U/S navigator box signal.

The motion model itself can be considered as a parameterized elastic deformation field, which assigns a correction vector to the catheter position measured in a known respiratory and cardiac phase in order to compensate for organ motion. Such a deformation field could be determined using a non-patient specific motion model of the coronaries or can be acquired directly by measurements using the MTS. The beauty of learning the motion from MTS measurements is that no additional images have to be acquired and the motion model can be updated and refined during the intervention itself. The motion model and thus the motion compensation can locally and temporally be refined and enhanced by adding new or replacing old sample points during the intervention in real-time. This feature is especially valuable when approaching complex structures where increased accuracy is advantageous or when motion patterns change at a point in time, which would render the previous model partially inaccurate.

In phantom studies, the elastic motion model is driven by a simulated ECG signal and a respiratory sensor signal derived from ultrasonic diaphragm tracking as shown in Figure 11-10. For U/S based diaphragm tracking, a small 'navigator' window is located in the ultrasound B-mode image. The diaphragm position is then determined using image processing techniques.

Typical results from phantom studies using ECG together with QRS detection and U/S based diaphragm tracking to drive an MTS-determined elastic, refinable motion model are outlined in Figure 11-11. The used phantom[28] comprises a pneumatically driven dynamic heart phantom, which can simulate the motion of the left ventricle and the left coronary arteries due to heartbeat and respiration. It includes the possibility of selecting different heart rates and respiratory cycle length. The three-dimensional roadmap of the coronary arteries was obtained by gated 3D-rotational coronary angiography.

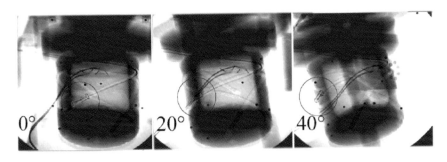

Figure 11-11. Motion-compensated 3D/2D image overlay of the tracked device (red circle) on the 3D roadmap and the X-ray fluoroscopy image at different gantry orientations.

In phantom studies[29], the accuracy of the navigation could be significantly improved. Residual motion turned out to be in the area of 1mm, enabling the unique identification of the vessel under examination.

6. SUMMARY AND DISCUSSION

Over decades, the main target in the cardiac catheterization laboratory has been the diagnosis and therapy of coronary artery disease. The main imaging modality applied for guidance has been and still is X-ray fluoroscopy. Although highly efficient, some major drawbacks arise from the ionizing radiation and especially from the two-dimensional projective nature of X-ray fluoroscopy, which might cause vessel foreshortening and vessel overlap. The ongoing trends of performing more complex transcatheter procedures such as treatment of multi-vessel diseases in the cath lab and the rise of new complex procedures such as PFO closures and valve repair and replacement demand improved guidance principles, preferably at lower dose levels.

Lower X-ray dose will be enabled by application-specific low-dose exposure protocols in combination with dedicated image processing techniques enabling noise-enhancement while conserving structures in the X-ray image or enabling local enhancement of structures by means of motion-compensation.

More complex procedures will be enabled by complementing X-ray fluoroscopy by three-dimensional morphological and functional imaging, likely in combination with advanced catheter localization and navigation techniques, which will utilize available images e.g. for roadmap based guidance. New interventional instruments providing intra-vascular and intra-cardiac imaging, while localizable by non line-of-sight localization techniques, will enter the field for improved interventional imaging and guidance.

Considering the current developments in medical imaging, due to the real-time and spatial resolution demands in intervention guidance, X-ray fluoroscopy will play a major role for the foreseeable future. However, new functionality will be introduced to increase the efficiency and efficacy of the procedures. Besides importing three-dimensional pre-interventional data, it is likely that the flexibility of recent X-ray system will be utilized for providing geometrically exact morphological information of the vessel lumen in 3D at high isotropic spatial resolution during the intervention. This information will improve the quantitative assessment of lesion dimensions and will enable the prediction of optimal projection angles providing minimal foreshortening and vessel overlap for a certain lesion. Roadmap-based techniques, either for dose reduction or improvement of the accuracy and efficacy of the procedures, will likely be introduced at a later stage, when the more complex procedures are clinically established and reliable registration and motion-compensation techniques will be available.

REFERENCES

1. R. Schrader, Indications and techniques of transcatheter closure of patent foramen ovale, *J Interv Cardiol* **16**(6), 543-51 (2003).
2. J.A. Condado, M. Velez-Gimon, Catheter-based approach to mitral regurgitation, *J Interv Cardiol* **16**(6), 523-34 (2003).

3.   J.M. Jones, W.J. Koch, Gene therapy approaches to cardiovascular disease, *Methods Mol Med* **112**, 49-57 (2005).

4.   J. Jago, A. Collet-Billon, C. Chenal, J.M. Jong, S. Makram-Ebeid, XRES - Adaptive enhancement of ultrasound images, *Medica Mundi* **46**(3), 36-41 (2002).

5.   J.Y. Meuwly, J. Thiran, F. Gudinchet, Application of Adaptive Image Processing Technique to Real-Time Spatial Compound Ultrasound Imaging Improves Image Quality, *Investigative Radiology* **38**(5), 257-262 (2003).

6.   P.J. Burt, E.H. Adelson, The Laplacian Pyramid as a Compact Image Code, *IEEE Trans Commun* **31**, 532-540 (1983).

7.   J.T. Maddux, O. Wink, J.C. Messenger, B.M. Groves, R. Liao, J. Strzelczyk, S.Y. Chen, J.D. Carroll, Randomized study of the safety and clinical utility of rotational angiography versus standard angiography in the diagnosis of coronary artery disease. *Catheter Cardiovasc Interv* **62**(2), 167-74 (2004).

8.   E. Kuon, P.N. Niederst, J.B. Dahm, Usefulness of rotational spin for coronary angiography in patients with advanced renal insufficiency, *Am J Cardiol* **90**(4), 369-373 (2002).

9.   B. Movassaghi, V. Rasche, M. Grass, M. Viergever, W. Niessen, A quantitative analysis of 3D coronary modeling from two or more projection images. *IEEE Trans Med Imag* **12**(23), 1517-1531 (2004).

10. S.Y.J. Chen, J.D. Carroll, 3-D Reconstruction of Coronary Arterial Tree to Optimize Angiographic Visualization, *IEEE Trans Med Imag* **19**(4), 318-336 (2000).

11. J.C. Messenger, S.Y. Chen, J.D. Carroll, J.E. Burchenal, K. Kioussopoulos, B.M. Groves, 3D coronary reconstruction from routine single-plane coronary angiograms: clinical validation and quantitative analysis of the right coronary artery in 100 patients, *Int J Card Imaging* **16**(6), 413-427 (2000).

12. G. Shechter, C. Ozturk, J.R. Resar, E.R. McVeigh, Respiratory motion of the heart from free breathing coronary angiograms. *IEEE Trans Med Imaging* **23**(8), 1046-1056 (2004).

13. V. Rasche, A. Buecker, M. Grass, R. Koppe, J. Op de Beek, R. Bertrams, R. Suurmond, H. Kuehl, R.W. Guenther, ECG-gated 3D-Rotational Coronary Angiography (3DRCA), *Proc CARS 2002,* 827-831 (2002).

14. C. Blondel, R. Vaillant, G. Malandain, N. Ayache, 3-D tomographic reconstruction of coronary arteries using a precomputed 4-D motion field, *Physics in Medicine and Biology* **49**(11), 2197-2208 (2004).

15. B. Movassaghi, V. Rasche, R. Florent, M.A.Viergever, W. Niessen, 3D reconstruction from calibrated motion-compensated 2D projections, *Proc CARS 2003, London*, 1079-1084 (2003).

16. M. Grass, R. Koppe, E. Klotz, P. Proksa, M.H. Kuhn, H. Aerts, J. Op de Beek, R. Kemkers, 3D Reconstruction of High Contrast Objects using C-Arm Image Intensifer Projection Data, *Computer Med Imaging Graphics* **23**(6), 311-321 (1999).

17. K.T. Vakharia, J.M. Mishell, T.A. Ports, Y. Yeghiazarians, A.D. Michaels, Determination of Adequate Stent Expansion: A Comparison of Quantitative Coronary Angiography, Intravascular Ultrasound, and Stent Boost Fluoroscopic Imaging, *SCAI C-45,* in press (2005).

18. F. Banovac, N. Glossop, D. Lindisch, D. Tanaka, E. Levy, S. Xu, K. Cleary, Liver Tumor Biopsy in a Respiring Phantom with the Assistance of a Novel Electromagnetic Navigation Device, *MICCAI 2002*, LNCS 2488, 200-207 (2002).

19. S.A. Ben-Haim, D. Osadchy, I. Schuster, L. Gepstein, G. Hayam, M.E. Josephson, Non-fluoroscopic, in-vivo navigation and mapping technology, *Nat Med* **12**, 1393-1395 (1996).

20. S.B. Solomon, P. White, D.E. Acker, J. Strandberg, A.C. Venbrux, Real-time bronchoscope tip localization enables three-dimensional CT-image guidance for transbronchial needle aspiration in swine, *Chest* **114**, 1405-1410 (1998).

21. S. Krüger, H. Timinger, R. Grewer, J. Borgert, Modality-integrated magnetic catheter tracking for x-ray vascular interventions, *Phys Med Biol* **50**, 581-597 (2005).

22. J. Krüger, A. Viswanathan, J. Borgert, N. Glossop, Y. Yang, B.J. Wood, An electro-magnetically tracked laparoscopic ultrasound for multi-modality minimally invasive surgery, *Proc CARS 2005, Berlin*, 746-751 (2005).

23. J. Borgert, S. Krüger, H. Timinger, J. Krücker, N. Glossop, A. Durrani, B.J. Wood, Respiratory Motion Compensation with Tracked Internal and External Sensors during CT Guided Procedures, *Proc CARS 2005, Berlin,* 577-582 (2005).

24. R.L. Ehman, J.P. Felmlee, Adaptive technique for high-definition MR imaging of moving structures, *Radiology* **173**, 225-63 (1989).

25. D. Manke, P. Rösch, K. Nehrke, P. Börnert, O. Dössel, Model evaluation and calibration for prospective respiratory motion correction in coronary MR angiography based on 3-D image registration, *IEEE Trans Med Imag* **21**, 1132-41 (2002).

26. G. Shechter, C. Ozturk, J.R. Resar, E.R.McVeigh, Respiratory motion of the heart from free breathing coronary angiograms, *IEEE Trans Med Imag* **23**, 1046-56 (2004).

27. B.U. Koehler, C. Hennig, R. Orglmeister, The principles of software QRS detection *IEEE Eng Med Biol* **21**, 42-57 (2002).

28. W. Sediono, O. Dössel, Heart Phantom: A Simple Elastomechanical Model of Ventricle, *Proc CARS 2002*, 1112 (2002).

29. H. Timinger, S. Krueger, J. Borgert, R. Grewer, Motion compensation for interventional navigation on 3D static roadmaps based on an affine model and gating *Phys Med Biol* **49**, 719-732 (2004).

Chapter 12

MRI-GUIDED FOCUSED ULTRASOUND
Apparatus for Noval Treatment of Breast Cancer

Chrit T.W. Moonen, Charles Mougenot
Université 'Victor Segalen Bordeaux 2', Bordeaux, France

Abstract: High Intensity Focused Ultrasound (HIFU) is the only known technology that can be used to generate local hyperthermia deep inside the human body in a non-invasive way. However, heat conduction and ultrasound energy absorption are difficult to predict in living tissue, and in particular in tumors, because of variations in blood flow and tissue composition. MRI guidance of the procedure allows in situ target definition and identification of nearby healthy tissue to be spared. It can then be used to provide continuous, precise temperature mapping during HIFU sonication for spatial and temporal control of the heating procedure based on automatic feedback to the HIFU apparatus. In addition, MRI also permits early evaluation of the efficacy of the treatment in situ. The principles of the combined MRI and focused ultrasound are reviewed, together with an overview of a novel platform for treatment of breast cancer.

Keywords: MRI, high intensity focused ultrasound, HIFU, thermo-therapy, breast

1.   INTRODUCTION

Local heating of tissues deep inside the body requires the use of a beam of electromagnetic or sound waves with the following characteristics: 1) deep penetration; 2) absorption by tissue transformed in heat; 3) harmless for tissues in the beam path; 4) ability to focus into a small region. Within the full spectrum of electromagnetic radiation and sound waves, only ultrasound and radiofrequency waves are capable of noninvasively depositing energy deep inside the human body without harming tissue in the beam path. Because of its short wavelength, ultrasound can be focused into a small, well-defined area of interest contrary to radiofrequency waves. Focused ultrasound is thus the only known technology that can be used to generate local hyperthermia non-invasively. The local temperature increase may serve

G. Spekowius and T. Wendler (Eds.), Advances in Healthcare Technology, 183-200.
© 2006 *Springer. Printed in the Netherlands.*

a wide variety of medical interventions such as ablation of tumoral tissue[1] or cardiac tissue to treat arrhytmias[2]. In addition, local hyperthermia has been suggested for local drug delivery with thermosensitive microcarriers[3], control of gene therapy using heat-sensitive promoters[4] and heat-activated chemotherapy[5]. The large potential in the field of neurosurgery and minimally invasive tissue ablation was realized as early as 1942[6]. Technological developments[7-9] have led to successful experimental research[10,11] and clinical trials in the oncology field[12]. The primary action mechanism of HIFU is through elevation of temperature although cavitation effects (microbubble formation at very high ultrasound pressure waves) may also be utilized for tissue destruction[13] and increased endothelial permeability for macro-molecular agents[14,15]. Transrectal focused ultrasound is gaining acceptance as a clinical application for prostate cancer[12,16]. Despite promising results in other tissues, clinical use of HIFU is still rather limited. However, the recent FDA approval for MRI guided Focused Ultrasound for treatment of uterine fibroids has accelerated interest in this technology for cancer treatment.

Since the primary effect is thermal, it is important to control the temperature evolution during the treatment. The temperature evolution is a function of heat deposition and heat diffusion. Both parameters can be spatially heterogeneous and may be affected by temperature increases. Heat deposition by HIFU depends on the local absorption of ultrasound waves. Blood hardly absorb ultrasound energy. The absorption of ultrasound by soft tissue depends on composition and on the actual wavelength. Therefore, accurate quantification of energy deposition by focused ultrasound and absorption by tissue is difficult to predict. Heat conduction also depends on tissue composition. Diffusion and perfusion processes may vary locally as a function of tissue architecture and tissue composition. Physiological events such as temperature-dependent perfusion increases may play a role[17]. In case of ablation procedures, tissue coagulation may significantly modify heat conduction as well as energy absorption. As a consequence, heat losses and energy absorption are difficult to predict in advance of the procedure. Therefore, the performance of HIFU therapeutic heating can be expected to be improved significantly with real time evaluation of the temperature distribution, and even more so with feedback control algorithms assuring adequate heating throughout the area of interest.

Of the different imaging modalities, MRI appears the ideal tool for guiding the non-invasive treatment by hyperthermia. Particular advantages of MRI are that the technique allows temperature mapping[18] as well as target definition, and may even provide an early evaluation of the therapeutic efficacy. Based on such considerations, Cline and colleagues[19] realized early on that the combination of MRI and HIFU would be a very promising tool.

Subsequently, the technology was further developed based on a prototype HIFU system integrated with a whole body MRI system in Boston[20,21]. This paper describes an overview of the state-of-the-art and the important advances made since the beginning of the technology, more than 10 years ago. Because of the severe technical difficulties associated with the merging of the distinct MR and ultrasound methodologies, the number of laboratories utilizing this approach is probably still limited, and clinical studies have only started to appear in the literature[22-27]. Early clinical studies have concentrated on the treatment of uterine fibroids[22,23]. In addition, preliminary studies on breast cancer have been published recently[24-27]. The enormous potential may lead to a fast growth in the MRI/HIFU area. We will briefly review here the technical aspects of focused ultrasound. The rest of the paper is devoted to the description of a novel platform for MRI guided Focused Ultrasound treatment of breast cancer developed at the University of Bordeaux.

2.   FOCUSED ULTRASOUND

Ultrasound is a form of mechanical energy that is propagated as a vibrational wave of particles within the medium at a frequency between about 20 kHz and 10 MHz. The oscillatory displacement of particles is associated with a pressure wave. The behavior of ultrasound waves in medium may be described in a similar way to that in optics. At tissue interfaces reflection of the wave occurs according to Snell's law depending on the wave velocity and the incident angle. The speed of ultrasound is about 1550 ms^{-1} for soft tissue, independent of the ultrasound frequency. In fatty tissue the average speed is only slightly lower (1480 ms^{-1}), whereas in air spaces a value of 600 ms^{-1} is found. In bone, the speed is much higher (between 1800 and 3700 ms^{-1})[28]. Ultrasound beams are usually generated electrically using piezoceramic plates outside the body and propagate inwards either longitudinally (as is the case for hyperthermia purposes) or transversely (called shear waves). Focusing of the longitudinal waves can be achieved using a spherical curvature of the plates, with a suitably designed lens system, or with a multi-element transducer with independent phase control for each element (Phased-Array transducer, see below). The interference of the multiple waves leads to an interference pattern. In a homogeneous medium, the phase of all waves is identical at the focal point, whereas outside the focal point the differences in phase lead to destructive interference and thus attenuation of the pressure wave. The minimum diameter of the focal area is thus given by the wavelength λ, which is equal to the speed divided by the frequency. For example, when using 1.5MHz ultrasound, the wavelength is approximately 1 mm in soft tissue. For a typical spherical transducer, the focal area is ellipsoidal, with the approximate dimensions[29]:

$$d_t = 1.417 \left[\frac{R}{2a} \right]$$

[1]

and

$$d_x = 7.17 \left[\frac{R}{2a} \right]^2,$$

[2]

where d_t and d_x are the width in the plane parallel to the transducer, and along the transducer axis, respectively. R and 2a are the radius of curvature and the diameter of the transducer, respectively. Focusing ultrasound waves requires a large acoustic window, unobstructed by air or bone, to reach the theoretical values above.

Ultrasound energy is attenuated in tissue due to processes of absorption and scattering. Whereas ultrasound absorption is proportional to the square of frequency in free liquids, it is approximately linearly proportional with frequency in tissue. In addition, ultrasound absorption in tissue is much more efficient than in free liquids or in blood. The mechanisms of ultrasound absorption in tissue have been reviewed previously[30]. The efficient energy absorption in soft tissue may be related to the friction between and in structures with dimensions of the order of the wavelength used. Overall, the attenuation of a plane wave may be described by an exponentially decaying function. The intensity I_x at depth x with respect to that at the original position (I_0) is given by

$$I_x = I_0 e^{-2\mu x}$$

[3]

where the symbol μ represents the attenuation coefficient of the wave amplitude per unit path length. For 1.5 MHz ultrasound waves, the intensity in soft tissues will drop to about 50% at 50 mm penetration.

In inhomogeneous media, the multiple wave reflections make it difficult to focus ultrasound waves in the area of interest since the wave phase and attenuation will be different according to their pathway from transducer to target. When using a multiple-element transducer, individual amplitude and phase modification is feasible for each element. The problem remains how to find an algorithm to adjust each transducer element to accomplish focusing. A possible solution has been described by Fink and colleagues based upon their so-called principle of temporal return of waves[31]. The technique relies on using first a short duration ultrasound burst from the area of interest (either using a small transmitter or an echogenic particle) and measuring the reflected waves at several locations outside the body. A temporal return of the received wave pattern, corrected for attenuation effects, leads in turn to exact focusing in the area of interest. Promising results have been obtained. However, the need to first use a transmitter in the area of interest may limit its practical use. Recently, phased-Array transducer technology was used to focus ultrasound through the skull into brain tissue[32,33]. Therefore, neurological applications of focused ultrasound appear technologically feasible although further developments are still necessary to accomplish focusing in a noninvasive way and to avoid any risk of heating at or near the skull.

A detailed recent review on focused ultrasound technology can be found elsewhere[34].

3. MAGNETIC RESONANCE IMAGING FOR GUIDANCE OF FOCUSED ULTRASOUND THERMOTHERAPY

Ideally, a thermotherapeutic treatment is preceded by precise 3D target definition, and localization of nearby tissue that must be spared. Then, with the tissue position unchanged, the thermal therapy should be performed with continuous temperature monitoring of target tissue and nearby tissue to be spared. The therapy will be continued until the appropriate thermal dose[35] is delivered to the entire target volume. Then, a first assessment of efficacy and possible complications should be carried out.

MRI offers specific advantages for each part of this procedure. It is well known that MRI offers superb soft tissue contrast, either without or with MR contrast agents. Tissue boundaries can be identified with high precision. The known coordinates can thus be used directly for image-guided therapeutic procedures.

During the thermal procedure, continuous temperature imaging can be performed with MRI using specific pulse sequences and data processing. Noninvasive, three-dimensional mapping of temperature changes is feasible with MR, and may be based on the relaxation time T_1[18], the diffusion coefficient (D)[36], or proton resonance frequency (PRF)[37] of tissue water. The use of temperature-sensitive contrast agents can provide absolute temperature measurements[38]. The principles and performance of these methods have been reviewed recently[39,40]. The excellent linearity and near-independence with respect to tissue type[41], together with good temperature sensitivity, make PRF based temperature MRI the preferred choice for many applications at mid to high field strength (≥ 1 T). The PRF methods employ RF-spoiled gradient echo imaging methods[42]. A standard deviation of less than 1°C, for a temporal resolution below 1s and a spatial resolution of about 2 mm, is feasible for a single slice for immobile tissues. Corrections should be made for temperature-induced susceptibility effects in the PRF method[43]. If spin echo methods are preferred, for example when field homogeneity is poor, the D and T_1 based methods may give better results. The sensitivity of the D method is higher that of the T_1 methods provided that motion artifacts are avoided and the trace of D (note that D is a tensor) is evaluated. Fat suppression is necessary for most tissues when T_1, D or PRF methods are employed[44]. The latter three methods require excellent registration to correct for displacements between scans since changes with respect to a reference are mapped. Motion artifacts can severely degrade the accuracy of MR temperature maps and must be carefully corrected[40].

MRI may also assess therapeutic efficacy and possible complications. For example, a hemorrhage can be demonstrated based on T2* changes. Edema formation can be described by T2 changes. Also diffusion and perfusion changes can be identified with specific MR methods[45]. Therefore, MRI may play a large role for in situ assessment of tissue changes. However, note also that many apoptotic processes may take up to 24 hours to become clearly detectable. Therefore, efficacy assessment immediately following therapy is still of rather limited use.

For guidance by MRI, the transducer is placed on or inside the patient bed. Because of the very high magnetic field, the use of non-ferromagnetic materials is mandatory. The confined space within the bore of the magnet makes it difficult to design a system that provides comfort to the patient as well an uninterrupted pathway for the ultrasound waves from transducer to target.

4. AUTOMATIC FEEDBACK COUPLING BETWEEN THE HIFU HEATING AND MR TEMPERATURE MAPPING

Optimal control of the temperature-based treatment requires regulation of the temperature. Recent developments have shown that rapid MR imaging, followed by on-line data processing, and real-time feedback to the focused ultrasound output[46], combined with new temperature regulation algorithms, may provide such control. The regulation of temperature evolution of the focal point was described based on temperature mapping and a physical model of local energy deposition and heat conduction. An important element in the stability of the regulator was the real-time evaluation of temperature gradients near the focal point. This was achieved by on-line calculation of the Laplacian from the temperature maps[47]. The following expression was used for automatic modification of the ultrasound output power *P(t)* in order to follow a predescribed time evolution of the temperature $\Theta(t)$:

$$P(t) = \frac{1}{\alpha_2(T_{max})}\left[\frac{d\Theta(t)}{dt} - \alpha_1(T_{max}) \cdot \nabla^2 T_{max}(t) + a \cdot [\Theta(t) - T_{max}(t)] + \frac{a^2}{4} \cdot \Delta(t)\right] \quad [4]$$

where α_1 and α_2 are the heat diffusivity in the tissue and the HIFU absorption coefficient, respectively. The maximum temperature is indicated as $T_{max}(t)$, and ∇^2 represents the Laplacian operator. Equation 4 resembles a classical PID (proportional, integral and derivative) type of temperature control, in which the term $\Theta(t)$-$T_{max}(t)$ is the difference between the measured and the planned temperature at time *t*, and $\Delta(t)$ the integral of the difference between the measured and the planned time evolution[47]. The parameter *a* is related to the characteristic response time t_r of the regulation loop ($a=2/t_r$). The objectives are that the temperature in the focal point should quickly reach the target value without overshooting or oscillating, and then remain constant for a user-defined period. It was demonstrated that the regulation system is insensitive to errors in estimates of ultrasound absorption and heat diffusion so long as the ratio of the two parameters is within a fairly large range. Therefore, the temperature trajectory of the focal point can be automatically regulated with a precision that is close to that of the precision of the temperature measurements at the focal point.

5. TREATMENT OF AN ENTIRE REGION OF INTEREST WITH MR FEEDBACK CONTROL OF THE HIFU PROCEDURE

Spatial control of temperature evolution during HIFU hyperthermia is necessary to guarantee the desired thermal dose in the volume of interest. Treatment of large volumes using a fixed focal point transducer was initially based on MR guidance of the complete heat treatment of a single point, followed by displacement of the HIFU focal point, and repeating the procedure until the target volume was covered[48]. Such a procedure necessitates long treatment times, and may leave 'gaps' between treated locations. Recently, Mougenot et al.[49] proposed an approach where the focal point was moved along multiple inside-out spiral trajectories covering the target region under continuous and maximal HIFU power for minimal treatment time. A complete PID control in the spiral plane provided stability and temperature uniformity within a large target region and followed closely predictions from simulations. It is evident that such methods can be even more useful when combined with phased array transducers that allow very fast (electronic) motion of a focal point. Therefore, upon multiple coverage of the target area, possible non-linear effects may be better corrected for. It should be kept in mind that simultaneous treatment of a large area of interest may lead to excessive near-field heating, and accumulation of undesired thermal dose in anterior and posterior areas with respect to the target region. Also, any motion of the transducer will lead to small modifications of the magnetic field even in the case of non-ferromagnetic material, and should be corrected for in particular when using the PRF method for temperature mapping.

The automated MRI feedback coupling to the HIFU heating relies on high speed, high SNR, temperature imaging. It has been shown that motion can severely degrade MR temperature mapping. Correction of motion artifacts, and acceleration of temperature mapping, is therefore an area of much interest in the further development of MRI guided HIFU. Recently, methods have been proposed ranging from the use of respiratory and/or cardiac triggering methods[50,51], the use of navigator echoes, and advanced post processing methods[40].

6.   NOVEL MRI-HIFU PLATFORM FOR TREATMENT OF BREAST CANCER

The platform developed for the treatment of uterine fibroids[22,23] has also been used for preliminary studies of breast cancer[24-27]. However, the long study duration, elongated focal point, and lack of real-time control may limit its use in clinical practice. Below, we describe a novel platform for MRI guided HIFU treatment of breast cancer with the following novel features:

- Enhanced safety by firing predominantly in a coronal plane avoiding heat deposition towards the rest of the body.
- Enhanced safety by providing real-time automatic control of the heating procedure.
- Enhanced efficacy by assuring adequate thermal dose throughout the region of interest.
- Drastically shortened treatment time due to heating of a large volume simultaneously due to volume temperature control.

Below, the system will be described in more detail. Figure 12-1 shows a diagram of the layout of the MRI-HIFU system. It shows the 1.5T MRI system (unmodified Intera system). A patient positioning system is placed on top of the standard bed and will be described below. The 256-element phased array transducer is placed inside the positioning system. The transducer is connected via a 256-channel impedance matching box with the main generator/amplifier positioned inside the Faraday cage and communicating with the HIFU computer by optical fiber. The generator/ amplifier is divided into 256 individual channels providing each 3Watt electrical output at 1.5 MHz with independent phase and amplitude control. Modification of amplitude and phase for all elements is achieved in less than 100 ms. Special attention is paid to the avoidance of interference with the MR detection frequency of 64 MHz. Temperature mapping is consistently achieved during HIFU without significant degradation of the temperature maps. The MR images are reconstructed using the standard Intera reconstructor and then sent as a set of complex data in real-time to the HIFU control computer. Rapid image processing then leads to the generation of temperature maps, followed by the calculation of the next set of amplitude and phase outputs for the 256 HIFU elements as well as the visualization of the latest temperature maps and thermal dose maps.

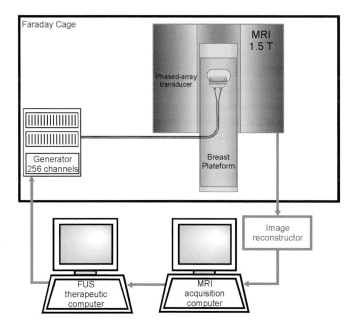

Figure 12-1. Layout of apparatus for focused ultrasound under MR guidance.

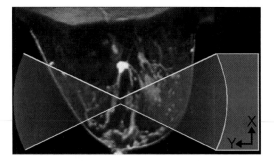

Figure 12-2. Enhanced safety by focusing predominantly in coronal orientation thus avoiding firing towards the body and avoiding inadvertent heating of other organs.

The patient is positioned prone on the table with the breast protruding into a gap of the positioning table. Below the table, the transducer can rotate around the breast in a coronal plane. Figure 12-2 shows the relative position of the breast and the HIFU transducer with the ultrasound beam highlighted indicating that the safety feature of avoiding firing towards the body and thus avoiding inadvertent heating of other tissues. Figure 12-3 shows the particular transducer geometry. Its overall shape is elliptical with 256 individual HIFU elements that are positioned in an optimized asymmetrical manner to minimize heat deposition in secondary lobes when the focal point is moved electronically away from its natural focal point.

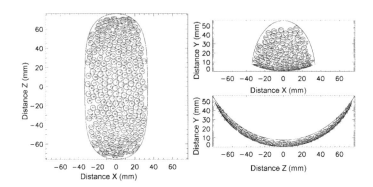

Figure 12-3. Transducer geometry with 256 elements in optimized asymmetrical compact disposition.

Figure 12-4 shows a diagram of the patient positioning system on top of the standard MR bed with the mechanical control at the inferior position. Figure 12-5 indicates the four motions of freedom under control of the operator by the three knobs and by the action of sliding the complete table along the magnet bore axis. The three knobs control a right-left displacement, a complete rotation of the transducer around the breast and a tilt of the transducer allowing a small deviation form the coronal plane. The latter tilt was preferred above an up-down displacement in order to avoid loss of available space in the magnet bore.

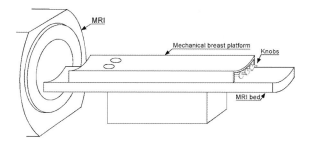

Figure 12-4. Global overview of the MRI with breast therapeutic platform. The function of the knobs is explained in Figure 12-5.

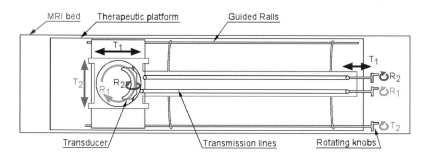

Figure 12-5. Mechanical breast therapeutic platform including 2 rotations and 2 translations. The four principal motions of freedom are controlled by the three knobs at the bottom and in addition the horizontal sliding of the complete platform.

Figure 12-6 shows photographs of (left) the inside of the patient positioning table with the elliptical HIFU transducer mounted on the rotating device viewed from the bottom, and (right) the inside of the breast gap with the transducer visible immediately beneath the gap as viewed from the top. Figure 12-7 shows (left) a photograph of the transducer together with the water reservoir serving as the interface between breast and transducer. The water reservoir is cooled continuously by pumping cooled water through four inlet and four outlet tubes as can be seen on the photograph and (right) on the corresponding MR image.

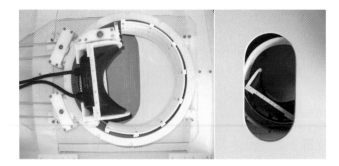

Figure 12-6. Bottom and top view of the phased array transducer inside the mechanical breast therapeutic platform. The transducer can rotate freely over 360° in the coronal plane.

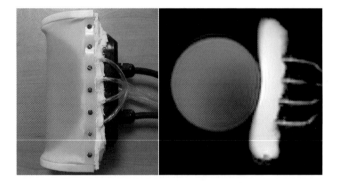

Figure 12-7. Phased array transducer with water reservoir and hydraulic cooling system (left), with four inlet and four outlet tubes visible in the MR image (right).

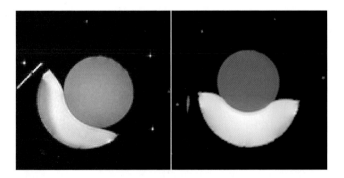

Figure 12-8. Transducer positioning from sulfate copper tubes allowing easy determination of the natural focal point of the system based on MR fiducials.

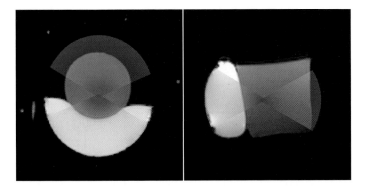

Figure 12-9. Membrane coupling check to assure complete water bath interface for HIFU with regard to aperture angle.

The HIFU coordinate system must be easily translated into the MR coordinate system. Figure 12-8 provides a convenient way to accomplish this using a set of fiducial markers positioned on the HIFU transducer. Four tube fiducials indicate the ZY plane with the focal point in the middle between the left and right markers. A fifth tube indicates the tilt of the transducer. Figure 12-9 allows easy checking of appropriate water interface covering the complete HIFU probe aperture.

Figure 12-10 shows the very large aperture (left) of the transducer and the relatively small height (6 cm). The simulations of the acoustic field shown in Figure 12-11 indicate a very small focal point of 1,60 x 0,48 x 1,28 mm. The small focal point excellent spatial definition of the heating as can be seen in the temperature maps of Figure 12-11 and thermal dose maps of Figure 12-12 obtained in a gel phantom.

7. DISCUSSION AND CONCLUSION

MRI guided HIFU allows an entirely non-invasive approach for local thermal therapies. The added value of MRI to the heating procedure by HIFU is evident. In situ target definition and identification by MRI of nearby healthy tissue to be spared can be followed by continuous, precise temperature mapping allowing spatial and temporal control of the heating procedure based on automatic feedback to the HIFU apparatus. An initial assessment of the efficacy of the intervention and possible complications may be performed immediately following therapy (albeit limited by the delayed effects of apoptosis and edema).

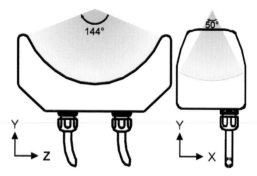

Figure 12-10. Large aperture angle induces a small focal point size.

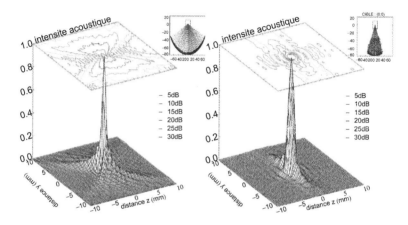

Figure 12-11. Simulations of the acoustic field: All the ultrasound energy is deposed into a coronal slice of 4mm. The focal point size is 0,48×1,28×1,6mm³.

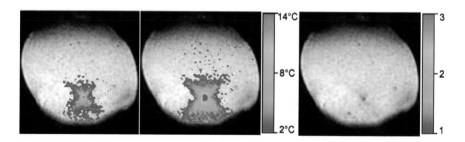

Figure 12-12. Left: Focal point shape from temperature acquired 5s and 15s after a heating procedure with 100 watt (electrical) of a gel composed of 2% agar and 1% of silicium powder. Right: Thermal dose after heating. The area exceeding the lethal dose threshold measures 2×2mm² in a single slice of 5mm.

The general principles of the technology have now been developed and feasibility on animal tissue and in clinical trials on uterine fibroids as well preliminary breast cancer protocols has been demonstrated. It is expected that phased-array ultrasound technology combined with increasing speed of temperature imaging will further help the development. The prototype system described here is expected to help in optimizing treatment strategy of breast cancer.

Significant technological challenges remain for widespread applications in other organs. In moving targets, temperature imaging is still hampered by motion problems despite recent advances. In addition, the focal point must accurately track the moving target. For brain, the major problem is the attenuation of ultrasound by the skull, and the difficulties to focus ultrasound waves to a precise location in the brain. However, recent progress has shown its feasibility. MRI guided focused ultrasound is practical with current technology in tissues that are accessible with a large acoustic window and that can be immobilized, e.g. breast, prostate and muscle. Based on the wealth of fundamental research and literature on alternative temperature controlled therapeutic approaches (local drug delivery, gene therapy, etcetera), it can be expected that, once a precise, non-invasive, spatial and temporal control of local hyperthermia is reliable, such alternative approaches may also soon be tested in the clinic.

REFERENCES

1. F.J. Fry, L.K. Johnson, Tumor irradiation with intense ultrasound, *Ultrasound Med Biol* **4**, 337-341 (1978).
2. S. Levy, Biophysical basis and cardiac lesions caused by different techniques of cardiac arrhythmia ablation, *Arch Mal Coeur Vaiss* **88**, 1465-1469 (1995).
3. J.N. Weinstein, R.L. Magin, M.B. Yatvin, et al., Liposomes and local hyperthermia, selective delivery of methotrexate to heated tumors, *Science* **204**, 188-191 (1979).
4. C. Rome, F. Couillaud, C.T. Moonen, Spatial and temporal control of expression of therapeutic genes using heat shock protein promoters, *Methods* **35**(2), 188-98 (2005).
5. M. Urano, M. Kuroda, Y. Nishimura, For the clinical application of thermochemo-therapy given at mild temperatures, *Int J Hyperthermia* **15**, 79-107 (1999).
6. J.G. Lynn, R.L. Zwemer, A.J. Chick, et al., A new method for the generation and use of focused ultrasound in experimental biology, *J Gen Physiol* **26**, 179-193 (1942).
7. J.Y. Chapelon, D. Cathignol, C. Cain, et al., New piezoelectric transducers for therapeutic ultrasound, *Ultrasound Med Biol* **26**, 153-159 (2000).
8. E.S. Ebbini, C.A. Cain, A spherical-section ultrasound phased array applicator for deep localized hyperthermia, *IEEE Trans Biomed Eng* **38**, 634-643 (1991).
9. F.J. Fry, Precision high intensity focusing ultrasonic machines for surgery, *Am J Phys Med* **37**, 152-156 (1958).
10. J.Y. Chapelon, J. Margonari, F. Vernier, et al., In vivo effects of high-intensity ultrasound on prostatic adenocarcinoma Dunning R3327, *Cancer Res* **52**, 6353-6357 (1992).

11. R.S. Foster, R. Bihrle, N.T. Sanghvi, et al., High-intensity focused ultrasound in the treatment of prostatic disease, *Eur Urol* **23**, 29-33 (1993).

12. A. Gelet A, J.Y. Chapelon, R. Bouvier, et al., Transrectal high-intensity focused ultrasound, minimally invasive therapy of localized prostate cancer, *J Endourol* **14**, 519-528 (2000).

13. F. Chavrier, J.Y. Chapelon, A. Gelet, et al., Modeling of high-intensity focused ultrasound-induced lesions in the presence of cavitation bubbles, *J Acoust Soc Am* **108**, 432-440 (2000).

14. M.D. Bednarski, J.W. Lee, M.R. Callstrom, et al., In vivo target-specific delivery of macromolecular agents with MR-guided focused ultrasound, *Radiology* **204**, 263-268 (1997).

15. K. Hynynen, N. McDannold, N.A. Sheikov, F.A. Jolesz, N. Vykhodtseva, Local and reversible blood-brain barrier disruption by noninvasive focused ultrasound at frequencies suitable for trans-skull sonications, *Neuroimage* **24**, 12-20 (2005).

16. C.G. Chaussy, S. Thuroff, High-intensive focused ultrasound in localized prostate cancer, *J Endourol* **14**, 293-299 (2000).

17. J.A. de Zwart, F.C. Vimeux, J. Palussiere, et al., On-line correction and visualization of motion during MRI-controlled hyperthermia, *Magn Reson Med*, in press (2005).

18. T.E. Dudar, R.K. Jain, Differential response of normal and tumor microcirculation to hyperthermia, *Cancer Res* **44**, 605-612 (1984).

19. D.L. Parker, V. Smith, P. Sheldon, et al., Temperature distribution measurements in two-dimensional NMR imaging, *Med Phys* **10**, 321-325 (1983).

20. H.E. Cline, J.F. Schenck, K. Hynynen, et al., MR-guided focused ultrasound surgery, *J Comput Assist Tomogr* **16**, 956-965 (1992).

21. H.E. Cline, K. Hynynen, R.D. Watkins, et al., Focused US system for MR imaging-guided tumor ablation, *Radiology* **194**, 731-737 (1995).

22. K. Hynynen, N.I. Vykhodtseva, A.H. Chung, et al., Thermal effects of focused ultrasound on the brain, determination with MR imaging, *Radiology* **204**, 247-253 (1997).

23. C.M. Tempany, E.A. Stewart, N. McDannold, B.J. Quade, F.A. Jolesz, K. Hynynen, MR imaging-guided focused ultrasound surgery of uterine leiomyomas, a feasibility study, *Radiology* **226**, 897-905 (2003).

24. J. Hindley, W.M. Gedroyc, L. Regan, et al., MRI guidance of focused ultrasound therapy of uterine fibroids, early results, *AJR Am J Roentgenol* **183**, 1713-1719 (2004).

25. D. Gianfelice, A. Khiat, M. Amara, A. Belblidia, Y. Boulanger, MR imaging-guided focused ultrasound surgery of breast cancer, correlation of dynamic contrast-enhanced MRI with histopathologic findings, *Breast Cancer Res Treat* **82**, 93-101 (2003).

26. D. Gianfelice, A. Khiat, Y. Boulanger, M. Amara, A. Belblidia, Feasibility of magnetic resonance imaging-guided focused ultrasound surgery as an adjunct to tamoxifen therapy in high-risk surgical patients with breast carcinoma, *J Vasc Interv Radiol* **14**, 1275-82 (2003).

27. D.F. Kacher, F.A. Jolesz, MR imaging-guided breast ablative therapy, *Radiol Clin North Am* **42**, 947-962 (2004).

28. D.B. Zippel, M.Z. Papa, The use of MR imaging guided focused ultrasound in breast cancer patients; a preliminary phase one study and review, *Breast Cancer* **12**, 32-38 (2005).

29. S.A. Goss, R.L. Johnston, F. Dunn, Comprehensive compilation of empirical ultrasonic properties of mammalian tissues, *J Acoust Soc Am* **64**, 423-57 (1978).

30. J.W. Hunt, Principles of ultrasound used for hyperthermia, *NATO ASI Series E* **127**, (Martinus Nijhoff Publishers, Boston, 1987).

31. F. Dunn, Ultrasonic attenuation, absorption, and velocity in tissues and organs, Vol. **453**, (NBS Spec Publ, Washington, 1976).
32. J.L. Thomas, F. Wu, M. Fink, Time reversal focusing applied to lithotripsy, *Ultrason Imaging* **18**, 106-121 (1996).
33. G.T. Clement, J. White, K. Hynynen, Investigation of a large-area phased array for focused ultrasound surgery through the skull, *Phys Med Biol* **45**, 1071-1083 (2000).
34. K. Hynynen, G.T. Clement, N. McDannold, N. Vykhodtseva, R. King, P.J. White, S. Vitek, F.A. Jolesz, 500-element ultrasound phased array system for noninvasive focal surgery of the brain, a preliminary rabbit study with ex vivo human skulls, *Magn Reson Med* **52**, 100-107 (2004).
35. A.L. Malcolm, G.R. ter Haar, Ablation of tissue volumes using high intensity focused ultrasound, *Ultrasound Med Biol* **22**, 659-69 (1996).
36. S.A. Sapareto, W.C. Dewey, Thermal dose determination in cancer therapy, *Int J Radiat Oncol Biol Phys* **10**, 787-800 (1984).
37. N. McDannold, K. Hynynen, D. Wolf, et al., MRI evaluation of thermal ablation of tumors with focused ultrasound, J *Magn Reson Imaging* **8**, 91-100 (1998).
38. D. Le Bihan, J. Delannoy, R.L. Levin, Temperature mapping with MR imaging of molecular diffusion, application to hyperthermia, *Radiology* **171**, 853-857 (1989).
39. Y. Ishihara, A. Calderon, H. Watanabe, et al., A precise and fast temperature mapping method using water proton chemical shift, *Proc SMRM, Berlin,* 4803 (1992).
40. S. Fossheim, K. Il'yasov, U. Wiggen, et al., Paramagnetic Liposomes as Thermo-sensitive Probes for MRI In Vitro Feasibility Studies, *Proc ISMRM, Philadelphia,* 725 (1999).
41. B. Quesson, J.A. de Zwart, C.T. Moonen, Magnetic resonance temperature imaging for guidance of thermotherapy, *J Magn Reson Imaging* **12**, 525-533 (2000)
42. B. Denis de Senneville, B. Quesson, C.T. Moonen, Magnetic Resonance Temperature Imaging, *Int J Hyperthermia*, in press (2005).
43. R.D. Peters, R.S. Hinks, R.M. Henkelman, Ex vivo tissue-type independence in proton-resonance frequency shift MR thermometry, *Magn Reson Med* **40**, 454-459 (1998).
44. J. De Poorter, C. De Wagter, Y. De Deene, et al., Noninvasive MRI thermometry with the proton resonance frequency (PRF) method, in vivo results in human muscle, *Magn Reson Med* **33**, 74-81 (1995).
45. R.D. Peters, R.S. Hinks, R.M. Henkelman, Heat-source orientation and geometry dependence in proton-resonance frequency shift magnetic resonance thermometry, *Magn Reson Med* **41**, 909-918 (1999).
46. J.A. de Zwart, F.C. Vimeux, C. Delalande, et al., Fast lipid-suppressed MR temperature mapping with echo-shifted gradient- echo imaging and spectral-spatial excitation, *Magn Reson Med* **42**, 53-59 (1999).
47. C.T. Moonen, P.C. van Zijl, J.A. Frank, et al., Functional magnetic resonance imaging in medicine and physiology, *Science* **250**, 53-61 (1990).
48. F.C. Vimeux, J.A. De Zwart, J. Palussiere, R. Fawaz, C. Delalande, Canioni P, N. Grenier, C.T. Moonen, Real-time control of focused ultrasound heating based on rapid MR thermometry, *Invest Radiol* **34**, 190-193 (1999).
49. R. Salomir, F.C. Vimeux, J.A. de Zwart, et al., Hyperthermia by MR-guided focused ultrasound, accurate temperature control based on fast MRI and a physical model of local energy deposition and heat conduction, *Magn Reson Med* **43**, 342-347 (2000).
50. N.J. McDannold, F.A. Jolesz, K.H. Hynynen, Determination of the optimal delay between sonications during focused ultrasound surgery in rabbits by using MR imaging to monitor thermal buildup in vivo, *Radiology* **211**, 419-426 (1999).

51. C. Mougenot, R. Salomir, J. Palussiere, N. Grenier, C.T. Moonen, Automatic spatial and7 temporal temperature control for MR-guided focused ultrasound using fast 3D MR thermometry and multispiral trajectory of the focal point, *Magn Reson Med* **52**, 1005-1015 (2004).
52. C. Weidensteiner, B. Quesson, B. Caire-Gana, N. Kerioui, A. Rullier, H. Trillaud, C.T. Moonen, Real-time MR temperature mapping of rabbit liver in vivo during thermal ablation, *Magn Reson Med* **50**, 322-330 (2003).
53. C. Weidensteiner, N. Kerioui, B. Quesson, B.D. de Senneville, H. Trillaud, C.T. Moonen, Stability of real-time MR temperature mapping in healthy and diseased human liver, *J Magn Reson Imaging* **19**, 438-46 (2004).
54. N. Vykhodtseva, V. Sorrentino, F.A. Jolesz, et al., MRI detection of the thermal effects of focused ultrasound on the brain, *Ultrasound Med Biol* **26**, 871-880 (2000).

Chapter 13

ADVANCES IN EXTERNAL BEAM RADIATION THERAPY

Towards Image-Guided and Adaptive Radiotherapy Using Multi-modal Imaging

Todd McNutt[1], Michael R. Kaus[2], Lothar Spies[2]

[1]*Johns Hopkins University, Baltimore, MD, USA;* [2]*Philips Research, Hamburg, Germany*

Abstract: Radiation therapy has advanced in the last decade fueled by the advancement of dose delivery (3D conformal, IMRT), computer processing, and medical imaging. Image processing techniques such as model-based image segmentation and deformable registration are becoming efficient enough for a clinical setting. Biological modeling based on nuclear medicine imaging is needed to provide a quantitative understanding of tumor biology and enable to identify regions of the tumor resistant to radiation, thereby, warranting a higher dose level. These imaging and processing techniques promise to advance radiotherapy with the ability to monitor the course of treatment by enabling image-guided radiotherapy and adaptive radiotherapy.

Keywords: Image guided radiotherapy, adaptive radiotherapy, ART, IMRT, molecular imaging, biological modeling, deformable image registration, image segmentation

1.   INTRODUCTION

Cancer is the second leading cause of death in the industrialized countries and the only major disease for which death rates are increasing. The demand for cancer care will increase over the decade as the aging of the baby boomer population drives a dramatic increase in the incidence of many cancers.

Approximately 60% of cancer patients are treated with external beam Radiotherapy (RT) at some point during management of their disease. The main goal of RT is to maximize the dose to the target while limiting the dose

G. Spekowius and T. Wendler (Eds.), Advances in Healthcare Technology, 201-216.

to nearby healthy organs ('risk organs'), in order to improve control of tumor growth and limit side effects.

Radiation therapy is primarily used to treat cancer by locally targeting radiation to the diseased tissue. Radiation beams are produced by medical linear accelerators. These devices are mounted on a gantry with a rotating couch to allow for many beam directions to be focused on the target volume. Sparing of normal tissues is accomplished in two fundamental ways: Geometric avoidance of normal tissues is accomplished by directing multiple beams at the target, thus delivering a high dose where the beams intersect at the target, and a relatively lower dose outside of the intersection. Biological sparing of normal tissue is accomplished by fractionating the therapy over several weeks, irradiating daily. The tumor tissue lacks repair mechanisms to repair DNA damage from the radiation, whereas normal tissues can repair minor DNA damage. Therefore, by fractionating the treatment, normal tissues are provided time to repair, thus biologically sparing the normal tissue.

In the late 1980s and 90s Computed Tomography (CT) based treatment planning became available due to the increased performance of computers. Both the imaging capabilities and the ability to compute radiation dose distributions on CT provided the framework for the modern 3D Radiotherapy Treatment Planning (RTP) system. These systems provide clinicians the ability to truly visualize and plan the treatments considering the true 3D nature of the problem.

Today, the current workflow for a patient begins with a CT simulation where the patient is immobilized with body molds and/or head masks. A CT scan is acquired and the patient is marked for repeated alignment with localization lasers in the treatment room. The treatment planning is then performed on the CT scan where beam geometries, energies, and collimation are determined, and the resultant dose distribution is computed. The treatments are then performed daily for several weeks. During the course of treatment, different imaging modalities are used to monitor the geometric setup of the patient to verify constancy in the patient position.

There have been many advances in the techniques used to deliver the treatment. Intensity Modulated Radiotherapy (IMRT) has allowed for each beam to be modulated, enabling dose distributions to carve out the target volume and spare normal tissues in the millimeter range. Several techniques and strategies have evolved and are in use today.

The research described in this chapter focus on the ability to accurately predict the dose and to precisely deliver the radiation to conform the dose to the target volume utilizing IMRT; the improvement in target and critical structure definitions through the use of multi-modality imaging; and the tools to enable the monitoring of the course of treatment to support image guided radiotherapy (IGRT) which provides daily alignment of the patient with soft tissue target volumes, and adaptive radiotherapy (ART) which provides the monitoring the treatment through repeat imaging for decision support on modifying the treatment strategy.

2. INTENSITY MODULATED RADIOTHERAPY

IMRT is a method to determine the optimal beam intensity pattern for each beam to deliver the dose distribution specified by a set of treatment objectives and constraints. Under IMRT, the paradigm of RT changes from specifying beam directions and apertures, to one where one specifies dose or biology based treatment objectives and the computer will optimize the modulated beam intensities to best deliver the treatment[1].

A typical target objective would be to deliver a uniform dose of 60 Gy in 30 fractions, and a typical critical structure objective would be to keep the dose below 25 Gy in more than 70% of the volume of the structure. Figure 13-1 shows a typical IMRT treatment.

The process of IMRT utilizes an inverse planning strategy that iteratively optimizes the intensity pattern of each beam to deliver the desired dose distribution defined by the objective functions. The intensity pattern of a beam is represented by a matrix of beamlets, each being a parameter of the treatment. The optimization process begins by initializing the intensity map (beamlets) of each beam to expose the target objective. Then the dose is computed for the set of beams. The treatment objective is evaluated, and the derivative of the objective with respect to each beamlet is determined. A new intensity map for each beam is determined by the optimization, and the dose is recomputed. This process is repeated until the improvement in the treatment objective between iterations is small indicating convergence to an ideal solution of intensity modulation.

Accurate dose calculation for RT is quite time consuming and is a difficult challenge for efficient IMRT planning. The convolution/super-position (C/S) dose engine in the Pinnacle[3] treatment planning system requires approximately 20 seconds per beam on a SunBlade 2000. This dose engine is quite accurate[2-9], but lacks the speed required for during IMRT optimization. In order to maintain the accuracy of the C/S method, and gain the speed required for IMRT, the Delta Pixel Beam dose computation method was developed[10]. This method uses a high-speed pencil beam dose computation method to get close to the desired solution in early iterations of the IMRT optimization. Then the C/S method is used to compute the dose for the interim solution. Following the C/S computation, the pencil beam method is used to modify the dose based on the change in intensity of the beam, leaving the majority of the dose computed by the more accurate C/S method.

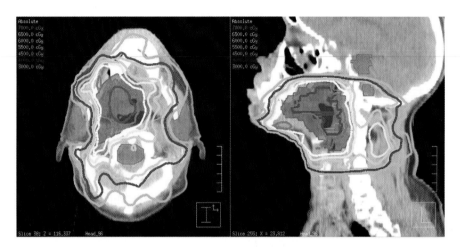

Figure 13-1. A 9-field IMRT treatment plan designed to deliver 60 Gy to the target volume (purple) and to spare the dose to the parotid glands (red) and the spinal cord and brainstem (green). The beams are equispaced in angle around the patient.

Once the intensity pattern of each beam is determined, it is converted into deliverable shapes by a multi-leaf collimator (MLC). Each beam will then be defined as a series of apertures defined by multiple MLC segments. Medical linear accelerators are equipped with MLC and deliver the set of MLC shapes automatically.

Newer methods in IMRT implemented in the Pinnacle[3] planning system include the ability to optimize the positions of each leaf of the MLC for each segment directly, rather than optimizing an intensity distribution for each beam, then later converting it to a set of MLC segments. By optimizing the leaf positions directly, the loss in desired treatment objective is reduced in the process.

IMRT provides a technique to conform the dose distribution tightly around a target volume while sparing the normal tissues. With this ability, the uncertainty in RT has been shifted to our ability to determine the desired target volumes, and the change in targets and critical structures over the course of RT.

3. MULTI-MODAL IMAGE PROCESSING TOOLS FOR TARGET AND STRUCTURE DEFINITION

Understanding the use of multi-modal image-based information for treatment design is an area of intensive research around the world. The contouring of risk organs and the target area in medical images is a fundamental planning step to optimize treatment parameters. Today, contours are drawn manually (with a mouse) on every image slice, which is an extremely time- and labor-intensive task. Particularly in the head and neck the process may take several hours. The merits of IMRT can only be exploited if this type of segmentation is achieved. The integration of additional image-based information acquired weekly or even daily into the RTP process will lead to an additional substantial increase in data and workload by an order of magnitude or more. Automated image segmentation technology is necessary to automatically contour risk organs and the tumor in order to make the improved process clinically feasible.

Target definition based on the structural appearance of the tumor in CT has limited accuracy in determining the true extent of the disease, and does not allow assessment of morphology and biological changes in response to fractionated treatment. For example, PET/CT promises to improve throughput and accuracy for head and-neck RT planning by minimizing the uncertainty of contouring by the identification of metabolically active areas in PET, while CT provides high resolution and anatomical context to address non-tumor-specific uptake in PET. Recent studies have used CT against Magnetic Resonance Imaging (MRI) or PET alone rather than together with registered structured imaging, and the current clinical practice is to draw contours on one modality and transfer the contours manually to the planning CT. The optimal technique for fusing image data to compensate for inconsist-encies between contours of different data sets remains controversially debated. Reproducible strategies for fusion of multi-modal contouring results and identification of conditions that exceed automated segmentation capacity are required.

Novel imaging agents such as fluoromisonidazole, [^{18}F] FMISO and others are becoming more widely available and are gaining clinical importance for radiotherapy applications[11]. These novel tracers probe deeply into the biological and molecular characteristics of a cancer. The tracer FMISO, for example, is a PET tracer that selectively binds to cells, which suffer from an undersupply of oxygen. The importance with respect to radiotherapy planning stems from the fact that so-called hypoxic cells may survive a radiation dose, which is lethal to cells with normal oxygen supply. This has wide-reaching clinical consequences, which will prompt molecular imaging guided targeting of cancers on sub-tumor level.

In this section key technologies required to pursue this strategy comprising segmentation, deformable registration and biological modeling are addressed.

3.1   Segmentation and deformable registration approaches

Image segmentation, at any level of automation or trained operator interaction, is difficult due to insufficient tissue contrasts, imaging artifacts, and the high inter- and intra-individual variability in shape and appearance of structures in the human body. Research efforts in image analysis and processing resulted in a well-established statement that segmentation of difficult cases cannot be done using image content alone, and some additional information is required[12,13].

A way to provide additional information to a segmentation algorithm is the use of prior knowledge about the shape of structures[14]. In medical image analysis, prior knowledge is represented, for example, in the form of an organ model, which includes information about both its shape as well as an organ-specific set of parameters specifying intensity range, gradient magnitude and direction, etc. When taking spatial relationships between different organs into account, this paradigm can be extended to organ constellations and even to whole regional anatomical atlases covering all structures of interest in particular body parts, which can automatically be adapted to the anatomy of individual patients.

Only few methods in the domain of automated organ segmentation for RTP that provide efficiency gain have been quantitatively proven to be accurate and robust so far. One can distinguish between three basic strategies in approaching this challenging problem: automation of 2D contouring aimed at robust detection of organ boundaries in 2D slices[15], 3D approaches based on deformable organ model adaptation[16,17], and methods based on adaptation of deformable atlases (images with labeled anatomy) to patient-specific image data[18].

Automated 2D delineation does not require substantial changes in the workflow compared to manual contouring to which the physicians are used. On the other hand, 3D shape context is not used at all by these methods, and this may negatively influence their robustness. In contrast, 3D delineation tools are potentially much more productive, since they simultaneously operate in several slices. Methods based on volumetric deformable atlas adaptation may be very useful, e.g. for delineation of 'invisible' structures, e.g. in the head and neck area. However, the results of delineation are dependent on the robustness of the image modality at hand, the underlying image registration algorithm and the validity of the deformation model.

Deformable image registration has been studied since the early 80's[19] and for many years, brain surgery and neurosciences have been the driving applications for developing an abundant number of techniques[20]. Despite the significant progress that has been made, deformable registration is still not clinically accepted and remains a challenging problem.

Registration algorithms are categorized into non-parametric and parametric methods[21]. In the non-parametric case the displacement-vector is estimated for each voxel. The reduced complexity in parametric approaches leads to efficient computation times, at the cost of fidelity in describing deformations. A classical example is landmark registration[22], where the new position for each voxel is interpolated or approximated from a given set of irregularly distributed points.

Another important choice is the deformation model, which can be purely geometric or physics-based. If the deformation process is due to physical processes, like in intra-patient registration, the use of physics-based deformation models aiming at describing real deformations may be advantageous over purely geometric transformations. Physics-based models are usually based on numerical[23] or analytical[24,25] solutions of the underlying equations of continuum mechanics.

A further classification of the registration techniques is the division into landmark-based, surface-based, and voxel-based methods. The first two groups provide the correspondences in the registered images between certain geometric entities, e.g. point landmarks or surfaces. The third group of methods maximizes voxel-based similarity between the images, i.e. information from the whole images contributes to the result.

In radiotherapy imaging, surface-based registration methods appear to be advantageous over voxel-based approaches. Surfaces of the relevant anatomical structures are available as output of the organ contouring. Based on this information, elastic tissue properties are assigned to the corresponding image regions[26]. Voxel-based image registration is difficult if the grey-value appearance of corresponding anatomical structures is not similar according to the definition of the similarity measure. This may not be the case in 4D CT of the thorax[27], but is more severe in longitudinal imaging of e.g. the rectum, where the gray-value appearance constantly changes due to peristalsis.

3.2 Biological modeling

As soon as functional or molecular images, such as PET or SPECT, and anatomical images are properly registered, the biological parameters relevant for defining a treatment, such as the radio-resistance across a tumor, have to be extracted. In the case of glucose metabolism as measured with FDG-PET this is not problematic. FDG, an analogue of glucose, accumulates in most tumors in a greater amount than it does in normal tissue, because tumor tissue growing faster and sugar uptake is thus greater.

It is best clinical practice to quantify glucose metabolism by calculating a so-called standard uptake value (SUV). SUV is the FDG-PET signal in a specific pixel or region divided by the amount of administered tracer and the patient's weight. The normalization shall eliminate the effect of patient size and weight on the detected signal. It provides a semi-quantitative measure to enable a better differentiation of an individual disease. It further enables a comparison of disease grades between different patients.

However, for tracers, which feature more complex reaction patterns, such as hypoxia imaging with FMISO, and which probe deeper into the molecular pathways of the tissue, a simple normalization does not always provide enough specific information. In such cases a more sophisticated modeling is wanted. Then uptake rates, reaction rates, residence times and washout-rates, which are not directly accessible from the images, need to be considered.

A pharmacokinetic analysis applied to time series of functional images can help quantify these parameters[28]. This technique deploys mathematical models, which describe the interactions of the tracer molecule with the tissue in time. The tissue is subdivided into compartments, which have by definition a similar tracer concentration-time behavior. Transfer of tracer from one to the other compartment and reverse is modeled via exchange rates.

These exchange rates often represent important kinetic information, e.g. the trapping rate of metabolized FMISO correlates with oxygen content, which are estimated in a consecutive optimization process by fitting measured time-activity curves to the model. Performed on a per voxel basis, this results in so-called parametric maps. Figure 13-2 shows a parametric map quantifying hypoxia in a lung cancer superimposed to an FMISO-PET image of the whole thorax region sampled at 2 hours after tracer injection. The modeling engine has been integrated into a Pinnacle[3] (Philips Medical Systems, Milpitas, Ca) research prototype ('BioGuide').

Once parametric maps of the relevant parameter are available, the transition to a dose has to be made. Radiobiological models can guide dose prescription and provide a means to optimize dose with respect to tumor cell kill and reduction of collateral damage[29]. Very recently a theoretical framework has been presented to quantitatively incorporate the spatial biology data, such as parametric maps, into IMRT inverse planning[30]. This or a similar framework in combination with parametric maps can be used to guide dose escalation dose to sub-tumor volumes while keeping the dose to critical structures at minimum. This could be a step further towards a safer and more effective radiotherapy.

4.   IMAGE GUIDED AND ADAPTIVE RADIOTHERAPY

In conventional RTP, risk organs and target areas are defined based on information that is currently limited to a single 3D anatomical CT image data set acquired at the onset of treatment design. This concept results in significant treatment uncertainties with irradiation of risk organs and reduced tumor coverage, see e.g. Mageras[31] and Chen[32] for review.

Natural processes in the body and response of normal and target tissue to the treatment result in significant inter- and intra-fractional geometrical changes. Intra-fractional geometric change occurs during radiation delivery due to breathing, cardiac motion, rectal peristalsis and bladder filling. Interfractional geometric change occurs in the extended time frame of fractionated radiotherapy (4-6 weeks), due to digestive processes, difference in patient setup, and treatment response like growth or shrinkage of the tumor or nearby risk organs (e.g. the parotids in head and neck treatment). These changes are only taken into account by population-based 'uncertainty' margins around the target area, which are often excessive and are applied to the structures identified before the therapy begins.

The concepts of adaptive radiotherapy (ART) and image-guided radiotherapy (IGRT) provide methods to monitor and adjust the treatments to accommodate the changing patient. ART is an off-line approach where the anatomical and biological changes are monitored over the course of treatment, and the treatment is modified when significant changes are identified. IGRT is typically an on-line concept where the patient or treatment plan is shifted or modified for each treatment. Both concepts require advanced image processing tools in order to be successful in clinical practice.

Additional imaging during the weeks of treatment is key to better understand and model these uncertainties. CT or kV cone-beam CT integrated into the treatment unit can provide patient-specific image-based quantitative surrogates of geometrical changes on the onset of a treatment fraction. Using the complementary strength of multi-modality imaging such as MRI providing superior soft-tissue contrast, and functional or molecular imaging such as PET, SPECT, MRI/MRS, can lead to improved target definition, and better understanding of the biological variations within the tumor that may affect response to the treatment. Finally, additional multi-modal imaging over the course of the treatment enables monitoring of target change over the course of therapy.

Integrating several image acquisitions over the course of treatment provides surrogates to compensate the change of risk organs and target areas. Besides the efficiency issue related to contouring, multi-modal image analysis requires estimating the correspondence between each voxel element of the multiple planning images. Estimating correspondences requires dedicated deformable image registration algorithms.

4.1   Concept for automated segmentation and deformable registration for adaptive IGRT

In order to manage a series of images from the same patient, an integrated concept of automated image segmentation and deformable image registration, in which an operator is provided with efficient algorithms that compute in the order of seconds, and a set of interactive tools to quickly access segmentation and registration results, and correct problematic areas if required.

The concept of automated organ segmentation proposed is a particular form of adapting deformable surface models[33]. Flexible surfaces are adapted to object boundaries by optimization of a measure expressing the goodness of the fit to image data in combination with certain constraints controlling the geometric properties of the surface.

To reduce the need for accurate initialization and reduce the problem of attraction to false boundaries, a framework of shape-constrained deformable model adaptation was developed[34], where prior knowledge obtained by a learning process[35] is embedded into an elastically deformable triangular mesh to compensate for the lack of reliable image content.

In the context of shape-constrained deformable models, a generic shape model is provided for each anatomical structure, i.e. a bladder model, a liver model, a lung model, etc. Since different structures consist of different tissue types (bone, soft tissue) with different imaging characteristics (grey value, contrast), organ-specific image features are used to diminish the risk for the model to be attracted by false image structures[16].

In an experimental validation study with 40 patient datasets, Pekar et al.[16] demonstrate that the method is suitable for clinical use for risk organs in the prostate area, i.e. bladder, rectum, and femoral heads, and significantly reduces the time for organ delineation compared to manual segmentation, with comparable segmentation accuracy in the order of 1-1.7 mm mean error. An example of the study is shown in Figure 13-3.

The ability to use deformable models efficiently for the segmentation of CT time series for prostate treatment planning was evaluated in Kaus et al.[36]. In order to increase the degree of automation and reduce the amount of interaction with each 3D volume in the image time series, an automated initial positioning strategy was developed based on the propagation of adapted surface meshes from one 3D image dataset to the next. The feasibility of this 4D approach was tested on a CT image time series taken from a single subject containing 16 3D CT datasets obtained at different days before and during treatment. Quantitative analysis demonstrated comparable results to the 3D interactive method for the femur and the bladder.

In another study, the tools were applied to the problem of risk organ segmentation in 4D CT imaging for lung tumor treatment planning[37]. The assessment was based on the 8 breathing phases of a patient's 4D CT dataset. Patient-specific models for the lungs, the heart, the spinal cord and the esophagus were generated by a clinical user on a Pinnacle[3] research prototype installed in the hospital, by manual contouring and triangulation of the first phase. The mesh adaptation algorithm was then carried out on the remaining 7 phases without further interaction. Accurate results were reported for all structures except for the esophagus, which is surrounded by soft tissue of similar grey value appearance.

When applying surface-based segmentation in a primary and a secondary dataset, a boundary mapping between the organ surfaces is automatically established through the correspondences between the mesh vertices. This information can be used for deformable image registration[38]. Essentially, a point-based deformable registration scheme is used, where the vertices of the triangular meshes act as corresponding control points. A spline function maps each control point in one image to the corresponding control point in the other image, while interpolating the mapping at all intermediate locations in the image.

Since the computation time increases linearly with the number of control points, only a subset of mesh vertices that is evenly distributed over the entire surface is used for the deformation. A reduction in the number of vertices (e.g. from 4000 to 80) reduces the computation time from hours to seconds on standard PC hardware with comparable surface registration accuracy.

In order to be clinically acceptable, the automated tools compute results in the order of seconds. Secondly, they support efficient editing, allowing the operator to quickly access and correct problematic areas if required. The user is provided with the ability to manipulate the model, thus interacting with both the segmentation of a structure and the deformable registration of a secondary image. For example, automated mesh adaptation, manual deformation of the mesh proportional to the translation of the mouse pointer, and re-sampling of a secondary image according to an updated deformable transform.

In contrast to manual slice-wise delineation, complete organ segmentation is possible within a few minutes. In addition, delineated structures are represented by smooth 3D shapes and not by stacked 2D slices, which avoids the common 'Christmas tree' effect by providing smooth surfaces.

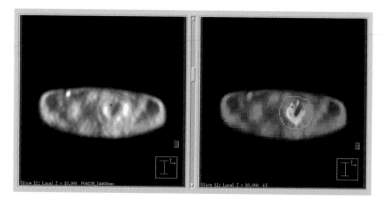

Figure 13-2. BioGuide plug-in is a research application running under Pinnacle3. The plug-in features a pharmacokinetic modeling engine and radiobiological modeling to improve target definition of an individual disease. Left window: FMISO-PET late time image with target contour in green. Right window: Same FMISO-PET image but with the corresponding parametric map (color coded) representing hypoxia for the tumor region superimposed.

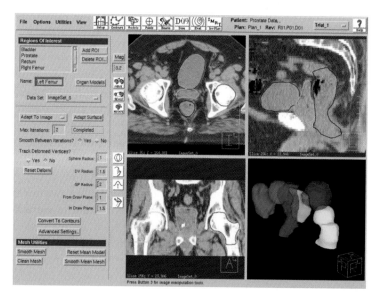

Figure 13-3. 3D model-based segmentation in CT of the target and the organs of risk. The image shows three orthogonal cross-sections, the contours where the surface meshes intersect the cross-sections (femur heads, bladder, rectum, prostate), and a rendering of the 3D surface models.

Unlike most voxel-based deformable registration schemes, surface-based registration is computationally efficient. In addition, because the deformation is controlled by surfaces that can be edited by an operator, it is possible to interact with the deformation algorithm, which is important in the context of clinical acceptance of a deformable registration algorithm.

Another important advantage of the presented approach is its generality. The organ database is currently being extended to other treatment areas such as breast, liver, lung, head and neck. Potentially, the method can be applied to other imaging modalities by using the principle of organ-specific image features[39].

4.2 Validation concepts for adaptive radiotherapy

In-treatment room kV cone-beam CT (CBCT) imaging is an emerging technology, which has still not reached the image quality of a conventional CT imaging regarding spatial resolution and soft tissue detectability.[40] Hence image processing techniques, which provide good registration and segmentation for conventional CT time series, may not be directly applicable to IGRT based on cone-beam volumetric imaging.

A test suite was designed to simulate the quantitative impact of CBCT imaging quality on the performance of image registration and segmentation techniques used to correlate treatment time images with planning images.[41] The result is measured with respect to improvements of the dose volume histograms. The main components of the test suite are:

- A simulation engine to transform the grey-values of conventional CT images to better match the imaging characteristics of CBCT, including effects such as beam quality, residual scatter, residual beam hardening, simulation of defect pixels, truncation, flat panel detector noise.
- The segmentation and registration algorithms such as described above.
- An inverse planning dose engine to create treatment plans and associated dose distributions based on the delineated target and organ at risks.
- A plan evaluation tool to create dose-volume histograms.

A first result suggested that rigid registration works robustly on CBCT even under low dose conditions. Moreover, an adaptation of the plan using a rigid correlation already improves the dose volume histogram.

5. SUMMARY

Radiation therapy (RT) has seen several advances in the past decade. Many improvements in computers, imaging and image post-processing technology have fueled much of these advancements. Sophisticated dose computation, 3D visualization and planning tools were enabled in software systems such as Pinnacle[3]. Intensity modulated radiotherapy was the next logical step and has provided the clinicians the ability to carve out dose distributions to treat desired targets while sparing normal structures.

The next round of advancements in RT include adaptive radiotherapy and image guided radiotherapy where the image based monitoring of the patient and treatment will enable correction of the treatment while the patient is on the table, or monitoring of the anatomical or biological changes in the patient prompting re-planning of the treatment if necessary.

These new techniques require substantial advances in image processing in the areas of model based image segmentation, deformable image registration and biological modeling. These tools will enable the evaluation of anatomical and biological changes in the patient and the accumulation of the true delivered doses to the tissues undergoing deformations during the course of RT.

Further evaluation of the biological and functional properties of the tissues in RT is enabling better definition of target volumes and improved knowledge of the effects of RT on biological function. Molecular imaging techniques have the potential to identify hypoxic regions of tissues, which are known to be resistant to RT, enabling the clinician to consider this in the prescription of doses. The knowledge of molecular imaging combined with intensity-modulated radiotherapy (IMRT) will give the clinician the ability to tailor the dose distribution to the anatomical target volumes as well as boost the dose to regions that are identified as either resistant to radiation, or regions known to contain high densities of tumor tissue.

As these techniques advance, radiotherapy departments will need to manage image-based data at an ever-increasing rate. Computers will continue to play a large role in advancing the practice of RT as well as other areas of medicine.

REFERENCES

1. J. Löf, H. Rehbinder, T. McNutt, and S. Johnson, P3IMRT Inverse planning optimization, *White Paper Publication, ADAC Laboratories (Philips)*, (Milpitas, CA 2002).
2. R. Mohan, C. Chui, and L. Lidofsky, Energy and angular distributions of photons from medical linear accelerators, *Med Phys* **12**, 592-597 (1985).

3. T.R. Mackie, J.W. Scrimger, and J.J. Battista, A convolution method of calculating dose for 15-MV Xrays, *Med Phys* **12**, 188-196 (1985).
4. T.R. Mackie, A.F. Bielajew, D.W.O. Rogers, et al., Generation of photon energy deposition kernels using the EGS Monte Carlo code, *Phys Med Biol* **33**, 1-20 (1988).
5. T.R. Mackie, P.J. Reckwerdt, T.R. McNutt, et al., Photon dose computations, *Proc AAPM Summer School, AAPM-College Park, MD* (1996).
6. A. Ahnesjo, P. Andreo, and A. Brahme, Calculation and application of point spread functions for treatment planning with high energy photon beams, *Acta Oncol* **26**, 49-56 (1987).
7. N. Papanikolaou, T.R. Mackie, C. Meger-Wells, et al., Investigation of the convolution method for polyenergetic spectra, *Med Phys* **20**, 1327-1336 (1993).
8. M.B. Sharpe and J.J. Battista, Dose calculations using convolution and superposition principles. The orientation of the dose spread kernels in divergent Xray beams, *Med Phys* **20**, 1685-1694 (1993).
9. T.R. McNutt, T.R. Mackie, P. Reckwerdt, et al., Calculation of portal dose images using the convolution/superposition method, *Med Phys* **23**(4), 527-535 (1996).
10. T.R. McNutt, Dose calculations Collapsed cone convolution and delta pixel beam, *White Paper Publication, ADAC Laboratories (Philips), Milpitas, CA* (1999).
11. J.D. Chapman, J.D. Bradley, J.F. Eary, et al., Molecular (functional) imaging for radiotherapy applications an RTOG symposium, *Int J Rad Onc Biol Phys* **55**(2), 291-301 (2003).
12. M. Kass, A and Witkin, D. Terzopoulos, Snakes active contour models, *Int J of Computer Vision* **1**(4), 321-331 (1988).
13. D.L. Collins, T.M. Peters, W. Dai, et al., Model-based segmentation of individual brain structures from MRI data, *Proc Vis Biomed Comp,* 10-23 (1992).
14. T.F. Cootes, A. Hill, C.J. Taylor, et al., The use of active shape models for locating structures in medical images, *Imag Vis Comp* **12**(6), 355-366 (1994).
15. L.S. Hibbard, Region segmentation using information divergence measures, *Proc MICCAI*, 554-561 (2003).
16. V. Pekar, T.R. McNutt, and M.R. Kaus, Automated model-based organ delineation for radiation therapy planning in the prostate region, *Int J Rad Onc Biol Phys* **60**(3), 973-980 (2004).
17. S. Pizer, P. Fletcher, S. Joshi, et al., Deformable M-reps for medical image registration, *Int J Comp Vis* **55**(2), 85-106 (2003).
18. P.F. D'Haese, V. Duay, R. Li, et al., Automatic segmentation of brain structures for radiation therapy planning, *Proc SPIE Medical Imaging*, 517-526 (2003).
19. R. Bajcsy and S. Kovacic, Multiresolution elastic matching, *Comp Vis Graph Imag Process* **46**, 1-1 (1982).
20. A. Toga (ed.), *Brain Warping,* (Academic Press, 1999).
21. J. Modersitzki, *Numerical methods for image registration,* (Oxford University Press, 2004).
22. F. Bookstein, Principal warps thin-plate splines and the decomposition of deformations, *IEEE PAMI* **11**, 567-585 (1989).
23. G. Christensen, R. Rabbitt, and M. Miller, Deformable templates using large deformation kinematics, *IEEE Trans Imag Process* **5**, 1435-1447 (1997).
24. M. Davis, A. Khotanzad, D. Flaming, et al., A physics-based coordinate transformation for 3D image matching, *IEEE Trans Med Imag* **16**(3), 317-328 (1997).
25. J. Kohlrausch, K. Rohr, and S. Stiehl, A new class of elastic body splines for nonrigid registration of medical images, *Proc BVM,* 164-168 (2001).
26. K. Brock, M. Sharpe, L. Dawson, et al., Accuracy of finite element model-based multi-organ deformable image registration, *Med Phys* **32**(6), 1647-1659 (2005).

27. T. Guerrero, G. Zhang, T. Huang, et al., Intrathoracic tumour motion estimation from CT imaging using the 3D optical flow method, *Phys Med Biol* **49**(2204), 4147-4161 (2004).
28. S. Huang, and M.E. Phelps, Principles of tracer kinetic modeling in positron emission tomography and audiography – principles and applications for the brain and heart, Raven Press, New York, 287-346 (1986).
29. G.G. Steel (ed), *Basic clinical radiobiology* (Oxford University Press, 2002).
30. Y. Yang, and L. Xing, Towards biologically conformal radiation therapy (BCRT) Selective IMRT dose escalation under guidance of spatial biology distribution, *Med Phys* **32**(6), 1473-1483 (2005).
31. G. Mageras (ed.), Management of target localization uncertainties in external beam therapy, *Seminars in Radiation Oncology* **15**(3) (2005).
32. G. Chen, T. Bortfeld (eds.), High-Precision therapy of moving targets, *Seminars in Radiation Oncology* **14**(1) (2004).
33. T. McInerney and D. Terzopoulos, Deformable models in medical image segmentation, *Med Imag Anal* **1**(2), 91-108 (1996).
34. J. Weese, M. Kaus, C. Lorenz, et al., Shape constrained deformable models for 3D medical image segmentation, *Proc IPMI,* 380-387 (2001).
35. M. Kaus, V. Pekar, C. Lorenz, et al., Automated 3D PDM construction from segmented images using deformable models, *IEEE Trans Med Imag* **22**(8), 1005-1013 (2003).
36. M.R. Kaus, T.R. McNutt, and V. Pekar, Automated 3D and 4D organ delineation for radiation therapy planning in the pelvic area, *Proc SPIE Medical Imaging*, 346-356 (2004).
37. D. Ragan, G. Starkschall, T. McNutt, et al., Semiautomated four-dimensional computed tomography segmentation using deformable models, *Med Phys* **32**(7), 2254-2261 (2005).
38. M.R. Kaus, V. Pekar, T.R. McNutt, et al., An efficient algorithm for image-based dose deformation and accumulation, *Med Phys* **32**(6), 1900 (2005).
39. M.R. Kaus, J. von Berg, J. Weese, et al., Automated segmentation of the left ventricle in cardiac MRI, *Med Imag Anal* **8**, 245-254 (2004).
40. D. Jaffray, Emergent technologies for 3-dimensional image-guided radiation delivery, *Seminars in Radiation Oncology* **15**, 15208-216 (2005).
41. M. Bal, L. Spies, and T. McNutt, Adapting treatment plan to organ motions and deformations using x-ray volumetric imaging, *Proc ESTRO*, abstract (2003).

Chapter 14

MOLECULAR IMAGING GUIDED RADIOTHERAPY
Imaging Resistance Factors and Response to Treatment

Kenneth A. Krohn[1] and Lothar Spies[2]

[1]*University of Washington, Seattle, WA, USA;* [2]*Philips Research, Hamburg, Germany*

Abstract: Assessment of tumor markers, including ones which determine the tumor's radiosensitivity and its response to radiation, are playing a pivotal role in future definition of radiotherapies. Two key characteristics, hypoxia and cell proliferation, as examples for dynamic imaging using two PET agents, FMISO and FLT, are addressed. Developmental pathways toward possibilities that exist to extract more quantitative information from these images are sketched. Furthermore, we propose how his information may be incorporated in radiotherapy planning.

Keywords: Molecular imaging, radiotherapy, tumor hypoxia, cell proliferation, FLT, FMISO, radiotherapy planning

1.   INTRODUCTION

Currently, several tumor characteristics are used to stage and grade a cancer and to predict its overall response to treatment, including its sensitivity to ionizing radiation. Some of these include size, site of growth, histology and certain biomarkers assayed in tissue or plasma samples. In addition, the overall health, age and performance parameters of the patient are also important factors to help define the appropriate treatment and to predict the response to a given therapy. However, even after the most aggressive radiotherapies, inter-patient response can be heterogeneous, local-regional failures are too high, and the five-year survival rates are variable. The underlying mechanisms of this heterogeneous response of patients with similar tumors to the same therapy are not adequately understood.

217

G. Spekowius and T. Wendler (Eds.), Advances in Healthcare Technology, 217-233.

Over the past years molecular imaging has made great advances to provide functional characterization at the sub-organ level using in-vivo assays. To some extent, this advance was triggered by novel molecules being labeled with radionuclides or other markers, which can probe and quantify aspects of molecular pathways characteristic of certain diseases. The most prominent imaging modalities being used for molecular imaging in the clinical setting are PET and SPECT. Traditionally FDG has been used for more than two decades to visualize glucose metabolism using PET. FDG-PET is of great significance in the diagnostic work-up of oncologic patients due to its sensitivity for a wide spectrum of neoplasms[1,2]. Whole-body scans are used for screening for metastatic disease. Tumor staging is significantly facilitated by FDG-PET as documented in several tumor entities[3] and it is being used increasingly to monitor response to treatment[4,5].

Recent advances in radiotherapy concern the development of Intensity Modulated Radiotherapy (IMRT) deploying inverse planning technologies in combination with advanced delivery equipment such as computer-controlled multi-leaf collimators[6]. This novel methodology has become widely available and is becoming part of routine clinical practice. IMRT provides unprecedented precision in 3D dose delivery, enabling dose escalation and organ sparring in the millimeter regime. Radiotherapy planning is based on CT information representing the anatomy of the region to be treated. The CT information is key since it correlates with the electron density of the tissue, which is needed to calculate the dose to be imparted by the megavoltage x-ray beam. MR images complement CT in cases where CT does not provide enough anatomic contrast, such as in the prostate, the female breast or in the brain. As opposed to its role in diagnosis and tumor characterization, the role of molecular imaging for treatment definition remains embryonic.

In 2000, Ling and coworkers[7] proposed the concept of biological target volume (BTV). The authors hypothesized that this BTV could be derived from biological images that represent metabolic, functional, physiologic, genotypic, and phenotypic data, to improve target delineation and dose delivery. Furthermore, they realized the potential of IMRT for intra-tumoral dose modulation using dose boosts for selected regions, for example areas that showed a higher radioresistance. This could be accomplished while sparring dose in radiosensitive regions, thus keeping the integral dose to the volume constant. They furthermore hypothesized that 'noninvasive biological imaging may provide the pertinent information to guide the painting or sculpting of the optimal dose distribution.' Since this landmark paper appeared, a few publications have emerged to develop Ling's theme. They can be divided into two categories: Papers of the first category have investigated how functional information can be used to improve target delineation, for example in cases where anatomical images give inconclusive results[8]. The second category comprises papers that investigate how molecular imaging can be used to better modulate a certain amount of integral dose to a target to closely adapt to intra-tumoral biology, for example non-uniformity of radiosensitivity. Recent examples demonstrate how functional information provided by SPECT and PET can be utilized to realize this adaptation[9-11]. To this end, an accurate quantification of intra-tumor biology is a prerequisite. Furthermore, a quantitative understanding of response measured by PET and SPECT is indispensable if treatment parameters or even treatment regimens have to be changed at an early stage.

This chapter is organized as follows: firstly, imaging assays for tumor hypoxia and cell proliferation as the most important tools for assessing tumor radioresistance and treatment response, respectively, are discussed. We focus on FMISO and FLT-PET imaging and elaborate what techniques are required to extract quantitative information. The chapter ends with a proposition how to incorporate quantitative tumor information into treatment definition.

2. IMAGING TUMOR MARKERS

The definition of molecular imaging is sometimes restricted to imaging specific molecular pathways, for example, cellular signaling and regulation. A more general definition would extend imaging to all of the molecular characteristics of a disease process that impact on planning appropriate therapy and following response to that therapy. Thus, we include in molecular imaging attempts to quantify with imaging the extent and spatial variance in numerous factors that affect resistance to therapy, including hypoxia, expression of multidrug resistance transporters, down-regulation of hormonal receptors, and methyl-alkyl transferase activity, as examples. In this chapter, hypoxia as one of the most imaged factors in resistance to therapy is addressed.

For imaging response to treatment, it is most useful to quantify common characteristics of the tumor phenotype. A benchmark essay by Hanahan and Weinberg[12] described six hallmarks of the cancer cell: Three are closely related as self-sufficiency in growth signals, insensitivity to anti-growth signals, and limitless replicative potential and the other three are invasion and metastasis, evading apoptosis and sustained angiogenesis. While molecular imaging strategies are being developed for each of these characteristics of the tumor phenotype, the general property of cellular proliferation is probably the most important way to quantify response to cancer therapy[13]. The death of a cancer cell often causes FDG uptake to go down, but the imaging signal can have a transient increase due to energy-intensive processes responding to the insult of therapy. In contrast, successful therapy will shut down cellular proliferation; the molecular machinery for DNA synthesis will halt. Thus, imaging proliferation is an unambiguous way to verify response to cytotoxic or cytostatic therapy[14].

2.1   Tumor hypoxia

The physiologic microenvironment of a tumor influences its response to therapy. For example, low levels of oxygen, perhaps as a result of poor vascularization in the tumor, reduce the cytotoxic effectiveness of ionizing radiation by about three-fold. The radiation oncology community has been aware of this for fifty years[15], but attempts to circumvent the cure-limiting effects of hypoxia have met with only very limited success[16]. To overcome radioresistance, strategies to target tumor hypoxia, an inherently heterogeneous phenomenon, are key. Hence, identification and quantification of hypoxic domains in a tumor may aid therapy definition, with the impact of a better cure that could be quantified as fewer local recurrences. One promising pathway to this goal is dose escalation on hypoxic tumor subvolumes, as proposed by Ling et al.[7]. The underlying hypothesis is that such a scheme may improve tumor control and reduce unwanted side effects.

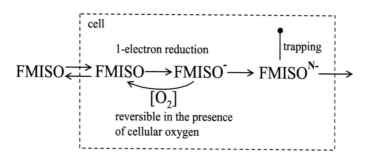

Figure 14-1. Reaction pathways of FMISO in a cell.

Many tracers for hypoxia imaging have been developed and tested to date[17]. Very few have made it into clinical trials with a significant number of patients. The most widely used agent is [^{18}F]-FMISO, fluoromisonidazole. It is a derivative of one of the earliest radiosensitizers used in clinical radiation oncology, the azomycin called misonidazole. The drug is bioreductively activated by electron transport, but the 1-electron reduction reaction to produce the nitro radical anion is reversible in the presence of oxygen in tissues. Addition of a second electron generates a bioreductive alkylation agent, a non-reversible reaction where the reduced FMISO binds quite indiscriminantly to macromolecules within the cell (Figure 14-1). The result is a positive image of FMISO at low levels of intracellular oxygen. Because there is a continuous gradient in oxygen tension in tissues, the contrast in FMISO images is only modest but the information content in terms of this important factor in resistance to ionizing radiation is large and is just becoming widely appreciated.

2.2 Cell proliferation

Measurement of cellular proliferation in tumors has played a key role in cancer research for many decades. The thymidine labeling index using tritiated thymidine, the only nucleoside that is exclusively incorporated into DNA, has long been the gold standard for quantifying changes in cellular growth in response to cancer therapy[18]. A decrease in cellular proliferation is one of the earliest events in response to successful cancer therapy. While the assay with tritium-labeled thymidine was applied to biopsy specimens, the advent of ^{11}C-labeled thymidine[19] opened the door for non-invasive imaging of this important measure of response to treatment.

Imaging cellular proliferation has a number of advantages over metabolic imaging with FDG-PET. Increased and uncontrolled cellular proliferation is a unique characteristic of tumors. In contrast, increased energy metabolism as measured by FDG is associated with a variety of other processes, included inflammation, multidrug resistance transporter function and apoptosis. Cellular proliferation changes earlier and is a more definitive indicator of successful response to treatment[20].

Imaging studies with [11C]-thymidine are proving useful for answering important questions in clinical research[21,22], but the procedure is complicated because of the abundance of metabolites and the short nuclear decay half-life. Therefore a series of non-metabolized thymidine analogs has been evaluated[23] and 3'-deoxy-3'-[18F]-fluorothymidine, FLT, was selected as a useful analogue agent for imaging cellular proliferation. FLT reacts with thymidine kinase 1, the cytosolic enzyme that produces the mono-phosphorylated nucleotide of FLT, but this molecule does not continue all the way to DNA synthesis because the fluorine substitution at the 3'-position terminates the polymerization chain. For FLT the rate-limiting step is thymidine kinase activity; for thymidine the rate is limited by DNA polymerase activity. Because these nucleoside analogs are not natural components of DNA, their uptake may not accurately reflect the synthetic rate of DNA. FLT and related radiopharmaceuticals still require more thorough validation studies. Nevertheless, Shields et al. published the first human image with FLT[24], and a dog image of FLT was recognized as 'Image of the Year' at the 1997 SNM[25]. Since that time publications involving FLT imaging have proliferated, along with attempts to further validate the interpretation of FLT images[14].

3.   QUANTIFICATION

The goal of quantitative data analysis in molecular imaging is to move from pictures to statistically defensible rate parameters that have a specific biological interpretation. The advantage of the positron emission signal is that it is quantitative and, with knowledge of the specific activity of the injectate, can be directly converted from imaging counts in a voxel to picomoles per volume. But this signal is a composite of the amount of tracer that was delivered to the imaged volume, the amount that was retained, and the amount that washed out or was otherwise metabolized. Because the relative contribution of these components varies from patient to patient and day to day, dynamic data analysis is a useful tool to resolve a series of dynamic images into a map of flux versus transport, for example[14]. The test-retest variability is better for modeled images than for simple dpm/voxel or SUV images.

Images of accurate electron densities provided by X-ray CT have formed the basis for accurate dose calculation, which is a prerequisite for treatment planning. Image distortions and artifacts in CT images propagate into sub-optimal treatment parameters, which eventually compromise treatment quality. A similar trend must be anticipated for molecular image information being used to guide dose prescription. Accurate and quantitative molecular parameters have the best potential to improve the quality of care in future applications. New technology that combines the biological information from PET and the anatomic information from CT in the same instrument will be important input for radiation treatment plans in the next decade.

3.1   Tumor hypoxia

The FMISO image potentially contains two complementary pieces of information: what volume or regions of the tumor are hypoxic and how hypoxic are these regions. At this time we do not know whether 'how much hypoxia' or 'how bad' is the more significant determinant of outcome. For quantification of the hypoxic volume from FMISO-PET images, a simple standard has been established by calculating a tissue-to-blood ratio, T:B, for each voxel. FMISO has a partition coefficient near unity so that the T:B ratio should be approximately one in well-oxygenated tissues. The numbers are normally extracted from late time images, commonly acquired between 90 to 120 min after tracer injection and ratioed to activity in a venous blood sample acquired at the imaging time. In an earlier work the tissue-to-muscle ratio was quantified and a value of 1.4 was considered as a practical level to discriminate between predominantly hypoxic versus normoxic tissue[26]. More recently a value of 1.2 for the tissue-to-blood ratio has been adopted as a discriminator[27]. The latter value was found representative because more than 99% of normal tissue does not show an uptake greater than 1.2 (Figure 14-2).

Thus, a simple analysis would describe the volume of pixels with T:B>1.2 as the hypoxic volume and the raw image would show the spatial heterogeneity of hypoxia in the tumor field. The highest pixel ratio, $T:B_{max}$, would then be a measure of the level of hypoxia and could be used to compare the level of hypoxia in patient images of FMISO before, during and after radiation therapy. For example, Koh et al.[26] used serial FMISO images in patients with lung cancer, who were being treated with photons, to observe the rate and extent of reoxygenation over the course of treatment.

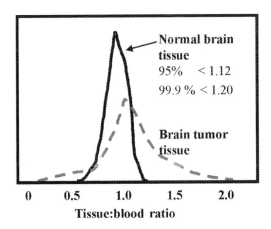

Figure 14-2. FMISO pixel histogram: Brain to blood (solid line) and tumor to blood (dashed line).

Alternative imaging agents for hypoxia are designed for more rapid plasma clearance via renal excretion. While this change in the radiopharmaceutical results in higher contrast images, it also introduces a component of blood flow into the data analysis. It is no longer valid to expect a constant ratio for all normoxic tissues at late times and so more complex analysis is required to distinguish effects of delivery (blood flow) from those of local retention (hypoxia).

Due to the high fraction of non-specific binding of FMISO in tissues, falsely indicating hypoxia, early attempts were made to extract kinetic parameters from time series of PET images. The suspicion was that non-specific binding might obscure the specific binding component, which is solely responsible for tracer accumulation and thus directly correlated with oxygen content. The hypothesis was that a compartmental model might offer advantages for discriminating non-specific from specific binding.[28] The compartmental model[29] was derived from a physiological picture, which modeled the various biological pathways of the tracer in tissue, such as uptake, retention and wash out of tracer and the pathways of chemically modified tracer molecules in the tissue (Figure 14-3). A parameter was identified, which quantifies the trapping rate of metabolized FMISO, termed κ_A. This parameter could be directly related to the oxygen concentration in the tissue. Having presented the full analysis, the work concluded that simple tissue-to-blood activity ratios correlate well with κ_A. They exemplified it for a human patient with a base of tongue squamous cell carcinoma, for whom they reported the following correlation: $T:B = 3.73 + 1.07 \cdot \log_{10}(\kappa_A)$, suggesting that the T:B ratio can be used as a surrogate for the oxygen concentration in the tissue. In Figure 14-4, we present results comparing T:B ratios and κ_A for recent data from patients with non-small cell lung cancer on a voxel basis[30]. The Philips Research pharmacokinetic modeling tool VOXULUS was employed for non-linear regression using a Levenberg-Marquardt algorithm with linear weights to estimate the free model parameters of the Casciari model (Figure 14-3).

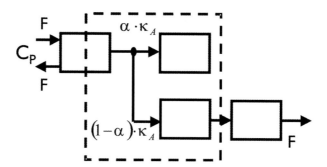

Figure 14-3. Compartmental model for FMISO transport and reaction rates in tissue. F is the flow rate of tracer from blood, C_P, into tissue and interstitial space. F also governs the transport of metabolized FMISO back to the blood. The dashed box indicates the compartments belonging to the cell. α is the branching ratio between trapped and washed-out FMISO metabolites. $\alpha \cdot \kappa_A$ is the rate of tracer trapped in the tissue.

Implementation of analytical solutions of the differential equations associated with the Casciari-model enabled processing of more than 50 voxel per second on a standard PC. The scatter plot suggests that the above relation may not always be an accurate representation of the trapping rate and consequently of hypoxia. By design, the kinetic model is able to discriminate between specific and non-specific binding, which might be an essential prerequisite for accurate quantification of hypoxia since the tracer's clearance is relatively slow and unbound tracer equilibrated with the vascular pool may always be present in the tissue even four hours after administration.

3.2 Cell proliferation

There is a substantial history on the modeling of nucleoside kinetics to infer DNA synthesis. Thymidine is incorporated into DNA via the salvage pathway, but not through the *de novo* pathway, and DNA synthesis from thymidine is substantially up regulated during early S-phase[14]. The approach to modeling [^{11}C]-thymidine metabolism is based on the pioneering work of Cleaver[31]. Thymidine nucleotides from both endogenous and exogenous sources freely mix within the intracellular DNA precursor pool and so relative utilization can be predicted based on the concentration of extracellular thymidine[32]. Unless there is a shortage of precursor, the rate of DNA synthesis depends on the 'proliferative state' of the tissue and not on the concentration of precursors; the flux of nucleotides through the precursor pool and into DNA is the rate of synthesis.

Thymidine in the body is rapidly degraded by thymidine phosphorylase into the pyrimidine nucleic acid, thymine, and deoxyribose. Thus, while a simple standard uptake value (SUV) or uptake ratio is easy to calculate for images derived from [^{11}C]-thymidine, it leads to a significant bias in estimating flux into DNA because it fails to account for the substantial level of metabolites that are in plasma and tissues. Using time-activity curves obtained from blood samples, kinetic parameters can be estimated by optimizing the fit of a model to the time course of tissue uptake measured by dynamic PET imaging and blood samples assayed for radioactive metabolites[33-35]. Since PET images integrate the entire radioactivity in a region, labeled metabolites affect quantitative interpretation of images from labeled thymidine, which is rapidly catabolized *in vivo*. In tumor imaging the approach of subtracting the metabolite background estimated from a reference tissue does not work because there is no tissue with sufficiently similar properties. To overcome this, a detailed model accounting for both thymidine and metabolites using data obtained from blood analysis was developed[33,34]. Animal studies were used to validate this model's ability to predict the time course of [^{11}C]-thymidine incorporation into DNA, and simulations and animal studies showed that this analysis provided reliable values for the pseudo-rate constant for DNA flux[36]. Preliminary results using a separate [^{11}C]-CO$_2$ injection to independently measure kinetics of this diffusible metabolite showed that compartmental analysis corrected for the metabolite background in the brain and separated the effects of transport and retention by DNA synthesis in the tumor[21].

PET images of cellular proliferation contain unique and clinically useful information. For example, Eary[21] compared PET imaging with [2-^{11}C]-thymidine, FDG, and MRI and found that thymidine showed different uptake in about half of the patients, indicating that different information was being obtained. Brain tumor images of thymidine showed promising results and an ability to distinguish active tumor from barrier effects that was superior to FDG. Thymidine has also been used to image high-grade sarcomas and small cell lung cancer and to monitor response to chemotherapy[20]. After successful therapy, the fractional decline in thymidine was greater than with FDG, suggesting that thymidine may be of particular value for measuring early response.

[2-^{11}C]-thymidine has also been used to evaluate response to new anti-cancer agents and to verify their mechanisms of action. For example, imaging was used in a small study of patients receiving experimental inhibitors of thymidylate synthase, TS, the enzyme that supplies thymidine nucleotides via the *de novo* pathway. These drugs, typified by 5-fluorouracil, block the *de novo* pathway and should increase demand for utilization by the salvage pathway. Images showed increased thymidine retention in tumors after the administration of experimental inhibitors as compared to a pre-drug study[22]. Thymidine may be particularly helpful in evaluating response to experimental immunotherapy, where the high demand for energy during an immune response may result in confusing FDG images.

The literature on quantitative analysis of FLT images is much less advanced. The early human studies have focused on SUV data from FLT-PET imaging and correlations with the Ki-67 index[37]. However, in view of the advantages of full compartmental modeling that have been documented for [^{11}C]-thymidine, a more sophisticated analysis of FLT biodistribution kinetics is clearly warranted. Muzi and colleagues[38] have developed and evaluated a method based on the analogy between the biochemistry of FLT and thymidine. The model measures the retention of FLT-monophosphate generated by the phosphorylation of FLT by thymidine kinase 1, the initial enzyme in the salvage pathway. This model assumes a steady-state biosynthesis and incorporation of nucleotides into DNA because, unlike authentic thymidine, FLT nucleotides do not get incorporated into the DNA polymer. This analysis also assumes equilibrium between nucleoside levels in tissue and plasma and that the relative rates of FLT and thymidine phosphorylation can be approximated by direct analysis of *in vitro* samples. The resulting 2-compartment model fits the dynamic imaging data collected over 120 minutes and the metabolite-corrected blood curve. This model was able to distinguish FLT flux from FLT transport. A companion paper described the performance of the model for human data in patients with lung cancer[39]. In this report the flux constants for FLT phosphorylation in tumor, bone marrow (high flux) and muscle (low flux) were determined in a series of 17 patients, 18 tumors, and compared with an *in vitro* assay of proliferation, the Ki-67 index. Compartmental modeling results were also compared with simple model-independent measures of FLT uptake. This analysis lead to robust estimates of the flux constant for FLT that correlated with *in vitro* measure of proliferation for tumor, marrow and muscle. The correlation with SUV was considerably weaker, substantiating the concept that more detailed biochemical parameters from imaging are more useful. Further direct comparisons will be required to determine the fidelity of FLT flux as a proxy for thymidine flux, the gold standard for imaging cellular proliferation. This work will require sequential imaging studies with [^{11}C]-thymidine and [^{18}F]-FLT and should involve tumors with a range of histologies and it should also evaluate tumors that have been treated.

4. TREATMENT DEFINITION

Once tumor markers relevant for treatment definition are quantified, a translation into an optimal dose prescription is needed. The translation is associated with two major problems. Firstly, parametric images are relatively noisy. This is because they are estimated from a series of PET images, which individually feature a high noise level. It is not surprising that the corresponding parametric maps have noise levels of 10 to 20%. A direct translation of these parameters into dose would result in a similar or greater level of noise in the dose prescription. This additional noise may not only prolong the inverse planning procedure, but may produce sub-optimal treatment parameters. Furthermore, physiological or molecular parameters are not directly proportional to the therapy dose, which maximizes cell kill. Very recently, Yang and Xing[40] proposed a theoretical framework, which relates radiobiological parameters such as clonogen density, radiosensitivity, and cell proliferation rate to dose. They defined a tumor control probability (TCP) utilizing the linear-quadratic model[41] to represent the tumor clonogen survival. The dose is then derived from a maximization of the TCP under the restriction that the integral dose to the tumor volume is a constant. We refer here to their publication for further details.

An appropriate means to reduce noise is clustering, e.g. using a k-means classifier[42]. Normally, dose confidence levels are provided by modeling in addition to the dose levels. The total number of classes ideally adapts to the noise content and the dose range in the target to be prescribed. Two dose levels or classes can generally be discriminated in a noisy environment if the difference of the class-representatives ΔS is at minimum five times greater than the noise, represented by the standard deviation σ_S. This argumentation is based on the model of image detection, which states similar criteria for a reliable detection of a uniform object in a noisy background, namely that the ratio of signal difference and noise shall be greater than five, or $\Delta S / \sigma_S \geq 5$. Consequently, the number of dose classes can be determined in accordance with:

$$\# clusters = \frac{D_{max} - D_{min}}{\delta \cdot \sigma_D}, \qquad\qquad [1]$$

where $D_{max,min}$ are the maximum and minimum dose, respectively, of the target volume; σ_D is the confidence level or standard deviation of the dose and δ is a constant with a value of five or greater according to the aforementioned imaging criterion.

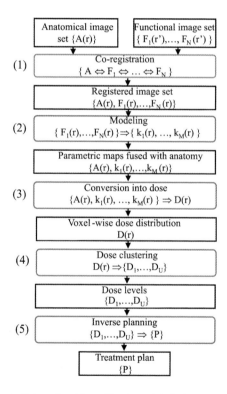

Figure 14-4. Flowchart of the algorithm. Numbers label the operation steps, which are described in the text.

To evaluate this strategy, the algorithm, illustrated in Figure 14-5, has been implemented as a research plug-in ('BioGuide') into a Pinnacle[3] treatment planning platform (Philips Medical Systems, Milpitas, CA, USA). It comprises the following main steps:

1. Co-registration of anatomical and functional image data cubes.
2. Kinetic modeling of disease or molecular parameters based on the provided functional information to create 3D parametric maps.
3. Translation of disease or molecular parameters into a voxel-based dose distribution for the target region and tolerance dose for the organs at risk.
4. Clustering of dose distributions into 'reasonable' sub-target and sub-tumor regions. Here operator interaction is indispensable to review and amend the automatically generated dose plateaus in the target and organ at risk.

Once the sub-tumor and sub-organ volumes have been generated and assigned to an appropriate dose level, inverse planning (step 5) can be executed to generate treatment parameters. A feasibility study for a prostate tumor featuring a non-uniform radioresistance was conducted to test the implementation. The algorithm yielded two distinct regions: for the more radioresistant region a 20% higher dose was prescribed than in the remaining tumor region. The study compares a standard treatment plan and one with adaptation to sub-tumor radioresistance. The result is shown in Figure 14-6.

5. SUMMARY AND OUTLOOK

Tumor hypoxia and cell proliferation are important parameters, which may allow characterization of tumor radio-resistance and response to radiotherapy. Accurate quantification of these parameters is a prerequisite if this novel information shall be optimally used for treatment definition. Kinetic modeling has the potential to provide the level of accuracy necessary. It has been discussed how a surrogate for the oxygen content in hypoxic tumors and the cell proliferation can be extracted from time series of PET images using the agents FMISO and FLT, respectively. Furthermore, a pathway how this information can be used to improve treatment definition and to enable sub-tumor dose sculpting has been presented.

Imaging and quantification of molecular markers will play an essential role in future radiotherapy planning. Technologies are emerging, which will allow processing and handling of quantitative molecular images in the radiotherapy planning suite, thereby facilitating clinical usage of these technologies. Certainly, much more clinical experience is needed before molecular imaging guided radiotherapy can be considered as a clinical reality.

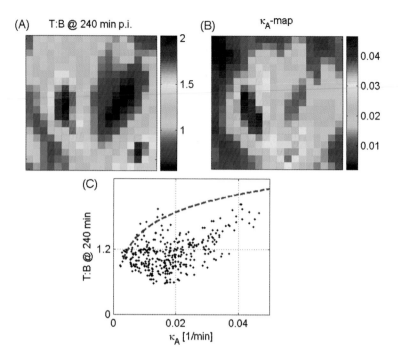

Figure 14-5. (A) T:B ratio at 240 min after tracer administration. (B) Parametric map of the rate constant K_A for the same region. The parameter α was kept fixed at 0.36 as suggested in the model[28]. (C) Scatter plot, T:B versus K_A, for lung cancer data (black dots) and the correlation hypothesized by Casciari[28] (red dashed line). (Data courtesy Dr. S.M. Eschmann, University of Tübingen).

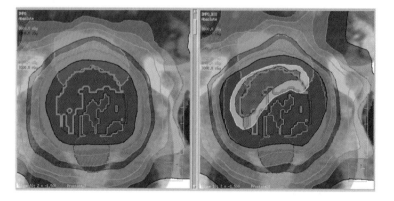

Figure 14-6. Standard prostate plan without (A) and with dose boosting (B) of a radioresistant sub-tumor region. The target volume is delineated in red color. The radioresistant sub-tumor region is delineated in green (contours are drawn in A and B).

ACKNOWLEDGEMENT

The PET program in cancer imaging at the University of Washington is generously supported by P01 CA42045 from the National Cancer Institute and S10 RR17229.

REFERENCES

1. G.J. Kelloff, J.M. Hoffman, B. Johnson et al., Progress and promise of FDG-PET imaging for cancer management and oncologic drug development, *Clin Cancer Res* **11**(8), 2785-808 (2005).
2. H. Van Tinteren, O.F. Hoekstra, F.F. Smit et al., Effectiveness of positron emission tomography in the preoperative assessment of patients with suspected non-small-cell lung cancer: the PLUS multicentre randomised trial, *Lancet* **359**(9315), 1388-93 (2002).
3. S.S. Gambhir, J. Czernin, J. Schwimmer, et al., A tabulated summary of the FDG PET literature, *J Nucl Med.* **43**(5 Suppl), 1S-93S (2001).
4. N.E. Avril, W.A. Weber, Monitoring response to treatment in patients utilizing PET, *Radiol Clin N Am* **43**, 189-204 (2005).
5. J.D. Schwarz, M. Bader, L. Jenicke et al., Early prediction of response to chemotherapy in metastatic breast camcer using sequential ^{18}F-FDG PET, *J Nucl Med* **46**(7), 1144-1150 (2005).
6. S. Webb, *Contemporary IMRT – Developing physics and clinical implementation,* (IOP Publishing Ltd, Bristol, 2005).
7. C.C. Ling, J. Humm, S. Larson et al., Towards multidimensional radiotherapy (MD-CRT): biological imaging and biological conformality, *Int J Radiation Oncology Biol Phys* **47**(3), 551-560 (2000).
8. K.S. Tralins, J.G. Douglas, K.J. Stelzer et al., Volumetric analysis of ^{18}F-FDG PET in glioblastoma multiforme: Prognostic information and possible role in definition of target volumnes in radiation dose escalation, *J Nucl Med* **43**(12), 1667-1673 (2002).
9. Y. Seppenwoolde, M. Engelsman, K. De Jaeger, et al., Optimizing radiation treatment plans for lung cancer using lung perfusion information, *Radiotherapy and Oncology* **63**, 165-177 (2002).
10. M. Alber, F. Paulsen, S.M. Eschmann et al., On biologically conformal boost dose optimization, *Phys Med Biol* **48**, N31-N35 (2003).
11. S.K. Das, M.M. Mifton, S. Zhou et al., Feasibility of optimizing the dose distribution in lung tumors using fluorine-18-fluorodeoxyglucose positron emission tomography and single photon emission computed tomography guided dose prescriptions, *Med Phys* **31**(6), 1452-1461 (2004).
12. D. Hanahan, R.A. Weinberg, The hallmarks of cancer, *Cell* **100**, 57-70 (2000).
13. C. Van de Wiele, C. Lahorte, W. Oyen et al., Nuclear medicine imaging to predict response to radiotherapy: A review, *Int J Radiation Oncology Biol Phys* **55**(1), 5-15 (2003).
14. D.A. Mankoff, A.F. Shields, K.A. Krohn, PET imaging of cellular proliferation, *Radiol Clin N Amer* **43**, 153-167 (2005).
15. R.H. Thomlinson, and L.H. Gray, The histological structure of some human lung cancers and the possible implications for radiotherapy, *Brit J Cancer* **9**, 537-549 (1955).

16. R.M. Sutherland, G.F. Whitmore, K.A. Krohn, in: *Prediction of Tumor Treatment Response*, edited by J.D. Chapman et al., 307-316 (Pergamon Press, New York, 1989).

17. J.G. Rajendran, and K.A. Krohn, Imaging hypoxia and angiogenesis in tumors, *Radiol Clin N Amer* **43**, 169-187 (2005).

18. R.B. Livingston, and J.S. Hart, The clinical applications of cell kinetics in cancer therapy, *Ann Rev Toxicol* **17**, 529-543 (1997).

19. D. Christman, E.J. Crawford, M. Friedkin et al., Detection of DNA synthesis in intact organisms with positron-emitting methyl-[C-11]-thymidine, *Proc Natl Acad Sci USA* **69**, 988-992 (1972).

20. A.F. Shields, D.A. Mankoff, J.M. Link et al., Carbon-11-thymidine and FDG to measure therapy response, *J Nucl Med* **39**, 1757-1762 (1998).

21. J.F. Eary, D.A. Mankoff, A.M. Spence et al., 2-[^{11}C]thymidine positron emission tomography of malignant brain tumors, *Cancer Res* **59**, 615-621 (1999).

22. P. Wells, E. Aboagye, R.N. Gunn et al., 2-[^{11}C]thymidine positron emission tomography as an indicator of thymidylate synthase inhibition in patients treated with AG337, *J Natl Cancer Inst* **95**, 675-682 (2003).

23. A.F. Shields, J.R. Grierson, S.M. Kozawa et al., Development of labeled thymidine analogs for imaging tumor proliferation, *Nucl Med Biol* **23**, 17-22 (1996).

24. A.F. Shields, J.R. Grierson, B.M. Dohmen et al., Imaging proliferation in vivo with [^{18}F]FLT and positron emission tomography, *Nature Med* **4**, 1334-1336 (1998).

25. H.N. Wagner, Jr., Molecular nuclear medicine: The best kept secret in medicine, *J Nucl Med Newsline* **38**, 15N-47N (1997).

26. W.J. Koh, J.S. Rasey, M.L. Evans et al., Imaging of hypoxia in human tumors with [^{18}F]FMISO, *Int J Radiation Oncology Biol Phys* **22**(1), 199-212 (1992).

27. J.G. Rajendran, D.C. Wilson, E.U. Conrad et al., [^{18}F]FMISO and [^{18}F]FDG-PET imaging in soft tissue sarcomas: correlation of hypoxia, metabolism and VEGF expression, *Eur J Nucl Med Mol Imaging* **30**, 695-704 (2003).

28. J.J. Casciari, M.M. Graham, J.S. Rasey et al., A modeling approach for quantifying tumor hypoxia with [^{18}F]fluoromisonidazole PET time-activity data, *Med Phys* **22**(7), 1127-1139 (1995).

29. S. Huang, M.E. Phelps, in: *Positron emission tomography and autoradiography – Principles and applications for the brain and heart*, edited by M.E. Phelps, J.C. Mazziotta, and H.R. Schelbert, 287-346 (Raven Press, New York, 1986).

30. S.M. Eschmann, F. Paulsen, M. Reimold et al., Prognostic impact of hypoxia-imaging with 18F-Misonidazole-PET in non-small cell lung cancer and head-and-neck cancer prior to radiotherapy, *J Nucl Med* **46**, 253-260 (2005).

31. J.E. Cleaver, Thymidine metabolism and cell kinetics, *Frontiers Biol* **6**, 43-100 (1967).

32. A.F. Shields, D.V. Coonrod, R.C. Quackenbush et al., Cellular sources of thymidine nucleotides: Studies for PET, *J Nucl Med* **28**, 1435-1440 (1987).

33. D.A. Mankoff, A.F. Shields, M.M. Graham et al., Kinetic analysis of 2-[carbon-11]-thymidine PET imaging studies: compartmental model and mathematical analysis, *J Nucl Med* **39**, 1043-1055 (1998).

34. J.M. Wells, D.A. Mankoff, M. Muzi et al., Kinetic analysis of 2-[^{11}C]thymidine PET imaging studies of malignant brain tumors: compartmental model investigation and mathematical analysis, *Molec Imaging* **1**, 151-159 (2002).

35. P. Wells, R.N. Gunn, M. Alison et al., Assessment of proliferation in vivo using 2-[^{11}C]thymidine positron emission tomography in advanced intra-abdominal malignancies, *Cancer Res* **62**, 5298-5702 (2002).

36. D.A. Mankoff, A.F. Shields, J.M. Link et al., Kinetic analysis of 2-[^{11}C]thymidine PET imaging studies: Validation studies, *J Nucl Med* **40**, 614-624 (1999).

37. H. Vesselle, J. Grierson, M. Muzi et al., In vivo validation of 3'-deoxy-3'-[^{18}F]fluoro-thymidine ([^{18}F]FLT) as a proliferation imaging tracer in humans: correlation of [^{18}F]FLT uptake by positron emission tomography with Ki-67 immunohistochemsitry and flow cytometry in human lung tumors, *Clin Cancer Res* **8**, 3315-3323 (2002).

38. M. Muzi, D.A. Mankoff, J.R. Grierson et al., Kinetic modeling of 3'-deoxy-3'-fluoro-thymidine in somatic tumors: mathematical studies, *J Nucl Med* **46**, 371-380 (2005).

39. M. Muzi, H. Vesselle, J.R. Grierson et al., Kinetic analysis of 3'-deoxy-3'-fluoro-thymidine PET studies: validation in patients with lung cancer, *J Nucl Med* **46**, 274-282 (2005).

40. Y. Yang, L. Xing, Towards biologically conformal radiation therapy (BCRT): Selective IMRT dose escalation under guidance of spatial biology distribution, *Med Phys* **32**(6), 1473-1483 (2005).

41. M.C. Joiner, S.M. Bentzen, in: *Basic clinical radiobiology*, G.G. Steel (ed.), 120-134, (Oxford University Press, New York, 2002).

42. R.O. Duda, P.E. Hart, *Pattern classification and scene analysis* (Wiley and Sons, New York, 1973).

PART IV: MOLECULAR MEDICINE

Chapter 15

MOLECULAR MEDICINE
A Revolution in Health Care

Hans Hofstraat

Philips Research, Eindhoven, The Netherlands

Abstract: 'Molecular' medicine, based on the use of molecular characteristics of disease, resulting from the recent progress in insight in the human genome and its function, will have a revolutionary impact on healthcare. Preventive and individualized healthcare will occupy an increasingly important place in the present medical practice, which is still predominantly based on symptomatic diagnosis and treatment. Elements of the concomitant paradigm shift in healthcare are early and more effective and successful treatment of disease with minimal side effects, and more effective follow-up post-therapy. Molecular Medicine has a very important technological component. The two main enabling technologies are molecular imaging, focused on identification of location and extent of the disease *in vivo*, in the patient, and molecular diagnostics, based on detection of biomarkers *in vitro*, in samples taken from the patient, generally blood. Both technologies and their integrated application in the disease 'Care Cycle', will be highlighted.

Keywords: Molecular medicine, molecular imaging, molecular diagnostics, bio-informatics, system biology, biomarker, biosensor, therapy, care cycle

1. INTRODUCTION

Advances in human genome research are opening the door to a new paradigm for practicing medicine that promises to transform healthcare. Personalized, 'molecular', medicine, the use of marker-assisted diagnosis, based on both *in vitro* testing and *in vivo* targeted imaging, and therapy planning, targeted therapies adapted to an individual's molecular profile, will impact the way drugs are developed and medicine is practiced[1,2]. In addition, patient care will be revolutionized through the use of novel approaches like determination of molecular predisposition, screening of individuals with an

G. Spekowius and T. Wendler (Eds.), Advances in Healthcare Technology, 235-246.

elevated risk profile, and by the exploitation of diagnostic, prognostic, pharmacogenomic and monitoring biomarkers. Although numerous challenges need to be met to make personalized medicine a reality, this approach will replace the traditional trial-and-error practice of medicine in due time by 'evidence-based' medicine (see Figure 15-1). Characteristics of molecular medicine are: early and faster diagnosis, better prognosis, and tailored therapy with higher efficacy and reduced side effects as compared to the present state-of-the-art. The basis for this revolution is the explosive growth in knowledge of the structure of the human genome, and its translation into the *functional* elements, the proteins. Key for the introduction of evidence-based medicine is the availability of advanced medical instrumentation, in particular for *in vitro* and *in vivo* diagnostics, and to support therapy, and advanced information technology to integrate the multiple and complex data streams generated, in support of clinical decision taking.

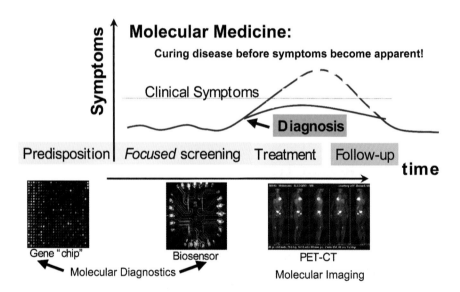

Figure 15-1. Molecular diagnostics and molecular imaging, coupled to therapy, will change the current practice of health care.

2. SYSTEM BIOLOGY AND BIOMARKERS

The next step, to relate the knowledge of the molecular translation cycle to onset, development and ultimately treatment of disease, is still extremely complex. It bases on insight into the genetic make-up of the individual, primarily given by hereditary factors, and laid down in the DNA, and subsequently transcribed by RNA into the proteins, the molecules which are instrumental in all major biological processes taking place in human cells, tissues and organs. Advances in technology have led to elucidation of the genetic make-up of, by now many, species, including humans, fueled by the ambitious human genome project. Similarly, efforts are going on to establish RNA patterns (the 'transcriptome') and – extremely challenging still – get insight into the range of proteins present (the 'proteome'). Knowledge of the genome, transcriptome and proteome by itself is not sufficient. Gaining insight into the functioning of protein signaling, and its impact on cell multiplication, interaction and transformation (stem cells) forms the main challenge of 'systems biology'. In systems biology or 'integrative' biology one tries to integrate all information available from genomics, transcriptomics, proteomics, the metabolic processes in our cells and organs ('metabolomics') in an effort to understand the intricate processes, which govern the human body – and provide the basis for understanding the origins of diseases. To establish the link to disease it is not sufficient to identify the primary genetic structures. In addition, we have to gain knowledge on the impact of 'environmental' factors, such as the effect of nutrition, lifestyle, our ambient, stress, etc. These external factors may have profound effects on the structure of the genome (e.g., modification of DNA by methylation, 'epigenetics'), and will translate into the proteome. Particularly understanding of these environmental factors is required to really get a handle on the origin of most diseases, and to be able to devise effective cures.

In an effort to reach this goal one tries to relate the wealth of information, which is available from patient samples (information from healthy and diseased tissue, generally comprising DNA, RNA, proteins and metabolites), to clinical information, with the aim to identify biomarkers – observables, which are characteristic for a particular disease, and can be used for early diagnosis. Such biomarkers can be discovered in bodily fluids, e.g. in blood or serum, so that they may be determined by *in vitro* diagnostic approaches, but also in tissue or organs, providing handles for targeted contrast agents, which can be visualized *in vivo* by making use of advanced imaging instrumentation. Specific biomarkers can be applied for early diagnosis and for monitoring of diseases, but they can also be used to accelerate the process of drug discovery and development: By using biomarkers as 'surrogate endpoints' in clinical trials drug effectiveness (and toxicology, or other side effects) can be detected much earlier than in the conventional practice, based on survival rate. The key to this data interpretation and analysis challenge is in linking the rich 'molecular' information to the relatively scarce patient data, which is furthermore complicated by the inherent biological variability. Bioinformatics here plays a central role. A diagrammatic representation of this complex process is presented in Figure 15-2. The main aims of the process are to identify characteristic and clinically validated biomarkers for disease, and to gain insight into the effects of external factors, like food or pharmaceuticals, on the individual human health status, defining the fields of nutrigenomics and pharma-cogenomics, and the effective implementation of personalized medicine. Chapter 17 describes the status of the use of biomarkers in their application for disease diagnosis and treatment.

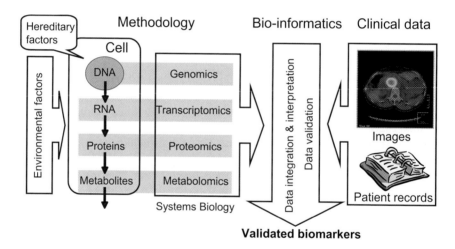

Figure 15-2. Validated biomarkers are key in the successful introduction of Molecular Medicine. Their identification requires the interpretation of large and complicated data sets, with the help of bio-informatics tools.

3.   OPPORTUNITIES OF MOLECULAR MEDICINE

The insight is growing in the molecular origin of disease. It becomes increasingly clear that the majority of life-threatening diseases has its origin, or at least is significantly influenced by, genetic effects. The sensitivity to all diseases that are the main causes of death, cardiovascular disease, cancer, diabetes, and infectious diseases (TBC, malaria, AIDS, etc.) is genetically determined to some extent. The same is true for the major debilitating diseases, which strongly influence the quality of life: Neuro-degenerative diseases (e.g., Alzheimer's, Parkinson's) and autoimmune diseases (like rheumatoid arthritis). Early detection of these diseases greatly improves the therapeutic success rate, leading to a prolongation of the healthy and productive lifespan of the individual, and treatment with fewer side effects. In addition it has a potential cost-containment effect as well: Particularly a shift in the onset of debilitating diseases results in a significant reduction of the very high personnel costs involved with nursing the patients.

Molecular medicine may completely change the healthcare 'industry'. Traditional medicine practice, based on trial-and-error, results both in under-treatment and over-treatment, multiple office visits, the need for drug monitoring, and frequent regimen changes. More than 100,000 deaths per year (USA alone) are attributed to adverse drug reactions[1]. A personalized approach of tailored care for every individual will become the standard. Introduction of targeted drugs, which block receptors in the membrane of tumor cells, for instance, may result in slowing down their proliferation or even in their elimination. Apart from more effective treatment, some cancer types may well be contained – effectively turning cancer in a manageable, 'chronic', disease. First successful targeted drugs have already been introduced. An example is the drug imatinib (Gleevec, by Novartis), developed after the discovery of a chromosome translocation creating a new gene structure, the abl-bcr gene, in chronic myeloid leukemia patients. Gleevec binds specifically to the abl-bcr protein, and can alleviate the leukemia in patients for whom other treatments have failed[3]. Other examples of targeted drugs are Herceptin (Genentech/Roche, indication: meta-static breast cancer), and the non-Hodgkin's lymphoma drugs Bexxar (GlaxoSmithKline), and Zevalin (BiogenIdec). All these drugs are based on monoclonal antibodies, which bind selectively to the tumor cells, and may be equipped with toxic substances to enhance their efficiency (e.g., in Bexxar radioactive ^{131}I is present to invoke radio immunotherapy). The targeted or 'smart' drugs are extremely expensive, for instance for treatment with Zevalin and Bexxar the cost of medication amounts to 25-30 k$ per patient. It is therefore also for financial reasons very important to identify those patients, which respond well to the medication prior to the treatment.

4.   TECHNOLOGY IS KEY

Molecular medicine is enabled by medical technologies, particularly by molecular diagnostics, applied for screening and monitoring to effect early detection, and by molecular imaging, relying on joint application of advanced imaging equipment and targeted and/or functional contrast agents (see Figure 15-3). Molecular imaging offers unique opportunities for combination with (targeted) therapy that can be much better planned and monitored with the help of advanced hardware and specifically developed software tools, which enable pharmacodynamic modelling. Typically, molecular diagnostics and molecular imaging will be applied in tandem, with the goal to provide tailored solutions for a wide range of diseases. A secondary opportunity may be the application of imaging techniques to advance and simplify the drug discovery and development process, driven by collaboration of pharmaceutical and biotech companies on the one hand, and medical technology companies on the other. The increasingly important role of medical technologies in molecular medicine offers opportunities to new entrants into this space, particularly to technology-rich companies.

Briefly, the two main technology areas will be discussed.

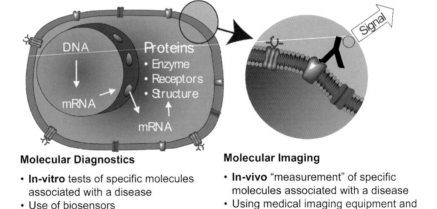

Molecular Diagnostics

• **In-vitro** tests of specific molecules associated with a disease
• Use of biosensors

Molecular Imaging

• **In-vivo** "measurement" of specific molecules associated with a disease
• Using medical imaging equipment and specific contrast agents

Figure 15-3. Molecular diagnostics and molecular imaging are the key technologies enabling molecular medicine. In both technologies characteristic and validated biomarkers are needed.

4.1 Molecular diagnostics and biosensors

In vitro diagnostic approaches will become indispensable for early diagnosis, for the selection of personalized therapy, and for effective follow-up, after completion of the treatment or to support maintenance of a chronic condition. A distinction should be made between techniques applied for the identification of genomic fingerprints and methods suitable for identification of particular biomarkers.

Genomic fingerprints thus far have been mostly applied to identify pathogens, particularly tests are commercially available for human papilloma virus, for various forms of the human immunodeficiency virus, and for hepatitis B and hepatitis C. Diagnostic products for infectious diseases therefore at present dominate the market. Detection is predominantly based on amplification of characteristic nucleotide sequences using the polymerase chain reaction (PCR), followed by a hybridization assay.

Increasingly, genomic fingerprints are utilized to assay the molecular make up of the host, rather than the pathogen, and are applied to phenotype individuals and hence to identify their predisposition to particular diseases or to tailor individual therapeutic interventions (e.g., selection of the appropriate dose of medication on the basis of metabolic characteristics). The thus obtained 'pharmacogenomic' fingerprints rely on the application of high-density arrays (e.g., the GeneChips provided by the American company Affymetrix, or the DNA Microarrays sold by, also US-based, Agilent). Typically, these high-density arrays contain many thousands of different oligonucleotide strings, which are located at different, well-known locations. The presence of complementary oligonucleotides in the sample can be measured optically, through sensitive detection of fluorescent labels; even single mismatches, so-called single nucleotide polymorphisms, can be identified. By careful execution of the measurement protocol also genetic expression profiles, highlighting upregulation or downregulation of certain parts of DNA or RNA can be made visible. The observed features can be applied for diagnostic classification, treatment selection and prognostic assessment.[4] In Figure 15-1 an image of (part of) a DNA 'chip' is shown. Other technologies gaining ground particularly for cancer diagnostics are in-situ hybridization and fluorescent in-situ hybridization.

Alternatively, the measurement can be focused on the identification of a (generally more limited) set of biomarkers. Biomarkers in general are proteins, which are triggered by the presence of a disease, such as membrane proteins, synthesized in response to disease (e.g., proteins, which signal apoptosis, or programmed cell death, or enzymes, which are released following a stroke or a myocardial infarction). Generally, well-established immunological techniques, such as the widely applied enzyme-linked immunosorbent assay ('ELISA'), are used for protein diagnostics, all based on the application of highly specific antibodies. For many diseases it is necessary to determine a multitude of proteins and, sometimes, additional biomarkers, which requires development of new methodologies (see Chapter 17). High throughput analysis of proteins can be applied for the detection of novel drug targets, diagnostic markers, and for the investigation of biological events[5]. Proteomics has the potential of becoming a very powerful tool in modern medicine, but still is strongly under development.

Another kind of biomarker is the presence of a particular kind of pathogen, which can be identified following the approach described above, so that immediately the cause of the infection and the optimal cure can be established.

Essential for the massive introduction of molecular diagnostics is the availability of cheaper and more accessible technologies. For applications, in which rapid turnaround times are important, in particular at the point-of-care (e.g., for diagnosis of a cardiovascular problem in the ambulance) rapid, simple and 'stand-alone' approaches are needed. Miniaturized, integrated, 'lab-on-a-chip' tools, based on microfluidic solutions and enabled by advances in micro- and nanotechnology, may serve this need. In Figure 15-1, a detail of Philips' very sensitive and integrated magnetic biosensor chip is shown, a true product of advanced microsystems technology[6].

In Chapter 21, a more detailed discussion of the developments in the use of proteins, and their application in health care, can be found, mainly focused on the application of mass spectrometry as technique to diagnose disease by simultaneous measurement of multiple proteins, as proteomic 'fingerprint'.

4.2   Molecular imaging and therapy

The possibilities offered by molecular imaging are impressive as well. Developments in medical imaging systems, increasingly integrating advanced, high-resolution, instruments with sophisticated data and image processing to provide ever increasing quality of information to the medical professional, go hand in hand with developments of sophisticated functional and targeted contrast agent[7,8]. Particularly, the advances in nuclear imaging technologies, such as Single Photon Emission Computed Tomography (SPECT) and Positron Emission Tomography (PET), extremely low concentrations of targets can be localized and quantified. These techniques can be utilized to visualize nanomolar or even picomolar concentrations of (radioactive) molecules, and can not only be applied for measurement of targeted contrast agents, but also for functional monitoring (e.g., measuring increased metabolic rates, related to tumor growth). Combination of the sensitive, but not very highly resolved nuclear imaging techniques with other imaging modalities, which do provide high-resolution morphological data, such as Computed Tomography (CT), leads to very powerful molecular imaging tools. Also in Magnetic Resonance Imaging (MRI) impressive improvements in sensitivity have been realized. By application of targeted nanoparticles, sub-micromolar concentrations of suitable contrast agents can be measured. Nanoparticles in general offer interesting opportunities as multifunctional platforms that can be used to accommodate, in addition to targeting units, both contrast agents and drugs, for targeted therapy[9].

An interesting opportunity of MRI is to use the imaging instrument directly, without the application of contrast agents, e.g. to measure brain activity. This so-called 'functional MRI' technique obviously has the advantage that truly non-invasive characterization can be done.

The introduction of Molecular Imaging approaches into the medical practice requires both instrumental and (bio)chemical advances. Chapter 16 on Molecular Imaging Systems addresses the first topic. The imaging agents, in a general sense are covered in Chapter 18, and the particular focus on the application of targeted nanoparticles in Chapter 19. Chapter 20 on molecular imaging with Annexin A5 provides a detailed account of the potential of *in vivo* medical imaging for tomorrow's healthcare, exemplified by the application of targeted contrast agents for the early identification of indications of cardiovascular disease.

5. IMPLEMENTATION: THE 'CARE CYCLE'

The full-fledged introduction of molecular medicine is the basis for an integrated approach of tomorrow's healthcare, with the following characteristics:

- Earlier detection of disease, by careful screening of people with elevated genetically inherited and/or lifestyle-related risks using highly specific biomarkers.
- Better diagnosis for better treatment, based on the individual patient's own biochemistry.
- Targeted and minimally invasive treatment with better efficacy and less side effects.
- This picture of the future is driven by technological advancements, but relies on important and challenging advancements in the biomedical sciences and in information technology as well.

It is Philips' ambition to address healthcare in an integrated fashion, addressing all aspects of the 'Care Cycle', as schematically depicted in Figure 15-4. The 'Care Cycle' approach starts with determination of the individual's predisposition to identify genetically inherited or lifestyle related risks using molecular diagnostics. It then moves to focused screening of people at risk, initially employing molecular diagnostic technologies, but in combination with molecular imaging for confirmation, localization and quantification, aiming at early detection of the onset of disease. Subsequently, when needed, individualized therapy is started, guided by treatment planning and monitoring of the therapeutic results with the aid of (molecular) imaging. In addition, imaging techniques can be invoked for minimally invasive treatment, providing more directed surgery and treatment. Finally, post-treatment molecular diagnostics and molecular imaging can be utilized to monitor for recurrence or for active containment of the disease. The proposed approaches, which of course need to be combined with established clinical procedures, lead to an explosive increase of data, both qualitative and quantitative (enabling more objective, 'evidence-based' medicine), which makes taking the right decisions more and more complex. Hence, attention needs to be paid to derive transparent information from the rich data sets, and help the physician to come to the right diagnosis and therapy. Philips has taken up this challenge and is developing 'Clinical Decision Support Systems' to serve this need.

First elements of molecular medicine have already been introduced into the clinical practice. Examples are screening for predisposition for breast cancer, which is offered by the company Myriad Genetics. Focused screening of women at risk may result in detection of breast cancer at an early stage, when it is still localized, with close to 100% treatment success. The Dutch start-up Agendia, based on the pioneering work of Laura van 't Veer and coworkers, has developed a tool for stratification of patients, based on 70 marker genes, allowing for the administration of the best treatment to the individual patient[10]. Philips Radiation Oncology Systems (PROS) provides innovative solutions to manage patient treatment, which include imaging, localization, simulation and planning of minimally invasive, image-guided procedures, and planning of conformal external beams for more effective radiation treatment. Genentech, finally, has developed a targeted, antibody-based, drug, which can be applied to cure women with metastasized breast cancer, provided they show overexpression of the Her2/Neu membrane receptor[11]. The company Vysis has developed a molecular diagnostic test to screen for this receptor, to identify those patients, which will benefit from the treatment[12].

Even though individual tests are available, it will take time to introduce molecular medicine throughout the care cycle. For many diseases no comprehensive insight is available into their origin, and no unambiguous biomarkers have yet been identified. To counter this challenge a tremendous effort is required, involving advanced academic research, together with contributions from pharmaceutical and biotech companies, and from medical technology companies, which should join forces to realize breakthroughs. At the same time it is crucial to link the increasing insights in the fundamental biochemistry of disease to clinical observations. In particular molecular imaging can play a crucial role in this translational challenge. Finally, the medical profession is (rightfully) conservative; therefore, convincing evidence for the efficacy of the Molecular Medicine approaches needs to be provided, before they will be accepted. The challenges have been recognized by NIH director Zerhouni, who identifies in his description of the NIH Roadmap the most compelling opportunities in three arenas: new pathways to discoveries, (highly multidisciplinary) research teams of the future, and re-engineering the clinical research enterprise[13].

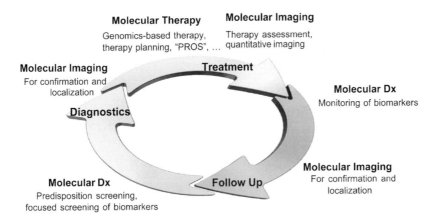

Figure 15-4. The future 'Care Cycle' of molecular medicine, based on the joint application of molecular diagnostics and molecular imaging to enable timely and targeted treatment.

My expectation is, however, that within the next decades an increasing number of molecular diagnostic and molecular imaging approaches will be introduced, providing molecular medicine care cycles for many important diseases.

REFERENCES

1. G.S. Ginsburg, and J.J. McCarthy, Personalized medicine: revolutionizing drug discovery and patient care, *Trends Biotechnol* **19**, 491-496 (2001).
2. R.I. Pettigrew, C.A. Fee, K.C. Li, Changes in the world of biomedical research are moving the field of 'personalized medicine' from concept to reality, *Nucl Med* **45**, 1427 (2004).
3. B.J. Druker, Imatinib alone and in combination for chronic myeloid leukemia, *Semin Hematol* **40**, 50-58 (2003).
4. R. Simon, Using DNA microarrays for diagnostic and prognostic prediction, *Expert Rev Mol Diagn* **3**, 587-595 (2003).

5. M. Fountoulakis, Proteomics in drug discovery: potential and limitations, *Biomed Health Res* **55**, 279-293 (2002).

6. M. Megens, M.W.J. Prins, Magnetic biochips: a new option for sensitive diagnostics, *J Magn Magn Mat* **293**, 702-708 (2005).

7. R. Weissleder, U. Mahmood, Molecular imaging, *Radiology* **219**, 316-333 (2001).

8. F.A. Jaffer, R. Weissleder, Molecular imaging in the clinical arena, *JAMA* **293**, 855-862 (2005).

9. S.A. Wickline, G. Lanza, Nanotechnology for molecular imaging and targeted therapy, *Circulation* **107**, 1092-1095 (2003).

10. L. van 't Veer, H. Dai, M. van de Vijver, Y.D. He, A.A.M. Hart, M. Mao, H.L. Petersar, K. van der Kooy, M.J. Marton, A.T. Witteveen, G.J. Schreiber, R.M. Kerkhoven, C. Roberts, P.S. Linsley, R. Bernards, S.H. Friend, Gene expression and profiling predicts clinical outcome of breast cancer, *Nature* **415**, 530-536 (2002).

11. 'Herceptin', or Trastuzumab humanized antibody in combination with paclitaxel; for therapeutic details and mode of action see www.gene.com.

12. PathVysion HER-2 DNA probe kit; www.vysis.com.

13. E. Zerhouni, Medicine. The NIH Roadmap, *Science* **302**, 63-64,72 (2003).

Chapter 16

MOLECULAR IMAGING SYSTEMS
Towards High Sensitive Detection of Molecular Processes for Early Diagnosis and Therapy

Tobias Schaeffter
Philips Research, Hamburg, Germany

Abstract: Molecular imaging is a new discipline in medicine that promises a paradigm shift in healthcare: from diagnosis and treatment of late symptoms, to the prevention and cure of diseases. In this chapter, the basic principles of molecular imaging are described. It is shown that molecular imaging requires imaging systems with high sensitivity. Basic principles of the different imaging modalities are described emphasizing the main factors that influence the sensitivity. Since the different imaging modalities can be considered as being complementary, the development of multi-modality systems is highly relevant for molecular imaging.

Keywords: Molecular imaging, PET, SPECT, optical, MRI, ultrasound, X-ray, sensitivity, multi-modality systems

1.   INTRODUCTION

The developments in molecular biology and genomics in the past decade have resulted in better understanding of the underlying processes of diseases. These new insights can cause a redefinition of diseases. Likewise, new diagnostic and therapeutic strategies will be designed to specifically target abnormal molecular pathways. Especially, many modern drugs stop or modulate molecular processes, whereas the assessment of the therapeutic effects caused by such drugs is still based upon the diagnosis of late symptoms, e.g. the size of tumors. The development of a molecular-based diagnosis could help to detect diseases in an early stage and to assess therapy effects more rapidly. Furthermore, the availability of molecular diagnostic techniques can also support the development and approval of new molecular

G. Spekowius and T. Wendler (Eds.), Advances in Healthcare Technology, 247-268.

therapies. In the long run, the development of molecular medicine (i.e. molecular diagnosis and therapy) could enable a paradigm shift from diagnosing and treating the late symptoms, to prevention or cure of diseases.

An important development in molecular medicine is the advancement of diagnostic imaging to assess disease-specific molecular information. This fast developing field of 'Molecular Imaging' aims at the early detection of pathological processes for better diagnosis and/or monitoring of therapies. Molecular imaging does not resolve the molecule's structure by employing ultra-high spatial resolution, but it aims at the 'exploitation of specific molecules as the source of image contrast'[1]. In principle all major diagnostic imaging techniques, like nuclear imaging, magnetic resonance imaging (MRI), ultrasound (US), X-ray and optical imaging, can be exploited for molecular imaging. In the following, the principle of molecular imaging will be introduced and the different imaging modalities will be discussed for their application in molecular imaging.

2.   PRINCIPLE OF MOLECULAR IMAGING

Already in an early stage of a disease, cells can show a number of pathological features: There may be specific mutations in one or a number of genes of the cell's DNA or the cells may show a different activity of gene expression, which results in an up- or downregulation of specific molecules in- or outside the cell. Molecular imaging aims at the detection and quantification of such molecules. Since the molecules themselves are too small to be imaged directly with non-invasive imaging techniques, targeted contrast agents are employed. In general, such a targeted contrast agent consists of a number of components (see Figure 16-1a): a ligand, a linker, a carrier and one or a number of labels. A ligand selectively binds to the target. This could be a peptide, aptamer, antibody or other small molecule. The linker connects the ligand to the carrier. Typical carrier substances are dendrimers[2], polymers[3], liposomes[4], perfluorcarbon nanoparticles[5] or fullerenes[6]. The carrier contains a number of labels, which influence the image contrast. The composition of the label depends on the imaging modality. For example, such a targeted label-compound could be a radioactive isotope for nuclear imaging[7], a fluorescent molecule for optical imaging[8], paramagnetic ions for MRI[9] or microbubbles[10] and/or nanoparticles[5] for ultrasound. Generally, there are two different interactions of targeted agents to detect molecular targets (see Figure 16-1b). First, a targeted agent can selectively bind to the molecular target (e.g. cell surface receptor). After clearance of the unbound contrast agent there is a one-to-one relation of agent and receptor. Therefore, the receptor density determines the number of targeted agents that can be imaged. Second, the targeted contrast agent could interact with molecules (e.g. enzymes) inside of cells resulting in trapping of the contrast agent inside the cell. An advantage of this approach is that an enzyme can trap a number of targeted agents. Therefore, over time, the contrast agent will accumulate in cells that contain the target molecule, i.e. this mechanism leads to an effective amplification of the signal. Another class of imaging agents is activatable or 'smart' agents. These are agents, in which the contrast mechanism could be switched 'on' and 'off', when the agent hits the molecular target[11,12].

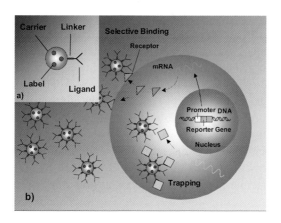

Figure 16-1. a) Components of targeted agents. b) Interaction of targeted agents: selective binding and trapping.

A critical step in utilizing molecular imaging is to define appropriate imaging targets and corresponding ligands. The definition of imaging targets depends on the existing scientific understanding of the disease. In some cases, targets and suitable ligands can be found in the existing scientific literature. Increasingly, high-throughput screening techniques, which incorporate data from genomic and proteomic screens, are being used to find molecules that are expressed at abnormally high or low levels in certain diseases. Most human diseases involve a number genes and proteins and the resulting over- or underexpression of molecules results from complex competing mechanisms influenced by genetics, environmental factors and the immune system. Therefore, it is often difficult to distinguish between molecules that are associated with the disease and those molecules, which are related to an immune response. Furthermore, the up- and down regulation of molecules is a dynamic process, i.e. diseases move through different stages and thus different types and levels of molecules are expressed. The identification of suitable targets is key for the development of targeted imaging agents and drugs. Currently available drugs are directed against approximately 500 molecular targets (45% of which are receptors; 30%, enzymes; and 25%, other targets), and it is estimated that potential future drug targets are in excess of 5,000–10,000[13]. A more detailed description of potential molecular targets can be found in the following Chapter 17.

In many cases, the accumulation of targeted imaging agents depends only on the proper selection of target-ligand combinations, but also on the physicochemical properties of the agent complex. After administration, a contrast agent will be distributed over and cleared from the body, which is called the pharmacokinetic of the agent. Characteristics like molecular weight, hydrophobicity and charge may cause a contrast agent to preferentially accumulate in certain cells or tissues. This passive targeting is for example used in the imaging of tumors, as the increased permeability of tumor vasculature allows macromolecules to extravasate and build up to a larger degree in tumor tissue[14]. Using targeted contrast agents does not mean that one can forget about passive targeting. A targeted contrast agent will still need to possess properties that enable it to reach its target. A detailed description of molecular imaging agents can be found in Chapter 18.

3.   MOLECULAR IMAGING SYSTEMS

Targeted contrast agents can be developed for different imaging modalities. The amount of image contrast caused by the agents depends on the underlying physical principle of the imaging modality, i.e. it depends on the type of the emitted energy and its interaction with the tissue. Imaging methods use either non-ionizing or ionizing radiation that interact with tissue at the molecular or atomic level, involving a variety of interaction mechanisms such as absorption, reflection, scattering and transmission. The type of energy involved and its interaction mechanisms determine not only the image contrast, but also the spatial resolution and sensitivity. Usually, these three properties depend on each other: even if the image has a very high signal-to-noise ratio (SNR), this is not useful unless there is a high enough contrast-to-noise ratio (CNR) to be able to distinguish between the accumulation of an agent and the background. The CNR depends also on the spatial resolution of the image. If the spatial resolution, (more precisely the full-width-half-maximum (FWHM) of the point spread function), is in the order of the size of the image feature, e.g. the accumulated contrast agent, then image blurring reduces the contrast significantly. In the following, the basic physical principles of the different imaging modalities are described, and the main factors that influence the sensitivity are discussed.

3.1 Nuclear imaging

Nuclear imaging is based on the detection of gamma rays that are emitted by radionuclides. Small amounts (typically nanograms) of radionuclides (e.g. ^{99m}Tc, ^{111}In, ^{123}I, ^{201}Tl, ^{11}C, ^{13}N, ^{15}O, and ^{18}F) are injected into the organism. In contrast to other imaging modalities like MRI, X-Ray or ultrasound, nuclear imaging does not provide morphology information but images the spatial distribution of radionuclides in the organism. This distribution strongly depends on the biological behavior of a radiopharmaceutical. Therefore, the development and synthesis of radiopharmaceuticals is key in nuclear imaging to obtain physiological, metabolic, and especially molecular information. Two main nuclear imaging techniques can be distinguished due to the use of different types of radionuclides: Single photon emitters decay under the emission of gamma rays with energies between 100 and 360 keV. Positron emitters decay under the emission of positrons that result in a pair of high-energy gamma rays (511 keV), after annihilation with an electron. The corresponding 3D imaging techniques are called single photon emission computed tomography (SPECT) and positron emission tomography (PET), respectively.

3.1.1 Single photon emission computed tomography (SPECT)

In SPECT, the injected radiopharmaceutical has accumulated in a suspicious region in the body. During the decay of the radionuclides, gamma rays are emitted in all directions. Some of the gamma rays are attenuated and scattered in the body. In order to detect the gamma rays a gamma camera is rotated around the body. The basic design of a gamma camera was described by Hal Anger in 1953[15], which mainly consists of three parts: a collimator, a scintillation crystal and a number of photomultipliers.

The collimator selects only those gamma rays that have a trajectory at an angle of 90° to the detector plane and blocks all others. The collimator is generally a lead structure with a honeycomb array of holes, where the lead walls (septa) are designed to prevent penetration of gamma rays from one hole to the other. The parallel hole collimator is the most widely used collimator. Other types of collimators can be used to magnify the size of an object on the image. A pinhole collimator is an extreme form of a converging collimator and allows magnifying small objects placed very close to the pinhole[16]. The disadvantage of collimators is the low efficiency of gamma ray utilization, because they absorb most of the emitted gamma rays.

The gamma rays that have passed through the collimator are converted into a detectable signal. Usually, a single sodium iodide crystal doted with thallium is used. When a gamma ray strikes this scintillation crystal, it loses energy through photoelectric interactions and, consequently, light is emitted. Overall, approximately 15% of the absorbed energy is converted into visible light. In order to convert the light signal into an electrical signal, photo-multipliers are closely coupled to the scintillation crystal. The position of the scintillation point is determined from the relative signal outputs of the photomultipliers using an Anger position network. In addition, the sum of the signals is proportional to the energy of the absorbed gamma rays, which can be used to differentiate between non-scattered and scattered gamma rays. Furthermore, energy windows can be used for simultaneous imaging of various tracers.

In SPECT, one or more gamma cameras are rotated around the patient. The camera acquires a number of planar images from different view angles in a 'stop-and-go' mode. Typically, 32 to 128 views are acquired to reconstruct a three-dimensional image of the object using a filtered backprojection algorithm. Usually, images with a numerical resolution of 64x64 and 128x128 are reconstructed. In order to improve the image quality in SPECT, the tissue attenuation has to be corrected for.

The spatial resolution in SPECT depends on a number of factors. Although the intrinsic resolution of the scintillator-photomultiplier combination is in the order of 3 mm, the practical resolution of gamma cameras is less and mainly limited by the collimator. The overall spatial resolution of clinical SPECT ranges from less than 1 cm to about 2 cm, depending on the collimator type and its distance from the gamma ray source. In dedicated animal systems, special collimators are used, such as pinhole collimators and their resolution can be below 3 mm.

The major applications of SPECT imaging are assessment of cardiac function, measurement of blood perfusion in various organs (e.g. heart, brain or lung), detection of tumors and measurement of renal function. SPECT has been successfully used in clinical oncology, e.g. for imaging of somatostatin receptors, which are overexpressed in many tumors[17].

3.1.2   Positron emission tomography (PET)

A different and more sophisticated nuclear imaging technique is positron emission imaging. The radiopharmeuticals used in this technique decay under the emission of positrons. The kinetic energy of emitted positrons depends on the radionuclide. The emitted positron travels a short distance (0.3-2 mm) within tissue until it is captured by an electron. The two particles annihilate and the mass of both particles is transformed into energy, i.e. into the generation of two γ-rays with an energy of 511 keV. These γ-rays can be detected by a detector system enclosing the object. The instrumentation design of PET is similar to SPECT. The main difference is that PET needs to detect significantly higher energies and the replacement of geometrical by electronic collimation requiring the design of a coincidence detection circuitry.

The theoretically achievable spatial resolution of most positron-emitters is in the order of 1mm, which depends on the energy of the positrons. However, the spatial resolution of practical PET systems is less. It mainly depends on the size of detector elements and is in the order of 4-8 mm for clinical systems and 2-4 mm for small bore animal systems (Fig. 16-2).

A major clinical application of PET is tumor imaging, since malignant cells have a higher rate of glucose metabolism, which results in increased uptake of radioactively labeled sugar (FDG). Recently, PET imaging was capable to image gene expression by using new reporter probes in small animals[18,19], and to monitor gene therapy in patients[20].

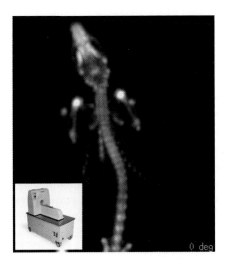

Figure 16-2. PET-image of a rat obtained with a dedicated small-bore PET system (Mosaic, Philips Medical Systems).

3.2 Sensitivity of nuclear imaging

The sensitivity of nuclear imaging depends on two independent factors: the properties of the contrast agent and the sensitivity of the detection system. In particular, the dose of the radiopharmaceutical will improve the SNR, whereas the effectiveness of the radiopharmaceutical, i.e. the degree of specific uptake at the site in comparison with the background, improves the CNR. The sensitivity of the detection system determines the amount of detectable γ-rays. Maximum detection efficiency is desirable to obtain maximum information with a minimum amount of radioactivity. In the following, the main factors that influence the sensitivity from the instrumental side will be described and trends to improve the sensitivity will be discussed.

3.2.1   Sensitivity of gamma-cameras (SPECT)

The sensitivity of a SPECT system depends on two major factors: the efficiency of the detector and the collimator efficiency. The detection efficiency refers to the rate of conversion of the emission from the radiation source into useful signals by the detector. This characteristic is affected by a number of factors[21]. First, the geometric efficiency with which the detector intercepts radiation emitted by the source. Second, the intrinsic absorption efficiency of the detector, which refers to the amount of radiation converted into output-signals. Third, the fraction of the output signals that are recorded by the energy-selective counting system that allows the differentiation between scattered and non-scattered radiation. The overall detection efficiency of the detector is the product of the individual factors.

The collimator performance is another major factor that influences the sensitivity of SPECT, which is affected by the type and geometry of the collimator. The collimator efficiency describes the fraction of γ-rays passing through the collimator per γ-ray emitted by the source. Typical values range[22] between 10^{-4} and 5×10^{-4}. As described above the collimator defines also the spatial resolution. Therefore, the resolution can only be improved at the expense of decreased collimator efficiency, or vice versa. The sensitivity of a SPECT with a general purpose parallel-hole collimator and for a small-volume source is in the order of 10^{-4} cps/Bq, i.e. around 0.01% events will be detected by the SPECT system. Typically, contrast agents with concentrations in the range of nM to pM can be detected with such a system.

In order to improve the sensitivity, the design of new SPECT systems targets at the above discussed factors. The development of new detector crystals aims at higher absorption efficiencies. An ideal crystal would have a high density and a large atomic number, which results in a high γ-ray detection efficiency. It must have a high light output and a high optical transparency to ensure efficient transmission of light. Another trend is the development of semiconductor detectors, like cadmium zinc telluride (CZT), which allow direct conversion of γ-ray into an electronic signal. Such a solid-state detection offers an improved energy resolution ensuring the elimination of Compton-scatter. An interesting design, is the 'SOLid STate Imager with Compact Electronics' (SOLSTICE)[23]. This system combines the direct gamma ray conversion through solid-state detectors with the better compromise offered by rotating slat collimators[24], which has a higher collimator efficiency. In contrast to conventional SPECT systems, plane integrals are measured due to the use of slat collimators.

3.2.2 Sensitivity of PET

The sensitivity of PET is determined mainly by the detection efficiency and the geometric efficiency. The main difference of PET compared to SPECT is that at two detector elements are involved in the coincidence detection and that no collimator is required. Therefore, the sensitivity of PET is proportional to the square of the intrinsic detector efficiency, i.e. the detector material is the critical component in PET. Typically, PET has much higher geometric efficiency than SPECT, because single and multi-detector rings are covering a large fraction of the total space angle. In addition, due to the higher energy of γ–rays in PET (511keV) the absorption by tissue is less relevant and more γ–rays will be detected.

The overall sensitivity of PET systems for a small volume source are in the order of 0.005 cps/sec (i.e. 0.5% events detected) for a single ring system and up to 0.1 cps/Bq (i.e. 10% events detected) for a multi ring system with 3D acquisition. Therefore, the sensitivity in PET can be up to 3 orders of magnitude higher than in SPECT, i.e. agents at concentration below pM can be detected. The critical component of PET tomographs is the scintillation crystal. Although γ–rays emitted in PET imaging can also be detected by sodium iodide crystals doted with thallium NaI(Tl), the sensitivity of these crystals is about 10-fold lower than that of other crystals. For instance, bismuth germanate (BGO), cerium doped gadolinium silicate (GSO) or cerium doped lutetium silicate (LSO) have higher detection efficiency. New detector materials, which have been used in particle physics, are currently tested for biomedical PET imaging[25]. Another way to improve the SNR is to measure and to exploit the differences in arrival times of γ–rays. This time-of-flight PET technique allows the location of the emission event within 4-10cm. Including these information can reduce the statistical uncertainty in the reconstructed image and thus a higher SNR, which can be one order of magnitude higher than in conventional PET.

3.3 Optical imaging

Optical imaging encompasses a large set of imaging technologies that use light from the ultraviolet to the infrared region to image tissue characteristics. These techniques rely on different contrast mechanisms like transmission, absorption, reflectance, scattering, luminescence and fluorescence. These mechanisms provide information on structure, physiology, biochemistry and molecular function. Naturally, these techniques currently are limited to surface imaging or experimental imaging in small animals, because the penetration depth of light is very limited. However, light within a small spectral window of the near infrared (NIR) region (600-900 nm) can penetrate more than 10 cm into tissue due to the relatively low absorption rates at these wavelengths[26]. The resolution of optical imaging is limited by the scattering of light: light photons propagating through tissue diffuse and follow random paths. Both, absorption and scattering are intrinsic contrast parameters of tissue that can be assessed by optical imaging. In 1929, Cutler developed a technique called transillumination[27]: light was shined on one side of a breast and the absorption behavior on the other side was examined. This approach is similar to projection X-ray imaging. However, compared to X-ray imaging, in transillumination the spatial resolution is significantly reduced due to the scattering of light photons. Because the absorption of hemoglobin depends on its oxygenation state, regions with increased vascularity could be detected with this technique. During the last decade, diffuse optical tomography (DOT) was developed[28]. In this technique, light is applied from different angles and scattered light is detected from all directions. In contrast to X-ray CT, in optical tomography proper modeling of the scattering process is essential. Typically, a numeric solution of the diffusion equation is used to describe the propagation of light photons in diffuse media and to predict the measurements of the experimental set-up.

Similar to nuclear imaging, optical imaging is a sensitive modality that can detect very low concentrations of an optical dye. In contrast to PET and SPECT, optical imaging does not involve ionizing radiation, the optical probes are in general stable, and the technologies are less expensive. Optical molecular imaging is developing fast in the field of small-animal imaging for contrast agent and pharmaceutical R&D. The considerable attenuation of light by tissue does not pose a large problem in mice. Two light generating principles can be differentiated: fluorescence and bio-luminescence. In fluorescence imaging a fluorescent probe (optical dye) is activated by an external light source and a signal is emitted at a different wavelength. In bio-luminescence imaging an enzymatic reaction is used as internal signal source. Luciferases are a class of enzymes (oxgenases) that emit light (bioluminescence) with broad emission spectra in the presence of oxygen. This reaction is responsible for the glooming-effect of fireflies. In contrast to fluorescence techniques, there is no inherent background signal in bio-luminescence imaging, which results in a high signal-to-background ratio and correspondingly in excellent sensitivity. However, bioluminescence imaging involves genetic engineering of the tissue of interest, hence, the method has only been applied in small animals so far[29].

The spatial resolution of optical tomography is rather poor and in the order of 5-10 mm, because there is strong scattering and the reconstruction problem is ill posed. In comparison with transillumination, diffuse optical tomography allows better quantification of absorption, scattering or fluorescence in three dimensions. Diffuse optical tomography has been applied in preclinical (mouse imaging) and clinical applications (breast imaging, Figure 16-3).

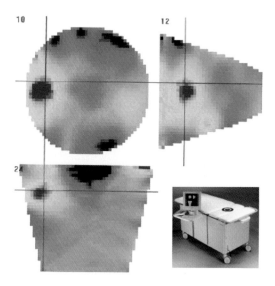

Figure 16-3. Cross sections of the right breast of a patient obtained with optical tomography (Philips Research Eindhoven). The strong attenuation (red) indicates the tumor.

3.3.1 Sensitivity of optical imaging

The sensitivity of optical tomography depends on a number of factors, like the light source (mercury lamp or laser), the detector and the reconstruction technique. In optical tomography, different types of lasers are used: continuous wave, modulated or short-pulse lasers. A continuous wave (CW) laser emits a steady beam of light, which results in a high sensitivity. Another method employs modulated laser light to correct for variations in attenuation. Pulsed laser emits laser light in an off-and-on manner. The application of such lasers allows the selection of ballistic photons, i.e. photons that are not or only weakly scattered, which arrive first on the other side. The shape of this distribution provides information about tissue optical parameters and allows improvement of the spatial resolution[30]. The sensitivity of optical imaging depends on the light source and especially on the detector. This can be avalanche photo-diodes or conventional CCD cameras. Cooling of CCD-cameras minimizes the dark current over the acquisition and thus improves the sensitivity. Improvement of CCD technology, specifically the introduction of back-thinned CCDs and anti-reflective coatings[31]. In addition, the sensitivity can be optimized through better optical coupling.

Another major factor influencing the sensitivity of optical tomography is the reconstruction algorithm, because the contrast-to-noise ratio of optical tomography is often influenced by background-artifacts rather than by noise. For reconstruction, typically, a numerical solution of the diffusion equation is used to describe the propagation of light photons in diffuse media and to predict the measurements of the experimental set-up (forward problem). Afterwards, model parameters are improved by using regression analysis, comparing the experimental data with the predictions of the forward approximation, resulting in images. The image quality can be improved by using advanced reconstruction techniques that apply spectral constraints of the chromophores and scattering spectra[32].

Optical tomography has a sensitivity similar to that of nuclear imaging. In particular, fluorescent phantoms at 100 femto-molar concentrations can be detected in a small the small-animal optical tomography scanner[33]. Theoretical considerations demonstrated that 100nM of agent should be detected with clinical scanners.

3.4   Magnetic resonance imaging

Magnetic resonance imaging (MRI) is a non-ionizing imaging technique with superior soft-tissue contrast, high spatial resolution and good temporal resolution. MRI is capable of measuring a wide range of endogenous contrast mechanisms that include proton density, spin-lattice relaxation time (T1), spin-spin relaxation time (T2), chemical shift, temperature and different types of motion, like blood flow, perfusion or diffusion. MRI has become the modality of choice in many preclinical and clinical applications, because it can provide structural and functional information.

MRI bases on the nuclear magnetic resonance (NMR) effect that was observed by Bloch and Purcell in 1946. Three basic requirements must be fulfilled to measure an MR-signal. First, the nucleus of interest must possess a nonzero magnetic moment. Typical nuclei are for instance hydrogen (1-H), phosphorus (^{31}P), carbon (^{13}C), sodium (^{23}Na) or fluorine (^{19}F). The second requirement is the presence of an external static magnetic field B_0. Typical field strengths for clinical MRI are between 0.23 and 3 Tesla, whereas they can be much higher for pre-clinical systems (4.7 Tesla, 7 Tesla and even higher than 10 Tesla). Due to the Zeeman effect, magnetic moments align under specific angles along or opposed to the external field B_0, resulting in a precessional movement of the magnetic moments. The precessional frequency, also called Larmor frequency, is given by $f_0 = \gamma B_0$, where γ is the gyromagnetic ratio, a constant for a given nucleus. Since an alignment parallel to the field is the lower energy state, it is preferred and slightly more nuclei will align along rather than opposed to the field. As a result, the tissue will exhibit a net magnetization, which is parallel to the external magnetic field and is called longitudinal magnetization. The amount of the net magnetization depends on the field strength and increases for higher magnetic fields. The third requirement is a time-varying magnetic field B_1 applied perpendicularly to the static B_0-field and which flips the longitudinal magnetization to an arbitrary angle (also called flip-angle) into the transversal plane. This precessing magnetization induces a voltage in a receive rf-coil.

The detected transverse magnetization does not remain forever, since two independent relaxation processes take place. First, the spin-lattice relaxation describes how fast the longitudinal magnetization recovers after applying the B_1-pulse. The rate of the recovery process is determined by the relaxation time T_1. Secondly, the spin-spin relaxation describes how fast the transversal magnetization loses its coherence and thus decays. The rate of dephasing is determined by the relaxation time T_2. In addition to spin-spin interactions, dephasing between the coherently precessing magnetic moments can also be caused by B_0-field inhomogeneities. As a result, an apparently stronger relaxation process is visible, which is called T_2^* relaxation. Both the spin-lattice relaxation time T_1 and the spin-spin relaxation time T_2 vary among different types of tissue. Furthermore, MR-contrast agents can be applied that shorten the relaxation times. In particular, the relaxation rate (the inverse of the relaxation time) is proportional to agent relaxivity and its concentration.

In order to distinguish signals from different spatial locations, magnetic field gradients are applied. Consequently, with the spatially varying field strength a spatially varying precessional frequency is connected. Typical values of the spatial resolution of clinical scanners are in the order of 0.5-1 mm. Higher resolution can be obtained at higher field strengths due to the better SNR (Figure 16-4a). High-resolution imaging of small animals on clinical MR-scanners is possible using dedicated rf-coils to increase the sensitivity. With these coils a spatial resolution of about 100 μm can be achieved (Figure 16-4b). A higher spatial resolution than the 100 μm for clinical scanners is possible in dedicated animal MR-scanners that operate at a higher magnetic field strength (e.g. 7 Tesla) and which apply strong gradients.

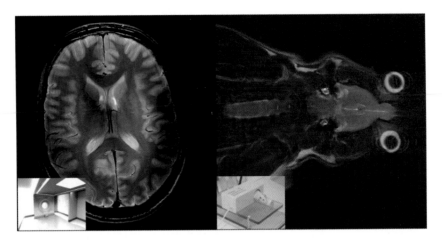

Figure 16-4. (a) Brain image (0.25mm res.) obtained on 7T clinical MR-scanner (Philips Medical Systems). (b) Rat image (100μm res.) obtained on a 3T clinical MR scanner image (Courtesy G. Adam UKE Hamburg) using a dedicated rf-coil (Philips Research Hamburg).

3.4.1   Sensitivity of MRI

The sensitivity of MR depends on the properties of the nucleus to be imaged, instrumental aspects and the way the measurement is performed. As stated above, the different nuclei possess different gyromagnetic ratios resulting in a different sensitivity. For instance, the gyromagnetic ratio of hydrogen is the largest of all nuclei. Obviously hydrogen has a high abundance in biological tissues. Fluorine-19 is one of the most sensitive of the NMR nuclei (about 80% of the gyromagnetic ratio of ^{1}H). However, there are no endogenous compounds that give detectable ^{19}F signals *in vivo*. Therefore, exogenous ^{19}F containing compounds have to be used. For example, ^{19}F NMR was used to identify patients who respond to the chemotherapy fluorouracil[34]. Recently, ^{19}F NMR was performed using Fibrin-targeted perfluorcarbon nanoparticles to study[35]. Carbon-13 has a low natural abundance, and has a much lower intrinsic sensitivity than ^{1}H NMR. Therefore, in the absence of isotopic enrichment, ^{13}C signals are very weak. Recently a new technique has been proposed to increase the sensitivity of ^{13}C NMR by using hyper-polarization[36].

The sensitivity of MRI strongly depends on the MR-instrument used. For instance, the higher the value of B_0 results in a higher signal. The sensitivity depends also strongly on the rf-coil used for detection. In particular, the geometry of the coil should cover the region of interest while keeping the volume small for a minimal patient noise contribution.

The sensitivity of contrast agent detection strongly depends on the contrast-to-noise ratio. The image contrast is primarily affected by the differences in relaxation times, the proton density and on the type and parameters of the MR-measurement sequence. The limit of the agent detection can be approximated from typical values of tissue relaxation rates and of the MR-agent relaxivity. For instance the relaxation rates of tissue are in the order of $1/s$, whereas the typical value relaxivity of Gd-DTPA agents is in the order of 4 $(mM\ s)^{-1}$. Assuming that 10% change in relaxation rates $(\Delta R_1 = 0.1/s)$ results in a detectable image contrast, the corresponding detectable agent concentration (of Gd-DPTA) is in the order of 25μM. Recently, a nanoparticle emulsion was proposed that was loaded with around 100.000 Gd-DTPA molecules, resulting in a relaxivity of about 10^6 $(mM\ s)^{-1}$. It was shown that such an agent allows detection of epitopes with a picomolar concentration[37]. The same considerations can be applied to super-paramagnetic agents that influence the R_2 and R_2^* values. These agents have a larger relaxivity of about 100 $(mM\ s)^{-1}$. The local contrast agent concentration can be determined by measuring the spatial distribution (map) of the relaxation rates. As mentioned above, this value is strongly influenced by B_0-inhomogeneity. Recently, a method was developed that allows correction of the B_0-inhomogeneity from the image data improving the accuracy of the relaxation rate map[38]. In addition, it was shown that approved iron-oxide agents concentrations could be quantified, at approx. 40μM concentration. A higher sensitivity is possible with a carrier increasing the relaxivity of the agent.

3.5 Ultrasound imaging

Ultrasound imaging is a noninvasive, portable and relatively inexpensive imaging modality, which is used extensively in the clinic. An ultrasound transducer (also called scanhead) sends short pulses of a high frequency sound wave (1-10 MHz) into the body. At interfaces between two types of tissue the wave will be refracted and part of the sound wave is reflected back due to Snell's law. How much is reflected depends on the densities of the respective tissues, and thus the speed of the sound wave within the different tissues. In addition, parts of the sound wave are also backscattered from small structures at tissue boundaries or within the tissue. The transducer not only sends the wave into the body but also receives part of the reflected and/or backscattered wave, also named echo.

An ultrasound image consists of a number of lines, where each line can be obtained in less than 100 μs. Therefore, an image consisting of 100 lines can be obtained in less than 10 ms, which means that real time imaging is possible. In addition to imaging morphology, ultrasound is also capable of measuring the velocity of blood in circulation using the Doppler effect. In several instances, the contrast in ultrasound is not high enough. For these applications, gas-filled microspheres (microbubbles) can markedly enhance US-contrast via two different mechanisms. The first mechanism is resonance of microbubbles that expand and contract in an ultrasound field. At the resonant frequency, strong signals are generated at multiples of the transmitted frequency, also called harmonics. The second mechanism bases on differences in the acoustic impedance and thus increases the back-scattering[39].

The spatial resolution of an ultrasound system depends on the scan and frequency used. For clinical systems the (axial) resolution in the order of 1-2 mm at 1 MHz and 0.3 mm at 5 MHz. For dedicated animal scanheads and/or systems operating at higher frequencies (up to 50 MHz) a much higher spatial resolution (below 100µm) can be obtained (Figure 4.5).

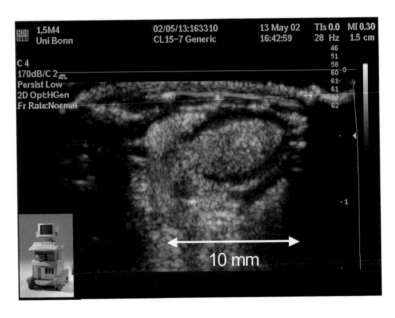

Figure 16-5. A microbubble contrast agent provides a high contrast between blood (white) and myocardium (Courtesy of K. Tiemann, University of Bonn, Germany).

3.5.1   Sensitivity of ultrasound

The sensitivity of ultrasound depends on the intensity and the frequency of the ultrasound pulse transmitted. The higher the intensity, the higher is the amplitude of the detected signals. However, there are safety limits for the ultrasound intensity, because the deposition of energy results in generation of heat within tissue. The sensitivity of ultrasound can also be improved by using contrast agents. For instance microbubbles can be detected by using harmonic or pulse inversion[40] ultrasound imaging. Furthermore, the targeted microparticles can also be detected due to the enhanced scattering. The low inherent echogenicity of particles when in suspension is a feature that allows for differentiation of the bound, targeted nanoparticles from those circulating freely in the body[39]. A sensitive detection of microbubbles is based on the stimulated acoustic emission effect (SAE), which occurs after destruction of microbubbles during Doppler ultrasound imaging. This sensitive particle acoustic quantification (SPAQ) allows quantification of SAE-signals based counts with high accuracy. In particular, it was shown that the technique is capable to detect a single microbubble[41]. The technique has been applied to quantify treatment effects of autoimmune encephalomyelitis by using targeted microbubble in an animal model[42].

3.6 X-ray imaging

X-ray imaging is a transmission-based technique, in which X-rays from a source pass through the patient and are detected on the opposite side of the patient. The contrast in the image arises from the different attenuation of X-rays in different tissues and the amount of absorption depends on the tissue composition. For example, dense bone matter will absorb many more X-rays than soft tissues, such as muscle and fat. In planar X-ray, the line integral of the spatially dependent attenuation is measured and the resulting intensity is displayed in a two-dimensional image. However, it is difficult to interpret overlapping layers of soft tissue and bone structures on such a projection image. In order to resolve such three-dimensional structures, X-ray computed tomography (CT) is used, which generates cross-sectional, two-dimensional images of the body. Therefore, an X-ray tube and a detector are rapidly rotated 360° around the object within 0.3 to 1 s. Modern CT scanners use a number (16-64) of detector rows, which allows the simultaneous measurement of multiple slices.

The spatial resolution in X-ray CT depends on the focal spot of the X-ray tube and the size of the detector elements. The spatial resolution of a clinical CT scanner is less than 0.5 mm in the center of the CT scanner. The spatial resolution of dedicated small animal scanners is much higher[43] and in the order of 20 μm. The major advantage of X-ray CT is its ease of use ('push-button-technology') for acquiring large 3D datasets with structural information at a very high spatial resolution. The disadvantage of X-ray CT is the use of ionizing radiation, which can lead to cell death or to cancer due to genetic mutations.

3.6.1   Sensitivity of X-ray imaging

The sensitivity of X-ray depends on the properties of the object and the major instrument components. The size of the object determines the number of X-rays that can be detected due to attenuation and of Compton-Scattering. The current of the X-ray tube determines number of photons emitted, which is inversely correlated to the noise of an image. The acceleration voltage of the X-ray tube determines the energy of the X-rays. Higher energy X-rays penetrate an object to a greater degree, thus, the amount of signal reaching the detector is increased. However, the energy of the X-rays determines also the contrast of the image. If high-energy X-rays are used, then Compton scattering is the dominant interaction, which is independent from the atomic number. Therefore, the contrast is reduced considerably.

The overall sensitivity of X-ray CT for the detection of contrast agents is in the mM range. In particular, it was shown that release of a iodine-based contrast agent (Iohexol) can be quantitatively monitored. Optimization of CT acquisition parameters yielded a sensitivity of about 0.4 mM for this agent[44]. A more sensitive detection (up to one order higher) of contrast agents can be achieved by k-edge imaging[45].

Table 16-1. Properties of the different imaging modalities

Modality	Sensitivity	Resolution	AQ-Time
X-ray-CT	$\approx 10^{-4}$M	<500 μm	≤Seconds
Animal CT		<50 μm	
SPECT	$\approx 10^{-10}$ M	5-20 mm	<Hours
Animal SPECT		1-3 mm	
PET	$\approx 10^{-12}$ M	4-10 mm	<Hours
Animal PET		2-4 mm	
Ultrasound	single bubble	100μm – 1mm	<Seconds
Animal Ultrasound		40μm	
MRI	10^{-6} - 10^{-12}M	250 μm – 1 mm	≤Minutes
Animal MRI		<100μm	
Optical Imaging	$\approx 10^{-10}$ M	100 μm –10 mm	Seconds

4.   CONCLUSION

Biomedical imaging modalities differ with respect to the image content, their sensitivity, spatial resolution and time resolution (see Table 16-1). It is obvious that X-ray based imaging can provide a high spatial resolution, but lack of sensitivity. Whereas nuclear imaging and optical techniques have a high sensitivity, but both provide a poor spatial resolution. Magnetic resonance and ultrasound have a medium spatial resolution and sensitivity. In general, the different imaging modalities provide different information and thus can be considered as being complementary rather than competitive. Therefore, it is very useful to combine modalities. This can be done by image registration or by using integrated systems. Nowadays, clinical PET-CT and SPECT-CT scanner combinations are commercially available (Figure 16-6), whereas other configurations like PET-MR[46] and DOT-MR[47,48] are tested in research. Besides the integration of different modalities into one system, a common table can be used to exchange the patient or animal rapidly and reproducibly. Each of the modalities or the combination of modalities have shown their potential value in molecular imaging applications. However, although molecular imaging has potentially a huge impact on healthcare, it is still in its infancy. The key for molecular imaging is the development and approval of targeted imaging agents. The specific properties of these new agents demand the development of highly sensitive detection and accurate quantification techniques. As the field is inter-disciplinary, a close collaboration between pharmaceutical companies, developers of contrast agents and vendors of imaging equipment is necessary. The coming years will show, how fast molecular imaging systems find their way into clinical practice.

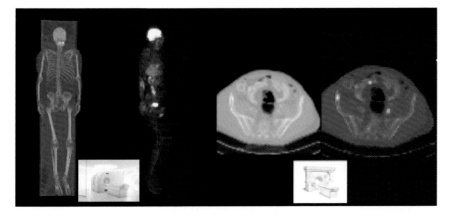

Figure 16-6. Left: Whole- body screening of metastasis using a combined PET-CT scanner (Gemini, Philips Medical Systems). Right: Lymph-node detection with a SPECT-CT scanner (Precedence, Philips Medical Systems).

REFERENCES

1. R. Weissleder, Molecular imaging: exploring the next frontier, *Radiology* **212** (3), 609-614 (1999).
2. E.C. Wiener, M.W. Brechbiel, H. Brothers, R.L. Magin, O.A. Gansow, D.A. Tomalia, P.C. Lauterbur, Dendrimer-based metal chelates: a new class of magnetic resonance imaging contrast agents, *Magn Reson Med* **31**, 1-8 (1994).
3. G. Schuhmann-Giampieri, H. Schmitt-Willich, T. Frenzel, W.R. Press, H.J. Weinmann, In vivo and in vitro evaluation of Gd-DTPA-polylysine as a macromolecular contrast agent for magnetic resonance imaging, *Invest Radiol* **26**, 969-974 (1991).
4. E. Unger, D.K. Shen, G.L. Wu, T. Fritz, Liposomes as MR contrast agents: pros and cons, *Magn Reson Med* **22**, 304-308 (1991).
5. G.M. Lanza, K.D Wallace, M.J Scott, W.P Cacheris, D.R Abendschein, D.H Christy, A.M Sharkey, J.G Miller, P.J Gaffney, S.A Wickline, A novel site-targeted ultrasonic contrast agent with broad biomedical application, *Circulation* **95**, 3334-3340 (1996).
6. M. Mikawa, H. Kato, M. Okumura, M. Narazaki, Y. Kanazawa, N. Miwa, H. Shinohara, Paramagnetic water-soluble metallofullerenes having the highest relaxivity for MRI contrast agents, *Bioconjug Chem* **12**, 510-514 (2001).
7. V. Sharma, G. Luker, D. Piwnica-Worms, Molecular imaging of gene expression and protein function in vivo with PET and SPECT, *J Magn Reson Imaging* **16**, 336-351 (2002).
8. W.C.W. Chan, D.J. Maxwell, X.H. Gao, R.E. Bailey, M.Y. Han, S. Nie, Luminescent quantum dots for multiplexed biological detection and imaging, *Curr Opin Biotechnol* **13**, 40-46 (2002).
9. S. Aime, C. Cabella, S. Colombatto, S.G. Crich, E. Gianolio, F. Maggioni, Insights into the use of paramagnetic Gd(III) complexes in MR-molecular imaging investigations, *J Magn Reson Imaging* **16**, 394-406 (2002).
10. J.R. Lindner, Molecular imaging with contrast ultrasound and targeted microbubbles, *Nucl Cardiol* **11**, 215-221 (2004).
11. C. Bremer, C.H. Tung, R. Weissleder, In vivo molecular target assessment of matrix metalloproteinase inhibition, *Nat Med* **7**, 743-748 (2001).
12. A.Y. Louie, M.M. Huber, E.T. Ahrens, U. Rothbacher, R. Moats, R.E. Jacobs, S.E. Fraser, T.J. Meade, *Nat Biotechnol* **18**, 321-325 (2000).
13. R. Weissleder, U. Mahmood, Molecular imaging, *Radiology,* **219**, 316-333 (2001).
14. Y. Matsumura, H. Maeda, A new concept for macromolecular therapeutics in cancer chemotherapy: mechanism of tumoritropic accumulation of proteins and the antitumor agent smancs, *Cancer Res* **46**, 6387-6392 (1986).
15. H.O. Anger, Radioisotope cameras, in: *Instrumentation in nuclear medicin*, edited by G.J. Hine, Vol. 1, 485-552 (Academic Press, New York, 1967).
16. F.J. Beekman, D.P. McElroy, F. Berger, S.S. Gambhir, E.J. Hoffman, S.R. Cherry. Towards in vivo nuclear microscopy: iodine-125 imaging in mice using micro-pinholes. *Eur J Nucl Med Mol Imaging* **29**, 933-938 (2002).
17. Y. Menda, D. Kahn, Somatostatin receptor imaging of non-small cell lung cancer with 99mTc depreotide, *Semin Nucl Med* **32**, 92-96, (2002).
18. J.G. Tjuvajev, G. Stockhammer, R. Desai, H. Uehara, K. Watanabe, B. Gansbacher, R.G. Blasberg. Imaging the expression of transfected genes in vivo, *Cancer Res* **55**, 6126-6132 (1995).
19. S.S. Gambhir, J.R. Barrio, L. Wu, M. Iyer, M. Namavari, N. Satyamurthy, E. Bauer, C. Parrish, D.C. MacLaren, A.R. Borghei, L.A. Green, S. Sharfstein, A.J. Berk, S.R. Cherry, M.E. Phelps, H.R. Herschman. Imaging of adenoviral-directed herpes simplex virus type 1 thymidine kinase reporter gene expression in mice with radiolabeled ganciclovir, *J Nucl Med* **39**, 2003-2011 (1998).

20. A. Jacobs, J. Voges, R. Reszka, M. Lercher, A. Gossmann, L. Kracht, C. Kaestle, R. Wagner, K. Wienhard, W.D. Heiss, Positron-emission tomography of vector-mediated gene expression in gene therapy for gliomas, *Lancet* **358**, 727-729 (2001).

21. S. R. Cherry, J. Sorenson, M. Phelps, Physics in Nuclear Medicine, Chapter 11, 3rd Edition Saunders (2003).

22. J.A. Sorenson, Quantitative measurement of radioactivity in vivo by whole body counting, *Instrumentation of Nuclear Medicine*, edited by G.J. Hine, J.A Sorenson, Vol 2, 311-348 (New York, Academic Press, 1974).

23. D. Gagnon, G.L. Zeng, J.M. Links, J.J. Griesmer, F.C. Valentino, Design considerations for a new solid-state gamma-camera: Soltice, *IEEE Nuclear Science Symposium*, Vol 2, 1156-1160 (2001).

24. S. Webb, M.A. Flower, R.J. Ott, Geometric Efficiency of a Rotating Slat-Collimator for Improved Planar Gamma- Camera Imaging, *Phys Med Biol* **38**, 627-638 (1993).

25. P. Lecoq, New Scintillating materials for PET scanners, *Proc Calorimetry in Particle Physics*, 262-273 (2002).

26. W.F. Cheong, S.A. Prahl, A.J. Welch, A review of the optical properties of biological tissues, *IEEE J Quantum Electronics* **26**, 2166-2185 (1990).

27. M. Cutler, Transillumination as an aid in the diagnosis of breast lesions, *Surg Gynecol Obstet* **48**, 721-729 (1929).

28. S.R. Arridge. Optical tomography in medical imaging, *Inverse Problems* **15**, 41-93 (1999).

29. P.R. Contag, I.N. Olomu, D.K. Stevenson, C.H. Contag, Bioluminescent indicators in living mammals, *Nat Med* **4**, 245-247 (1998).

30. D. Grosenick, H. Wabnitz, H. H. Rinneberg, K. T. Moesta, P. M. Schlag, Development of a time-domain optical mammograph and first in vivo applications, *Applied Optics* **48**, 2927-2943, (1999).

31. C.H. Contag, M.H.Bachmann, Advances in in vivo bioluminescence imaging of gene expression, *Ann Rev Biomed Eng* **4**, 235-260 (2002).

32. S. Srinivasan, B.W. Pogue, S. Jiang, H. Dehghani, K.D. Paulsen, Spectrally constrained chromophore and scattering near-infrared tomography provides quantitative and robust reconstruction, *Applied Optics* **44**, 1858-1869 (2005).

33. V. Ntziachristos, R. Weissleder, Charge-coupled-device based scanner for tomography of fluorescent near-infrared probes in turbid media, *Med Phys* **29**, 803-809 (2002).

34. C.A. Presant, W. Wolf, M.J. Albright, K.L. Servis, R. Ring, D. Atkinson, R.L. Ong, C. Wiseman, M. King, D. Blayney, Human tumor fluorouracil trapping: clinical correlations of in vivo 19F nuclear magnetic resonance spectroscopy pharmacokinetics, *Clin Oncol* **8**, 1868-73 (1990).

35. A.M. Morawski, P.M. Winter, X. Yu, R.W. Fuhrhop, M.J. Scott, F. Hockett, J.D. Robertson, P.J. Gaffney, G.M. Lanza, S.A. Wickline, Quantitative 'magnetic resonance immunohistochemistry' with ligand-targeted (19)F nanoparticles, *Magn Reson Med* **52**, 1255-1262 (2004).

36. K. Golman, J.H. Ardenkjaer-Larsen, J.S. Petersson, S. Mansson, I. Leunbach. Molecular imaging with endogenous substances, *Proc Natl Acad Sci USA* **100**, 10435-10439 (2003).

37. A.M. Morawski, P.M. Winter, K.C. Crowder, S.D. Caruthers, R.W. Fuhrhop, M.J. Scott, J.D. Robertson, D.R. Abendschein, G.M. Lanza, S.A. Wickline Targeted nanoparticles for quantitative imaging of sparse molecular epitopes with MRI, *Magn Reson Med* **51**, 480-486 (2004).

38. H. Dahnke, T. Schaeffter, Limits of detection of SPIO at 3.0 T using T2 relaxometry, *Magn Reson Med*, **53**, 1202-1206 (2005).

39. M.S. Hughes, J.N. Marsh, C.S. Hall, R.W. Fuhrhop, E.K. Lacy, G.M. Lanza, S.A. Wickline, Acoustic characterization in whole blood and plasma of site-targeted nanoparticle ultrasound contrast agent for molecular imaging, *J Acoust Soc Am* **117**, 964-972 (2005).

40. M. Averkiou, J. Powers, D. Skyba, M. Bruce, S. Jensen, Ultrasound contrast imaging research, *Ultrasound Q* **19**(1), 27-37 (2003).

41. M. Reinhardt, P. Hauff, A. Briel, V. Uhlendorf, R.A. Linker, M. Maurer, M. Schirner, Sensitive particle acoustic quantification (SPAQ): a new ultrasound-based approach for the quantification of ultrasound contrast media in high concentrations, *Invest Radiol* **40**, 2-7 (2005).

42. M. Reinhardt, P. Hauff, R.A. Linker, A. Briel, R. Gold, P. Rieckmann, G. Becker, K.V. Toyka, M. Maurer, M. Schirner, Ultrasound derived imaging and quantification of cell adhesion molecules in experimental autoimmune encephalomyelitis (EAE) by Sensitive Particle Acoustic Quantification (SPAQ), *Neuroimage* **16**, 267-278 (2005).

43. E.L. Ritman, Micro-computed tomography-current status and developments, *Annu Rev Biomed Eng* **6**, 185-208 (2004).

44. A. Szymanski-Exner, N.T. Stowe, K. Salem, R. Lazebnik, J.R. Haaga, D.L. Wilson, J. Gao, Noninvasive monitoring of local drug release using X-ray computed tomography: optimization and in vitro/in vivo validation, *J Pharm Sci* **92**, 289-296 (2003)

45. H Elleaume, A.M. Charvet, S. Corde, F. Est`eve, J. F. Le Bas, Performance of computed tomography for contrast agent concentration measurements with monochromatic x-ray beams: comparison of K-edge versus temporal subtraction, *Phys Med Biol* **47**, 3369-3385 (2003).

46. P.K. Marsden, D. Strul, S.F. Keevil, S.C. Williams, D. Cash, Simultaneous PET and NMR, *Br J Radiol* **75**, 53-59 (2002).

47. V. Ntziachristos, A.G. Yodh, M. Schnall, B. Chance, Concurrent MRI and diffuse optical tomography of breast after indocyanine green enhancement, *Proc Natl Acad Sci USA* **97**, 2767-2772 (2000).

48. H. Xu, R. Springett, H. Dehghani, B.W. Pogue, K.D. Paulsen, J.F. Dunn, Magnetic-resonance-imaging-coupled broadband near-infrared tomography system for small animal brain studies, *Applied Optics* **44**, 2177-2188 (2005).

Chapter 17

BIOMARKERS IN DISEASE DIAGNOSIS AND TREATMENT
Integration of Biomarkers to Improve Patient Care

Ralf Hoffmann
Philips Research, Eindhoven, The Netherlands

Abstract: The concept of biomarkers is becoming more relevant in disease diagnosis and prognosis, as well as in pharmaceutical drug development. The particular role of these biomarkers is to improve the early diagnosis of human disorders, to give an individual prognosis of the stage and progression of a diagnosed disease, and to predict and monitor the effectiveness of an applied therapy. In medical compound development, their main impact will be on the prediction of adverse and toxic effects, and clinical efficacy of new chemical entities in man.

Keywords: Biomarkers, molecular markers, molecular diagnostics, molecular imaging, therapy, drug development, integration of biomarkers

1. RELEVANCE OF BIOMARKERS

In 2001, the Human Genome Consortium presented the first draft of the human genome sequence, and provided a final update of the draft sequence three years later[1,2]. Despite the enormous promise of its clinical relevance, the impact of the human genome sequence in terms of benefit in treating human disorders turned out to be limited, until we better understand how a genome translates into a phenotype and which changes on the molecular level give rise to a pathology on the macroscopic level.

Knowledge of the human genome sequence will accelerate the identification of genes, whose function is associated with a human disease. Several approaches can lead to the discovery of novel human disease genes, e.g., genetic linkage analysis[3], or expression profiling of transcripts or their corresponding protein products in the context of pathological conditions[4,5].

G. Spekowius and T. Wendler (Eds.), Advances in Healthcare Technology, 269-285.
© 2006 *Springer. Printed in the Netherlands.*

Although we have seen a huge increase in knowledge of molecular biology of life, we still do not understand very well how to translate this plethora of information into relevant clinical applications. For instance, many putative biomarkers have been described for use in different medical applications and diseases, including different tumor disorders[6-14], neurological[15-17] and metabolic[18] as well as cardiovascular[19,20] conditions. However, most are not well accepted among clinicians, with the exception of a fairly low number of partly long-known molecules like PSA (Prostate Specific Antigen). This is consistent with the observation that the number of newly developed diagnostic assays based on new biomarkers seems to be declining over the last decade[21], despite the fact that an increasing number of entries in Medline in the context of the biomarkers and biomarker concepts can be found.

A recent investigation of Medline, while searching for publications including the term biomarker* (in titles and abstracts) between the period of 1995 - 2005, resulted in approximately 6000 records (only items with English abstract and work on humans have been selected).

Further investigation of these hits (Figure 17-1), showed that the terminology of biomarker(s) was used in 1995 in only <100 publications, whereas in 2004, we already counted around 1250 relevant entries, and it seems that this number is still increasing in 2005 (data not shown). When looking further into the context of the use of a biomarker concept, we identified a fairly significant number of records in the area of diagnostics (Dx) as well as therapeutics (Tx), whereas the number of citations in the context of imaging (Im) was only starting to increase in 2001/2002. This brief analysis at least indicates that the interest in the biomarker concept and terminology in the context of disease diagnosis and treatment has been strongly increasing during the last decade (although it should be noted that other terminology may have been used in similar research before 1995).

2.   BIOMARKER CONCEPT: DEFINITIONS

As the interest in the concept of biomarkers for diagnosis and treatment of diseases is growing over the last years, a number of different definitions on the types and application of biomarkers have been used. Many terms with partly overlapping meaning like molecular markers, biological markers, biomarkers, diagnostic markers, surrogate markers, etc can be found in the relevant literature.

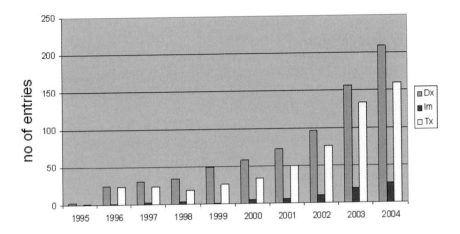

Figure 17-1. Medline entries 1995 - 2005 including the term ' biomarker*' in title or abstract (see text). Note that the presented analysis does obviously not cover all publications on biological markers - the intention was to get an idea on the introduction and use of the biomarker concept during the last decade. Dx - Diagnostics, Im - Imaging, Tx - Therapeutics.

In order to improve the discussion towards a consensus around types of biomarkers and use of the biomarker concepts in diagnosis or treatment of a disease, the NIH Biomarker Definitions Working Group suggest the use of the following definition[22]: *"Biological marker (biomarker): A characteristic that is objectively measured and evaluated as an indicator of normal biological processes, pathogenic processes, or pharmacological responses to a therapeutic intervention".*

This broad definition of the term biomarker indicates that the nature of a biological marker can be rather diverse, ranging from a specific gene transcript, a peptide or a protein, which have been measured as being deregulated during the progression into a pathological status, but can also be an identified genetic mutation, or a physiological process by itself.

Typical examples of protein biomarkers include CA 125 (ovarian cancer), CA 15-3 and CA 27-29 (breast cancer), CEA (ovarian, lung, breast, pancreas, and gastrointestinal tract cancers), PSA (prostate cancer), or Aß42, (phospho)-tau (Alzheimer's Disease), CRP (Inflammation). Other examples would be blood pressure, LDL cholesterol, HIV load, FDG-PET imaging in Alzheimer's Disease, tumor shrinkage, bacterial/viral/fungal culture and sensitivity (infectious diseases), glucose, hemoglobin A1c (diabetes), or intra-ocular pressure (glaucoma).

Equally important in the context of biomarker concepts is the definition of the terms 'clinical endpoint' as well as 'surrogate endpoint'. According to the 'NIH Biomarkers Definitions Working Group', the expressions clinical and surrogate endpoints are defined as[22]:

A **clinical endpoint** is a characteristic or variable that reflects how a patient feels, functions, or survives. Clinical endpoints are distinct measurements or analyses of disease characteristics observed in a study or a clinical trial that reflect the effect of a therapeutic intervention. Clinical endpoints are the most credible characteristics (e.g., survival, myocardial infarction, stroke, recurrence of cancer, etc) used in the assessment of the benefits and risks of a therapeutic intervention (e.g., application of a drug, surgery, device, etc) in randomized clinical trials.

A **surrogate endpoint** is a characteristic that is intended to substitute for a clinical endpoint. A surrogate endpoint is expected to predict clinical benefit (or harm or lack of benefit) based on epidemiological, therapeutic, patho-physiologic, or other scientific evidence. The term *surrogate endpoint* applies primarily to endpoints in therapeutic intervention trials.

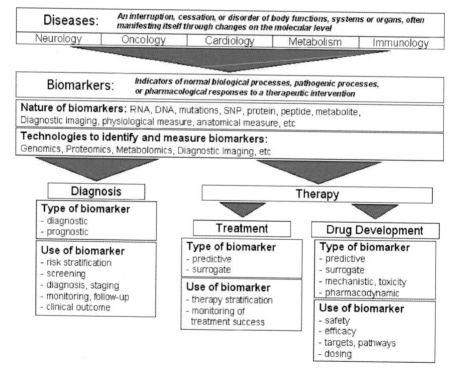

Figure 17-2: Overview of the types and use of biomarkers in diagnosis and treatment of disorders, as well as in drug development. The types of the biomarkers used for the detection of diseases are mostly diagnostic and prognostic, whereas in the area of treatment and compound development, the types of implemented biomarkers are predictive, surrogate, as well as mechanistic (including toxicity) and pharmacodynamic.

According to those definitions, several types of biomarkers can be distinguished related to their use in diagnostics of diseases, or therapeutic treatment, and pharmaceutical drug development (Figure 17-2)[23]:

Diagnostic biomarker:	Indicates the presence (and stage) of a disease
Prognostic biomarker:	Indicates the future behavior of a disease
Predictive biomarker:	Indicates the relative response to a treatment
Surrogate biomarker:	Substitutes for a clinical endpoint
Mechanistic biomarker:	Sndicates an effect on a desired target pathway
Toxicity biomarker:	Indicates a potentially toxic/adverse effect
Pharmacodynamic biomarker:	Indicates the highest effective dose of a drug

3. BIOMARKERS IN DIAGNOSTICS

Although the nature of a biomarker can be very diverse, ranging from an RNA or DNA sequence, a genetic mutation, a metabolite, an anatomical or physiological measurement, a diagnostic image, the protein biomarkers belong to the most relevant biochemical biomarkers in the clinical routine today.

Currently, there is enormous interest in the identification and validation of novel protein biomarkers for the early diagnosis of all kinds of tumor diseases, neurodegenerative disorders, cardiovascular conditions, and others. In particular, the introduction of what is usually referred to as 'Clinical Proteomics' has led to a dramatic increase in studies on clinical material like different types of body fluids (serum, plasma, urine, saliva, etc) for the presence of novel proteins or a multitude of proteins, which give a highly sensitive and specific indication if a pathological condition has developed in the past.

Until recently, a biomarker was a single event measurement, e.g. the putative presence of a disease was based on the detection and quantification a single protein like PSA in Prostate Cancer diagnosis.

Although the clinical introduction of PSA as a molecular marker has significantly impacted the diagnosis of Prostate Cancer[24], there are still major concerns in view of the specificity to discriminate between a benign and malignant prostate condition. It turned out in many clinical studies that the specificity (the probability that a diagnostic test result will be negative when the disease is not present) of PSA testing is relatively poor (in the order of 20-50%, depending on the details of the investigation)[25-27]. The expression of PSA is not a tumor-specific event, as its level can also be significantly increased in different benign conditions of the prostate, e.g.

hyperplasia, or inflammation. Obviously, the power of this biomarker molecule to discriminate between a malignant and a benign condition of the prostate organ is very low, and in consequence, a lot of false-positive results are generated based on solely PSA measurements in a serum sample of a patient.

According to a recent calculation[28], currently 8% of the male US population has increased PSA levels of >4 ng/ml, which is an indication to take a tissue biopsy from the prostate. In 2004, this would lead to the detection of around 760,000 malignancies compared to ca. 2,300,000 men (from a total of approx. 3 million men between the ages of 45 and 74) undergoing unnecessary biopsy due to low specificity of PSA testing.

Another serious problem with PSA has been reported to be in men with PSA levels <4 ng/ml, which so far has been considered as of low risk for Prostate Cancer[29]. Around 15% of men in this group were found to have malignancies in their prostate, from which another 15% showed advanced disease. There seems to be at least a significant risk of having a prostate tumor, even if the measured protein level in serum is below the usually used lower cut-off limit of 4 ng/ml PSA.

Therefore, there is a very strong interest for the search of proteins with an increased diagnostic power to discriminate between healthy/benign conditions versus malignancies of the male prostate. There is a whole range of proteins being suggested as potential biomarkers in prostate cancer care[9,30], but none of these has yet been successfully introduced into the clinical practice.

Only very recently, new technologies have been introduced into the biomarker discovery research, raising the possibility to not only identify single proteins as potential indicative event, but rather searching through the measured parameters for a combination of molecules, defining a diagnostic fingerprint or pattern[31]. The conceptual idea is that the individual proteins, coding for such a fingerprint, are not necessarily significant events to discriminate, e.g., a healthy from a diseased state, but the combination of these parameters will lead to a finally robust clinical assay. Using combinations of several biomarkers can help to make a diagnostic test more robust against the usual variability of diagnostic tests applied to a commonly quite heterogeneous patient population. Furthermore, single-events often suffer from technical errors, including sample variability in collection and preparation, measurement and instrumental errors, etc.

Several approaches suitable for the identification of novel biomarkers or biomarker fingerprints have been applied to patient body fluids (like urine, serum, plasma, prostatic fluid) to find improved answers for the diagnosis of prostate cancer (but also of many other diseases), in particular to improve the discrimination between benign and malignant lesions. The technologies ranges from 2-DE (2-dimensional gel electrophoresis)[32-34], and SELDI (Surface Enhanced Laser Desorption Ionization)[35-37], to 2-D LC-MS (2-dimensional Liquid Chromatography coupled to Mass Spectrometry)[38].

Some first results obtained using the SELDI approach to identify biomarker profiles for diagnosis of Prostate Cancer indicate that it may be feasible to improve the diagnostic sensitivity and specificity by applying a multi-marker technology. Several studies reported sensitivities up to 95%, and specificities up to 97% [39-41].

It has to be mentioned however, that, according to a recent investigation[42], the individual results of different studies on Prostate Cancer profiling by SELDI, come to diverse models regarding the discrimination between the different types of samples analysed (e.g., normal vs. benign vs. malignant). The diagnostic value of each described fingerprint is therefore unclear, and has to wait for further validation on larger, multi-centered studies.

4. BIOMARKERS IN THERAPY

The pharmaceutical industry is currently facing a tremendous challenge, as the number of FDA approved new chemical entities (NCEs) has been considerably declining over the last 15 years[43]. The exact reason for this is not fully understood. Most common explanations are that companies have to deal with very complex disorders, with an increasing number of novel targets, or with currently not fully explored targets with an inherently bigger risk of failure, together with a limited range of predictive tools for decisions early in the development process, and finally, ever more demanding regulatory authorities.

Interestingly, the diagnostic industry seems to be in a quite analog situation as it has been reported that the number of newly developed and approved serum or plasma protein based diagnostic tests has been dropping in a similar way as the number of novel NCEs in the pharmaceutical industry over the last 15 years[21]. Also in the diagnostic area, it is speculated that the complexity of human physiology decreases the chances of success to accurately diagnose the status of a disease by using the body fluid level of a (single) protein.

Looking at the different reasons for attrition (or success) rates of a pharmaceutical development, three general trends are emerging[43]:

- Currently, the major reasons for compound failure are issues with clinical safety and/or toxicology (attrition rate ca. 10% and 15%, respectively), and lack of clinical efficacy (ca. 30% attrition rate).

- The attrition rate due to issue with PK (pharmacokinetics) and/or bioavailability has been dramatically decreased over the last 15 years from approx. 40% to now 10%.
- Whereas the average success rates from clinical phase 1 to achieve regulatory registration in different investigated indications is about 11%, there are significant differences between success rates of individual therapeutic areas like oncology and CNS (5-7%) versus, e.g., cardiovascular diseases or arthritis/pain (15-20%).

It seems that for diseases, where animal models are reasonably well able to represent the complex behavior of the human patho-physiology, the probability of a successful drug development is higher compared to those disorders, where valid and predictive animal models are lacking (e.g., CNS, oncology) - these areas are much more susceptible to attrition of a development compound.

Furthermore, whereas the prediction of *in vivo* characteristics of chemicals, like PK/bioavailability[44], which can be relatively well simulated by use of *in vitro* systems, has been clearly improved over the last decade this has not been achieved for the prediction of drug efficacy in man based on cell culture systems or animal models. A similar situation exists for the prediction of clinical safety/toxicology of compounds to be used in man.

This indicates, that the difficulty to predict the complex behavior of the human physiology, in particular with respect to expected negative or positive effects of a developmental compound, is currently the major hurdle for improvements in the drug development chain.

As the development of predictive biomarkers seems to be an attractive solution for these obstacles, it has to be mentioned that only relatively few biomarkers so far are accepted as being useful as surrogate endpoints in clinical trials. This is (again) mostly due to the fact that a single biomarker can hardly represent all possible effects of a therapeutic intervention in a very complex system like the human body.

Thus, it seems to be an obvious choice to go for multiple-biomarker strategies to predict clinical compound efficacy, as well as safety and toxicological aspects. Some first successful examples have emerged over the last few years already. For instance a recent study demonstrated that, based on a set of the expression values of a multitude of genes, it was possible to correctly classify >30 approved drugs used in three different therapeutic areas in CNS, namely antidepressants, antipsychotics, and opioid drugs. The analysis was performed on primary human neuronal cell cultures. It was possible to predict the correct drug class from those compounds, which has been excluded from the original training set with an accuracy in the higher 80% range[45]. It has to be noted that the used CNS compounds are often highly related in terms of chemical structure as well as pharmacology, even for compounds used in different therapeutic areas (e.g., antidepressants and antipsychotics).

Also in the area of prediction of hepatotoxicity quite a number of recent reports were able to underscore the relevance of genomic and proteomic technologies to identify profiles or patterns of events, which are able to predict the toxicity of known hepatotoxicants in cultured primary human hepatocytes[46-50].

A very important aspect to be considered in this context is that the power of predicting desired or undesired effects of compounds by *in vitro* profiling technologies strongly depends on the breadth of the represented effects in the input training set: only those effects (desired or undesired), which are elicited by the chemicals in the group of drugs used for the selection of predictive biomarker patterns, can later be predicted for a test compound. This is in particular true for the prediction of therapeutic effects, as they are normally related to a very specific molecular mechanism. For instance, the numerous medications used today in the treatment of psychotic disorders, are mostly directed towards the dopamine D2 receptor. It has been shown in different reports that these compounds demonstrate a good correlation between their specific affinity to the dopamine D2 receptor and their antipsychotic potential[51,52]. In the case of antidepressive treatments, the molecular target of many developments in this area is focused around the serotonergic neurotransmitter system (e.g., the SSRI - Selective Serotonine Reuptake Inhibitors).

Furthermore, it has been shown that the activation of a specific molecular target leads to expression of characteristic down-stream effects. In consequence, the algorithms that are used to predict clinical efficacy for a certain drug can classify only those compounds, which induce similar up-stream and down-stream events compared to already known chemicals in the related therapeutic area. Drugs with a fully new mechanism of action cannot be recognized as belonging to a class of therapeutic compounds within the training set. This gives some clear limitations on the potential power of the biochemical marker profile approach to predict clinical efficacy in man.

In the case of biochemical markers, which are predictive for toxicologically adverse effects e.g. in the liver, this might be a slightly different situation. The toxic events of many pharmacologically active compounds have been characterized in the past. It is therefore expected that there is a relatively good chance that the induced toxicity of any new chemical entity tested is already (at least partially) represented within the chemical space of existing pharmaceutical drugs. In consequence, screening a large number of compounds with a known toxicity profile may suffice to prepare the learning tools of the used classification algorithms so that they can pick up all relevant potential toxic side effects by the selection of an appropriate gene/protein profile.

5.   INTEGRATED BIOMARKER APPROACH

As the underlying pathology of the development and progression of many human disorders is a very complex and dynamic process with many parameters changing temporally and spatially, depending on the stage of the disease, the concept of integrating several biomarkers of different types to more accurately diagnose and treat a human disorder will become more relevant in healthcare and disease management.

The main driving force for this development is that it cannot be expected that a single biomarker (or a biomarker pattern) will deliver an accurate diagnosis or prognosis of a disease and its outcome, and at the same time can predict the effectiveness of an applied therapeutic treatment.

Furthermore, the number of different possible treatment options for a certain disease makes it very unlikely that a single biomarker is able to represent all potential subsequent effects on the physiological or molecular level. For instance, in Alzheimer's Disease (AD), the major treatment concepts, which are currently under development in the pharmaceutical industry, are targeting the cholinergic neurotransmitter system on the one hand, and the amyloid plaque cascade on the other (Figure 17-3)[53].

Still, the most prominent target system is the CNS acetylcholine neurotransmitter pathway, not only in terms of numbers of development compounds, but in particular also concerning the development stage, which is far more advanced compared to other developments (not shown). Strongly increasing since a few years are the numbers of compounds to prevent the generation of beta-amyloid plaque deposition in some relevant brain regions. Although a few other targets are under therapeutic development for treatment of AD, the cholinergic and the amyloid pathways nearly contribute 2/3 of all compounds in clinical phases (Figure 17-3).

However, as the suggested cholinergic and amyloid cascades involve molecular targets from quite different neurological cells as well as different receptors or enzymes, it is easy to imagine that different biomarkers would be necessary in order to prove the effectiveness of a specific treatment in an individual patient. In the first case, the *in vivo* imaging of the forebrain cholinergic neurons by, e.g., targeting the nicotinic acetylcholine receptors, or the non-invasive monitoring of the activity of the acetylcholinesterase could be a way to follow treatment efficacy[54-58]. In the latter case, the direct imaging extra-cellular senile plaques by amyloid binding compounds may deliver a relevant biomarker for treatment monitoring[59-63].

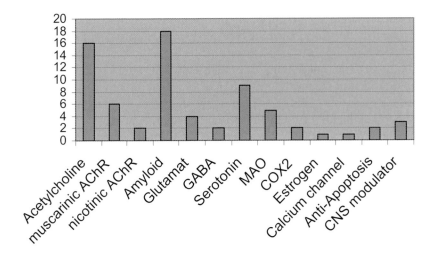

Figure 17-3. Lines of treatment options in AD, currently under development in the pharmaceutical industry (only compounds shown, which are at least in clinical phase 1).

In the case of early diagnosis of AD, the situation with respect to a useful biomarker is again different. The pathology of Alzheimer's Disease is characterized by the reduction of neurons in the temporal and frontal cortex, as well as the development of different extra- and intracellular depositions, in particular beta-amyloid (senile) plaques and neurofibrillary tangles[64]. However, the definitive diagnosis of AD is currently not possible in living subjects and is done by means of pathological examination of post-mortem biopsy material based on criteria established by the National Institute on Aging, and the Consortium to Establish a Registry for Alzheimer's Disease (CERAD). Furthermore, neurodegenerative disorders are characterized by the fact, that patients remain asymptotic for many years after the pathological disease process has already started.

A variety of imaging-based as well as biochemical biomarkers have been studied over the last years in order to improve the positive predictive value for early diagnosis of AD and the differential diagnosis versus related dementia disorders. On the imaging side, this includes measurements like volumetric MRI of the complete brain and specific brain areas, like the hippocampus[65,66], MR spectroscopy[67-69], and PET imaging of amyloid plaques or inflammatory processes[70,71]. Only recently, the Centers for Medicare and Medicaid Services (CMS) approved FDG-PET for the differential diagnosis of AD for reimbursement in the USA[72].

On the biochemical path, a whole range of different putative biomarkers has been suggested in the past[15-17,73,74]. Although, some of these biomarkers like beta-amyloid or the tau proteins seem to be involved in the pathological processes leading to AD, none of the currently discussed components are able neither to fully describe the different stages nor to predict the progression of the disease. Very recently, also a biomarker approach based on a fingerprint consisting of a multitude of serum proteins has been proposed to have diagnostic value in AD[75].

A very relevant clinical problem in the diagnosis of Alzheimer's Disease is only partially addressed by the currently available biomarkers - namely the differential diagnosis between AD and other forms of dementia. This is very relevant, as around one third of all dementia cases in elderly are accounted to conditions other than AD. Highly relevant among diseases to be discriminated from AD are for instance vascular dementia, frontotemporal dementia, Lewy body dementia, depression-related dementia, and some others. Although the clinical symptoms are similar, the molecular pathology of these disorders is quite different compared to AD, which has important implications for treatment decisions.

There is increasing evidence from recent studies that the latent (asymptomatic) stage of AD, which may develop very slowly and unrecognized over several decades, is progressing into MCI (Mild Cognitive Impairment) first, before moving into a more advanced stage of mild AD[76,77]. MCI compared to AD is characterized in that patients show less prominent cognitive deficits. There is still quite some debate on the exact definition of MCI, and in particular on the question of how many MCI patients will progress into AD, or if MCI can be a stable condition in some patients. There is some believe that virtually all patients with MCI may have pathological features of AD, whereas others do more believe that only a certain percentage of MCI patients will finally progress into Alzheimer's Disease pathology[78,79]. One recent study supporting the latter view has followed up a number of MCI patients and could show that around 10% of all patients yearly progressed into AD characteristics[80]. However, it is virtually impossible to predict, which patient is going to progress from MCI to AD and which MCI patients will be staying stable with their mild cognitive effects. This is obviously important information, as it is generally believed that an early treatment with available therapeutics today (i.e., mainly acetylcholinesterase inhibitors) may attenuate the progression of AD more effectively as compared to the usual (often too late) start of medication. This generates an urgent need to develop biomarkers, which are able to predict the progression into AD from early or pre-stages of this disease.

Figure 17-4 shows a schematic outline of the possible integration of different types of biomarkers in the clinical care of Alzheimer's Disease. During (late) asymptomatic phases of the disease or during phases of MCI, i.e., pathological changes have already become manifest but no or only mild clinical symptoms can be diagnosed, it is very likely that only a combination of several biomarkers on the psychological, biochemical, as well as on the neuro-imaging level can deliver an accurate diagnosis of an existing neurodegenerative process, a differential diagnosis of AD vs. related disorders, as well as a predictive value for the progression of MCI into AD, or into other forms of dementia.

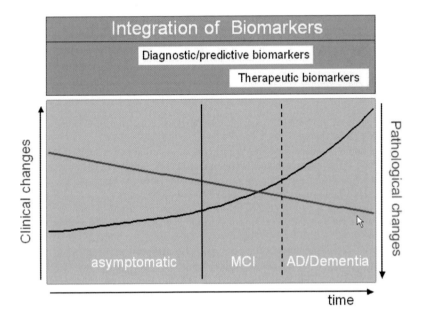

Figure 17-4. Integration of biomarkers in AD care (modified according to [76,77]). For details see text.

The usefulness of a biomarker for monitoring of therapeutic efficacy of an applied treatment clearly depends on the diagnosis and prognosis of the disease progression (e.g., AD vs. other forms of dementia), as well as the choice of a specific type of treatment (e.g., cholinergic vs. amyloid).

6. CONCLUSIONS

The concept of biomarkers to support the diagnosis of diseases, as well as the to support the development of therapeutic drugs is becoming more evident as our knowledge on the underlying molecular mechanisms of diseases is increasing.

The nature of biomarkers can be very diverse, ranging from a biochemical marker (e.g., DNA, RNA, protein, metabolite) to a physiological measurement like blood pressure. Non-invasive *in vivo* imaging is strongly emerging as one important nature of a relevant biomarker.

Different types of biomarkers exist, depending on their usefulness in diagnosis of diseases, or in pharmaceutical drug development (e.g., diagnostic, prognostic, surrogate, mechanistic, etc).

However, due to the complexity of many diseases, only the integration of different types of biomarkers will lead to an improved patient treatment on a personalized basis.

REFERENCES

1. E.S. Lander et al., Initial Sequencing and Analysis of the Human Genome. *Nature* **409**, 860-921 (2001).
2. International Human Genome Sequencing Consortium, Finishing the euchromatic sequence of the human genome, *Nature* **431**, 931-945 (2004).
3. M. Eriksson et al., Recurrent de novo point mutations in lamin A cause Hutchinson-Gilford progeria syndrome, *Nature* **423**, 293-298 (2003).
4. T.J. Aitman et al., Identification of Cd36 (Fat) as an insulin-resistance gene causing defective fatty acid and glucose metabolism in hypertensive rats, *Nat Genet* **21**(1), 76-83 (1999).
5. K. Mirnics et al., Analysis of complex brain disorders with gene expression microarrays: schizophrenia as a disease of the synapse, *Trends Neurosci* **24**, 479-486 (2001).
6. W.J., Gradishar, The future of breast cancer: the role of prognostic factors, *Breast Cancer Res Treat* **89**(Suppl1), S17-26 (2005).
7. L. Van't Veer, et al., Gene Expression Profiling of Breast Cancer: A New Tumor Marker, *J Clin Oncol* **23**, 1631-1635 (2005).
8. S. Braun et al., Circulating and disseminated tumor cells, *J Clin Oncol* **23**, 1623-1626 (2005).
9. J.V. Tricoli et al., Detection of Prostate Cancer and Predicting Progression: Current and Future Diagnostic Markers, *Clin Cancer Res* **10**(12), 3943-3953 (2004).
10. R.M. Huber et al., Molecular Oncology - Perspectives in Lung Cancer, *Lung Cancer* **45**(Suppl2), S209-213 (2004).
11. C. Muller-Tidow et al., Genome-wide screening for prognosis-predicting genes in early-stage non-small-cell lung cancer, *Lung Cancer* **45**(Suppl2), S145-150 (2004).
12. R.J. Fischer et al., Validation of molecular and immunological factors with predictive importance in lungs cancer, *Lung Cancer* **45**(Suppl2), S151-161 (2004).
13. J. Agrawal et al., Colon cancer screening strategies, *Curr Opin Gastroenterol* **21**, 59-63 (2005).
14. N.P. Crawford et al., Tumor Markers and Colorectal Cancer: Utility in Management, *J Surg Onco* **84**, 239-248 (2003).
15. H. Hampel et al., Core biological marker candidates of Alzheimer's disease - perspectives for diagnosis, prediction of outcome and reflection of biological activity, *J Neural Transm* **111**, 247-272 (2004).

16. R.A. Frank et al., Biological markers for therapeutic trials in Alzheimer's disease Proceedings of the biological markers working group; NIA initiative on neuroimaging in Alzheimer's disease, *Neurobiology of Aging* **24**, 521-536 (2003).

17. M.C. Irizarry, et al., Biomarkers of Alzheimer's Disease in Plasma, *NeuroRx* **1**, 226-234 (2004).

18. I. Schulte et al., Peptides in body fluids and tissues as markers of disease, *Expert Rev Mol Diagn* **5**, 145-157 (2005).

19. L.W. Dobrucki et al., Cardiovascular Molecular Imaging, *Semin Nucl Med* **35**, 73-81 (2005).

20. E.M. Tuzcu et al., Atherosclerosis imaging: Intravascular ultrasound, *Drugs* **64**(Suppl2), S1-7 (2004).

21. N.L. Anderson et al., The Human Plasma Proteome, *Molecular & Cellular Proteomics* **1**, 845-867, (2002).

22. Biomarkers Definitions Working Group. Biomarkers and surrogate endpoints: preferred definitions and conceptual framework. *Clin Pharmacol Ther* **6**(3), 89-95 (2001).

23. M. Baker, In Biomarkers we trust?, *Nat Biotechnol* **23**(3), 297-304 (2005).

24. R.J. Ablin., Prostate-specific antigen: chronology of its identification, *Oncology* **12**(7), 1016 (1998).

25. A.F. Prestigiacomo et al., A comparison of the free fraction of serum prostate specific antigen in men with benign and cancerous prostates: the best case scenario, *J Urol* **156**(2), 350-354 (1996).

26. W.J. Catalona et al., Prostate cancer detection in men with serum PSA concentrations of 2.6 to 4.0 ng/mL and benign prostate examination. Enhancement of specificity with free PSA measurements, *JAMA* **277**(18), 1452-1455 (1997).

27. W.J. Catalona et al., Use of the percentage of free prostate-specific antigen to enhance differentiation of prostate cancer from benign prostatic disease: a prospective multicenter clinical trial, *JAMA* **279**(19), 1542-1547 (1998).

28. W.E. Grizzle et al., The Early Detection Research Network surface-enhanced laser desorption and ionization prostate cancer detection study: a study in biomarker validation in genitourinary oncology, *Urologic Oncology: Seminars and Original Investigations* **22**, 337-343 (2004).

29. I.M. Thompson et al., The influence of finasteride on the development of prostate cancer, *New Eng J Med* **349**(3), 215-224 (2003).

30. C. Kumar-Sinha et al., Prostate cancer biomarkers: a current perspective, *Expert Rev Mol Diagn* **3**(4), 459-470 (2003).

31. V.E. Bichsel et al., Cancer proteomics: from biomarker discovery to signal pathway profiling, *Cancer J* **7**(1), 69-78 (2001).

32. P.K. Grover et al., Analysis of prostatic fluid: evidence for the presence of a prospective marker for prostatic cancer, *Prostate* **269**(1), 12-18 (1995).

33. P.K. Grover et al., High resolution two-dimensional electrophoretic analysis of urinary proteins of patients with prostatic cancer, *Electrophoresis* **18**(5), 814-818 (1997).

34. A.W. Partin et al., Nuclear matrix protein patterns in human benign prostatic hyperplasia and prostate cancer, *Cancer Res* **53**(4), 744-746 (1993).

35. L.H. Cazares, et al., Normal, benign, preneoplastic, and malignant prostate cells have distinct protein expression profiles resolved by surface enhanced laser desorption/ionization mass spectrometry, *Clin Cancer Res* **8**(8), 2541-2552 (2002).

36. L.L. Banez, et al., Diagnostic potential of serum proteomic patterns in prostate cancer, *J Urol* **170**(2), 442-446 (2003).

37. S. Lehrer et al., Putative protein markers in the sera of men with prostatic neoplasms, *B J U Int* **92**(3), 223-225 (2003).

38. M.E. Wright et al., Mass spectrometry-based expression profiling of clinical prostate cancer, *Molec Cell Proteomics* **4**(4), 545-554 (2005).

39. E.F. Petricoin et al., Serum proteomic patterns for detection of prostate cancer, *J Natl Cancer Inst* **94**(20), 1576-1578 (2002).

40. B.L. Adam et al., Serum Protein Fingerprinting Coupled with a Pattern-matching Algorithm Distinguishes Prostate Cancer from Benign Prostate Hyperplasia and Healthy Men, *Cancer Res* **62**, 3609-3614 (2002).

41. Y. Qu et al., Boosted decision tree analysis of surface-enhanced laser desorption/ ionization mass spectral serum profiles discriminates prostate cancer from noncancer patients, *Clin Chem* **48**(10), 1835-1843 (2002).

42. E.P. Diamandis, Mass Spectrometry as a Diagnostic and Cancer Biomarker Discovery Tool, *Mol Cell Proteomics* **3**, 367-78 (2004).

43. I. Kola, Can the pharmaceutical industry reduce attrition rates?, *Nat Rev Drug Discovery* **3**(8), 711-715 (2004).

44. D.D. Breimer et al., Relevance of the application of pharmacokinetic-pharmacodynamic modelling concepts in drug development, *Clin Pharmacokinet* **32**(4), 259-267 (1997).

45. E.C. Gunther at al., Prediction of clinical drug efficacy by classification of drug-induced genomic expression profiles in vitro, *Proc Natl Acad Sci* **100**(16), 9608-9613 (2003).

46. A.J. Harris et al., Comparison of basal gene expression profiles and effects of hepatocarcinogens on gene expression in cultured primary human hepatocytes and HepG2 cells, *Mutat Res* **549**(1-2), 79-99 (2004).

47. Q. Huang et al., Gene expression profiling reveals multiple toxicity endpoints induced by hepatotoxicants, *Mutat Res* **549(1-2)**, 147-167 (2004).

48. A.N. Heinloth et al., Gene expression profiling of rat livers reveals indicators of potential adverse effects, *Toxico Sci* **80(1)**, 193-202 (2004).

49. G. Steiner et al., Discriminating different classes of toxicants by transcript profiling, *Environ Health Perspect* **112**(12), 1236-1248 (2004).

50. R.G. Ulrich et al., Overview of an interlaboratory collaboration on evaluating the effects of model hepatotoxicants on hepatic gene expression, *Environ Health Perspect* **112**(4), 423-427 (2004).

51. P. Seeman et al., Dopamine receptor sequences. Therapeutic levels of neuroleptics occupy D2 receptors, clozapine occupies D4, *Neuropsychopharmacology* **7**(4), 261-284 (1992).

52. P. Seeman et al., Brain receptors for antipsychotic drugs and dopamine: direct binding assays, *Proc Nat Acad Sci* **72**(11), 4376-4380 (1975).

53. Thomson Scientific, Investigational Drugs Databases; http://www.iddb.com.

54. W. Sihver et al., Ligands for in vivo imaging of nicotinic receptor subtypes in Alzheimer brain, *Acta Neurol Scand* **176**(Suppl), S27-33 (2000).

55. A. Nordberg, Functional studies of cholinergic activity in normal and Alzheimer disease states by imaging technique, *Prog Brain Res* **145**, 301-310 (2004).

56. W. Sihver et al., Development of ligands for in vivo imaging of cerebral nicotinic receptors, *Behav Brain Res* **113**(1-2), 143-157 (2000).

57. V.L. Villemagne et al., Imaging nicotinic acetylcholine receptors with fluorine-18-FPH, an epibatidine an, *J Nucl Med* **38**(11), 1737-1741 (1997).

58. A. Horti et al., Fluorine-18-FPH for PET imaging of nicotinic acetylcholine receptors, *J Nucl Med* **38**(8), 1260-1265 (1997).

59. A. Nordberg, PET imaging of amyloid in Alzheimer's disease, *Lancet Neurol* **3**(9), 519-257 (2004).

60. Y. Wang et al., Development of a PET/SPECT agent for amyloid imaging in Alzheimer's disease, *J Mo Neurosci* **24**(1), 55-62 (2004).

61. E.D. Agdeppa, et al., In vitro detection of (S)-naproxen and ibuprofen binding to plaques in the Alzheimer's brain using the positron emission tomography molecular imaging probe, *Neuroscience* **117**(3), 723-730 (2003).

62. M.P. Kung et al., Binding of two potential imaging agents targeting amyloid plaques in postmortem brain tissues of patients with Alzheimer's disease, *Brain Res* **1025**(1-2), 98-105 (2004).

63. W.E. Klunk et al., Imaging brain amyloid in Alzheimer's disease with Pittsburgh Compound-B, *Ann Neuro* **55**(3), 306-319 (2004).

64. L.I. Binder et al., Tau, tangles, and Alzheimer's disease, *Biochim Biophys Acta* **1739** (2-3), 216-23 (2005).

65. C.R. Jack et al., MRI as a biomarker of disease progression in a therapeutic trial of milameline for AD, *Neurology* **60**(2), 253-260 (2003).

66. N.C. Fox et al., Presymptomatic hippocampal atrophy in Alzheimer's disease. A longitudinal MRI study, *Brain* **119**(6), 2001-2007 (1996).

67. A. Lin et al., Efficacy of proton magnetic resonance spectroscopy in neurological diagnosis and neurotherapeutic decision making, *NeuroRx* **2**(2), 197-214 (2005).

68. A. Falini et al., A whole brain MR spectroscopy study from patients with Alzheimer's disease and mild cognitive impairment, *Neuroimage* **26**(4), 1159-1163 (2005).

69. P.J. Modrego et al., Conversion from mild cognitive impairment to probable Alzheimer's disease predicted by brain magnetic resonance spectroscopy, *Am J Psychiatry* **162**(4), 667-675 (2005).

70. A. Cagnin et al., In vivo detection of microglial activation in frontotemporal dementia, *Ann Neurol* **56**(6), 894-897 (2004).

71. M.R. Turner et al., Evidence of widespread cerebral microglial activation in amyotrophic lateral sclerosis: an [11C](R)-PK11195 positron emission tomography study, *Neurobiol Dis* **15**(3), 601-609 (2004).

72. http://www.cms.hhs.goc/mcd/viewdecicionmemo.asp?id=104.

73. T. Sunderland et al., Evidence of widespread cerebral microglial activation in amyotrophic lateral sclerosis: an [11C](R)-PK11195 positron emission tomography study, *J A M A* **289**(16), 2094-2103 (2003).

74. S. Brettschneider et al., Decreased Serum Amyloid β1-42 Autoantibody Levels in Alzheimer's Disease, Determined by a Newly Developed Immuno-Precipitation Assay with Radiolabeled Amyloid β1-42 Peptide, *Biol Psychiatry* **57**, 813–816 (2005).

75. O. Carrette et al., A panel of cerebrospinal fluid potential biomarkers for the diagnosis of Alzheimer's Disease, *Proteomics* **3**, 1486-1494 (2003).

76. P.J. Nestor at al., Advances in the early detection of Alzheimer's Disease, *Nat Rev Neurosci* **5**(Suppl), S31-S41 (2004).

77. S.T. DeKosky et al., Looking Backward to Move Forward: Early Detection of Neurodegenerative Disorders, *Science* **302**, 830-834 (2003).

78. J.C. Morris et al., Cerebral amyloid deposition and diffuse plaques in "normal" aging: Evidence for presymptomatic and very mild Alzheimer's disease, *Neurology* **46**(3), 707-719 (1996).

79. J.C. Morris et al., Pathologic correlates of nondemented aging, mild cognitive impairment, and early-stage Alzheimer's disease, *J Mo Neurosci* **17**, 101-118 (2001).

80. R.C. Petersen, Mild cognitive impairment: transition between aging and Alzheimer's disease, *Neurologia* **15**(3), 93-101 (2000).

Chapter 18

MOLECULAR AGENTS FOR TARGETED IMAGING AND THERAPY
Trends and Concepts in Agent Development

Holger Grüll and Marc S. Robillard
Philips Research, Eindhoven, The Netherlands

Abstract: Molecular Imaging allows the visualization of biological processes *in vivo*, offering new chances for healthcare with respect to early diagnosis and improved therapy. The new field of molecular imaging has been boosted by more sensitive imaging systems and the emergence of targeted imaging agents that home in on molecules of interest. This chapter describes the principles of molecular imaging and the different strategies to design targeted agents. Each imaging modality offers certain strong points but also shortcomings, which impact targeted agent design and their potential area of application.

Keywords: Molecular imaging, nuclear imaging, magnetic resonance imaging, ultrasound, contrast agents, imaging agents, therapy

1.   INTRODUCTION

Diagnosis of disease is today largely based on rather non-specific imaging of morphological changes in the human body, mainly using Computed Tomography (CT), Magnetic Resonance Imaging (MRI), or UltraSound (US). CT, US and MRI provide anatomical and functional information of the human body, where image contrast is a result of differences in absorptive, acoustic or magnetic tissue properties, respectively. All three modalities can also be used in combination with contrast agents to enhance contrast between healthy organ tissue and pathological lesions. The two nuclear imaging modalities Positron Emission Tomography (PET) and Single Photon Emission Computed Tomography (SPECT) always rely on radiolabeled pharmaceuticals to generate images. In

G. Spekowius and T. Wendler (Eds.), Advances in Healthcare Technology, 287-304.

nuclear imaging, an abnormal biodistribution of radiopharmaceuticals rather than morphological information indicates pathology.

Molecular Imaging takes diagnostic imaging one step further: molecular imaging is commonly defined as the *in vivo* imaging of biological processes at a molecular level, which is achieved with the help of targeted contrast agents homing in on specific biological molecules in the body[1]. In principle, all building blocks of a cell can be exploited as targets for molecular imaging[2], e.g. mRNA, enzymes, proteins, or glycoproteins present on the cell membrane as shown in Figure 15-3. The underlying idea is not at all new: for over 100 years biological research has been making use of specific optical and radioactive imaging agents to study biological processes on a molecular basis. However, the term *Molecular Imaging* was only introduced with the application of this concept in animals and humans. Mainly MRI, US, and the two nuclear imaging modalities are used for molecular imaging, where each modality offers certain advantages and trade-offs in spatial and temporal resolution, and sensitivity[3]. CT has so far not been used due to its limited sensitivity and the radiation burden for the patient.

2.   CONTRAST AGENT DEVELOPMENT

The development of a targeted contrast agent comprises several steps. First, suitable markers or pathways (see Chapter 17) that are associated with a disease need to be identified. Only in rare cases is a disease associated with a single gene, enzyme or protein, which is either absent or altered. Most diseases originate from a complex aberration of gene expression, cellular pathways and an altered proteome. Useful targets for molecular imaging are either highly over-expressed molecules, which can be directly targeted by a contrast agent, or up-regulated pathways, which can be exploited to accumulate a contrast agent in the diseased cell. The next step is the development of a targeting ligand, which specifically and selectively binds to the marker with an optimal affinity. Typical targeting ligands are antibodies or fragments thereof, peptides, aptamers, or small organic molecules. Finally, the targeting moiety is linked to a contrast or signal-providing unit, such as a paramagnetic ion for MRI or a radioactive isotope for PET or SPECT (Figure 18-1). However, modification of the targeting ligand may not disturb or alter its affinity to the target. Most agents are administered intravenously and have to meet a couple of requirements: non-toxic, stable under *in vivo* conditions, high uptake in the lesion with rapid systemic clearance from non-target tissue and blood. The ratio of uptake and clearance determines the contrast to noise ratio between a pathology and the surrounding healthy tissue. High uptake can be obtained when a contrast agent is effectively internalized by malignant cells. In case of radiolabeled agents, the physical half-life of the isotope needs to match the kinetics of the targeted biological process. The fate of a contrast agent inside a living system is summarized by its ADME parameters, which stands for Adsorption, Distribution, Metabolism, and Excretion. Medicinal chemistry provides ways to manipulate these ADME parameters to optimize the performance of a contrast agent similar to lead compound optimization in drug development. Though some properties of targeted contrast agents can be tested *in vitro* using cell assays before proceeding to animal studies, the prediction of the ADME parameters is difficult, making animal experiments for contrast agent testing and optimization a necessity.

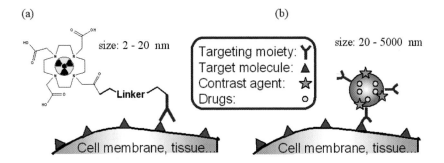

Figure 18-1. (a) direct labeling of a targeting ligand; (b) scaffold carrying targeting ligands, contrast agents and drugs.

Targeted contrast agents are always made up out of three essential elements: the targeting ligand or moiety, a contrast or signal providing part, and a spacer to connect these two. The most straightforward examples are found in nuclear imaging, where often a targeting ligand is labeled with a radioactive isotope (Figure 18-1a). This can be done either directly via a covalent bond with atoms such as [18]F (e.g. in FDG, Figure 18-2), or via a multivalent chelator group such as DTPA (e.g. octreotide, Figure 18-3) or DOTA, which can hold radioactive metal isotopes such as ^{111}In and [68]Ga (Figure 18-1a). Another strategy in the design of contrast agents is to use a scaffold, which can be loaded with multiple targeting ligands and many contrast providing groups to increase sensitivity, but also drugs for a simultaneous treatment (Figure 18-1b). Typical carriers are dendrimers, micelles, liposomes, nanoparticles, or polymers. Although these scaffolds allow a toolbox approach that can be tailored for different applications in molecular medicine, the trade-off comes with the increased size and a more complicated biodistribution of these constructs.

3.   NUCLEAR IMAGING

SPECT imaging uses radiopharmaceuticals with an isotope that decays under gamma radiation emission. The newer and increasingly popular modality is PET imaging with positron emitting radiopharmaceuticals. In general, SPECT enables imaging of biological processes with slow kinetics (in the order of hours to days), e.g. antibody-based imaging, because of the generally longer physical half-lives of the radionuclides. Most nuclides do not have to be produced by a cyclotron and are therefore more readily available and cheaper. The most commonly used SPECT radionuclide ^{99m}Tc ($t_{1/2}$ = 6.0 h) is commercially available via the ^{99}Mo/^{99m}Tc generator, which allows a convenient and decentralized preparation of radiopharmaceuticals in every hospital. Another advantage of SPECT is that multi-isotope procedures can be performed simultaneously using tracers that emit gamma radiation of different energy. In comparison, all PET nuclides effect the same mono-energetic gamma radiation (511 keV) upon positron annihilation and are therefore indistinguishable for the detector[4,5]. Most SPECT nuclides are metal ions, which can be conjugated to targeting molecules using a metal-chelating functionality. The subsequent chelate labeling chemistry with the metal nuclide is usually straightforward and easily implemented in a kit format for hospital-based 'shake-and-shoot' preparation.

PET has an approximately two to three orders of magnitude higher sensitivity than SPECT[4,6]. PET has a better temporal resolution and - at least for most clinical applications today - a better spatial resolution, and offers the possibility for quantitative kinetic measurements. PET nuclides have shorter half-lives than SPECT nuclides, and most have to be cyclotron-produced. There is, however, increasing interest in ^{68}Ga ($t_{1/2}$ = 68 min) and ^{82}Rb ($t_{1/2}$ = 1.3 min), which are can be obtained via a generator[5]. The most popular PET nuclides are the small organic atoms ^{18}F and ^{11}C that can readily replace naturally occurring atoms, producing less or no perturbation to the biochemical behavior of the radiolabeled parent molecule. These tracers will follow the same pharmacokinetic pathway of the parent molecule from which it was derived and will provide quantitative information about that pathway and ADME parameters. Because of the small size and high sensitivity of organic PET nuclides, they are the nuclides of choice in tracers that have to cross the cell membrane or the blood brain barrier. The shorter half-lives do give rise to more complicated synthetic requirements with respect to the labeling chemistry: fast reactions, high yields, no or little purification. The main advantage of Nuclear Imaging over other imaging modalities is the high sensitivity[4,7]. Extremely low concentrations are sufficient to delineate a lesion based on its biological characteristics, circumventing any pharmacological effect.

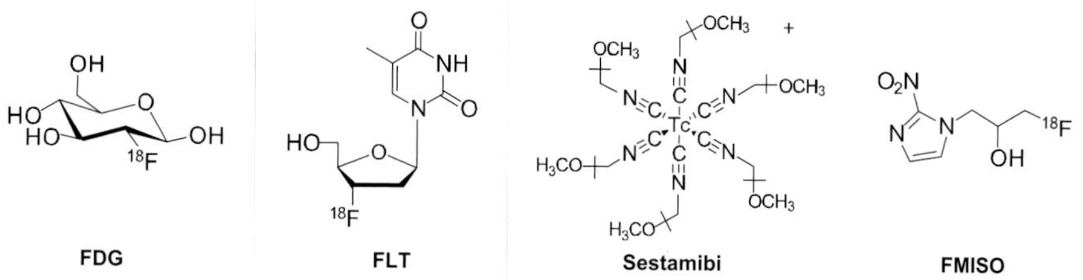

Figure 18-2. Structure of FDG, FLT, ^{99m}Tc-Sestamibi and ^{18}F-FMISO.

Furthermore, because there is almost no background radiation, nuclear imaging inherently has a high signal to noise ratio. Due to the small size of the label, the availability of radionuclides of biologically relevant elements (^{11}C), and its sensitivity, nuclear imaging is the only modality that can be used in combination with all types of targeting agents (metabolic substrates, small organic molecules, peptides, macromolecules, antibodies, nanoparticles, liposomes, polymers, RNA) to image all types of targets (genes, intracellular processes, protein and receptor expression).

Disadvantages are the use of ionizing radiation, and the fact that radioactivity decays. The latter means that an image has to be recorded within several half-lives of the nuclide, while there usually still is a non-specific background signal present in an image due to non-specific binding of radiotracers, residual radiotracer in the circulation and routes of excretion[3].

3.1 Nuclear imaging and therapy

The use of one targeting device in combination with different radioactive isotopes offers the combination of imaging with therapy. For targeted radiotherapy, cytotoxic β emitters, such as ^{90}Y or ^{188}Re have been extensively studied. The path length of β particles is several mm (i.e. 10-100 cell diameters), which permits crossfire to poorly accessible cells or antigen-negative cells. ^{90}Y has a high energy, which makes it suitable for irradiation of larger tumors. The absence of gamma emission by ^{90}Y precludes imaging of its *in vivo* biodistribution. Here, either the gamma emitter ^{111}In or the positron emitting analog ^{86}Y can be used as a surrogate for tracing the biodistribution[5,8,9]. Based on their similar chemical properties, ^{99m}Tc can be used as a matched pair isotope with ^{188}Re, where ^{99m}Tc-labeled agents are used as a tracer to confirm tumor targeting and to predict dosimetry for the ^{188}Re-labeled therapeutic.

3.2   Nuclear imaging agents

Nuclear imaging agents range from small molecules, such as simple metal complexes, receptor ligands or enzyme substrates, to big constructs, such as monoclonal antibodies, proteins or polymers[10]. Since much of nuclear imaging has to do with the properties of the targeting device, in this overview we have categorized several exemplary imaging agents by molecule type.

General building blocks of the cell: A wide range of tracers has been designed that target a general cellular process that is upregulated during a disease such as cancer. These processes include glucose metabolism, DNA synthesis, protein synthesis, and membrane synthesis. The corresponding probes are based on glucose, nucleosides, amino acids, and choline[4,5]. Two examples are given below.

The most successful PET tracer on the market is [^{18}F]-fluoro-deoxyglucose (FDG, Figure 18-2), a glucose analog. Like glucose, FDG is transported into cells by a glucose transporter and is rapidly converted into FDG-6-phosphate. However, as FDG lacks a hydroxyl group at the 2-position, it cannot undergo further phosphorylation and is trapped within the cell. Tumor cells have a higher glucose uptake than healthy cells and FDG accumulation is therefore also elevated, allowing the visualization of malignant lesions in a patient against a background uptake in normal tissue.

The same holds for 3-deoxy-3-[^{18}F]fluorothymidine (FLT, Figure 18-2), which is still under clinical investigation. FLT is the labeled analog of the nucleoside thymidine. Cell proliferation is increased in cancer, which leads to an increased DNA replication and therefore to an increased demand for nucleotides.

Small inorganic compounds: ^{99m}Tc-Sestamibi (Figure 18-2) is a myocardial perfusion SPECT agent. It is a lipophilic monovalent cation that enters the cell via diffusion, possibly through electrical potentials generated across the membrane bilayers. A region of myocardial tissue with poor blood flow (i.e. ischemic tissue) will take up less ^{99m}Tc-Sestamibi[10].

Small organic compounds: Small organic compounds comprise receptor ligands (i.e. estrogen and progesterone analogs), enzyme substrates, and many drugs. In cells with low oxygen content (hypoxic), nitroimidazoles can undergo biochemical reduction forming covalent bonds to intracellular protein thiols. In cells with normal oxygen content (normoxic), these compounds can freely enter and leave the cell. By being selectively trapped in hypoxic cells, the ^{18}F-labeled fluoromisonidazole (^{18}F–FMISO, Figure 18-2) has been used to distinguish normal from hypoxic tissues in ischemic myocardium as well as in hypoxic areas in tumors[7]. The latter is relevant for tumor radiation planning, as well as for assessment of anti-angiogenic drugs.

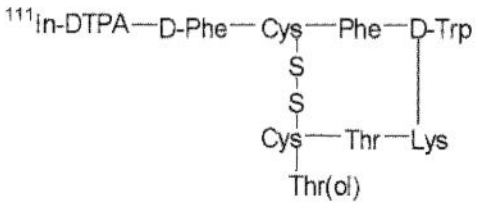

Figure 18-3. Example octreotide-based imaging agent: ^{111}In-DTPA-Octreotide (Octreoscan).

Peptides: Peptides have been primarily used to target cell-surface receptors[11]. Peptides have favorable pharmacokinetic characteristics, such as rapid uptake by target tissue and rapid blood clearance. However, their short biologic plasma half-life poses problems because peptides may decompose before they reach their target. That is why almost all peptide-based tracers are cyclic and/or contain one or more D-amino acids. Somatostatin is a linear peptide 14 amino acids long, involved in the release and regulation of several hormones[10]. Somatostatin receptors are present on the cell surface of many tissue types but are overexpressed (particularly the subtype SSTR2) in various types of cancer such as neuroendocrine tumors, making it a target for cancer diagnosis and treatment. As the peptide somatostatin itself has a short biological half-life of 2-3 minutes in blood, more stable cyclic analogs such as octreotide were developed (half-life 90-120 minutes in blood), which could be used for therapy. Octreotide and analogs have also been labeled with radionuclides to image SSTR2 positive primary and metastatic tumors in patients. An extensively studied example is ^{111}In-D-Phe-DTPA-octreotide (Octreoscan, Figure 18-3). This tracer is not only useful for detecting cancer, but also for monitoring therapy and therapy response. Radiotherapy can be performed with the β-emitting analog ^{90}Y-DOTA-Tyr(3)-octreotide.

Also ^{99m}Tc octreotide analogs have been developed, of which ^{99m}Tc-depreotide has become commercially available. The SPECT tracers are likely to be replaced by the upcoming PET analog with ^{68}Ga, which would allow detection of smaller lesions or lesions with a lower receptor expression[14]. Also, the β-emitter ^{177}Lu analog is gaining in popularity due to its favorable β energy for radiotherapy of smaller tumors and the fact that it is also a gamma emitter allowing imaging and therapy with the same compound[12,13]. Another interesting avenue is the use of [86]Y-octreotide for PET dosimetry studies before moving to therapy with the ^{90}Y analog[14].

Antibodies: The characteristic of monoclonal antibodies (MAbs) to recognize individual molecular disease-specific targets has also lead to applications in nuclear imaging. MAbs, which are used for imaging purpose are usually labeled with gamma-emitting radionuclides. The widely used CEA-scan consists of a ^{99m}Tc-labeled MAb that recognizes the tumor marker carcinoembryonic antigen over-expressed in recurrent and/or metastatic colorectal cancer[15].

In order to confirm tumor targeting by the therapeutic radiolabeled MAb (e.g. ^{90}Y-labeled Zevalin for Non-Hodgkin's lymphoma) and to estimate the radiation dose to tumor and normal organs before applying radioimmunotherapy (RIT), scouting procedures with diagnostic radiolabeled MAbs can be used (e.g. ^{111}In-labeled Zevalin)[16,17].

4.   MAGNETIC RESONANCE IMAGING

Today, contrast agents are used in almost 40% of all MRI examinations. As opposed to nuclear imaging, it is not the contrast agent itself that can be imaged but the effect it has on the T_1 or T_2 relaxivity of water in its direct surroundings. This effect leads either to a signal increase (T_1 agents) or to a signal void (T_2 agents) in the MR image[18]. Paramagnetic T_1 agents are usually based on Gadolinium, while T_2 agents have a small superparamagnetic iron oxide (SPIO) core. Direct imaging of agents with MRI is only feasible if the agents contain an atom with a resonance frequency significantly different from that of water protons, such as [19]F. So far only non-targeted T_1 and T_2 agents are approved for clinical use.

4.1   Targeted imaging with paramagnetic agents

Paramagnetic contrast agents carry an atom with one or more unpaired electrons leading to a magnetic moment. This magnetic moment interacts with the magnetic moment of a polarized water proton nucleus changing its T_1 and T_2 relaxation. The most popular ion is Gd^{3+}, which exhibits a strong magnetic moment thanks to 7 unpaired electrons. As free Gd^{3+} is toxic, the ion is complexed with a chelating molecule such as DTPA or DOTA to render it safe for medical use (see Figure 18-4). Most of all paramagnetic FDA approved T_1 contrast agents are based on derivatives of DOTA or DTPA containing Gd. The chelate occupies 8 coordination sites of the Gd-ion, leaving only one accessible for water.

The efficiency of a MRI contrast agent in shortening the relaxation times T_1 and T_2 of water is expressed in terms of its relaxivity, r_1 and r_2, given in units of $(mmol/l \cdot s)^{-1}$. Typically, small mono-molecular Gd-Chelates such as Gd-DTPA or Gd-DOTA have a relaxivity of $r_1 = 4$ $(mmol/l \cdot s)^{-1}$ at 1.5 Tesla[18]. The observed $T_{1,obs}$ and $T_{2,obs}$ relaxation times of a tissue containing a contrast agent consist each out of two contributions, where $1/T_{1,d}$ corresponds to the diamagnetic relaxation rate in the absence of a paramagnetic substance and a second term, which increases with increasing concentration of the contrast agent[19].

$$1/T_{i,obs} = 1/T_{i,d} + r_i \cdot [Gd], \quad \text{where } i = 1,2 \qquad\qquad [1]$$

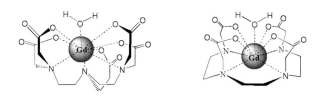

Figure 18-4. (Left) Gd-DTPA (Magnevist); (Right) Gd-DOTA (Dotarem).

Differences in relaxation times and proton density between tissues can be visualized using MRI. Typically, most tissues have a T_1 in the order of 1s, while the T_2 is around 0.1s. The image contrast depends on T_1 and T_2 differences between tissues and on parameters of the MR pulse sequence, such as repetition time, echo time and flip-angle. The presence of a contrast agent in one of the tissues shortens T_1 and T_2, which will therefore increase image contrast. An observable image contrast requires roughly a 10% difference in T_1 and/or T_2 between two tissues. Using eq. [1], the detection limit for a Gd-DTPA or Gd-DOTA can be estimated to be on the order of 25 µmol/l[20,21].

Above calculation also implies that the limit of detection can be decreased by either increasing the ionic relaxivity of an agent or by increasing the Gd concentration in a tissue. The former approach inspired intense chemical research in agents with a higher relaxivity.

The theory of relaxivity can be modeled using the Solomon-Bloembergen-Morgan equations[18,19]. Certain parameters strongly affect the relaxivity such as the number of interaction sites between Gd and water (q), the tumbling or rotation rate of a Gd-complex (τ_r), the water exchange rate (τ_m) and the magnetic field strength itself.

The relatively low relaxivity of small mono-molecular Gd-chelates such as Gd-DTPA or Gd-DOTA is mainly due to their fast rotational tumbling, which leads to ca. a factor 20 lower relaxivity than theoretically possible. Slowing down the rotational tumbling by conjugating the Gd-chelate either non-covalently via adsorption, or covalently to a large carrier can significantly increase the ionic relaxivity. Today, some new contrast agents exploiting that strategy are close to approval. The blood pool agent MS 325 non-covalently adsorbs on human serum albumin, which leads to a significant increase in relaxivity due to slower tumbling[22]. Gadomer-17 is an agent that has 24 Gd-DOTA attached to a polylysine-based dendrimer, which leads to a strong increase of the relaxivity[23].

Increasing relaxivity alone will not be sufficient for molecular imaging. Keeping in mind typical marker concentrations (e.g. cell surface receptors) in the order of pmol/l to nmol/l, even the saturation of all binding sites with a ligand carrying one or a few Gd-chelates is usually not sufficient to provide a signal[24]. One signal amplification strategy is use of a targeted carrier system decorated with a large number of Gd-contrast agents (Figure 18-1, 5).

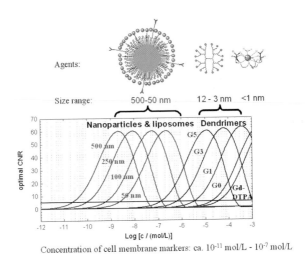

Figure 18-5. Calculated Contrast to Noise ratio (CNR) for different carrier systems carrying increasing numbers of Gd-chelates. The MRI signal intensity is calculated using a spin echo sequence[21]. The CNR increases with increasing carrier concentration, passes through a max. and subsequently decreases due to an increasing T_2 shortening. Parameters from [21,26,28].

Typical carriers are dendrimers[25,26], liposomes[27,28], or emulsion nano-particles[29]. Due to the high number of Gd-chelates attached to the carrier, the relaxivity per carrier is enormously increased. Figure 18-5 shows a calculation of the contrast to noise ratio between two tissues, where one tissue contains a varying amount of carrier particles, which are loaded with an increasing number of Gd-contrast agents. For example, a dendrimer of generation 5 (G5) carries 64 Gd-chelates[26], whereas a liposome of 500 nm can potentially accommodate up to $3 \cdot 10^6$ Gd-chelates. The number of Gd-chelates that can be accommodated on a carrier thus increases with its size. The graph shows that at least dendrimers of a generation 5 are needed for targeted imaging. More promising for molecular imaging are targeted liposomes or microemulsion nanoparticles, where one binding event increases the net Gd-chelate concentration by up to 6 orders of magnitude. The detection limit for these agents is in the picomol/l to nanomol/l range. The downside of this approach is the trade-off between increasing sensitivity and an increasing agent size, which hinders extravasation. The latter limits the potential medical application, as basically only markers can be targeted that are accessible via the vascular system (e.g. thrombosis, unstable plaque, or angiogenesis). Targeting cell surface markers of a solid tumor, which requires efficient extravasation into the interstitial space, is more promising with nuclear imaging agents.

Above concepts were recently applied to image microthrombus formation. Microthrombus formation along the intimal surface of a vulnerable plaque is an early warning for a more severe plaque rupture. Imaging of microthrombi in risk patients may offer an opportunity to intervene in time to prevent e.g a stroke or ischemic attack. Fibrin is abundantly present at high concentration in a thrombus. Targeting of fibrin is one of the rare examples where binding of a small targeting moiety linked to a few Gd-chelates is enough to render a fibrin clot visible in MRI[30]. The targeting moiety is a peptide with strong affinity for fibrin, which was conjugated to 4 Gd-chelates. *In vitro* analysis of the thrombi showed a Gd concentration of ca. 74 µmol/l. Another approach to image fibrin is the use of fibrin-targeted perfluorocarbon-based emulsion particles, which carry up to 50.000 Gd-chelates (see Chapter 19). The emulsion particles can be detected at a high pmol/l concentration thanks to the enormous relaxivity per particle[31]. The same type of emulsion particles were successfully used to target the receptor $\alpha_v\beta_3$, which is over-expressed on the endothelium of growing microvessels during angiogenesis[32].

4.2 Targeted imaging with superparamagnetic agents

Superparamagnetic agents are based on small mono- or polycrystalline iron oxide particles in the range of 4-10 nm in diameter usually consisting out of magnetite (Fe_3O_4) or maghemite ($\gamma\text{-}Fe_2O_3$). The detection limit for these T_2 agents can be estimated following the same approach as taken above for T_1 agents. The minimal detectable ionic concentration of iron in one imaging voxel is about 25 µmol/l, which is comparable to the detection threshold for gadolinium[33,34]. That limit of detection corresponds to roughly 3 nmol/l iron oxide particles assuming monodisperse 7 nm sized magnetite cores. The core particle is stabilized with a polymer layer for which polysaccharides are often used. The hydrodynamic diameter including coating varies between 20-100 nm.

Targeting ligands can be attached to the coating of iron oxide particles for targeted imaging of receptors. Artemov et al.[35] showed targeting of the HER-2/neu receptor, which is over-expressed on the surface of breast cancer cells, using a streptavidin-coated iron-oxide particle in combination with the biotinylated antibody Herceptin in a pretargeting approach. Several other receptors like $a_v\beta_3$ and vascular adhesion molecules were also successfully imaged using iron oxide-based targeted agents[36].

Growing interest over the past years in stem cell therapy promoted the use of iron oxide agents for non-invasive cell tracking. Before implantation, cells can be loaded *in vitro* with a sufficiently high concentration of iron-oxide to allow MR imaging. Of importance is to choose the imaging voxel small enough to ensure an iron concentration that is above the detection limit per voxel volume[33,34,36].

4.3   Trends in MRI contrast agents

Recently, a new class of 'smart' agents emerged. These respond with an increase of their relaxivity to (a change in) local metabolic activities and conditions, such as enzymes, pH, or ion-concentration[37]. These agents are always based on Gd-chelates with a low initial relaxivity due to e.g. a blocked 9th coordination site (q=0), fast rotation, or an unfavorable water exchange time τ_m. The underlying mechanism is a change of q, τ_r, or τ_m upon activation by the target, which leads to an increase of the relaxivity[37]. Imaging of enzyme activity is the most promising application as one enzyme can activate a large number of agent molecules. However, the concentration of activated agents still needs to exceed the required minimum detection limit according to Eq.1, which is especially challenging for imaging enzymes within a cell or within the extra-cellular matrix. Another very promising class of agents makes use of the Chemical Exchange Saturation Transfer (CEST) effect. Here, an external RF pulse is used to switch the contrast on and off, modulating the water proton intensity in the vicinity of the CEST agent. Differential scans taken with contrast 'on' and 'off' could eliminate background signal allowing for a better localization of the agent. CEST agents can also be engineered to respond to parameters such as pH. The latter allows an assessment of hypoxia, which occurs in some tumors or after an ischemic attack and is an important parameter for subsequent therapy planning[37,38].

Targeted microemulsion nanoparticles (250 nm mean diameter) filled with perfluorooctylbromide can also be used for ^{19}F-MR imaging. Marowski et al.[39] showed *in vitro* using fibrin-targeted nanoparticles that ^{19}F-MR imaging achieves a comparable sensitivity and limit of detection as the above approach based on T_1 agents. The advantage of fluorine is that it lacks any background signal, as there is no endogenous fluorine present in the soft tissue of a human body. A T_1 or T_2-agent accumulation at a lesion provides only a hot spot or a signal void, respectively, in an MR image. This can be easily missed within the natural contrast variations of the surrounding tissue. In that sense, ^{19}F-MR is comparable to nuclear imaging, and the perfluorocarbon nanoparticles should be regarded as a tracer or imaging agent rather than a contrast agent.

5.   ULTRASOUND

Most ultrasound contrast agents are basically microbubbles that consist of an interior gas phase stabilized by an appropriate shell[40]. Their size is usually in the range between 1 to 5 μm, which allows passing through the pulmonary capillary bed. Microbubbles are strongly echogenic due to their large acoustic impedance mismatch with the surroundings. The response of an ultrasound contrast agent to an acoustic field depends on the applied mechanical index (MI), which is in simple terms proportional to the peak pressure of the acoustic wave divided by the square root of its frequency. At a low mechanical index (MI<0.1), the particles show Rayleigh scattering of the impinging wave, which increases with the sixth power of the particle radius and is dampened with increasing shell stiffness and gas density of the interior phase. At intermediate mechanical index (0.1<MI<0.5), micro-bubbles start to strongly resonate in the sound field, also producing higher harmonics, which can be exploited using higher harmonic imaging. Increasing the mechanical index further (i.e. MI>0.5) can lead to disruption of the agents, releasing the trapped interior phase[41]. That event produces not only a strong characteristic signal, but can also be used for therapeutic application, such as drug delivery[42].

Microbubbles are stabilized mainly using sugar derivatives, phospho-lipids layers or polymer shells. The latter are characterized by excellent stability at higher mechanical index. The usage of a hydrophobic gas, such as SF_6 or perfluorocarbons, greatly enhances the stability as it efficiently prevents dissolution of the interior gas in blood. The breakthrough to prepare highly stable microbubbles finally enabled targeted imaging with ultrasound, as the agents need to circulate long enough in the blood for efficient accumulation at the target site to take place. Furthermore, binding to the target should be strong enough to resist shear force in the blood vessel[43].

A different class of targeted ultrasound contrast agents is based on a perfluorocarbon emulsion[44]. These particles with a mean diameter of 250 nm are considerably smaller than microbubbles allowing them to extravasate to a certain extent. Their smaller size also makes them more resistant to pressure and mechanical stress. Due to their low inherent echogenicity, these particles do not increase the echogenicity of the blood, but become visible only upon accumulation at a pathological site[45].

5.1 Applications of ultrasound contrast agents

Typical applications of ultrasound contrast agents are echo signal enhancement of the blood pool, which can be used for quantification of the cardiac perfusion in echocardiography or perfusion measurements in organs. Some agents show a preferential biodistribution, which leads to passive targeting of a certain organ such as the liver. This passive targeting allows a better diagnosis and staging of e.g. liver metastasis and hepatocellular carcinomas. Besides organs, ultrasound contrast agents can also passively attach to cells such as leukocytes and lymphocytes, which internalize the microbubbles via phagocytosis. As white blood cells travel to sites of inflammation, this process can be exploited to image inflammation[46,47].

Active targeting of microbubbles has always been done for markers that are over-expressed on the endothelium and are accessible via the vascular system, such as inflammation, thrombosis or angiogenesis.

Inflammation processes associated with atherosclerosis induce an over-expression of certain cell adhesion molecules such as P-Selectin and ICAM-1, which mediate the adhesion of leucocytes to the endothelium, followed by their transport to the site of inflammation inside the lumen. Both P-Selectin as well as ICAM-1 were explored with targeted microbubbles for their use as surrogate markers for inflammation. Villanueva et al.[48] demonstrated selective binding of microbubbles targeted with an antibody against ICAM-1 *in vitro*. Weller et al.[49] showed similar *in vitro* results with rat cells as well as *in vivo* ultrasonic detection in the setting of acute cardiac allograft rejection.

One of the earliest examples of targeted ultrasound agents was reported by Lanza et al.[44] using above described perfluorocarbon-based emulsions to target fibrin in combination with an avidin/biotin pretargeting scheme. Unger et al.[50] used targeted lipid-shelled microbubbles to visualize a thrombus. *In vivo* experiments in canine models showed an increase in intensity of the ultrasonic image of clots upon agent binding with the possibility to also dissolve the clot with the help of ultrasound-induced bubble cavitation.

Angiogenesis, the formation of new microvessels, is a response to ischemia, which is associated with many diseases. Endothelial cells of an angiogenic blood vessel differ from mature endothelial cells by a variety of over-expressed molecules on the cell surface. Especially the integrin receptor $\alpha_v\beta_3$ is well studied in the context of targeted imaging of angiogenesis with ultrasound contrast agents[51,52]. *In vitro* studies showed that the cyclic peptide arginine-glycine-aspartic acid (cRGD) can be incorporated onto microbubbles for successful targeting of $\alpha_v\beta_3$. In this respect, Dayton et al.[52] published interesting results showing that contrast agents bound to a target provide a different acoustic response compared to contrast agents free in solution. Meanwhile, the first *in vivo* studies have appeared showing successful targeting of $\alpha_v\beta_3$ with microbubbles[53].

5.2   Microbubbles in therapy

The role of ultrasound is firmly established in diagnostic imaging. Over the last years, many new therapeutic applications of ultrasound in combination with microbubbles emerged. Especially the use of ultrasound for more efficient thrombolysis is intensively being investigated. Ultrasound alone is already beneficial in promoting thrombolysis, however, studies of

Birnbaum et al.[54] in canine models showed that cavitation of microbubbles in the vicinity of the clot helps to dissolve the thrombus.

Ultrasound-induced microbubble cavitation can enhance the permeability of cell membranes[55], can lead to a rupture of microvessels[56] and significantly enhances extravasation of nanoparticles[57]. All of the above effects can enhance drug uptake or promote gene delivery[58], when drugs or genes are co-injected systemically together with microbubbles or carried as cargo by the microbubbles[42]. The payload can be delivered upon ultrasound-induced cavitation at the location of interest or delivery can be combined with a targeting approach.

6. CONCLUSION

Molecular Imaging is an exciting new field, which will have a tremendous impact on future healthcare. Applications of molecular imaging range from earlier disease diagnosis to better staging, and from more accurate therapy planning to improved follow-up care. Crucial for success are well-designed and validated imaging and contrast agents, which allow selective and specific visualization of diseases. The development of imaging agents will go hand in hand with the development of targeted therapeutics. Some examples in research already show a combination of both worlds using the same carrier system. Yet, the step from preclinical animal trials to human applications in the clinic has still to be taken.

REFERENCES

1. H.R. Herschmann, Molecular Imaging: Looking at Problems, Seeing Solutions, *Science* **302**, 605 (2003).
2. T.F. Massoud, S.S. Gambhir, Molecular imaging in living subjects: seeing fundamental biological processes in a new light, *Genes Dev* **17**, 545-580 (2003).
3. S.R. Cherry, In vivo molecular and genomic imaging: new challenges for imaging physics, *Phys Med Biol* **49**, R13-R48 (2004).
4. M.G. Pomper, D.A. Hammoud, Positron emission tomography in molecular imaging, *IEEE Engin Med Biol* **23**, 28-37 (2004).
5. *Handbook of Nuclear Chemistry, Vol. 4*, edited by A.Vértes, S.Nagy, Z.Klecsár (Kluwer Academic Publishers, Dordrecht, 2003).
6. S.S. Gambhir, Molecular imaging of cancer with positron emission tomography, *Nature Rev Cancer* **2**, 683-693 (2002).
7. F.G. Blankenberg, Molecular imaging with single photon emission computed tomography, *IEEE Engin Med Biol* **23**, 51-57 (2004).
8. J.A. Carrasquillo, J.D. White, C.H. Paik, A. Raubitschek, N. Le, M. Rotman, M.W. Brechbiel, O.A. Gansow, L.E. Top, P. Perentesis, J.C. Reynolds, D.L. Nelson, T.A. Waldmann, Similarities and differences in In-111- and Y-90-labeled 1B4M-DTPA antiTac monoclonal antibody distribution, *J Nucl Med* **40**, 268-276 (1999).

9.   A. Lövqvist, J.L. Humm, A. Sheikh, R.D. Finn, J. Koziorowski, S. Ruan, K.S. Pentlow, A. Jungbluth, S. Welt, F.T. Lee, M.W. Brechbiel, S.M. Larson, PET imaging of Y-86-labeled anti-Lewis Y monoclonal antibodies in a nude mouse model: Comparison between Y-86 and In-111 radiolabels, *J Nucl Med* **42**, 1281-1287 (2001).

10. *Handbook of Radiopharmaceuticals – Radiochemistry and Applications*, edited by M.J. Welch, C.S. Redvanly (Wiley, Chichester, 2003).

11. S. Liu, D.S. Edwards, Fundamentals of receptor-based diagnostic metalloradiopharmaceuticals, *Top Curr Chem* **222**, 259-278 (2002).

12. M. de Jong, D. Kwekkeboom, R. Valkema, E.P. Krenning, Radiolabelled peptides for tumor therapy: current status and future directions, *Eur J Nucl Med* **30**, 463-469 (2003).

13. M. de Jong, W.A.P. Breeman, R. Valkema, B.F. Bernard, E.P. Krenning, Combination radionuclide therapy using Lu-177- and Y-90-Labeled somatostatin analogs, *J Nucl Med* **46**, 13S-17S (2005).

14. W.P. Li, L.A. Meyer, C.J. Anderson, Radiopharmaceuticals for positron emission tomography imaging of somatostatin receptor positive tumors, *Top Curr Chem* **252**, 179-192 (2005).

15. L.S. Zuckier, G.L. DeNardo, Trials and tribulations: Oncological antibody imaging comes to the fore, *Semin Nucl Med* **27**, 10-29 (1997).

16. T.E. Witzig, L.I. Gordon, F. Cabanillas, M.S. Czuczman, C. Emmanouilides, R. Joyce, B.L. Pohlman, N.L. Bartlett, G.A. Wiseman, N. Padre, A.J. Grillo-López, P. Multani, C.A. White, Randomized controlled trial of yttrium-90-labeled ibritumomab tiuxetan radioimmuno-therapy versus rituximab immunotherapy for patients with relapsed or refractory low-grade, follicular, or transformed B-cell non-Hodgkin's lymphoma, *J Clin Onco* **20**, 2453-2463 (2002).

17. G.L. DeNardo, M.E. Juweid, C.A. White, G.A. Wiseman, S.J. DeNardo, Role of radiation dosimetry in radioimmunotherapy planning and treatment dosing, *Crit Rev Oncol Hemato* **39**, 203-218 (2001).

18. A.E. Merbach, E. Tóth, *The Chemistry of Contrast Agents* (Wiley & Sons, 2001).

19. P. Caravan, J.J. Ellison, T.J. McMurry, R.B. Lauffer, Gadolinium chelates as MRI contrast agents: structure, dynamics, and applications, *Chem Rev* **99**, 2293-2352 (1999).

20. E.T. Ahrens, U. Rothbächer, R.E. Jacobs, S.E. Fraser, A model for MRI contrast enhancement using T1 agents, *Proc Natl Acad Sci* **95**, 8443-8448 (1998).

21. A.M. Morawski, P.M. Winter, K.C. Crowder, S.D. Caruthers, R.W. Fuhrhop, M.J. Scott, J.D. Robertson, D.R. Abendschein, G.M. Lanza, SA. Wickline, Targeted nanoparticles for quantitative imaging of sparse molecular epitopes with MRI, *Magn Reson Med* **51**, 480-486 (2004).

22. P. Caravan, N.J. Cloutier, M.T. Greenfield, S.A. McDermid, S.U. Dunham, J.W.M. Bulte, J.C. Amedio, R.J. Looby, R.M. Supkowski, W. DeW. Horrocks, T.J. McMurry, R.B. Lauffer, The interaction of MS-325 with human serum albumin and its effect on proton relaxation rates, *J Am Chem Soc* **124**, 3152-3162 (2002).

23. G.M. Nicolle, E. Tóth, H. Schmitt-Willich, B. Radüchel, and A.E. Merbach, The impact of rigidity and water exchange on the relaxivity of dendritic MRI contrast agents, *Chem Eur J* **8**, 1040-1048 (2002).

24. A.D. Nunn, KE. Linder, MF. Tweedle, Can receptors be imaged with MRI agents?, *Q J Nucl Med* **41**, 155-162 (1997).

25. H. Kobayashi, M.W. Brechbiel, Dendrimer-based macromolecular MRI contrast agents: characteristics and application, *Molecular Imaging* **2**, 1-10 (2003).

26. S. Langereis, Q.G. de Lussanet, M.H.P. van Genderen, W.H. Backes, E.W. Meijer, Multivalent contrast agents based on Gadolinium-diethylenetriaminepentaacetic acid-terminated poly(propyleneimine) dendrimers for magnetic resonance imaging, *Macromolecules* **37**, 3084-3091 (2004).

27. R.W. Storrs, F.D. Tropper, H.Y. Li, C.K. Song, D.A. Sipkins, J.K. Kuniyoshi, M.D. Bednarski, H.W. Strauss, K.C. Li, Paramagnetic polymerized liposomes as new recirculating MR contrast agents, *J Magn Reson Imaging* **5**, 719-724 (1995).

28. W.J Mulder, G.J. Strijkers, A.W. Griffioen, L. van Bloois, G. Molema, G. Storm, G.A. Koning, K. Nicolay, A liposomal system for contrast-enhanced magnetic resonance imaging of molecular targets, *Bioconjug Chem* **15**, 799-806 (2004).

29. G.M. Lanza, P. Winter, S. Caruthers, A. Schmeider, K. Crowder, A. Morawski, H. Zhang, M.J. Scott, S.A. Wickline, Novel paramagnetic contrast agents for molecular imaging and targeted drug delivery, *Curr Pharm Biotechnol* **5**, 495-507 (2004).

30. E. Spuentrup, B. Fausten, S. Kinzel, A.J. Wiethoff, R.M. Botnar, P.B. Graham, S. Haller, M. Katoh, E.C. Parsons, W.J. Manning, T. Busch, R.W. Günther, A. Buecker, Molecular MRI of atrial clots in a swine model, *Circulation* **112**, 396-399 (2005).

31. S. Flacke, S. Fischer, M.J. Scott, R.J. Fuhrhop, J.S. Allen, M. McLean; P. Winter, G.A. Sicard, P.J. Gaffney, S.A. Wickline, G.M. Lanza, Novel MRI contrast agent for molecular imaging of fibrin, *Circulation* **104**, 1280-1285 (2001).

32. A.H. Schmieder, P.M. Winter, S.D. Caruthers, T.D. Harris, T.A. Williams, J.S. Allen, E.K. Lacy, H. Zhang, M.J. Scott, G. Hu, .JD. Robertson, S.A. Wickline G.M. Lanza, Mol. MR imaging of melanoma angiogenesis with alphanubeta3-targeted paramagnetic nanoparticles, *Magn Reson Med* **53**, 621-627 (2005) and references therein.

33. H. Dahnke T. Schaeffter, Limits of Detection of SPIO at 3.0 T Using T_2^* Relaxometry, *Magn Reson Med* **53**, 1202-1206 (2005).

34. C. Heyn, C.V. Bowen, B.K. Rutt, P.J. Foster, Detection treshold of single SPIO-labeled cells with FIESTA, *Magn Reson Med* **53**, 312-320 (2005).

35. D. Artemov, N. Mori, B. Okollie, and Z.M. Bhujwalla, MR molecular imaging of the Her-2/neu receptor in breast cancer cells using targeted iron oxide nanoparticles, *Magn Reson Med* **49**, 403-408 (2003).

36. J.W.M. Bulte, DL. Kraitchman, Iron oxide MR contrast agents for molecular and cellular imaging, *NMR Biomed* **17**, 484-499 (2004).

37. T.J. Meade, A.K. Taylory, S.R Bull, New magnetic resonance contrast agents as biochemical reporters, *Curr Op Neurobiol* **13**, 597-602 (2003).

38. S. Aime, A. Barge, D. Delli Castelli, F. Fedeli, A. Mortillaro, F.U. Nielsen, and E. Terreno, Paramagnetic lanthanide(III) complexes as pH-sensitive chemical exchange saturation transfer (CEST) contrast agents for MRI applications, *Magn Reson Med* **47**, 639-648 (2002).

39. A.M. Morawski, P.M. Winter, X. Yu, R.W. Fuhrhop, M.J. Scott, F. Hockett, J.D. Robertson, P.J. Gaffney, G.M. Lanza, SA. Wickline, Quantitative 'magnetic resonance immunohistochemistry' with ligand-targeted (19)F nanoparticles, *Magn Reson Med* **52**, 1255-1262 (2004).

40. A.L. Klibanov, Ultrasound contrast agents: development of the field and current status, *Top Cur Chem* **222**(II), 73-106 (2002).

41. N. de Jong, A. Bouakaz, and F.J. Ten Cate, Contrast harmonic imaging, *Ultrasonics* **40**, 567-573 (2002).

42. P.A. Dijkmans, L.J.M. Juffermans, RJP. Musters, A. van Wamel, F.J. Ten Cate, W. van Gilst, C.A. Visser, N. de Jong, O. Kamp, Microbubbles and ultrasound: from diagnosis to therapy, *Eur J Echocardiography* **5**, 245-256 (2004).

43. A.L. Klibanov, Targeted delivery of gas-filled microspheres, contrast agents for ultrasound imaging, *Adv Drug Del Rev* **37**, 139-157 (1999).

44. G.M. Lanza, K.D. Wallace, M.J. Scott, W.P. Cacheris, D.R. Abendschein, D.H. Christy, A.M. Sharkey, J.G. Miller, P.J. Gaffney, S.A. Wickline, A novel site-targeted ultrasonic contrast agent with broad biomedical application, *Circulation* **94**, 3334-3340 (1996).

45. M.S. Hughes, J.N. Marsh, C.S. Hall, R.W. Fuhrtop, E.K. Lacy, G.M. Lanza, S.A. Wickline, Acoustic characterization in whole blood and plasma of site-targeted nanoparticle ultrasound contrast agent for molecular imaging, *J Acoust Soc Am* **117**, 964-972 (2005).

46. J.R. Lindner, P.A. Dayton, M.P. Coggins, K. Ley, J. Song, K. Ferrara, S. Kaul, Noninvasive imaging of inflammation by ultrasound detection of phagocytosed microbubbles, *Circulation* **102,** 531-538 (2000).

47. J.R. Lindner, P.A. Dayton, M.P. Coggins, K. Ley, J. Song, K. Ferrara, S. Kaul, Noninvasive ultrasound imaging of inflammation using microbubbles targeted to activated leukocytes, Circulation **102**, 2745-2750 (2000).

48. F.S. Villanueva, R.J. Jankowski, S. Klibanov, M. Pina, S.M. Alber, S.C. Watkins, G.H. Brandenburger, W.R. Wagner, Microbubbles targeted to intercellular adhesion molecule-1 bind to activated coronary artery endothelial cells, *Circulation* **98**, 1-5 (1998).

49. G.E.R. Weller, E. Lu, M.M. Csikari, A.L. Klibanov, D. Fischer, W.R. Wagner, and F.S. Villanueva, Ultrasound imaging of acute cardiac transplant rejection with microbubbles targeted to intercellular adhesion molecule-1, *Circulation* **108,** 218-224 (2003).

50. E.C. Unger, T.O. Matsunaga, T. McCreery, P. Schumann, R. Sweitzer, R. Quigley, Therapeutic applications of microbubbles, *Eur J Radiol* **42**, 160-168 (2002).

51. D.B. Ellegala, H. Leong-Poi, J.E. Carpenter, A.L. Klibanov, S. Kaul, M.E. Shaffrey, J. Sklenar, J.R. Lindner, Imaging tumor angiogenesis with contrast ultrasound and microbubbles targeted to $\alpha_v\beta_3$, *Circulation* **108**, 336-341 (2003).

52. P.A. Dayton, D. Pearson, J. Clark, S. Simon, P.A. Schumann, R. Zutshi, T.O. Matsunaga, K.W. Ferrara, Ultrasonic analysis of peptide- and antibody-targeted microbubble contrast agents for molecular imaging of alphavbeta3-expressing cells, *Molecular Imaging* **3**, 125-134 (2004).

53. H. Leong-Poi, J. Christiansen, P. Heppner P, C. Lewis, A. Klibanov, S. Kaul, J.R. Lindner, Assessment of endogenous and therapeutic arteriogenesis by contrast ultrasound molecular imaging of integrin expression, *Circulation* **111**, 3248-3254 (2005).

54. Y. Birnbaum, H. Luo, T. Nagai, M.C. Fishbein, T.M. Peterson, S. Li, D. Kricsfeld, T.R. Porter, R.J. Siegel, Noninvasive in vivo clot dissolution without a thrombolytic drug: recanalization of thrombosed iliofemoral arteries by transcutaneous ultrasound combined with intravenous infusion of microbubbles, *Circulation* **20**, 130-134 (1998).

55. A. van Wamel, A. Bouakaz, M. Versluis, N. de Jong, Micromanipulation of endothelial cells: ultrasound-microbubble-cell interaction, *Ultrasound Med Biol* **30**, 1255-1258 (2004).

56. R.J. Price, D.M. Skyba, S. Kaul, TC. Skalak, Direct in vivo visualization of intravascular destruction of microbubbles by ultrasound and its local effects on tissue, *Circulation* **98**, 290-293 (1998).

57. R.J. Price, D.M. Skyba, S. Kaul, T.C. Skalak, Delivery of colloidal particles and red blood cells to tissue through microvessel ruptures created by targeted microbubble destruction with ultrasound, *Circulation* **98**, 1264-1267 (1998).

58. H. Koike, N. Tomita, H. Azuma, Y. Taniyama, K. Yamasaki, Y. Kunugiza, K. Tachibana, T. Ogihara, and R. Morishita, An efficient gene transfer method mediated by ultrasound and microbubbles into the kidney, *J Gene Med* **7**, 108 – 116 (2005).

Chapter 19

TARGETED NANOPARTICLES FOR MOLECULAR IMAGING AND THERAPY
A Multi-Modality Approach to Molecular Medicine

Shelton D. Caruthers[1,2], Samuel A. Wickline[1], Gregory M. Lanza[1]

[1]*Washington University, St. Louis, MO, USA;* [2]*Philips Medical Systems, Cleveland, OH, USA*

Abstract: The emerging era of personalized medicine offers the potential for early diagnosis and, therefore, treatment of pathology close to onset. Molecular imaging will allow noninvasive phenotypic characterization of pathologies leading to segmentation of patients for custom-tailored therapy. Additionally, the application and efficacy of this targeted therapy will be monitored non-invasively via molecular imaging. Nanoparticulate agents are being intensively researched as formulation platforms for various targeted clinical applications. As exemplified by perfluorocarbon nanoparticles, these new agents in combination with the rapid innovations in imaging hardware and software will allow the emergence of new diagnostic and therapeutic paradigms.

Keywords: Perfluorocarbon nanoparticles, multimodality imaging, MRI, ultrasound, applications in cardiovascular and oncology, monitoring therapy effectiveness

1. INTRODUCTION

Recent advances in the interrelated fields of genomics, proteomics, molecular imaging and targeted drug delivery have prompted a paradigm shift in medical diagnosis and therapy from a 'one-size-fits-all' strategy to an approach tailored to the individual[1,2]. Requiring novel contrast agents, the general tactic of molecular imaging is to recognize and characterize presymptomatic, early disease, which otherwise would be difficult or impossible to detect using routine imaging techniques. In essence, the intent of biochemical imaging agents is to provide non-invasive assessments of pathology analogous to the use of immuno-histochemistry. However, such characterization is quite complex, requiring the simultaneous detection and

305

G. Spekowius and T. Wendler (Eds.), Advances in Healthcare Technology, 305-322.
© 2006 *Springer. Printed in the Netherlands.*

quantification of multiple epitopes, and thus far, molecular imaging agents have been primarily focused on detecting single biomarkers as a pathognomonic signature of disease. Nonetheless, techniques for cellular and molecular imaging have been developed, and are continually being improved, for virtually every imaging modality including nuclear[3,4], optical[4-6], CT[7,8], ultrasound[9], and MRI[10,11].

With specific examples of current and imminent applications, this chapter addresses molecular imaging using a liquid perfluorocarbon (PFC) nanoparticle platform that can be detected and quantified by multiple modalities and, through specific targeting, offers great potential for diagnosis, therapy, and monitoring.

2.   GENERALIZED PLATFORM FOR TARGETED MOLECULAR IMAGING

Success with molecular imaging contrast agents requires not only reaching and binding the specific target, but also being able to detect the agent once bound[12]. While optical[13,14] and nuclear[15,16] techniques are exquisitely sensitive to their agents, MRI, for instance, is not as sensitive. With MR molecular imaging agents (see Figure 19-1), a common theme is to deliver to important (but sparse) biochemical epitopes a large 'payload' of paramagnetic metal to overcome the scarcity. One example, dendrimers, can bear a vast number of metal atoms to a target site[17,18], but as yet, limited utility as a targeted agent *in vivo* has been established. Nanoparticles, due to their inherently great surface area, have been shown to be a more effective platform, with predominately two classes: liposomes[19-21] and emulsions[22,23].

2.1   Paramagnetic liposomes

Paramagnetic liposomes, initially instituted as an instrument to overcome the partial volume dilution problem, are vesicles with a lipid bilayer membrane that enclose hefty payloads of gadolinium in an aqueous volume. Unfortunately, for MRI applications, the limited water diffusivity across the liposomal membranes drastically reduces the efficacy of the paramagnetic chelates entrapped within[24,25]. More effectively, amphipathic paramagnetic chelates have been incorporated directly into lipid membranes[26,27], which improves interactions between the relaxation agent and surrounding water thus augmenting r_1 relaxivity.

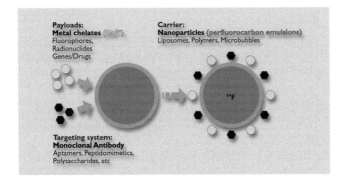

Figure 19-1. Generalized paradigm for targeted nanoparticle contrast agents. The core provides a skeleton onto which volumes of the targeting system, imaging 'payload' and even therapeutic agents can be placed. Such amplification strategies permit molecular imaging to be feasible when targeting sparse epitopes. (Reproduced by courtesy of *Medicamundi* [28]).

In 1998, Sipkins et al.[29] first reported a paramagnetic polymerized liposome targeted to $\alpha_v\beta_3$ for the detection of angiogenesis in a cancer tumor model. This biotinylated liposome system, complexed through avidin to a pre-targeted biotinylated antibody, provided early *in vivo* examples that sparse pathologic biomarkers were detectable via MR molecular imaging with 'ultraparamagnetic' particles. Later, Hood et al.[30], in a mouse melanoma model, reported a therapeutic application using a similar construct, again, targeted to the $\alpha_v\beta_3$-integrins of angiogenic blood vessels, to deliver a mutant Raf gene and thereby induce tumor regression.

2.2 Paramagnetic perfluorocarbon emulsions

The second major class of paramagnetic nanoparticles is emulsions, the most notable being a liquid perfluorocarbon-based emulsion that has been targeted to multiple cardiovascular and oncological markers[22,31-36].

PFC nanoparticles (see Figure 19-1), in contradistinction to bubbles and liposomes, consist of a liquid PFC core encapsulated by a phospholipid monolayer and can be functionalized for targeted molecular imaging by attaching homing ligands into this monolayer[31,35-37]. With typical nominal diameters of 200 to 300 nm, PFC nanoparticles are endowed with an enormous surface area to transport, and concentrate, payloads such as radioactive and/or paramagnetic metals to important vascular biomarker sites. This translates into, e.g. for the case of paramagnetic agents with ~100,000 gadolinium atoms per nanoparticle, particulate r_1 relaxivities greater than 2,000,000 (mM·s)$^{-1}$ at 1.5T[38].

While the surface area available for exploitation is an invaluable attribute, the core is also key. Owing to the properties of the perfluorocarbons in their core, PFC nanoparticles, unique from other oil-based emulsions, exhibit robust stability against handling, pressure, heat and shear. The liquid core, representing 98% by volume of the nanoparticle, can be any one of a number of PFCs (e.g., perfluorooctylbromide (PFOB), perfluoro-15-crown-5 ether (CE), perfluorodichlorooctane), with PFOB being the most commonly used. Thus, within the core of each PFOB nanoparticle, there is a concentration of roughly 100M of ^{19}F.

The carbon-fluorine bond is not only chemically and thermally stable, but also essentially biologically inert. Having been used for liquid ventilation, oxygen delivery and imaging, the biocompatibility of most liquid fluorocarbons has been well documented to be, even at extremely generous doses, innocuous and physiologically inactive[39,40]. Regarding pure fluorocarbons within the range of 460 – 520 MW, no toxicity, carcinogenicity, mutagenicity or teratogenic effects have been reported. A reversible increase in pulmonary residual volumes has been reported for very large doses of PFC emulsions (i.e., complete blood transfusion), in macaque, swine and rabbits, but this increase was not seen in mouse, dog or human[41-43]. PFC nanoparticle distribution and clearance data fit well into a biexponential function with a circulatory half-life in excess of one hour (300 min ± 110 min, Lanza et al., unpublished). The tissue half-life residencies range from 4 days for PFOB to as much as 65 days for perfluorotripropylamine. The fate of fluorocarbons is not metabolism, but rather gradual reintroduction by lipid carriers into the circulation, in dissolved form, where they are ultimately released in the lungs and exhaled[39].

3.   LIQUID PERFLUOROCARBON NANO-PARTICLES FOR TARGETED IMAGING AGENTS

3.1   Fibrin targeted nanoparticles

The first *in vivo* demonstration of adapting PFC nanoparticles for site-targeted molecular imaging was in the mid-1990's wherein the nanoparticles were homed to fibrin via an antifbrin monoclonal antibody and a three-step avidin-biotin technique[22] (see Figure 19-2). The contrast agent, bound to intravascular thrombus in canines, was detected with ultrasound imaging based on the inherent acoustic properties of liquid PFC nanoparticles[44-46].

Before Contrast   **After Contrast**

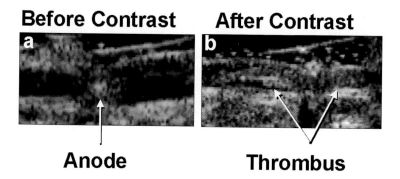

Anode   **Thrombus**

Figure 19-2. Ultrasound imaging of femoral artery thrombus before (a) and after (b) exposure to targeted PFC nanoparticles. The acute thrombus is poorly visualized with a 7.5-MHz linear-array, focused transducer. (a) The transmural electrode (Anode) and the wall boundaries of the femoral artery are clearly delineated. (b) After exposure to the targeted emulsion, the thrombus is easily visualized. (Reprinted with permission from *Circulation*[22]).

Later, this acoustic agent was further modified for MR molecular imaging by attaching gadolinium chelates onto the outer surface[47], and again applied not only toward the non-invasive *in vivo* detection of thrombi in canine models (see Figure 19-3) but also *in vitro* detection of microthrombi deposits in human endarterectomy specimens[37]. Although fibrin clots offer an abundance of binding sites that results in relatively easy detection on T1-weighted MR images, these 'ultraparamagnetic' nanoparticles are designed to have ample payloads (50,000 - 100,000 Gd-chelate molecules per nanoparticle)[38] such that minute concentrations (i.e., picomolar) of targeted agent can be conspicuously visualized[48].

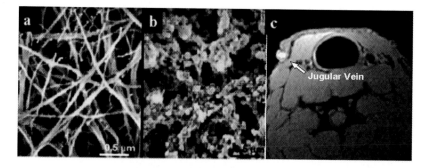

Figure 19-3. A scanning electron micrograph (a) shows the fibrin tendrils of a clot. Targeted nanoparticles densely decorate the fibrin (b), bringing >50,000 Gd chelates per binding site. The effect, in this canine model (c) is a marked enhancement (arrow), as compared to the control clot in the contralateral vein. (Reprinted with permission from *Circulation*[37]).

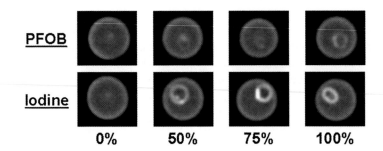

Figure 19-4. CT images of human plasma clots treated with either iodinated oil or PFOB nanoparticles targeted to fibrin. Radio-opaque particles were mixed with nanoparticles of safflower oil for graduation of targeted contrast effects. (Reprinted with permission from *Acad. Radiol.*[50]).

More recently, the fibrin-targeted nanoparticles have been imaged using CT. While PFOB, due mostly to the bromine, is radio-opaque, other emulsions have also been designed to be more conspicuous on CT. The first results of a fibrin-targeted nanoparticle molecular imaging agent were presented in 2003[49,50] wherein the CT agent provided a four-fold increase in contrast-to-noise between targeted and non-targeted fibrin clots *in vitro*. In Figure 19-4[50] the CT images of ~3mm-diameter fibrin clots demonstrate the graduation of attenuation as the amount of fibrin-targeted, iodinated nanoparticles is varied.

Regardless of modality, the ability to detect and localize non-invasively the exposed fibrin associated with fissured atherosclerotic plaque is of great value in discerning the difference between plaques that are restricting the lumen but stable versus those at greater risk for catastrophic rupture[51-53]. Current standards call for therapeutic intervention when the luminal narrowing exceeds 50%, but ironically, it is often those plaques of more moderate grade that rupture leading to stroke or heart attack and frequently sudden death[54-56]. Furthermore, while the detection of lumenally-exposed fibrin may prove useful as a *sine qua non* for unstable plaque, others[55,57] have shown that angiogenesis within the vasa vasorum is also a requirement for growth and development of atherosclerotic plaques, but at a far earlier stage than rupture. Thus, molecular imaging of angiogenesis offers a portal to observe early atherosclerosis, in addition to other important pathologies.

3.2   Molecular imaging of angiogenesis

Just as physicians and scientists interested in cardiovascular diseases are keen to detect and manage angiogenesis, so are many others in fields such as oncology and rheumatology. Angiogenesis is a complex process with many biomarkers, but one molecular signature, the $\alpha_v\beta_3$ integrin, has attracted significant attention as a target[58-63]. The $\alpha_v\beta_3$ integrin, which plays a critical part during the formation of new blood vessels[64], is expressed on activated endothelial cells but not on mature quiescent cells of established vessels[58]. Thus, $\alpha_v\beta_3$ is a popular recipient for angiogenesis-targeted applications.

The utility of paramagnetic PFC nanoparticles to image the expression of $\alpha_v\beta_3$ on angiogenic vessels associated with not only early atherosclerosis but also nascent tumors[58-61,63,65,66] has been ascertained *in vivo* [28,34-36,67].

As an example, atherosclerotic rabbits fed high cholesterol diets for eighty days develop early expansion of the vasa vasorum in the adventia of coronaries and aortic arteries, which continues to fuel plaque progression as the diffusional limits from the arterial lumen are exceeded. If these rabbits are then given intravenous injections of $\alpha_v\beta_3$-targeted paramagnetic nanoparticles, significant MRI signal enhancement can be detected (heterogeneously distributed) along the aorta (see Figure 19-6); whereas little signal enhancement can be seen in the aortas of animals receiving a control diet[36]. These findings were corroborated with histology.

Importantly, the specificity of nanoparticle binding was verified through competitive blockade experiments wherein high-avidity $\alpha_v\beta_3$-targeted non-paramagnetic nanoparticles (i.e., invisible on MRI) were injected in excess into hypercholesterolemic rabbits to saturate the binding sites. When $\alpha_v\beta_3$-targeted paramagnetic nanoparticles were later injected, no significant enhancement was detected[36] (see Figure 19-5)– thus confirming that T1-weighted MRI signal enhancement was due to the specific binding of paramagnetic nanoparticles to the $\alpha_v\beta_3$ marker of angiogenesis resulting from early-stage atherosclerotic disease.

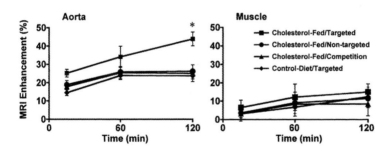

Figure 19-5. Analysis of angiogenesis from data of Figure 19-6 as MRI signal enhancement from the entire aorta (left) and skeletal muscle (right) after treatment with either $\alpha_v\beta_3$-targeted (squares and diamonds) or nontargeted (circles) paramagnetic nanoparticles in cholesterol-fed or control diet groups. In atherosclerotic rabbits, the enhancement at two hours is significantly greater (P<0.05) than all other groups, which remained virtually unchanged. Importantly, if $\alpha_v\beta_3$-integrins are pre-saturated with non-paramagnetic nanoparticles, the signal enhancement is competitively blocked (triangles). (Reprinted with permission from *Circulation*[36]).

Besides atherosclerosis, cancer is an important disease in which angiogenesis plays a vital role and is widely targeted for molecular imaging. As a model of breast cancer, Vx-2 tumors were implanted into the hindlimb of New Zealand white rabbits and the induced neovasculature was imaged with MRI twelve days later with intravenously–injected $\alpha_v\beta_3$-targeted paramagnetic nanoparticles[35]. Using a clinical 1.5T MRI and dedicated surface receive coils, high-resolution 3D T1-weighted images were acquired dynamically to track the accumulation of nanoparticles within the tumor versus the surrounding musculature. For the two hours imaged, the signal intensity increased as a function of time with the final targeted contrast enhancement of the neovasculature having increased 126% over baseline, twice the change in MR signal due to passive extravascular leakage alone. The neovascular-related signal enhancement was heterogeneous and typically located asymmetrically around the tumor capsule, at interfaces between tumor and muscle, and in neighboring vasculature (see Figure 19-7). Again, *in vivo* competitive binding experiments, wherein the $\alpha_v\beta_3$-integrins were pre-saturated with targeted non-paramagnetic nanoparticles then followed by $\alpha_v\beta_3$-targeted paramagnetic nanoparticles, demonstrated receptor specificity of the targeted agent.

Further substantiating these findings are similar studies, with equivalent results and histological corroboration, in a tumor model of human melanoma (C-32) implanted into athymic mice[34]. The Vx-2 model has also been repeated with $\alpha_v\beta_3$-integrin-targeted nanoparticles adapted for nuclear imaging with dramatic increases in detection sensitivity. Using single pinhole, planar nuclear imaging, Figure 19-8 presents an image of a Vx-2 tumor following $\alpha_v\beta_3$-targeted ^{99m}Tc nanoparticles. Note the prominent contrast enhancement of the tumor as well as enhancement of the testis and epiphyseal heads of long bones in the leg. In these young rabbits, angiogenesis is a prominent and natural feature of the maturing epididymis (which is highly vascular) and the growth plates of the long bones. All sites are specifically targeted and identified by the expression of $\alpha_v\beta_3$-integrin, which is not seen in the mature vasculature of the muscle and surrounding tissues. $\alpha_v\beta_3$-Integrin targeted ^{111}In nanoparticles have also shown significant promise with similar *in vivo* findings.

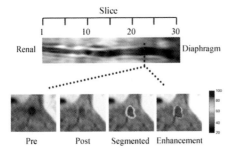

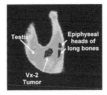

Figure 19-6. In vivo MR images of hyperlipidemic rabbit aorta. (Top) From renal artery to diaphragm, the vessel wall enhances heterogeneously due to the $\alpha_v\beta_3$ targeted nanoparticles. (Bottom) Transverse images before (Pre) and after (Post) nanoparticles, after segmentation of the vessel wall (Segmented), and the final image (Enhancement) with color encoding of the percent enhancement resulting from the contrast agent bound to the marker of angiogenesis in this model of early atherosclerosis. (Reprinted with permission from *Circulation*[36]).

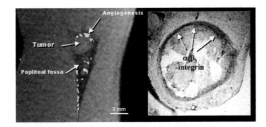

Figure 19-7. In this Vx-2 tumor model, the T1-weighted MR signal enhancement from the $\alpha_v\beta_3$-targeted paramagnetic nanoparticle is overlaid on the baseline image (left). The integrin is expressed heterogeneously around the 3mm tumor capsule and other nearby areas of angiogenesis. The histology (right) corroborates the heterogeneous distribution of $\alpha_v\beta_3$-integrin (dark stain). (Reproduced by courtesy of *Medicamundi*[28]).

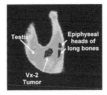

Figure 19-8. Planar nuclear image of Vx-2 tumor in the hind limb of a rabbit following $\alpha_v\beta_3$-targeted ^{99m}Tc nanoparticles. Note the prominent contrast enhancement of the tumor as well as other areas of natural angiogenesis in this young, maturing rabbit.

4.   THERAPEUTIC PERFLUOROCARBON NANOPARTICLES

As briefly presented above, the capability to target and image specific molecular biomarkers with perfluorocarbon nanoparticles provides the unique opportunity to 1) segment patient populations for the presence and severity of disease, 2) deliver potent individualized therapy directly to disease sites, and 3) monitor the treatment response through noninvasive imaging[33,68]. This emerging paradigm of personalized medicine has been demonstrated in several animal models using targeted therapeutic nanoparticles[33,69], which are laced with therapeutic agents either by dissolving lipophilic drugs into the phospholipid monolayer or by fixing lipophobic drugs onto the outer surface with a lipophilic anchor. The drugs, then, are transferred to targeted cells via 'contact facilitated drug delivery,' wherein the transfer of lipids and associated drugs between the nanoparticle monolayer and the cell membrane is enabled by ligand-directed binding[10,33,70] (see Figure 19-9). In contrast, nanoparticles that do not bind (i.e., non-targeted) retain greater than 90% of their apportioned drug. Lanza et al.[33] elucidated this concept first *in vitro* demonstrating that targeted therapeutic nanoparticles (delivering, e.g., paclitaxel) had a significant effect on smooth muscle cell proliferation, whereas non-targeted therapeuctic nanoparticles had no effect.

Contact Facilitated Drug Delivery

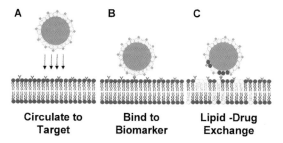

A	B	C
Circulate to Target	Bind to Biomarker	Lipid -Drug Exchange

Figure 19-9. Schematic representation of contact-facilitated drug delivery. Phospholipids and drug within the perfluorocarbon nanoparticle surfactant exchange with lipids of the target membrane through a convection process rather than diffusion, as is common among other targeted systems. Without the stable membrane contact, enabled through specific binding, drug is not released from the particle. (Reprinted with permission from *J Nucl Cardiol*[70]).

An *in vivo* example of targeted nanoparticle drug delivery is that performed by Winter et al.[69] in atherosclerotic rabbits, which, when fed high cholesterol diets, develop early neovascular expansion of the vasa vasorum, which fuels plaque progression[71,72]. Delivered intravenously, $\alpha_v\beta_3$-targeted paramagnetic nanoparticles laden with fumagillin, a potent antiangiogenic drug also known in its water soluble form as TNP-470[73], markedly pruned the nascent vessels from the vasa vasorum when measured one week later (using drug-free $\alpha_v\beta_3$-targeted paramagnetic nanoparticles as described in the previous section) (See Figure 19-10). Hyperlipidemic rabbits given 'control' nanoparticles (i.e., $\alpha_v\beta_3$-targeted paramagnetic nanoparticles without drug) at baseline had no change in angiogenic vessel density when imaged one week after treatment. Moreover, nontargeted fumagillin nanoparticles also had no significant effect on the neovasculature – again, substantiating that without 'contact facilitated drug delivery' little drug is released from the nanoparticles into the circulation. By way of corroboration, histological assessments showed that the level of angiogenesis in those animals receiving targeted drug-carrying nanoparticles was significantly reduced in comparison with the vasa vasorum expansion noted in rabbits receiving non-targeted or targeted drug-free nanoparticles. It is interesting to note that the total injected drug dosage of fumagillan associated with these $\alpha_v\beta_3$-targeted therapeutic nanoparticles was about 50,000 times lower than the total cumulative dose given orally in previous studies[73] with similar outcomes. This mechanism of locally concentrating drug via site-targeted delivery, coupled with the virtual absence of drug release unless bound, provides therapeutic nanoparticles with enormous potential for achieving results while reducing side effects.

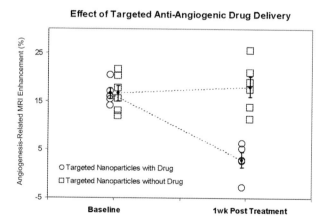

Figure 19-10. Using $\alpha_v\beta_3$-targeted paramagnetic nanoparticles allows both the detection of angiogenesis and the delivery of anti-angiogenic therapy. At the time of treatment (baseline) the level of angiogenesis is the same in both groups of cholesterol-fed atherosclerotic rabbits. One week after the single treatment, the effect of the drug is clear, but animals receiving drug-free nanoparticles exhibit no therapeutic effects. (Reprinted with permission from [74]).

5.   QUANTIFICATION OF PERFLUOROCARBON NANOPARTICLES

The examples above have shown that not only can specific biomarkers be explicitly visualized through the use of targeted nanoparticles, but they can also be the sole recipients of locally-intensified drug delivery. Moreover, the follow-up monitoring of therapeutic efficacy has been exemplified. But with this new archetype of particulate drug delivery, where serum levels of drug are meaningless, new models of measuring and predicting therapeutic effects will be required[10,75]. Perhaps the best method will be simply to quantify non-invasively the amount of drug amassed at binding sites. Thus, the unique ability to image quantitatively these therapeutic nanoparticles would be of incalculable benefit for determining local drug concentrations and developing new pharmacokinetic models of drug transport and personalized response. Furthermore, given the complexity of pathology, the ability to independently interrogate *multiple* biomarkers would greatly facilitate the phenotyping of disease and allow better prediction and monitoring of individualized response to therapy. Depending on the imaging modality, PFC nanoparticles can be quantified in a variety of manners.

Some modalities are inherently quantitative. The detection of nanoparticles labeled with radioisotopes, for example, gives an absolute number of counts per minute. MRI, on the other hand, gives images with relative signal intensity simultaneously weighted by a multitude of factors. Even so, Winter et al., in the hyperlipidemic rabbit study[69], were able to observe a relationship between initial T1-weighted signal enhancement at the time of treatment with targeted paramagnetic therapeutic nanoparticles and the resultant reduction in angiogenesis.

More precise, however, would be traditional techniques rooted in quantitative MR imaging such as T1 mapping[76], etc. In typical MRI, contrast agents interact with their immediate milieu resulting in changes in both T1 and $T2^*$ relaxation phenomena of the hydrogen nuclei. For well-behaved systems, these effects can be modeled to predict signal intensity as a function of contrast agent concentration. This approach has been described by Morawski et al.[48] for predicting the minimum concentration of targeted paramagnetic nanoparticles with known relaxivities that must be bound within an imaging voxel to produce conspicuous enhancement. Importantly, this group also used T1 measurement techniques in combination with these models to calculate the number of tissue-factor-targeted nanoparticles bound to smooth muscle cells in culture. This algorithm, while more precise than quantifying from signal intensity alone, remains limited by assumptions about relaxivities, water exchange rates, molecular geometries, and other confounding effects.

An alternative to modeling or measuring signal change as a function of contrast agent concentration would be to measure the agent directly, i.e., detecting a unique signal that otherwise would not be present. In the case of PFC nanoparticles, that alternative exists with the nuclei of [19]F. Actually, fluorine is a strong candidate for MR spectroscopy and imaging because ^{19}F, with a spin ½ nucleus and a natural abundance of 100%, has a gyromagnetic ratio close to that of ^{1}H and a relative sensitivity 83% that of [1]H. With essentially no ^{19}F in the human body, there is no background signal. Additionally, owing to its nine electrons, ^{19}F has a greater range and sensitivity to its environment via chemical shift than hydrogen does. This is the foremost reason ^{19}F MRI has been used in a wide variety of applications such as the study of tumor metabolism[77-79], the mapping of physiologic pO_2 tension[80-82], and the characterization of liquid ventilation[83,84].

After exploring the minimum detection limits of PFC nanoparticles with ^{19}F spectroscopy[48], Morawski et al.[85] went on to employ ^{19}F spectroscopy and imaging at 4.7T to quantify the varying amounts of PFC nanoparticles bound to *in vitro* clots and in human endarterectomy samples. Extending for the first time this application to clinical systems and utilizing rapid steady-state imaging techniques[86], ^{19}F image-based quantification of fibrin-bound nanoparticles was demonstrated. Further, this group demonstrated simultaneous independent detection and imaging of multiple unique species of PFC nanoparticles in varying volumes (see Figure 19-11).

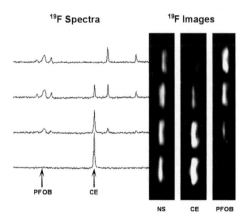

Figure 19-11. [19]F MR spectroscopy and imaging of liquid PFC nanoparticles bound to fibrin clots. The four ^{19}F spectra (left) acquired from the corresponding four clots (right) demonstrate the changing concentrations of the two nanoparticles applied. The three ^{19}F images (right), which have no proton background, represent three 'weightings' of the same four clots. Without selectivity (NS), all clots have high signal. Employing a species-selective excitation allows independent visualization of the bound CE or PFOB nanoparticles.

6.   CONCLUSION

The synergistic combination of targeted drug delivery and molecular imaging has revolutionary potential. PFC nanoparticles, homed to specific biomarkers, provide the non-invasive tools to characterize pathology at the molecular level. With the promise of extending to a multi-spectral palette, this technique offers the potential to characterize phenotypically the biochemical nature or therapeutic sensitivity of disease. Furthermore, image-based confirmation and measurement of localized drug delivery and serial monitoring of biomarker response permits tailored treatment. Coupling the rapid developments in nanotechnology, genomics, proteomics, molecular biology, and imaging systems has catalyzed the multi-disciplinary field of molecular imaging, thus helping to usher in the era of personalized medicine.

REFERENCES

1. R.I. Pettigrew, C.A. Fee, K.C. Li, Changes in the world of biomedical research are moving the field of "personalized medicine" from concept to reality, *J Nucl Med* **45**(9), 1427 (2004).
2. R. Weissleder, U. Mahmood, Molecular imaging, *Radiology* **219**(2), 316-333 (2001).
3. S.H. Britz-Cunningham, S.J. Adelstein, Molecular targeting with radionuclides: state of the science, *J Nucl Med* **44**(12), 945-1961 (2003).
4. H.R. Herschman, Molecular imaging: looking at problems, seeing solutions, *Science* **302**(5645), 605-608 (2003).
5. R.Y. Tsien, Imagining imaging's future, *Nat Rev Mol Cell Biol* (Suppl), S16-21 (2003).
6. C. Bremer, V. Ntziachristos, R. Weissleder, Optical-based molecular imaging: contrast agents and potential medical applications, *Eur Radiol* **13**(2), 231-243 (2003).
7. P.M. Winter, H.P. Shukla, S.D. Caruthers et al., Molecular imaging of human thrombus with computed tomography, *Journal of the American College of Cardiolog* **43**(5, Supplement 1), A10 (2004).
8. A. Bergman, Hepatocyte-specific contrast media for CT. An experimental investigation, *Acta Radiologica* **411**(Suppl), 1-27 (1997).
9. G.M. Lanza, S.A. Wickline, Targeted ultrasonic contrast agents for molecular imaging and therapy, *Curr Probl Cardiol* **28**(12), 625-653 (2003).
10. S.A. Wickline, G.M. Lanza, Molecular imaging, targeted therapeutics, and nanoscience, *J Cell Biochem* **39**(Suppl), 90-97 (2002).
11. S.A. Wickline, G.M. Lanza, Nanotechnology for molecular imaging and targeted therapy, *Circulation* **107**(8), 1092-1095 (2003).
12. R. Weissleder, Molecular imaging: exploring the next frontier, *Radiology* **212**(3), 609-614 (1999).
13. G. Choy, P. Choyke, S.K. Libutti, Current advances in molecular imaging: noninvasive in vivo bioluminescent and fluorescent optical imaging in cancer research, *Molecular Imaging: Official Journal of the Society for Molecular Imaging* **2**(4), 303-312 (2003).
14. S. Achilefu, Lighting up tumors with receptor-specific optical molecular probes, *Technol Cancer Res Treat* **3**(4), 393-409 (2004).

15. S.R. Cherry, In vivo molecular and genomic imaging: new challenges for imaging physics, *Phys Med Biol* **49**(3), R13-48 (2004).

16. V. Sharma, G.D. Luker, D. Piwnica-Worms, Molecular imaging of gene expression and protein function in vivo with PET and SPECT. *Journal of Magnetic Resonance Imaging* **16**(4), 336-351 (2002).

17. H. Kobayashi, M.W. Brechbiel, Dendrimer-based nanosized MRI contrast agents, *Curr Pharm Biotechnol* **5**(6), 539-549 (2004).

18. A. Quintana, E. Raczka et al., Design and function of a dendrimer-based therapeutic nanodevice targeted to tumor cells through the folate receptor, *Pharmaceutical Research* **19**(9), 1310-1316 (2002).

19. K.C. Li, M.D. Bednarski, Vascular-targeted molecular imaging using functionalized polymerized vesicles, *Journal of Magnetic Resonance Imaging* **16**(4), 388-393 (2002).

20. G. Navon, R. Panigel, G. Valensin, Liposomes containing paramagnetic macromolecules as MRI contrast agents, *Magnetic Resonance in Medicine* **3**(6), 876-880 (1986).

21. E.C. Unger, T. Porter, W. Culp, R. Labell, T. Matsunaga, R. Zutshi, Therapeutic applications of lipid-coated microbubbles, *Advanced Drug Delivery Reviews* **56**(9), 1291-1314 (2004).

22. G. Lanza, K. Wallace, M. Scott et al., A novel site-targeted ultrasonic contrast agent with broad biomedical application, *Circulation* **94**, 3334-3340 (1996).

23. B.A. Moffat, G.R. Reddy, P. McConvilee et al., A novel polyacrylamide magnetic nanoparticle contrast agent for molecular imaging using MRI, *Molecular Imaging: Official Journal of the Society for Molecular Imaging* **2**(4), 324-332 (2003).

24. S.L. Fossheim, A.K. Fahlvik, J. Klaveness, R.N. Muller, Paramagnetic liposomes as MRI contrast agents: influence of liposomal physicochemical properties on the in vitro relaxivity, *Magnetic Resonance Imaging* **17**(1), 83-89 (1999).

25. S.H. Koenig, Q.F. Ahkong, R.D. Brown 3rd et al., Permeability of liposomal membranes to water: results from the magnetic field dependence of T1 of solvent protons in suspensions of vesicles with entrapped paramagnetic ions, *Magnetic Resonance in Medicine* **23**(2), 275-286 (1992).

26. C.W. Grant, S. Karlik, E. Florio, A liposomal MRI contrast agent: phosphatidylethanol-amine-DTPA, *Magnetic Resonance in Medicine* **11**(2), 236-243 (1989).

27. G.W. Kabalka, M.A. Davis, E. Holmberg, K. Maruyama, L. Huang, Gadolinium-labeled liposomes containing amphiphilic Gd-DTPA derivatives of varying chain length: targeted MRI contrast enhancement agents for the liver, *Magnetic Resonance Imaging* **9**(3), 373-377 (1991).

28. G.M. Lanza, R. Lamerichs, S. Caruthers, S.A. Wickline, Molecular imaging in MR with targeted paramagnetic nanoparticles, *Medicamundi* **47**(1), 34 – 39, (2003).

29. D.A. Sipkins, D.A. Cheresh, M.R. Kazemi, L.M. Nevin LM, M.D. Bednarski, K.C. Li, Detection of tumor angiogenesis in vivo by alphaVbeta3-targeted magnetic resonance imaging, *Nat Med* **4**, 623-626 (1998).

30. J.D. Hood, M. Bednarski, M. Frausto et al., Tumor regression by targeted gene delivery to the neovasculature.[see comment], *Science* **296**(5577), 2404-2407 (2002).

31. G. Lanza, C. Lorenz, S. Fischer et al., Enhanced detection of thrombi with a novel fibrin-targeted magnetic resonance imaging agent, *Acad Radiol* **5**(suppl 1), S173-S176, (1998).

32. G.M. Lanza, D.R. Abendschein, C.S. Hall et al., Molecular imaging of stretch-induced tissue factor expression in carotid arteries with intravascular ultrasound, *Investigative Radiology* **35**(4), 227-234 (2000).

33. G.M. Lanza, X. Yu, P.M. Winter et al., Targeted antiproliferative drug delivery to vascular smooth muscle cells with a magnetic resonance imaging nanoparticle contrast

agent: implications for rational therapy of restenosis, *Circulation* **106**(22), 2842-2847 (2002).

34. A.H. Schmieder, P.M. Winter, S.D. Caruthers et al., Molecular MR imaging of melanoma angiogenesis with alphanubeta3-targeted paramagnetic nanoparticles, *Magn Reson Med* **53**(3), 621-627 (2005).

35. P.M. Winter, S.D. Caruthers, A. Kessner et al., Molecular imaging of angiogenesis in nascent Vx-2 rabbit tumors using a novel alpha(nu)beta3-targeted nanoparticle and 1.5 tesla magnetic resonance imaging, *Cancer Res* **63**(18), 5838-5843 (2003).

36. P.M. Winter, A.M. Morawski, S.D. Caruthers et al., Molecular imaging of angiogenesis in early-stage atherosclerosis with alpha(v)beta3-integrin-targeted nanoparticles, *Circulation* **108**(18), 2270-2274 (2003).

37. S. Flacke, S. Fischer, M. Scott et al., A novel MRI contrast agent for molecular imaging of fibrin:implications for detecting vulnerable plaques, *Circulation* **104**, 1280 –1285 (2001).

38. P.M. Winter, S.D. Caruthers, X. Yu et al., Improved molecular imaging contrast agent for detection of human thrombus, *Magn Reson Med* **50**(2), 411-416 (2003).

39. S.F. Flaim, Pharmacokinetics and side effects of perfluorocarbon-based blood substitutes, *Artif Cells Blood Substit Immobil Biotechnol* **22**(4), 1043-1054 (1994).

40. A.J. McGoron, R. Pratt, J. Zhang, Y. Shiferaw, S. Thomas, R. Millard, Perfluorocarbon distribution to liver, lung and spleen of emulsions of perfluorotributylamine (FTBA) in pigs and rats and perfluorooctyl bromide (PFOB) in rats and dogs by 19F NMR spectroscopy, *Artif Cells Blood Substit Immobil Biotechnol* **22**(4), 1243-1250 (1994).

41. M. Krafft, Fluorocarbons and fluorinated amphiphiles in drug delivery and biomedical research, *Adv Drug Del Rev* **47**, 209-228 (2001).

42. L.C. Clark Jr., R.E. Hoffmann, S.L. Davis, Response of the rabbit lung as a criterion of safety for fluorocarbon breathing and blood substitutes, *Biomater Artif Cells Immobilization Biotechnol* **20**(2-4), 1085-1099 (1992).

43. A.M. Police, K. Waxman, G. Tominaga, Pulmonary complications after Fluosol administration to patients with life-threatening blood loss, *Crit Care Med* **13**(2), 96-98 (1985).

44. C.S. Hall, J.N. Marsh, M.J. Scott, P.J. Gaffney, S.A. Wickline, G.M. Lanza, Temperature dependence of ultrasonic enhancement with a site-targeted contrast agent, *J Acoust Soc Am* **110**(3 Pt 1), 1677-1684 (2001).

45. M.S. Hughes, J.N. Marsh, C.S. Hall et al., Acoustic characterization in whole blood and plasma of site-targeted nanoparticle ultrasound contrast agent for molecular imaging, *J Acoust Soc Am* **117**(2), 964-972 (2005).

46. J.N. Marsh, C.S. Hall, S.A. Wickline, G.M. Lanza, Temperature dependence of acoustic impedance for specific fluorocarbon liquids, *J Acoust Soc Am* **112**(6), 2858-2862 (2002).

47. X. Yu, S.K. Song, J. Chen et al., High-resolution MRI characterization of human thrombus using a novel fibrin-targeted paramagnetic nanoparticle contrast agent, *Magn Reson Med* **44**(6), 867-872, (2000).

48. A.M. Morawski, P.M. Winter, K.C. Crowder et al., Targeted nanoparticles for quantitative imaging of sparse molecular epitopes with MRI, *Magn Reson Med* **51**(3), 480-486 (2004).

49. H.P. Shukla, P.M. Winter, M.J. Scott et al., Thrombus-Targeted Nanoparticulate Molecular Imaging Agent for Computed Tomography, *Mol Imaging* **2**(3), 280 (2003).

50. P.M. Winter, H.P. Shukla, S.D. Caruthers et al., Molecular Imaging of Human Thrombus with Computed Tomography, *Academic Radiology* **12**(5, Suppl 1), 9-13 (2005).

51. M.J. Davies, A.C. Thomas, Plaque fissuring–the cause of acute myocardial infarction, sudden ischaemic death, and crescendo angina, *Br Heart J* **53**(4), 363-373 (1985).

52. C. Lendon, G.V. Born, M.J. Davies, P.D. Richardson, Plaque fissure: the link between atherosclerosis and thrombosis, *Nouv Rev Fr Hematol* **34**(1), 27-29 (1992).

53. M. Naghavi, P. Libby, E. Falk et al., From vulnerable plaque to vulnerable patient: a call for new definitions and risk assessment strategies: Part I., *Circulation* **108**(14), 1664-1672 (2003).

54. J.A. Ambrose, M.A. Tannenbaum, D. Alexopoulos et al., Angiographic progression of coronary artery disease and the development of myocardial infarction, *J Am Coll Cardiol* **12**(1), 56-62 (1988).

55. S. Ojio, H. Takatsu, T. Tanaka, et al., Considerable time from the onset of plaque rupture and/or thrombi until the onset of acute myocardial infarction in humans: coronary angiographic findings within 1 week before the onset of infarction, *Circulation* **102**(17), 2063-2069 (2000).

56. K. Yokoya, H. Takatsu, T. Suzuki et al., Process of progression of coronary artery lesions from mild or moderate stenosis to moderate or severe stenosis: A study based on four serial coronary arteriograms per year, *Circulation* **100**(9), 903-909 (1999).

57. K.S. Moulton, K. Vakili, D. Zurakowski et al., Inhibition of plaque neovascularization reduces macrophage accumulation and progression of advanced atherosclerosis, *Proc Natl Acad Sci U S A* **100**(8), 4736-4741 (2003).

58. P.C. Brooks, S. Stromblad, R. Klemke, D. Visscher, F.H. Sarkar, D.A. Cheresh, Antiintegrin alpha v beta 3 blocks human breast cancer growth and angiogenesis in human skin, *J Clin Invest* **96**(4), 1815-1822 (1995).

59. R. Falcioni, L. Cimino, M.P. Gentileschi et al., Expression of beta 1, beta 3, beta 4, and beta 5 integrins by human lung carcinoma cells of different histotypes, *Exp Cell Res* **210**(1), 113-122 (1994).

60. B. Felding-Habermann, B.M. Mueller, C.A. Romerdahl, D.A. Cheresh, Involvement of integrin alpha V gene expression in human melanoma tumorigenicity, *J Clin Invest* **89**(6), 2018-2022 (1992).

61. C.L. Gladson, D.A. Cheresh, Glioblastoma expression of vitronectin and the alpha v beta 3 integrin, Adhesion mechanism for transformed glial cells, *J Clin Invest* **88**(6), 1924-1932 (1991).

62. J.S. Kerr, S.A. Mousa, A.M. Slee, Alpha(v)beta(3) integrin in angiogenesis and restenosis, *Drug News Perspect* **14**(3), 143-150 (2001).

63. P.G. Natali, C.V. Hamby, B. Felding-Habermann et al., Clinical significance of alpha(v)beta3 integrin and intercellular adhesion molecule-1 expression in cutaneous malignant melanoma lesions, *Cancer Res* **57**(8), 1554-1560 (1997).

64. M.H. Corjay, S.M. Diamond, K.L. Schlingmann, S.K. Gibbs, J.K. Stoltenborg, A.L. Racanelli, alphavbeta3, alphavbeta5, and osteopontin are coordinately upregulated at early time points in a rabbit model of neointima formation, *J Cell Biochem* **75**(3), 492-504 (1999).

65. B.P. Eliceiri, D.A. Cheresh, Role of alpha v integrins during angiogenesis, *Cancer J* **6**(Suppl3), S245-249 (2000).

66. A.N. Tenaglia, K.G. Peters, M.H. Sketch Jr., B.H. Annex, Neovascularization in atherectomy specimens from patients with unstable angina: implications for pathogenesis of unstable angina, *Am Heart J* **135**(1), 10-14 (1998).

67. S.A. Anderson, R.K. Rader, W.F. Westlin et al., Magnetic resonance contrast enhancement of neovasculature with alpha(v)beta(3)-targeted nanoparticles, *Magn Reson Med* **44**(3), 433-439 (2000).

68. T.L. Chenevert, C.R. Meyer, B.A. Moffat et al., Diffusion MRI: a new strategy for assessment of cancer therapeutic efficacy, *Mol Imaging* **1**(4), 336-343 (2002).

69. P.M. Winter, S.D. Caruthers, S.A. Wickline, G.M. Lanza, Molecular Imaging and Targeted Drug Delivery in Cardiovascular Disease with Paramagnetic Nanoparticles, *Mol Imaging* **3**(3), 188 (2004).

70. G.M. Lanza, P.M. Winter, S.D. Caruthers et al., Magnetic resonance molecular imaging with nanoparticles, *J Nucl Cardiol* **11**(6), 733-743 (2004).

71. K.S. Moulton, Plaque angiogenesis: its functions and regulation, *Cold Spring Harb Symp Quant Biol* **67**, 471-482 (2002).

72. Y. Zhang, W.J. Cliff, G.I. Schoefl, G. Higgins, Immunohistochemical study of intimal microvessels in coronary atherosclerosis, *Am J Pathol* **143**(1), 164-172 (1993).

73. K.S. Moulton, E. Heller, M.A. Konerding, E. Flynn, W. Palinski, J. Folkman, Angiogenesis inhibitors endostatin or TNP-470 reduce intimal neovascularization and plaque growth in apolipoprotein E-deficient mice, *Circulation* **99**(13), 1726-1732 (1999).

74. S.D. Caruthers, P.M. Winter, S.A. Wickline, G.M. Lanza, Targeted Magnetic Resonance Imaging Contrast Agents, in: *Magnetic Resonance Imaging: Methods and Biologic Applications Vol. 124,* edited by P.V. Prasad, 387-399 (Humana Press, Totowa, 2005).

75. H. Harashima, S Iida, Y. Urakami, M. Tsuchihashi, H. Kiwada, Optimization of antitumor effect of liposomally encapsulated doxorubicin based on simulations by pharmacokinetic/pharmacodynamic modeling, *J Control Release* **61**(1-2), 93-106 (1999).

76. D.C. Look, D.R. Locker, Time saving in measurement of NMR and EPR relaxation times, *Rev Sci Instrum* **41**(2), 621-627 (1970).

77. H. Ikehira, F. Girard, T. Obata et al., A preliminary study for clinical pharmacokinetics of oral fluorine anticancer medicines using the commercial MRI system 19F-MRS, *Br J Radiol* **72**, 584-589 (1999).

78. H. Schlemmer, M. Becker, P. Bachert et al., Alterations of intratumoral pharacokinetics of 5-fluorouracil in head and neck carcinoma during simultaneous radiochemotherapy, *Cancer Res* **59**, 2363-2369 (1999).

79. W. Wolf, C. Presant, V. Waluch, 19F-MRS studies of fluorinated drugs in humans, *Adv Drug Deliv Rev* **41**, 55-74 (2000).

80. U. Noth, P. Grohn, A. Jork, U. Zimmermann, A. Haase, J. Lutz, 19F-MRI in vivo determination of the partial oxygen pressure in perfluorocarbon-loaded alginate capsules implanted into the peritoneal cavity and different tissues, *Magn Reson Med* **42**, 1039-1047 (1999).

81. S. Hunjan, D. Zhao, A. Canstandtinescu, E. Hahan, P. Antich, R. Mason, Tumor oximetry: demonstration of an enhanced dynamic mapping procedure using fluorine-19 echo planar magnetic resonance imaging the Dunning prostate R3327-At1 rat tumor, *Int J Radiat Oncol Biol Phys* **49**, 1097-1108 (2001).

82. X. Fan, J. River, M. Zamora, H. Al-Hallaq, G. Karczmar, Effect of carbogen on tumor oxygenation: combined fluorine-19 and proton MRI measurements, *Int J Radiat Oncol Biol Phys* **54**, 1202-1209 (2002).

83. M. Huang, Q. Ye, D. Williams, C. Ho, MRI of lungs using partial liquid ventilation with water-in-perfluorocarbon emulsions, *Magn Reson Med* **48**, 487-492 (2002).

84. S. Laukemper-Ostendorf, A. Scholz, K. Burger et al., 19F-MRI of perflubron for measurement of oxygen partial pressure in porcine lungs during partial liquid ventilation, *Magn Reson Med* **47**, 82-89 (2002).

85. A.M. Morawski, P.M. Winter, X. Yu et al., Quantitative "magnetic resonance immunohistochemistry" with ligand-targeted (19)F nanoparticles, *Magn Reson Med* **52**(6), 1255-1262 (2004).

86. S.D. Caruthers, A.M. Neubauer, F.D. Hockett et al., In vitro demonstration using 19F magnetic resonance to augment molecular imaging with paramagnetic perfluorocarbon nanoparticles at 1.5T, *Invest Radiol* **41**, in press (2006).

Chapter 20

MOLECULAR IMAGING WITH ANNEXIN A5
The Molecular Basis for the Success of Annexin A5 as a Molecular Imaging Probe

Chris Reutelingsperger and Leonard Hofstra
University Maastricht, Maastricht, The Netherlands

Abstract: Molecular imaging strives to visualize processes on the molecular and cellular level *in vivo*. Understanding these processes supports diagnosis and evaluation of therapeutic efficacy on an individual basis and makes, thereby, personalized medicine possible. Programmed cell death (PCD) has evolved in the past decade as an important target for Molecular Imaging not only because of its involvement in a number of diseases but also because of the availability of the probe annexin A5. This chapter highlights aspects of PCD and reviews the development and significance of annexin A5 as a Molecular Imaging probe within the preclinical and clinical arenas.

Keywords: Molecular imaging, programmed cell death, annexin A5, personalized medicine, cardiovascular diseases, oncology

1.   INTRODUCTION

Molecular Imaging (MI) is a rapidly emerging discipline, the main objectives of which are to allow early diagnosis of diseases and to guide therapy and patient management[1]. MI aims to visualize processes at the molecular and cellular level *in vivo* by using specific and intelligent probes. In contrast to conventional imaging techniques, such as computer tomography (CT) and/or magnetic resonance imaging (MRI), both aiming to visualize the anatomical or physiological consequences of a disease, MI focuses on the visualization of the molecular and cellular fingerprints of an awakening or existing disease. MI depends on the one hand on the knowledge about disease-specific targets and on the other hand on labeled

323

G. Spekowius and T. Wendler (Eds.), Advances in Healthcare Technology, 323-336.
© 2006 *Springer. Printed in the Netherlands.*

probes that exhibit sufficient sensitivity and specificity for these targets *in vivo*.

Programmed cell death (PCD) is an orchestrated form of cell suicide that plays a fundamental role in physiology as well as in pathology of the multi-cellular organism[2]. Acute myocardial infarction, heart failure and the unstable atherosclerotic plaque for example are characterized by increased PCD[3-5]. Tumor growth in cancer can occur because the balance between cell proliferation and PCD is disturbed in favor of proliferation. Anti-cancer therapies such as radiation and chemotherapy appear to be effective if they induce PCD in cancer cells[6]. These aspects combined render PCD into an attractive cellular process to be measured by MI.

PCD has been studied intensively at the molecular and cellular level over the past two decades. These investigations unraveled a large set of molecules and their biochemical mechanisms underlying PCD. The cell surface expression of the phospholipid phosphatidylserine (PS) appeared to be a common denominator of the various forms of PCD for most cell types and cell death inducing triggers[7]. Annexin A5 (anxA5) binds with high affinity to cell surface expressed PS. This feature together with its physicochemical properties have turned anxA5 into a widely used MI-probe for the visualization of PCD *in vitro* and *in vivo* in animal models and patients using various imaging modalities.

This chapter treats aspects of PCD and anxA5 in conjunction with its development and properties as an MI-probe for preclinical and clinical applications.

2.   PROGRAMMED CELL DEATH

2.1   The different forms of PCD

Upon the discovery of apoptosis[2] a generalized model of cell death arose in which two forms were the protagonists. Necrosis was recognized as the common insult-induced type of cell death, characterized by cell swelling, membrane rupture and subsequent release of cellular constituents into the environment invoking undesirable inflammation. Its counterpart, apoptosis, was perceived to embody a highly organized mode of cell suicide executed by a group of proteases called caspases, the activities of which underlie the apoptotic morphological and biological features[8]. The most obvious are cyto-plasmic shrinkage, chromatin condensation, DNA degradation, membrane blebbing, subsequent formation of apoptotic bodies, and, importantly, no inflammatory response. Extensive investigations over the past decade have demonstrated that this model was too simplistic to maintain.

Research has revealed a considerable overlap between necrosis and apoptosis. For instance, cells undergoing apoptosis (which is an energy-consuming process) appear to have the ability to switch to necrosis upon energy depletion[9,10], whereas the opposite may also occur when the noxious stimulus driving a cell into necrosis is removed before the end. If insufficient damage occurs to continue the necrotic process, the cell may initially survive to perish later on from its injuries through apoptosis[11]. Interestingly, it has also been shown that extracellular signals triggering PCD may result in both apoptotic and necrotic phenotypes of cell death, depending on cell type or cellular content[12]. This not only implies that both modes might be closely intertwined, but moreover that necrosis can be the result of a regulated initiation of cell death, in contrast to the widely perceived notion of necrosis as a passive process following damage.

In 2001, Leist and Jäättelä pointed out that caspases, the central executioners of apoptosis, are not always involved in PCD[13]. In fact, species lacking caspases display apoptosis-resembling cell death too. Combined with the discovery of other proteases being capable of mediating cell death, this led them to suggest a less rigid model, in which cell death is regarded a hybrid event on the gliding scale between two extremes, i.e. apoptosis and necrosis[13]. The precise mode of cell death is determined by the resultant of cell type, stimulus and competition of different PCD mechanisms. This model provides a new paradigm for studying cell death and its modes of appearance and, thereby, creates a challenge for MI.

2.2   Phosphatidylserine, the ubiquitous flag of PCD

Early work revealed that the membrane of the erythrocyte is characterized by a phospholipid asymmetry over the two leaflets of the bilayer. Phosphatidylserine (PS), a negatively charged aminophospholipid, is predominantly found in the inner leaflet that faces the cytosol. The outer leaflet that is in contact with the environment contains predominantly phosphatidylcholine and sphingomeylin while PS is almost completely lacking. The PS asymmetry results from the ATP-dependent action of the aminophospholipid translocase that transports PS from the outer to the inner leaflet[14]. Inspired by this early work the group of Devaux showed that nucleated cells also have a PS-asymmetry and mechanisms to generate and maintain this asymmetry that are similar to those operating in erythrocytes[15].

In 1992 Valerie Fadok and co-workers reported that PS becomes exposed on the surface of apoptotic lymphocytes where it functions as a flag towards phagocytes, which respond to the signaling flag by engulfing the dying cell[16,17]. Using fluorescent analogs of PS it was demonstrated that activation of apoptosis is accompanied by the inhibition of the aminophospholipid translocase and the activation of the scramblase. The combined action results in the surface expression of PS whilst the plasma membrane integrity remains intact[18].

The first experiments following the landmark paper of Fadok et al. focused primarily on apoptosis and revealed that PS expression is ubiquitous in the sense that cells regardless of the cell type and the cell death inducing trigger express PS at their cell surface *in vitro*[7] as well *in vivo*[19]. In addition, PS expression during apoptosis appears to be phylogenetically conserved[20]. It not only occurs in mammals but also in plants, flies and worms indicating that the PS signature of the dying cell is of vital importance to a multicellular organization.

Apoptosis is the major form of cell death but it is not the only way to the demise of cells occurring in multicellular organisms (see section 2.1). In addition to classic apoptosis, cells may also die from necrosis, mitotic catastrophe, or autophagy[6,21]. Dependent on cell type and environmental context, PCD, thus, may present in many different forms that can have distinguishing and overlapping morphological and biochemical features. Within the complex environment of the whole tissue PCD may even start in one form and transform in another. Recent research has revealed that all the PCD forms known so far share surface expression of PS as a common denominator. Apoptosis, necrosis, mitotic catastrophe and autophagy are all characterized by the surface expression of PS[22-25]. This feature renders PS into an attractive target for MI of PCD to understand pathogenesis, support diagnosis and assess therapeutic efficacy. In 1994 the group of Reutelingsperger discovered that the protein annexin A5 can be employed as an MI probe to visualize PCD *in vitro* and *in vivo*.

3.   ANNEXIN A5

3.1   Annexin A5, a phosphatidylserine binding member of the annexin family

Annexin A5 (AnxA5) was originally discovered in human umbilical cord arteries as a strong anticoagulant protein. AnxA5 appeared to exert its anticoagulant action through a high affinity binding to PS expressing membranes, which catalyze certain procoagulant reactions[26]. Molecular and physicochemical investigations revealed that anxA5 belongs to a large family of proteins, termed the annexins, that share structural and functional features[27].

AnxA5 is a single chain protein that is not glycosylated and has no intramolecular disulfide bridges. It binds in the presence of calcium-ions to PS containing membranes with a Kd of less then 10^{-9}M [28,29]. Its affinity for phospholipids such as phosphatidylcholine and sphingomyeline is two orders of magnitude lower. The calcium need of anxA5 for binding to PS resides within the range of 0.1 - 2 mM, which is the level of ionized calcium in the extracellular compartments of mammals.

The tertiary structure of anxA5 has been resolved as well as the calcium binding sites and the phospholipid binding side[30]. AnxA5 is a monomer in solution but when it binds to PS it forms homo-trimers through protein-protein interactions. The trimers organize subsequently into a carpet of interacting trimers covering the PS expressing membrane surface[31]. These biological and physicochemical properties render anxA5 into an ideal probe for MI of PCD.

3.2 Annexin A5, the ideal probe for molecular imaging of programmed cell death

The anxA5-affinity assay to measure PCD of B-lymphocytes *in vitro* by flow cytometry and fluorescence microscopy was firstly published in 1994[32]. The assay was rapid and simple. The cells were incubated with fluorescently-labeled anxA5 in the presence of calcium ions during 5-10 minutes. AnxA5 did not bind to viable cells but bound to cells that were in the various phases of apoptosis (Figure 20-1).

AnxA5 appears to recognize apoptotic cells regardless of the cell-type and the cell death inducing trigger[7,33-36]. The next important step of its development as an MI probe was made by the group of Vermeij-Keers. They showed elegantly that biotinylated anxA5, when injected into the blood stream of the living mouse embryo ex utero, only bound to apoptotic cells and not to living cells[20,36]. These studies revealed the ability of anxA5 to discriminate between living and dying cells in the complex environment of the whole tissue at the ambient calcium concentration. This understanding firmly established the basis for anxA5 as an MI probe to measure PCD *in vivo*.

AnxA5 was labeled with a variety of reporters to allow visualization of PCD *in vivo* employing different imaging modalities such as optical-[37,38], nuclear-[39], ultrasound- (Johan Verjans, personal communication) and magnetic resonance imaging[40].

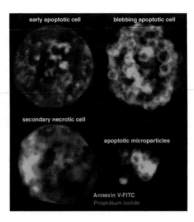

Figure 20-1. Confocal scanning laser microscopy of Jurkat cells that were triggered to execute apoptosis with anti-Fas antibody. The cells were incubated with anxA5-FITC and the membrane permeability probe propidium iodide. The various phases of apoptosis are distinguishable using this imaging protocol.

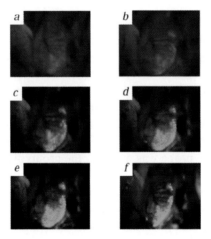

Figure 20-2. These panels show the time course of binding of Oregon-Green labeled anxA5 following ischemia and reperfusion of the mouse heart *in vivo*, as assessed by optical imaging. Ischemia is induced by ligation of the LAD, which is one of the main coronary arteries. To achieve restoration of flow (reperfusion) the ligature around the LAD is released. This model strongly mimics the clinical setting of patients with acute myocardial infarction, who are treated by reperfusion. During ischemia (A and B) slight uptake of the Oregon-Green labeled anxA5 is visible in the area risk of the heart. However, after the on set of reperfusion (C = 2 minutes after reperfusion), anxA5 binding to the area at risk rapidly increases (D = 8 minutes after reperfusion, and E = 20 minutes after reperfusion). No further increase in binding of anxA5 is seen after 20 minutes following reperfusion (F = 45 minutes after reperfusion). These data indicate that reperfusion is a strong trigger for the induction of PCD in the heart.

Altogether the *in vitro* and *in vivo* studies created the expectation that the anxA5 imaging protocol would be the first MI protocol that could be applied to unmet medical needs in the clinical arena.

4. MOLECULAR IMAGING OF PROGRAMMED CELL DEATH IN THE CLINICAL ARENA WITH ANNEXIN A5

4.1 Cardiovascular diseases

One of the most prominent unmet clinical needs in cardiovascular medicine is the development of heart failure. Heart failure affects millions of patients in the Western world and is associated with a low quality of live and a high risk of dying. The major cause for heart failure is the occurrence of acute myocardial infarction. Experimental models have shown that loss of cardiomyocytes following myocardial infarction is caused by the activation of PCD of the cardiomyocytes. Measurement of PCD in the heart may, hence, offer understanding of the processes leading to heart failure and may provide the opportunity for the early detection of patients at risk to develop heart failure.

Preclinical investigations showed that the anxA5 imaging protocol measures the PCD of cardiomyocytes in a mouse model of acute myocardial infarction[37] (Figure 20-2).

The first demonstration of MI of PCD in a clinical setting was in patients with acute myocardial infarction using Technetium-labeled anxA5 and SPECT analysis[41]. This study showed extensive binding of technetium labeled anxA5 in the area at risk in the left ventricle on day one (Figure 20-3). These data suggest that at least part of the heart cells in the infarct area undergo PCD, indicating that cell death of these cells may be prevented by cell death inhibiting compounds. The area of uptake of anxA5 correlated well with the defect seen on perfusion imaging of the heart on day 3 after acute myocardial infarction, suggesting that the uptake of anxA5 as seen on day one indeed indicates loss of cells and infarction.

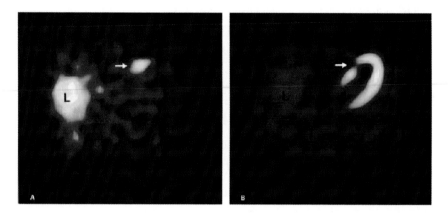

Figure 20-3. Transectional SPECT images of a patient with acute myocardial infarction who was injected with Technetium-labeled anxA5 on day 1 immediately after the start of reperfusion (left panel) and with Technetium-labeled Sestamibi, which is a perfusion imaging agent, on day 3 (right panel). Enhanced uptake of Technetium-labeled anxA5 is seen in the anterior wall of the heart (arrow), indicating PCD of heart cells in this area. Perfusion imaging on day 3 of this patient shows a defect at exactly the same site. L indicates the liver.

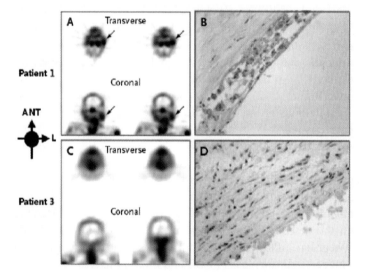

Figure 20-4. Panels A and C show the SPECT imaging of Technetium-labeled anxA5 in patient 1 with a recent TIA (A) and patient 3, who had no TIA 3 months before imaging (C). Patient 1 shows enhanced uptake at the side of the symptomatic carotid artery (arrows) whereas patient 3 does not reveal enhanced uptake. Panel B shows the histologic analysis of the unstable carotid artery plaque of patient 1, characterized by macrophage infiltration and anxA5 staining (brown staining). Panel D illustrates the histologic analysis of the carotid artery plaque of patient 3 showing a stable phenotype and an absence of anxA5.

The substrate leading to myocardial infarction consists in 90% of the cases of rupture of an unstable atherosclerotic plaque in a coronary artery. So far, the medical community has not been able to succeed in developing diagnostic tools to recognize patients at risk to undergo acute vascular events, such as acute myocardial infarction. Rupture of unstable atherosclerotic lesions is also the main mechanism leading to stroke in patients with carotid artery lesions. Extensive research in the last two decades has shown that unstable plaques are defined by a high content of inflammatory cells such as macrophages and apoptotic cells. Therefore, MI of PCD may also provide an attractive target for the identification of unstable atherosclerotic lesions.

The group of Narula showed the feasibility of detection of plaque instability in a rabbit model of atherosclerosis using Technetium-labeled anxA5[42]. These data reveal that the extent of anxA5 uptake in the atherosclerotic lesions in the aorta of high fat treated rabbits correlates well with the complexity of the lesions and the content of inflammatory and apoptotic cells (Figure 20-5).

The preclinical data suggest that targeting apoptotic cells in atherosclerotic lesions may be a way to identify patients at risk to undergo acute vascular events. In a preliminary clinical study it was shown that the anxA5 imaging protocol may also be able to identify plaque instability in patients[43]. Two different patient groups with significant carotid artery stenosis were investigated in the atherosclerosis imaging study. In one group, patients with a recent transient ischemic attack (TIA), a sign of clinical plaque instability, were investigated and in a second group patients with a remote history of a TIA were included. In the patients with a recent TIA enhanced uptake of Technetium-labeled anxA5 was observed at the site of the symptomatic carotid artery lesion, which was confirmed by histologic analysis of the surgically removed stenotic lesions (Figure 20-4). In addition, a patient with carotid artery stenosis and no TIA in the past 3 months did not show enhanced uptake of anxA5.

These data strongly suggest that clinical identification of patients at risk of undergoing stroke and/or TIA may be possible with the MI protocol using Technetium-labeled anxA5.

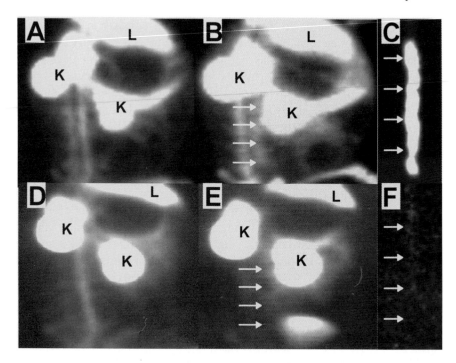

Figure 20-5. Nuclear imaging of apoptosis in experimental atherosclerosis in the rabbit using Technetium-labeled anxA5. Panel A shows the image at the time of injection of anxA5. Some blood pool activity is visible. Panel B shows the image taken 2 hours after injection. Enhanced uptake can be seen in de aortic region. Panel C is the *ex vivo* image of the atherosclerotic aorta. Focalized uptake of anxA5 is clearly visible. Histologic analysis confirmed the binding of anxA5 to apoptotic macrophages in the atherosclerotic lesions. Panels D-F are the images of the control animal. No enhanced uptake of anxA5 is visible, at the time of injection (D), two hours after injection (E) and *ex vivo* (F). K and L indicate the kidney and liver respectively.

4.2   Oncologic diseases

In oncology the MI of PCD may have two important clinical benefits. Firstly, MI of PCD may help to diagnose the malignancy of tumors that are not eligible for taking biopsies either by inaccessibility or by imposing an unacceptable risk to the patient when taking the biopsy. Intracardiac tumors are examples of such type of tumors. A preliminary clinical study demonstrated the feasibility of MI of intracardiac tumors using the Technetium-labeled anxA5[44]. This study also indicated that the anxA5 imaging protocol may differentiate between malignant and benign tumors. A larger clinical study should substantiate and confirm this hypothesis.

Secondly, MI of PCD may help to evaluate the efficacy of anti-cancer therapy shortly after the start of the therapy. Current common practice comprises the evaluation of efficacy after the treatment has been completed. Thus, patients bear the risk to suffer from possibly ineffective therapy over a relatively long period of time. Since effective radiation and chemotherapy cause one or another form of PCD in the tumor shortly after the start of the therapy, MI of PCD using anxA5 may allow the evaluation of efficacy much earlier in the time course of therapy. Thus, ineffective therapies can be aborted much sooner and can be replaced much quicker by other therapies that have a chance of being effective. The first evaluations of cancer therapy based on anxA5 uptake in patients showed promising results[45-48], although significant additional clinical research is still required. The potential gains from this application involve aspects of time, cost and reduction of unnecessary side-effects.

5. FUTURE PERSPECTIVES

MI of PCD using anxA5 has made the successful transition from the *in vitro* settings via the preclinical arena into the clinical arena. In the latter, the SPECT imaging protocol using Technetium-labeled anxA5 is the only protocol currently being applied. Continued work on MI of PCD indicate that in the future also other imaging modalities will be available for application in the clinical arena. Recent findings show that it is feasible to label anxA5 with PET probes[49-51], thus allowing PET/CT imaging of PCD. This will not only yield high resolution images but will also combine biological information with anatomical structures. This can be of importance for the evaluation of atherosclerotic plaques situated in the coronary arteries.

Other anxA5 conjugates may find their way to the clinic for imaging of PCD with non-nuclear modalities such as ultrasound and magnetic resonance imaging.

In the case of ultrasound imaging it is possible to add the function of targeted drug delivery by the inclusion of drugs into the anxA5-conjugated echo-bubbles. The concept of targeted drug delivery using anxA5 has become even more attractive not only from the experiences with anxA5 as an MI-probe but also from the recent findings that anxA5 opens a novel portal of cell entry[52]. These novel insights create the paradigm "Seek, Enter and Act" for anxA5 in which the acting can be cell rescuing in for example myocardial infarction and heart failure, and cell killing in for example cancer. Tuning the action can be accomplished by the choice of drugs that will be attached to anxA5.

The drug targeting concept of anxA5 is a logical extension of the MI-experience and bears a great clinical promise for the diagnosis and treatment of cardiovascular and oncologic diseases.

REFERENCES

1. R. Weissleder, U. Mahmood, Molecular imaging, *Radiology* **219**, 316-333 (2001).
2. J.F. Kerr, A.H. Wyllie et al., Apoptosis: a basic biological phenomenon with wide-ranging implications in tissue kinetics, *Br J Cancer* **26**, 239-257 (1972).
3. S. Garg, L. Hofstra et al., Apoptosis as a therapeutic target in acutely ischemic myocardium, *Curr Opin Cardiol* **18**, 372-377 (2003).
4. S. Garg, J. Narula et al., Apoptosis and heart failure: clinical relevance and therapeutic target, *J Mol Cell Cardiol* **38**, 73-79 (2005).
5. V.E. Stoneman, M.R. Bennett, Role of apoptosis in atherosclerosis and its therapeutic implications, *Clin Sci* **107**, 343-354 (2004).
6. J.M. Brown, L.D. Attardi, The role of apoptosis in cancer development and treatment response *Nat Rev Cancer* **5**, 231-237 (2005).
7. S.J. Martin, C.P. Reutelingsperger et al., Early redistribution of plasma membrane phosphatidylserine is a general feature of apoptosis regardless of the initiating stimulus: inhibition by overexpression of Bcl-2 and Abl, *J Exp Med* **182**, 1545-1556 (1995).
8. M.O. Hengartner, The biochemistry of apoptosis, *Nature* **407**, 770-776 (2000).
9. M. Leist et al., Intracellular adenosine triphosphate (ATP) concentration: a switch in the decision between apoptosis and necrosis, *J Exp Med* **185**, 1481-1486 (1997).
10. Y. Eguchi, S. Shimizu, Y. Tsujimoto, Intracellular ATP levels determine cell death fate by apoptosis or necrosis, *Cancer Res* **57**, 1835-1840 (1997).
11. R.A. Gottlieb et al., Reperfusion injury induces apoptosis in rabbit cardiomyocytes, *J Clin Invest* **94**, 1621-1628 (1994).
12. T. Vanden Berghe et al., Differential signaling to apoptotic and necrotic cell death by Fas-associated death domain protein FADD, *J Biol Chem* **279**, 792579-33 (2004).
13. M. Leist, M. Jaattela, Four deaths and a funeral: from caspases to alternative mechanisms, *Nat Rev Mol Cell Biol* **2**, 589-598 (2001).
14. R.F. Zwaal, A.J. Schroit, Pathophysiologic implications of membrane phospholipid asymmetry in blood cells, *Blood* **89**, 1121-1132 (1997).
15. A. Zachowski, A. Herrmann et al., Phospholipid outside-inside translocation in lymphocyte plasma membranes is a protein-mediated phenomenon, *Biochim Biophys Acta* **897**, 197-200 (1987).
16. V.A. Fadok, D.R. Voelker et al., Exposure of phosphatidylserine on the surface of apoptotic lymphocytes triggers specific recognition and removal by macrophages, *J Immunol* **148**, 2207-2216 (1992).
17. R.A. Schlegel, P. Williamson, Phosphatidylserine, a death knell, *Cell Death Differ* **8**, 551-563 (2001).
18. B. Verhoven, R.A. Schlegel et al., Mechanisms of phosphatidylserine exposure, a phagocyte recognition signal, on apoptotic T lymphocytes, *J Exp Med* **182**, 1597-1601 (1995).
19. S. Van den Eijnde, L. Boshart et al., Phosphatidylserine plasma membrane asymmetry in vivo: a pancellular phenomenon which alters during apoptosis, *Cell Death Differ* **4**, 311-316 (1997).

20. S.M. van den Eijnde, L. Boshart et al., Cell surface exposure of phosphatidylserine during apoptosis is phylogenetically conserved, *Apoptosis* **3**, 9-16 (1998).

21. H. Okada and T.W. Mak, Pathways of apoptotic and non-apoptotic death in tumour cells, *Nat Rev Cancer* **4**, 592-603 (2004).

22. G. Brouckaert, M. Kalai et al., Phagocytosis of necrotic cells by macrophages is phosphatidylserine dependent and does not induce inflammatory cytokine production, *Mol Biol Cell* **15**(3), 1089-1100 (2004).

23. C.W. Wang, D.J. Klionsky, The molecular mechanism of autophagy, *Mol Med* **9**(3-4), 65-76 (2003).

24. Y.W. Eom, M.A. Kim et al., Two distinct modes of cell death induced by doxorubicin: apoptosis and cell death through mitotic catastrophe accompanied by senescence-like phenotype, *Oncogene* **24**(30), 4765-4777 (2005).

25. D. Arnoult et al., On the evolutionary conservation of the cell death pathway: mitochondrial release of an apoptosis-inducing factor during Dictyostelium discoideum cell death, *Mol Biol Cell* **12**, 3016-3030 (2001).

26. C.P. Reutelingsperger, G. Hornstra et al., Isolation and partial purification of a novel anticoagulant from arteries of human umbilical cord, *Eur J Biochem* **151**, 625-629 (1985).

27. S.E. Moss, R.O. Morgan, The annexins, *Genome Biol* **5**, 219 (2004).

28. H.A. Andree, C.P. Reutelingsperger et al., Binding of vascular anticoagulant alpha (VAC alpha) to planar phospholipid bilayers, *J Biol Chem* **265**, 4923-4928 (1990).

29. J.F. Tait, D. Gibson et al., Phospholipid binding properties of human placental anticoagulant protein-I, a member of the lipocortin family, *J Biol Chem* **264**, 7944-7949 (1989).

30. R. Huber, J. Romisch et al., The crystal and molecular structure of human annexin V, an anticoagulant protein that binds to calcium and membranes, *Embo J* **9**(12), 3867-3874 (1990).

31. F. Oling, W. Bergsma-Schutter et al., Trimers, dimers of trimers, and trimers of trimers are common building blocks of annexin a5 two-dimensional crystals, *J Struct Biol* **133**, 55-63 (2001).

32. G. Koopman, C.P. Reutelingsperger et al., Annexin V for flow cytometric detection of phosphatidylserine expression on B cells undergoing apoptosis, *Blood* **84**, 1415-1420 (1994).

33. C.H. Homburg, M. de Haas et al., Human neutrophils lose their surface Fc gamma RIII and acquire Annexin V binding sites during apoptosis in vitro, *Blood* **85**, 532-540 (1995).

34. I. Vermes, C. Haanen et al., A novel assay for apoptosis. Flow cytometric detection of phosphatidylserine expression on early apoptotic cells using fluorescein labelled Annexin V, *J Immunol Methods* **184**, 39-51 (1995).

35. M. van Engeland, L.J. Nieland et al., Annexin V-affinity assay: a review on an apoptosis detection system based on phosphatidylserine exposure, *Cytometry* **31**, 1-9 (1998).

36. S.M. van den Eijnde, J. Lips et al., Spatiotemporal distribution of dying neurons during early mouse development, *Eur J Neurosci* **11**, 712-724 (1999).

37. E.A. Dumont, C.P. Reutelingsperger et al., Real-time imaging of apoptotic cell-membrane changes at the single-cell level in the beating murine heart, *Nat Med* **7**(12), 1352-1355 (2001).

38. V. Ntziachristos, E.A. Schellenberger et al., Visualization of antitumor treatment by means of fluorescence molecular tomography with an annexin V-Cy5.5 conjugate, *Proc Natl Acad Sci USA* **101**, 12294-12299 (2004).

39. F.G. Blankenberg, P.D. Katsikis et al., In vivo detection and imaging of phosphatidylserine expression during programmed cell death, *Proc Natl Acad Sci U S A* **95**(11), 6349-6354 (1998).

40. D.E. Sosnovik, E.A. Schellenberger et al., Magnetic resonance imaging of cardiomyocyte apoptosis with a novel magneto-optical nanoparticle, *Magn Reson Med* **54**, 718-724 (2005).

41. L. Hofstra, I.H. Liem et al., Visualisation of cell death in vivo in patients with acute myocardial infarction, *Lancet* **356**(9225), 209-212 (2000).

42. F.D. Kolodgie, A. Petrov et al., Targeting of apoptotic macrophages and experimental atheroma with radiolabeled annexin V: a technique with potential for noninvasive imaging of vulnerable plaque, *Circulation* **108**(25), 3134-3139 (2003).

43. B.L. Kietselaer, C.P. Reutelingsperger et al., Noninvasive detection of plaque instability with use of radiolabeled annexin A5 in patients with carotid-artery atherosclerosis, *N Engl J Med* **350**, 1472-1473 (2004).

44. L. Hofstra, E.A. Dumont et al., In vivo detection of apoptosis in an intracardiac tumor, *JAMA* **285**(14), 1841-1842 (2001).

45. T. Belhocine et al., Increased uptake of the apoptosis-imaging agent (99m)Tc recombinant human Annexin V in human tumors after one course of chemotherapy as a predictor of tumor response and patient prognosis, *Clin Cancer Res* **8**, 2766-2774 (2002).

46. R.L. Haas et al., In vivo imaging of radiation-induced apoptosis in follicular lymphoma patients, *Int J Radiat Oncol Biol Phys* **59**, 782-787 (2004).

47. H. Vermeersch, D. Loose et al., 99mTc-HYNIC Annexin-V imaging of primary head and neck carcinoma, *Nucl Med Commun* **25**(3), 259-263 (2004).

48. M. Kartachova, R.L. Haas et al., In vivo imaging of apoptosis by 99mTc-Annexin V scintigraphy: visual analysis in relation to treatment response, *Radiother Oncol* **72**(3), 333-339 (2004).

49. H.G. Keen, B.A. Dekker et al., Imaging apoptosis in vivo using 124I-annexin V and PET, *Nucl Med Biol* **32**, 395-402 (2005).

50. K.J. Yagle, J.F. Eary et al., Evaluation of 18F-annexin V as a PET imaging agent in an animal model of apoptosis, *J Nucl Med* **46**, 658-666 (2005).

51. S. Zijlstra, J. Gunawan et al., Synthesis and evaluation of a 18F-labelled recombinant annexin-V derivative, for identification and quantification of apoptotic cells with PET, *Appl Radiat Isot* **58**, 201-207 (2003).

52. H. Kenis, H. van Genderen et al., Cell surface-expressed phosphatidylserine and annexin A5 open a novel portal of cell entry, *J Biol Chem* **279**(50), 52623-52629 (2004).

Chapter 21

PROTEOMICS FOR DIAGNOSTIC APPLICATIONS
The Convergence of Technology and the Resulting Challenges

Gordon R. Whiteley
National Cancer Institute - Frederick, Gaithersburg, MD, USA

Abstract: The emergence of proteomics in the post-genomic era has led to a resurgence in the study of and use of proteins for disease diagnosis. While the number of new protein markers has declined over the past 5 years, the use of new and exciting tools such as mass spectrometry, separation techniques and bioinformatics has fueled a search for markers and diagnostic patterns of markers that show great promise. The complexity of validation of these markers and panels of markers is a considerable challenge but the potential exists for the laboratory diagnosis of diseases for which there is no currently available lab test. This new era of proteomic diagnostics will continue to revolutionize our diagnostic arsenal and improve patient outcomes.

Keywords: Proteomics, biomarkers, mass spectrometry, bioinformatics

1. INTRODUCTION

The use of proteins for diagnosis of disease has been in practice for many decades. During the last half of the last century, numerous new markers for disease were discovered in blood. Originally, these were detected by immunological techniques such as immunodiffusion, radioimmunoassay (RIA), hemagglutination, precipitation techniques and enzyme linked immunosorbent assay (ELISA). There were several significant discoveries that advanced this field. The development of the monoclonal antibody by Kohler and Milstein[1] gave the specificity to diagnostic immunoassays that was only dreamed of in earlier years. Innovative techniques such as the use of fluorescent substrates and electrochemiluminescence have further enhanced sensitivity of immunoassays. Discovery of new proteins expanded

337

G. Spekowius and T. Wendler (Eds.), Advances in Healthcare Technology, 337-348.

the list of analytes being approved for use in the diagnostic lab. Some of these such as CEA were initially greeted with very high hopes for their diagnostic capabilities but proved to be less specific than originally hoped and their approved use has been limited. Others such as troponin have proven to be extremely powerful diagnostic tools.

Over the past few years, the discovery and approval of new biomarkers has diminished dramatically. Even with detection technologies that are sensitive the approval of new analytes for diagnosis by the FDA has declined[2] as shown in Figure 21-1.

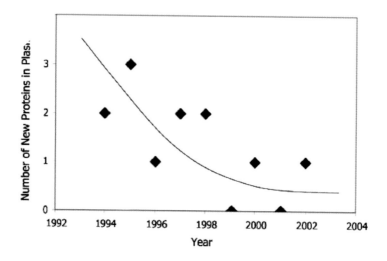

Figure 21-1. The declining rate of introduction of new protein tests. The data are plotted to indicate the rate of introduction of new protein analytes in FDA-approved clinical tests (From: N.L. Anderson, N.G Anderson, *MCP* **1**(11), 845-67, 2002).

This decline could be due to several factors: the discovery of the high abundance disease markers is probably nearly complete, the diseases now being researched are more complex and will require a series of markers for diagnosis or we are looking in the wrong place in serum for the presence of these markers or a combination of the above factors.

In the past few years, there have been significant advances in many scientific areas that have led to the new field of proteomics. These advances in the areas of computer science and computing power, computerized databases and database management, separation technologies, biology, and mass spectrometry to name a few have come together to provide tools that are leading to a new wave in disease diagnosis and management. It is the convergence of these diverse technical areas that has demonstrated the possibilities this technology can yield for disease diagnosis through an identification and understanding of the source and function of new disease markers previously overlooked because of their lack of sensitivity and or specificity or fraction in the serum or tissue.

The progress of the 13 year long human genome project[3] led naturally to the study of the products of the genes – the proteins. Although some of the techniques used in proteomics had been developed years before and the term 'proteomics' had been coined originally in 1994, it was not until 1999 that the term became commonly used in literature[4]. Proteomics was defined as referring "to the study of the proteome using technologies of large-scale protein separation and identification". One popular separation technique had been described in the mid 1970's and this was 2 dimensional or 2D gels[5]. The use of 2D gels for protein separation followed by digestion of the proteins into fragments and then analysis of the fragments by mass spectrometry gave an identification of proteins through peptide mass fingerprinting. At the time, there was also talk of making an entire catalog of proteins in the same way the human genome project had made a catalog of genes. However, the challenge remained to identify proteins that were expressed in disease and not in unaffected groups.

In the mid 1990's, the technique of laser capture microdissection was described[6]. This allowed for the separation of diseased cells from neighboring normal cells in tissue and a comparison of these two groups of cells could be done in order to determine if the protein content had changed and certain pathways had been triggered disease. The separation was done using a laser activated adhesive coated film that was placed over a tissue section. The cells were examined by a pathologist and diseased cells identified. A laser was then fired that activated the adhesive properties of the coated film and the cells were physically lifted from the slide. The process was then repeated on a second piece of adhesive film but normal cells were picked this time providing a control that matched the diseased cells in every way except for the protein content that had been activated.

Another key development at about the same time was the commercialization of the surface enhanced laser desorption ionization (SELDI) technology by Ciphergen (www.ciphergen.com). This technology is based on the fractionation of serum on the same surface that is used as the target for matrix enhanced surface desorption ionization (MALDI). The protein arrays consist of a metal surface that has been coated with active binding groups. The variety of groups (anionic exchange, cationic exchange, metal binding surfaces) allows for binding of different fractions from the serum and unbound fractions are then washed away. An energy absorbing matrix is then added directly to this surface and it is then used as the laser target in a mass spectrometer that has been specifically developed to handle these arrays. The surfaces are configured on arrays – 8 spots to an array and a bioprocessor holds12 arrays to give the configuration of a 96 well microtiter plate. This configuration is one familiar with biologists and one that has several robotic and other tools available for sample processing. The arrays are then fed into a low resolution but high sensitivity mass spectrometer that is easy to operate and has software that makes interpretation familiar with not only spectral views but also a 'gel' view that displays data in a manner familiar to biologists. Thus the tools available to biologists now included mass spectrometry.

2. DISCOVERING NEW APPLICATIONS

With these advances came an explosion of potential diagnostic tests analytes, test principles and procedures. One of the earlier publications described the combination of laser capture microdissection and SELDI to demonstrate differences between cancer cells and neighboring normal cells in tissue sections[7]. In this publication, tissue sections had been stained and were microdissected into a lysis buffer. An aliphatic reverse phase SELDI biochip was used to capture proteins from solubilized cancer cells or solubilized control normal cells. The proteins were then crystallized with matrix and mass spectrometry spectra were gathered. A comparison of the spectra from the tumor cells as compared to the normal cells clearly showed differences in up regulation and down regulation of several proteins. This was observed in several conditions including colon cancer, liver cancer, and in prostate cancer where differences were seen when comparing normal cells, prostatic intraepithelial neoplasia cells, tumor cells and stromal cells. The suggestion was made here that protein fingerprinting of early disease lesions was possible based on the differences seen in both spectral and gel views of these cells.

The next step in the process was to extend this finding into looking for these differences in serum. In 2002, the first publication to suggest that serum might indeed carry these differences and these could be observed by mass spectrometry was published[8]. In this publication, a series of sera from ovarian cancer patients and cancer free women were examined by SELDI and the resulting spectra were used to train a computer algorithm to recognize the differences between the two groups. The pattern was then used to classify 116 additional patient samples – 50 with cancer and 66 from cancer free women including several with benign disease such as ovarian cysts. The results of this study were remarkable giving a 100% sensitivity including 18 patients with stage I disease and 95% specificity. This study was followed by similar findings in a wide range of diseases including prostate cancer[9], breast cancer[10], renal cancer[11], pancreatic cancer[12], and ovarian cancer[13]. In addition, there was also activity in detection of other diseases such as cardiac disease using this technique[14].

However, there was much criticism of this method both from the bioinformatics side[15] as well as the biological perspective[16]. The use of bioinformatic methods that were random such as genetic algorithms and thus did not always give absolute reproducibility of patterns was the basis of some criticism. Further refinement of raw spectrum (data processing) was thought to be primitive and needed improvement. Biologically, it was also felt that the source of these peptides that made up patterns was necessary in order to confirm that they were actually associated with the disease being studied. In addition, the reproducibility of the mass spectrometers themselves was at question and whether they could ever be robust enough to be used as a diagnostic device had yet to be answered. Only through rigorous validation of the method could this question be answered.

As part of the investigation process and as biologists gained more experience and confidence in using mass spectrometry, a higher resolution instrument was evaluated. While this still used the SELDI-TOF principle and a source manufactured by Ciphergen, the instrument measuring the time of flight was the ABI Q-star which is a quadrapole time of flight instrument. This instrument is able to resolve individual peaks observed in the Ciphergen SELDI instrument into several peaks. Furthermore, the instrument's higher resolution was not subject to drift observed in the Ciphergen mass spectrometer. A repeat evaluation of the ovarian cancer study samples reported earlier was done using this system and the results gave a 100% sensitivity and specificity in the sample group tested[17]. While a genetic algorithm with a self-organizing map was used and several patterns were generated, there were at least 4 that gave this excellent result. Furthermore, the overlap of several ions in these patterns indicated their importance in the diagnostic test. The increase in the specificity would be important in further use of the technique because of the low incidence of ovarian cancer in the general population. While the 100% correlation would be ideal, it was noted that this was in a limited number of samples and would need to be further developed and validated in a much larger study in order to be considered as the basis for a diagnostic system.

The bioinformatics analysis of data has also received much attention. It is known that more than 300 groups have downloaded the data from the original Petricoin ovarian study done in 2002 and analyzed it in detail from several points of view. Many of these groups were able to reproduce the original results while some groups believed that the original analysis was flawed. Several suggestions have been made in terms of preprocessing data and analysis including the posting of data in its raw form[18] to allow different preprocessing methods to be properly evaluated. However, it was pointed out that communication between those analyzing the data and those who produced the data is essential because of the possibility of a mis-interpretation of results based on a mis-understanding of the purpose of the experiment[19]. Currently there are multiple data analysis and classification tools in use and being developed both commercially and in academic settings.

In addition to bioinformatics solutions that involve computer algorithms, data visualization tools have been and are continuing to be developed to allow for the handling of large data sets in a manner that can be analyzed by the human eye. The use of these tools can help reduce datasets to simplify the computer process or can be used in an iterative process with bioinformatics tools to confirm patterns as is shown in Figure 21-2[27]. In this example, the initial data is examined for quality and any spectra that are found to be of low total ion current for example are eliminated. The entire dataset consisting of all spectra from all patients are then imported into a visualization tool and are colorized by disease group. Using the visualization tool, certain areas are selected as showing discriminating characteristics through visual examination of the data in three dimensions: intensity, mass/charge value and disease group. These areas are then selected and fed to computer algorithms for the selection of individual discriminating values. These values are then confirmed by examining individual spectra from both the disease and normal groups. The process ensures the presence of a pattern rather than artifacts and has been valuable in studies where patterns are difficult to find using bioinformatics tools or where over-fitting can occur.

The next development in proteomics as a diagnostic tool was to determine the principle of the test. As part of this work, the source of diagnostic peptides needed to be reconciled. Basic questions had been raised: why such a small source as an early stage tumor could provide sufficient quantity in the blood by mass spectrometry and why were the small peptides not excreted in the urine as quickly as they accumulated? The answer lay in the discovery that diagnostic protein fragments and peptides appeared to be associated with large and abundant carrier proteins such as albumin[20]. In this publication, the authors capture albumin out of serum, washed and then caused peptides to dissociate from the albumin through the use of 50% acetonitrile. After a 30mw size exclusion separation, the peptides were examined by mass spectrometry. What was found was a large number of low molecular weight peptides that had been associated with albumin. Identification of some of these peptides has shown their identity to be known linked to cancer such as P53 and BRCA1 and 2. It was proposed that the albumin's long half-life (19 days) acted as a concentrating and protecting molecule carrying the peptides and preventing clearance by the kidneys[21].

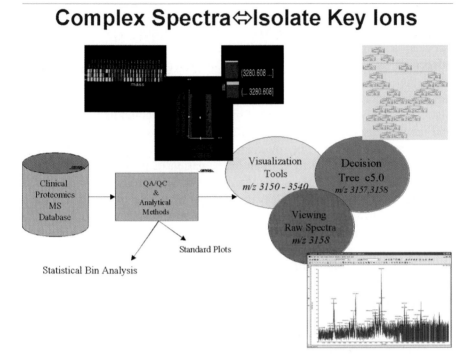

Figure 21-2. Data Visualization as an Aid to Data Analysis (From: D.Johann et al., *Ann N Y Acad Sci* **1022**, 299, 2004).

This discovery led to the enrichment for albumin in proteomics – the antithesis of that had been done previously. Commercialization of a biomarker enrichment method using the principle of albumin capture has recently been done by PerkinElmer in collaboration with Viva Sciences (www.perkinelmer.com). This method has been optimized as a discovery tool in a 96 well format including albumin capture, elution and dissociation of peptides from albumin, capture and concentration in a C18 Zip plate and direct deposition on a PerkinElmer disposable target plates to be read in the ProTOF orthogonal MALDI instrument. An evaluation of the method for the discovery of a pattern for Alzheimer's disease has been reported[25] and a pattern for ovarian cancer diagnosis[26]. The instrument has the high resolution properties in combination with the ability to scale up discovery. This combination should allow for the large validation studies that will be required to both verify and validate a pattern for disease diagnosis. It is anticipated that the scale of such studies will need to be massive not only to convince skeptics of the validity of patterns as well as to convince the regulatory agencies that these patterns are effective and should be approved as diagnostic tests.

While proteomic patterns have been widely reported, another tactic in the use of proteomics for diagnosis has been biomarker discovery. A connection between a diagnostic marker and its function in the disease has been advocated by some as a necessary step in order to validate the use of a biomarker in disease diagnosis. In this case, the proteomics approach would not result necessarily in a test itself but would be used as a discovery platform for biomarkers or panels of biomarkers that could be used to detect and monitor disease. One example of this approach is the work of Zhang et al[22] where biomarkers for ovarian cancer were discovered using the Ciphergen proteomic platform in an investigation of patients from multiple centers. The three biomarkers identified were apolipoproteinA1, a truncated form of transthyretin and a cleavage fragment of inter-α-trypsin inhibitor heavy chain H4. The addition of these three biomarkers as a panel to CA125 improved the sensitivity and specificity of CA125 alone for detection of disease. The panel approach has been used in diseases such as thyroid disease for many years but the application of this approach to heterogeneous diseases such as cancer is now being investigated and in theory has a sound scientific basis.

In addition to diagnosis, the possibility of disease progression and treatment monitoring has been an attractive use of proteomics technology. The field of individualized medicine is an area that could predict a patient's response to a therapy thereby guiding the treating physician rather than waiting to see if a patient responds to a therapy[21]. Disease progression could also be monitored by an analysis of changes in an individual's proteomic pattern over time and looking for changes in targeted points in the spectra or by the isolation and identification and quantitation of individual proteins in serial samples. This is currently done in a primitive way in the quantitation of antibodies in infectious disease over the course of time or with tumor markers such as CEA in selected cancers where the initial diagnosis yields an elevated level that is monitored during treatment in serial samples. The mass spectrometry tool is particularly powerful at discrimination of post-translational modifications that take place in the course of disease and this is generally difficult in immunoassays. A combination of the two techniques has been investigated[23] and could prove to give the advantages of purification by a binding reaction followed by the resolution of the subtle differences in the binding entities by mass spectrometry.

Table 21-1. Recommended Practices for Clinical Applications of Protein Profiling by MALDI TOF Spectrometry.

1. PREANALYTICAL

- Evaluate optimum patient preparation
- Identify optimum procedures for specimen collection and processing
- Analyze specimen stability
- Develop criteria for specimen acceptability

2. ANALYTICAL

- Prepare calibrators for mass, resolution, and detector sensitivity
- Use internal standards
- Automate specimen preparation
- Optimize methods to yield highest possible signals for peaks of interest
- Identify sequences of peaks of interest
- Develop calibration materials for components of interest
- QC: prepare/identify at least two concentrations of control material
- Evaluate reproducibility (precision)
- Evaluate limits of detection and linearity
- Evaluate reference intervals
- Evaluate interferences such as hemolysis, lipemia, renal failure, acute-phase responses
- Develop materials or programs for external comparison/proficiency testing of analyzers

3. POSTANALYTICAL

- Analyze each spectrum to identify peaks before applying diagnostic algorithms
- Develop criteria for the acceptability of each spectrum based on peak characteristics
- Use peaks rather than raw data as the basis for diagnostic analysis
- Use caution in interpretation of peaks with m/z <1200
- Select peaks with high intensities and sample stability for diagnosis
- Select approximately equal numbers of peaks that increase and decrease in intensity as diagnostic discriminators
- In developing a training set for diagnosis, careful clinical classification of patients is essential
- Clinical validity depends on having a typical rather than highly selected population of patients
- The number of training specimens should be at least 10 times the number of measured values
- Any clinical application should use a fixed training set and algorithm for analysis
- Any analysis should provide a numerical value
- Diagnostic performance should be evaluated with ROC curves to select cutoffs
- A sensitivity analysis should be performed of the necessary precision for accurate diagnostic performance
- There should be QC procedures for daily verification of software performance

*Adapted from G.L. Hortin[24].

3.   DELIVERING THE PROMISE

All of these new technologies have opened up the possibility for improved diagnostic tests for a wide variety of diseases. However the validation and regulatory challenges are quite great. The validation of a mass spectrometry pattern diagnostic would require the validation and integration of systems and technologies as diverse as proteomics itself: Reagents and the chemistry behind them, robotics processors, mass spectrometers, operational software and diagnostic software along with the clinical end including the sample handling and transport, sample stability and a host of other factors[24].

However, the power and potential of the technology will drive the continued innovation, validation and eventual commercialization of the area of proteomics and the eventual arrival of these techniques in the clinical lab will give tools for improved patient outcomes.

ACKNOWLEDGEMENTS

The author would like to thank the NCI/FDA Clinical Proteomics Program staff, both past and current, and the staff of the Clinical Proteomics Lab for their support and insight.

The content of this publication does not necessarily reflect the views or policies of the Department of Health and Human Services, nor does mention of trade names, commercial products, or organization imply endorsement by the U. S. Government. This project has been funded in whole or in part with Federal funds from the National Cancer Institute, National Institutes of Health, under Contract No. NO1-CO-12400.

REFERENCES

1.   G. Kohler, C. Milstein, Continuous cultures of fused cells secreting antibody of predefined specificity, *Nature* **256**, 495 (1975).
2.   N.L. Anderson and N.G. Anderson, The Human Plasma Proteome, *MCP* **1**(11), 845-67, (2002).
3.   E.S. Lander, L.M. Linton et al, International Human Genome Sequencing Consortium. Initial sequencing and analysis of the Human Genome, *Nature* **409**(6822), 860-921, (2001).
4.   Abbott, Proteomics, transcriptomics: what's in a name?, *Nature* **202**, 715-716, (1999).
5.   L. Anderson, N.G. Anderson, High resolution two-dimensional electrophoresis of human plasma proteins, *Proc Natl Acad Sci USA* **74**, 5421-5425 (1977).
6.   M.R. Emmert-Buck, R.F. Bonner, P.D. Smith, R.F. Chauqui, Z. Zhuang, S.R. Goldstein, R.A. Weiss, L.A., Liotta, Laser capture microdissection, *Science* **274**, 998-1001 (1996).

7. C.P. Paweletz, J.W. Gillespie, D.K. Ornstein, N.L. Simmone, M.R. Brown, K.A. Cole, Q.H. Wang, J. Huang, N. Hu, T.T Yipe, W.E. Rich, E.C. Kohn, W.M. Linehan, T. Weber, P. Taylor, M.R. Emmert-Buck, L.A. Liotta, E.F. Petricoin, Rapid Protein Display Profiling of Cancer Progression Directly from Human Tissue Using a Protein Biochip, *Drug Dev Research* **49**, 34-42 (2000).

8. E.F. Petricoin, A.M. Ardekani, B.A. Hitt, P.J. Levine, V.A. Fusaro, S.M. Steinberg, G.B. Mills, C. Simone, D.A. Fishman, E.C. Kohn, L.A. Liotta, Use of Proteomic Patterns in Serum to identify Ovarian Cancer, *Lancet* **359**, 572-577 (2002).

9. E.F. Petricoin, D.K. Ornstein, C.P. Paweletz, A. Ardekani, P.S. Hackett, B.A. Hitt, A.Velassco, C. Trucco, L. Weigand, K. Wood, C.B. Simone, P.J. Levine, W.M. Linehan, M.R. Emmert-Buck, S.M. Steinberg, E.C. Kohn, Serum Proteomic Patterns for Detection of Prostate Cancer, *JNCI* **94**, 1576-1578 (2002).

10. J. Li, Z. Zhang, J. Rosenzweig, Y.Y. Wang, D.W. Chan, Proteomics and bioinformatics approaches for identification of serum biomarkers to detect breast cancer *Clin Chem* **48**, 1296-1304 (2002).

11. Y. Won, J.J. Song, T.W. Kang, J.J. Kim, B.D. Han, S.W. Lee, Pattern analysis of serum proteome distinguishes renal cell carcinoma from other urologic diseases and healthy persons, *Proteomics* **3**, 2310-2316 (2003).

12. S. Bhattacharyya, E.R. Siegel, G.M- Petersen, S.T. Chari, L.J. Suva, R.S. Haun, Diagnosis of Pancreatic Cancer Using Serum Proteomic Profiling, *Neoplasia* **6**, 674-686 (2004).

13. K.R. Kozak, W.A. Malaika, S.M. Pusey, F. Su, M.N. Luong, S.A. Luong, S.T. Reddy, R. Farias-Eisner, Identification of biomarkers for ovarian cancer using strong anion-exchange ProteinChips: Potential use in diagnosis and prognosis, *PNAS* **100**, 12343-12348 (2003).

14. J. Marshall, P. Kupchak, W. Zhu, J. Yantha, T. Vrees, S. Furesz, K. Jacks, C. Smith, I. Kireeva, R. Zhang, M. Takahashi, E. Stanton, G. Jackowski, Processing of Serum Proteins Underlies the Mass Spectral Fingerprinting of Myocardial Infarction, *J Proteome Res* **2**, 361-372 (2003).

15. K.A. Baggerly, J.S. Morris, K.R. Coombes, Reproducibility of SELDI-TOF protein patterns in serum: comparing datasets from different experiments, *Bioinformatics* **20**, 777-785 (2004).

16. E.P. Diamandis, Analysis of Serum Proteomic Patterns for Early Cancer Diagnosis: Drawing Attention to Potential Problems, *JNCI* **96**, 353-356 (2004).

17. T.P. Conrads, V.A. Fusaro, S. Ross, D. Johann, V. Rajapakse, B.A. Hitt, S.M. Steinberg, E.C. Kohn, D.A. Fishman, G. Whiteley, J.C. Barrett, L.A. Liotta, E.F. Petricoin, T.D. Veenstra, High-resolution serum proteomic features for ovarian cancer detection, *Endocrine Related Cancer* **11**, 163-178 (2004).

18. K.A. Baggerly, J.S. Morris, J. Wang, D, Gold, L.C. Xiao, K.R. Coombes, A comprehensive approach to the analysis of matrix-assisted laser desorption/ionization-time of flight proteomics spectra from serum samples, *Proteomics* **3**, 1667-1672 (2003)

19. L.A. Liotta, M. Lowenthal, A. Mehta, T.P. Conrads, T.D. Veenstra, D.A. Fishman, E.F. Petricoin, Importance of Communication Between Producers and Consumers of Publicly Available Experimental Data, *JNCI* **97**, 310-314 (2005).

20. A. Mehta, S. Ross, M.S. Lowenthal, V. Fusaro, D.A. Fishman, E.F. Petricoin, L.A. Liotta, Biomarker amplification by serum carrier protein binding, *Disease Markers* **19**, 1-10 (2003,2004).

21. L.A. Liotta, M. Ferrari, E. Petricoin, Written in Blood, *Nature* **425**(6961), 905 (2003).

22. Z. Zhang, R.C. Base, Y. Yu, J. Li, L.J. Sokol, A.J. Rai, J.M. Rosenzweig, B. Cameron, Y.Y. Want, X.Y. Meng, A. Berchuck, C. Haaften-Day, N.F. Hacker, H.W.A. Bruijn,

A.G.J. Zee, I.J. Jacobs, E.R. Fung, D.W. Chan, Three Biomarkers Identified from Serum Proteomic Analysis for the Detection of Early Stage Ovarian Cancer, *Cancer Res* **64**, 5882-5890 (2004).

23. D. Nedelkov, R.W. Nelson, Surface plasmon resonance mass spectrometry: recent progress and outlooks, *Trends in Biotech* **21**, 301-305 (2003).
24. G.L. Hortin, Can Mass Spectrometric Protein Profiling Meet Desired Standards of Clinical Laboratory Practice?, *Clin Chem* **51**, 3-5 (2005).
25. M.F. Lopez, A. Mikulsdis, S. Kuxzdzal, A. Bennet. et al, High Resolution Serum Proteomic Profiling of Alzheimer Disease Samples Reveals Disease-Specific, Carrier-Protein-Bound Mass Signatures, *Clin Chem* **51**(10), in press (2005).
26. M.S. Lowenthal, A.I. Mehta, K. Frogale, R.W. Bandle et al., Analysis of Albumin-Associated Peptides and Proteins from Ovarian Cancer Patients, *Clin Chem* **51**(10), in press (2005).
27. D.J. Johann, M.D. McGuigan, A.R. Patel, S. Tomav, S. Ross, T.P. Conrads, T.D. Veenstra, D.A. Fishman, G.R. Whiteley, E.F. Petricoin, L.A. Liotta, Clinical Proteomics and Biomarker Discovery, *Ann N Y Acad Sci* **1022**, 295-305 (2004).

PART V: MEDICAL INFORMATICS

Chapter 22

MEDICAL INFORMATION TECHNOLOGY
Recent Advances and Research Trends

Charles Lagor[1], William P. Lord[1], Nicolas W. Chbat[1], J. David Schaffer[1], Thomas Wendler[2]

[1]*Philips Research, Briarcliff Manor, NY, USA;* [2]*Philips Research, Hamburg, Germany*

Abstract: Information technology (IT) has been applied in different medical areas in the past 40 years. Although many IT applications are technically mature enough to be used, they are still not present in hospitals. In this chapter, we give an overview of the current status of IT in medicine, as well as the future directions that we believe IT will take. Our approach in writing this chapter is to view IT from the perspective of three groups of users: clinicians, researchers, and patients. Given that healthcare lags behind other industries in terms of adopting IT, we also discuss the challenges that need to be overcome.

Keywords: Information technology (IT), medical informatics, computers in medicine

1.   INTRODUCTION

Approximately 40 years ago, Information Technology (IT) was first applied in health care. The vision back then was to use IT to improve the patients' outcomes. Since then the vision has not changed. Ultimately any endeavor involving medical IT, whether it be developing a program to help physicians select the optimal antibiotic treatment or designing a web page with health care information, is directed towards this vision.

Implementing medical IT in clinical settings, however, never was an easy undertaking. To demonstrate the benefits of IT a certain critical mass of patients' data had to be collected first. Most hospitals were not willing to invest in a hospital information system whose return of investment seemed uncertain. Clinicians resisted the introduction of IT into the wards, because they saw no value in IT and they felt that IT would disrupt their workflow. On the technical side, it was hard to model medical information and

349

G. Spekowius and T. Wendler (Eds.), Advances in Healthcare Technology, 349-366.

knowledge to be interpretable for computers. Medical information is sometimes fuzzy and ambiguous. Medical knowledge is incomplete on the one hand, but expands dramatically on the other hand.

Despite the difficulties that IT has had in medicine, a scientific discipline – medical informatics – had emerged by the 1970's. This discipline studied the storage, the retrieval, and the processing of patient data for clinical problem-solving and decision-making. It was inherently interdisciplinary drawing on the principles from other fields such as computer science, social science, and the clinical sciences. Medical informatics kept expanding rapidly. In recent years, the term 'healthcare informatics' has been introduced to encompass disciplines such as dental informatics, pharmaceutical informatics, nursing informatics, and public health informatics. It has been modified even further to 'healthcare bioinformatics' to include bioinformatics (see Chapter 26).

Through the constant efforts of researchers in the field, there is now an increasing awareness that IT is necessary to solve some of the major health care problems of today. Many adverse events that occur in hospitals, for example, are preventable with the assistance of computers[1]. Computers could help in maintaining the high quality of health care at a lower cost. This is of particular interest in an increasingly aging population that will put a stress on current health care resources. The importance of medical IT has also been understood at a political level. The US government created the new position of National Health Information Coordinator in 2004[2]. The ambitious goal is to provide electronic health records for most Americans within the next decade. In the same time frame, the National Health Service in the United Kingdom wishes to provide IT on a national scale to more than 30,000 general practitioners and 300 hospitals[3].

In this chapter, we will give a broad overview of medical IT. We will describe recent advances and trends of selected areas and put some of them in a historical perspective. Our goal is to show the great variety and the huge potential of medical IT.

2.   AREAS OF RESEARCH

In this section, we discuss various areas of medical informatics research and development. We have grouped the areas according to who the main user of each area is. We identified three users: clinicians, researchers, and patients. We are aware that other users, such as administrators or librarians, exist. In addition, we realize that one area can have multiple users. For example, an electronic patient record is not only of interest to clinicians, but also to patients or administrators. Given the breadth of the field, however, we attempted to provide a more general classification.

2.1 Areas directed at clinicians

2.1.1 Electronic patient record

The successful implementation of many IT solutions in medicine depends on an existing IT infrastructure, i.e. a departmental information system or even better an Electronic Patient Record (EPR). The EPR is a repository for electronically stored data of a patient's health status and health care[4]. Synonyms include the 'electronic medical record', the 'electronic health record', or the 'computer-based patient record'. An electronic patient record system can provide functions to improve the quality and the efficiency of health-care delivery. Examples of the EPR's functionality are providing reminders and alerts, offering access to multiple clinicians at the same time, or linking knowledge sources to the patients' data. Traditional paper-based medical records lack such functions.

Although a few pioneering medical centers have demonstrated how computers could support health care, most hospitals are cautious in adopting EPRs in their clinical settings[5]. The clinical environment proves to be a very difficult place to implement IT solutions. Clinicians resist IT, because they feel that computers disrupt their workflow patterns and do not support them in their work. Boards of directors dismiss clinical IT solutions, because they cannot see any return of investment in terms of revenue. Given the difficulties in implementing IT in the health industry, it is not surprising that only less than 20% of U.S. hospitals have implemented electronic patient records and 9.6% have implemented computerized physician order entry[6].

Nevertheless there is a good reason to believe that the number of hospitals with an EPR will increase within the next decade. Hospitals face major challenges such as reducing preventable adverse events, maintaining a high level of health care at low costs, or managing increasing amounts of patients' data. It is hard to imagine how these problems can be overcome without an EPR. In addition to internal motivations to adopt IT, there are also incentives outside of the hospitals. In the U.S., for example, hospital approval organizations, such as the Leapfrog Group (a consortium of Fortune 500 companies and other organizations that provide health benefits) or the Joint Commission on Accreditation of Healthcare Organizations (a not-for-profit organization that sets standards for measuring health care quality), require hospitals to adopt IT. Furthermore, the U.S. government is strongly committed to building a national health information infrastructure[2].

2.1.2   Medical decision support

One of the major focuses of medical informatics research is medical or clinical decision support. Storing clinical data in an electronic format as opposed to a paper format alone does not justify the computerization of the medical record. One of the major values of electronically stored data comes from their ability to enable clinical decision support; i.e. helping clinicians to make the correct choices and to avoid errors. Medical decision support systems are discussed in detail in Chapter 25.

2.1.3   Workflow management

The challenging situation of rapid changes in the health care system, such as shrinking budgets and increasing demands to increase the quality of services, calls for solutions that not only help handling data but improving the organization of work. Optimizing and automating processes and better utilization of all kind of resources becomes essential for meeting medical and commercial targets of health care institutions. Workflow technology is one way to organize more efficient and provide better service quality. In a radiology department, for instance, a typical goal will be to better utilize imaging equipment (higher throughput), while simultaneously improve the essential performance indicators such as time to report delivery for referring physicians.

Workflow management is a technology[7] that enables health institutions like hospitals to automate parts of routine medical business processes, based on models of underlying processes and organizations. These explicit models, designed according to the needs and policies of an institution, are kept in separate administrative databases. They are instantiated and enacted at run-time by workflow engines. These engines have to be embedded in information systems infrastructures[8].

There are a number of research challenges associated with workflow management. How to integrate workflow engines in data driven healthcare IT infrastructures has to be further explored. On the methodology side, we need to understand how to design workflow management principles that serve very well defined, structured processes (as represented by a pre-ordered X-ray examination in Radiology), as well as flexible, ad-hoc case processing (such as emergency cases). Commercially, workflow engines as base technology and kernels of workflow management solutions are available from a number of vendors.

2.1.4 Natural language processing

As pointed out in section 2.1.2, a major value of electronic data is to enable clinical decision support. In order for computers to provide decision support, they must be able to 'understand' the clinical data. Numeric data, such as laboratory test results, pose no problem for computers, since it is straightforward to attribute a specific meaning to a numeric input. For example, one can specify that an input with a value greater than 5.2 indicates a potassium value above the normal range. Text data, on the other hand, are challenging for computers, because a word has a specific meaning only within the context of other words. Consider the meaning of the word 'cold' in the following sentences.

"The patient claimed that she had a *cold* last week."
"The patient's extremities were *cold*."

To humans it is clear that the word 'cold' means something different in each sentence. This so seemingly easy task of understanding the meaning of words, however, is extremely difficult to program in a computer.

Given the complex task of programming computers to understand humans, the scientific discipline of computational linguistics has emerged, in which natural language is investigated from a computational perspective. A subfield of computational linguistics is Natural Language Processing (NLP), which deals with the processing and the manipulation of natural language. In this chapter we will use the term NLP in the context of understanding natural language, however, NLP encompasses other topics as well, such as the generation of natural language.

The first peer-reviewed articles on the applications of NLP in medicine were published in the late 1970's. The main goal of applying NLP in medicine was (and still is) to abstract medical concepts from electronically stored free text reports. Initially, NLP research focused on radiology[9,10], because the reports in this specialty were structured and contained a well-defined vocabulary. At the same time, radiology was complex enough to provide value for clinical decision support and research. This research showed that NLP applications were as accurate in extracting certain medical concepts as physicians[11]. In recent years, NLP has expanded to other clinical problems. For example, in the area of biosurveillance NLP has been applied during the Winter 2002 Olympics in Salt Lake City, Utah, to monitor potential disease outbreaks as a result of a bioterrorist attack[12]. Another trend is to use NLP for detecting adverse events[13], in particular in discharge summaries[14].

The potential of NLP has also been realized in the industry. We expect that an increase in commercially available NLP products will catalyze the availability of other medical IT products, in particular medical decision support applications.

2.1.5   Applying information technology in imaging

Information technology (IT) is an integral part of imaging modalities such as computer tomography. In this section, however, we will focus on using IT to help physicians interpret various images. In the past 20 years, computer-aided detection (CAD) of suspicious findings in images has been developed to improve the physicians' sensitivity (true positive rate) and specificity (true negative rate). CAD has been deployed in different areas – detecting pulmonary nodules in radiographs, or detecting intracranial aneurysms in magnetic resonance angiograms, to name a few. The benefits of CAD, such as identifying cancers at an earlier stage or reducing the number of biopsies, still need to be shown. With continuous improvements in the accuracy, however, CAD will enable the computer-aided diagnosis (CADx) of lesions on an image. Chapter 24 covers CAD and CADx in the area of lung nodule detection.

2.2   Areas directed at researchers

2.2.1   Data mining

Modern computerized medical practices, at least in developed countries, produce large amounts of data. Here we exclude the growing volume of bio-molecular data that is the topic of bioinformatics (see Chapter 26). These data are believed to contain (hide) valuable patterns that could improve healthcare deliver if they could be discovered. Since the early 1990s this (and other domains with similar data explosions) has given rise to the field of knowledge discovery from data (KDD)[15].

The steps in a medical data mining exercise usually involve: 1) identify a problem (question) and a dataset to study, 2) extract and 'clean' the data 3) exploratory analyses 3) pattern/knowledge discovery. This may be considered hypothesis generation. If the findings are deemed novel and important, then one also needs to consider 4) validation or hypothesis testing.

Cios and Moore discuss at length the unique nature of medical data and the issues that come into play when attempting to mine it[16]. Medical data are voluminous and heterogeneous; they include numerical values like lab test results, categorical values like diagnoses, signals, like ECGs, images, and structured or, more likely, unstructured text like physicians notes. The importance and difficulty of the step of assembling and cleaning the data cannot be overestimated. Images provide their own challenges and are the subject of extensive research into computer aided detection (CAD) and diagnosis (CADx, see Chapter 24). An additional challenge for medical data mining is that most of these data were collected for purposes of patient care and not explicitly for mining. This gives rise to substantial issues with missing data, but perhaps more subtly to issues about statistical inference: what population of patients or clinical sites may the sample be considered to represent?

Exploratory analyses usually at least include descriptive statistics such as means, variances, and ranges for the individual variables. Further analyses include principle component or factor analyses that try to reduce the number of variables to consider. Clustering is also applied in an attempt to gain insights into how the sample is distributed. Graphic visualizations are employed to exploit the pattern perception abilities of the human eye and to make the patterns intelligible.

More sophisticated pattern recognition algorithms from statistics and machine learning are also being vigorously applied. The simplest tests for association are contingency tables and the chi square statistic. Supervised learning is the approach wherein a given set of correctly classified examples is used to derive a predictive model. Artificial neural networks, decision trees, genetic programming, support vector machines, Bayesian classifiers, nearest neighbor classifiers, fuzzy and rough sets, and rule-induction algorithms are some of the more popular methods. One step beyond the classification task is the regression task wherein the outcome to be predicted is not a class membership, but a numerical value. Another approach is to attempt to derive a causal model usually in the form of a Bayesian network. These models are often applied to the task of predicting the outcome of a considered intervention. Such models have clear application to clinical decision support systems (see Chapter 25).

Validation of discovered patterns or models often involves the use of an independent dataset, presumed to be representative of the same population as the original learning data. An even more trustworthy (though much more expensive) approach involves a prospective clinical trial.

Medical data mining will continue to be vigorously pursued as the quality and quantity of electronic medical data continue to grow. We are optimistic that security and privacy issues will be addressed, although the current state of affairs suggest otherwise to some. Data and terminology standards will greatly assist this effort.

2.2.2   Bioinformatics

It is widely recognized that the past twenty years has ushered in a new era in molecular biology. The mapping of the human genome is just the first step. New measurement technologies like gene microarrays and mass spectroscopy applied to proteins have been accompanied by new algorithms and applied to virtually ever aspect of understanding these new data. Optimism is running high that these approaches will soon be applied in the clinic giving us new tool against many of our most challenging diseases like cancer, immune and neurodegenerative disorders. Given its importance among the new horizons in healthcare technology bioinformatics is discussed in its own chapter (see Chapter 26).

2.2.3   Grid technology

A grid is a type of parallel or distributed computer system. It enables the sharing, selection, and aggregation of geographically distributed 'autonomous' computing resources on demand, depending on their availability, capability, performance, cost and users' quality-of-service requirements.

Compute grids were the initial focus of researchers, discovering untapped processing power, sharing the process load across many computers and enabling scientists to attack large problems faster. The primary focus was on the ability to break large problems into properly sized problems and then reliably distribute, track and reassemble them into solutions.

Another type of grid is called a data grid (or information grid). It relies on the same compute grid technologies, but requires additional standards to manage dynamic or large distributed repositories.

Since applications drive the use and configuration of an appropriate grid structure, there is in fact no single grid architecture, but rather there are 'middleware' tools that manage federated resources. The middleware layer finds and registers resources and then balances the demand across the different resources in an attempt to meet the needs of many simultaneous users. Standards, commercial software and services, and open software toolkits have emerged, thus making Compute and data grid applications feasible today.

An example of a medical application supported by compute grid technology is the work on functional brain imaging and white matter fiber tractography to image areas in the brain that are active during specific tasks, visualize the connecting pathways among these brain structures, and show the clinical pathology[17]. White fiber tracking is an indirect medical imaging technique, based on diffusion weighted imaging that allows for the extraction of the connecting pathways among brain structures. The time to run such an application can amount to many hours without compute grid technology. Therefore, in order to introduce this application to routine clinical practice there is a need for increasing the throughput without decreasing the quality of the solution. This can be achieved by parallelization and compute grids.

A project called 'caBIG' (cancer Biomedical Informatics Grid) is a good example of how a data grid can be a powerful medical research tool[18]. The ultimate goal of the caBIG project is the creation of a platform that connects the entire cancer research community and provides tools for knowledge discovery (data mining) and information sharing. Nodes of the caBIG are striving to understand disease pathogenesis, improve diagnoses and advance treatment for cancer. The caBIG platform will be a common, extensible informatics platform that integrates diverse data types and supports interoperable analytic tools. This platform will allow research groups to tap into the rich collection of emerging cancer research data while supporting their individual investigations.

Dozens of significant research and commercial medical applications of compute and data grids exist. It is likely that as the use of grid technology grows we will also see a shift towards Application Service Provider (ASP) based business models. This combination will allow the cash starved medical industry to focus on delivering their product: Healthcare, and not information technology.

2.2.4   Models and simulation

Models and simulations are important elements in Medical IT for they enable us to deepen our understanding of physiology and ultimately improve clinical outcomes.

There are different classes of models. 'Mechanistic' models include physiological models, which - depending on the context - are also known as medical models or biomedical models. In this class, the mechanisms (biophysics, biochemistry, and physiology) that underlie physiological systems and human health conditions are represented mathematically. Other modeling classes exist such as 'black-box' models, which use input and output data only and no underling mechanism information, 'gray-box', causal, stochastic, Markov, finite element, and others. Often, a model is a combination of different types of modeling classes.

The aforementioned model classes attempt to describe the transport, regulation, or function of one or more of the following properties of a physiological system: chemical, mechanical, electrical, diffusive, thermal, hydraulic, rheological, and others. Hence, these models may assume different names: pharmacokinetic, metabolic, hemodynamic, etc., depending on which properties are modeled. Almost all fields of medicine are touched by these models including virology, infectious diseases, epidemiology cardiopulmonary, orthopedics, neurology, endocrinology, ophthalmology, and many others.

The applicability of physiological modeling spans the following areas:

- **Research:** Where hypotheses are tested and new ones are formulated to further the knowledge of human physiology and health conditions.
- **Teaching and training:** Where healthcare givers, trainees, and medical students study, test, and simulate different clinical and emergency scenarios.
- **Medical diagnosis and prognosis:** Where a pathophysiological condition can be predicted or prognosed so appropriate actions can be taken, or where a support to that decision is generated and given to the clinician as an aid in the diagnosis process. This application field is a current area of work, and involves intelligent monitoring and advanced medical systems.
- **Medical industry:** Physiological modeling is increasingly becoming a core step of the engineering design process in pharmaceuticals, as well as medical devices and systems industries.

An interesting application that is gaining momentum is the field of human (or mannequin) simulators, which are comprehensive models of parts of human physiology and related health conditions. They are used for education, training and research in cardiopulmonary resuscitation, cardiology skills, anesthesia clinical skills, and crisis management. They exist either as software or embedded in a physical mannequin with limited actuation. Some of the known products are in the field are: Anesthesia Simulator-Consultant (ASC), Comprehensive Anesthesia Simulation Environment (CASE), Cardiopulmonary Resuscitation (CPR), and others.

Some recent work is focusing on integrative modeling, in which different models are combined. These can be horizontal integrative models, ones that include more than one physiological system (e.g. cardiovascular system linked with a respiratory system), or vertical integrative, ones that model on the organ as well its tissue and molecular levels. These have recently started to benefit from fields in engineering and applied mathematics that have been steadily maturing ever since the 1940's, such as multivariable feedback control theory, signal processing, and nonlinear dynamics. The mathematical sophistication reached in these fields lends itself naturally for multi-system modeling that can deal with nonlinearities as well as parameters that are time-varying (with age and health condition, for instance). These new mathematical tools offer a formulation that can apply across scales in physiology, and hence present ease for vertical integration. This is a new field of research work that is very promising in propelling physiological modeling into new levels. A few research groups are working in this field[19-21]. There is also an international effort to describe the human organism quantitatively: the Physiome project[22]. Further, a hybrid combination of the aforementioned tools along with the fields of optimization and soft computing is a promise for the advancement of physiological modeling.

2.3 Areas directed at patients

2.3.1 Consumer health information

Of the three focus areas discussed in this chapter, those directed at patients have the shortest history. This is not surprising, because patients traditionally had a passive role in their own health care. Medical knowledge was perceived as being too hard to understand and so the physician's authority was not questioned. In the past decades, however, society has become more health conscious and patients are actively seeking answers to their own medical problems. As a result, patients are increasingly using electronic health services.

The most notable example of an electronic health service is the health information that is available through the Internet. Consumers are using the Internet not only to solicit health information for themselves, but also for their friends and families[23]. Initially, there has been concern that the Internet could be a platform for information that is misleading or harmful[24], however, this concern is probably overestimated. There are numerous web sites, such as healthfinder (www.healthfinder.gov) or NetWellness (www.Netwellness .org), in which patients can be assured of quality information[25]. The National Library of Medicine has even developed a site called the 'Genetics Home Reference'[26] to help consumers understand genetic conditions. In addition, patients do not shy away from querying sites such as PubMed (www.ncbi.nlm.nih.gov/entrez/query.fcgi), which are directed towards health care professionals and researchers.

Despite the increasing usage of health information resources via the Internet, those that who could benefit from such services most are the least likely to have an access to them[27-29]. Factors such as cost, geographic location, speed of connection, literacy, cultural preferences or experience with computers contribute to this dilemma. These factors probably explain why there still is a digital divide by race, ethnicity, and socioeconomic status among electronic health care consumers. Different possibilities for reducing the digital divide are being explored. One area, for example, deals with understanding and promoting health literacy[30].

Clearly, the goal for the future is to make health information resources accessible to as many consumers as possible. As the bandwidth of Internet connections increase, video servers could enhance current health web pages with a rich multimedia content. Patients will be better informed about their own disease and they will probably be more active in their own treatment. They will have a better 'working relationship' with their physicians. As a result, the number of unnecessary tests or adverse events would decrease.

2.3.2   Empowering patients

There are different ways in which technology can give patients more control over their own health. In the previous section, we discussed how health care information would help patients to be more active in their own treatments. In this section, we will discuss additional possibilities for empowering patients.

One type of patient-centered technologies centers on capturing information. An example of allowing patients to provide information is the asthma kiosk at the Children's Hospital of Boston[31]. This touch screen multimedia computer was designed to help parents provide health related information on their children, who suffered from asthma. An evaluation of the system showed that the information provided by the parents was not only as accurate but also much more complete than the information provided by physicians[32]. Particularly in busy settings such as emergency departments these kiosks would be of value, because often physicians have little time to conduct an extensive interview. As a consequence, important information may be missed. Kiosks that provide an unaided self-entry of patients' data may therefore become a common sight in future.

Another area in which patients could have more control over their data is the personal health record (PHR). The PHR is a web-based application in which patients can enter information about their diagnosis, their medications, their laboratory test, and other clinical data. The American Health Information Management Association offers a free PHR (www.myphr.com). There are also commercial sites such as WebMD (www.webmd.com) that offer PHRs with additional tools to help patients manage their health. An evaluation of various PHRs in 2002, however, indicated that PHRs still might exhibit a limited functionality[33]. Further research is warranted to evaluate whether certain sites have improved. Another approach could be giving patients an online access to their electronic patient record (EPR). Studies on how patients perceive the usefulness of an online access to the EPR provide conflicting evidence[34,35]. Nevertheless, there seems to be the consensus that clinical data must be presented in such a way that patients recognize their health status.

2.3.3 Remote communication

The third area directed at consumers that we would like to discuss is remote communication. We use this broad term to refer to any electronic means by which patients can communicate health-related issues with others. The advantages of communicating health related problems electronically include not having to leave the house (which may be an issue for disabled people), asking delicate questions anonymously, or obtaining answers from individuals who one would not have met otherwise. Consider a patient suffering from tinnitus of unknown origin. Since all the possible causes have been excluded, her physician may have reached the limits of medical knowledge. Faced with a distressing ear ringing for the rest of her life, she joins a newsgroup of patients who suffer from the same problem. She realizes that she is not alone with such a problem and she learns how others have tried to cope with their situation.

The patients-physician relationship could also benefit from electronic communication technologies. Physicians are sometimes so busy that they have little time to communicate extensively with their patients face-to-face. As a result, patients may not feel heard. An asynchronous mode of communication such as e-mails may greatly enhance the communication between physicians and patients[36,37]. The physicians could answer e-mails at a quieter period of the day. There are a number of concerns that need to be addressed, as e-mails are becoming a more popular way of communicating. Physicians may be overburdened with too much e-mail. They could address this problem by providing an e-mail service through a web page that limits the size of e-mails. For longer messages the web page would advise the patients to seek advise through regular communication channels such as the telephone. The questions of cost need to be investigated. On the one hand, physicians spend time on answering e-mails. On the other hand, electronic communication may reduce the number of visits. Finally, there are questions about ensuring the patients' privacy, maintaining the confidentiality of clinical information, and covering medicolegal aspects.

The remote communication methods that come closest to a physician visit involve audio or video. There are different models on how to employ these media. The Department of Medicine at the Boston Medical Centre has developed a computer-based telecommunication system, which provides automated consultations via the telephone[38]. The system has been successfully used to monitor patients with chronic diseases and to encourage health behavior changes. At Columbia University, New York, a telemedicine system for educating diabetes patients has been piloted[39]. The system provides functionalities for synchronous videoconferencing and for transmitting self-monitored blood glucose and blood pressure data. Although the systems impact on diabetes care is still being evaluated, the initial funding for four years has been extended by another four years. Another way to deploy telemedicine is to use the TV set instead of the computer as a means of videoconferencing. Philips uses this approach in the Motiva system, which was designed to help congestive heart failure patients modify their health behavior. Patients use their TV sets to receive personal charts and educational videos tailored to their needs. In addition, they manage their own health by tracking vital signs, such as weight, heart rate, heart rhythm, and blood pressure, with wireless measurement devices. A pilot study on 30 patients showed that the patients felt that the Motiva system had a positive impact on their health behavior, and now a large-scale study with 620 chronic heart failure patients is planned in Europe.

3.   CHALLENGES

There are many IT applications that are technically advanced enough to be implemented; yet they are still far from being an integral part of the clinical routine. The main reason for not having yet integrated feasible IT applications in healthcare can be summarized in one word: *Integration*. Consider, for example, a computer application that calculates a patient's risk of bleeding when placed on an anticoagulant drug. As a standalone application into which clinicians first would have to enter a whole list of parameters, such as age, previous history of bleeds, or other medications, this application is of limited value. Most likely, the clinicians would not be motivated to devote part of their busy schedule to entering data into a computer just to have one question answered. Even if they were motivated, they might still forget to use the system for most of the patients on anticoagulants. Integrated into a physician order entry application of an electronic patient record, however, the application could have a high value. The parameters needed by the application would already be present in the EPR, so that entering the parameters would not be necessary. Furthermore, the clinicians would not have to remind themselves of using the application, because the program would make itself noticeable as soon as the physician would order an anticoagulant for someone who is at a high risk of bleeding.

The above example illustrates that in order to integrate an application into the clinical routine, it should be integrated into an information system (a departmental information system or ideally a hospital information system). The information system itself must be successfully integrated into the clinical routine. As pointed out in the introduction and in section 2.1.1, however, not that many hospitals have a successfully integrated information system. The challenge here is mainly a socioeconomic one, because stakeholders focus more on perceived disadvantages (low return of investment, no clinical support) than on potential benefits (reduction of adverse events, optimizing patient care). To shift the focus, disadvantages must be minimized and benefits must be clearly demonstrated. Although this is easier said than done, we would like to provide some examples of incentives that could help overcome certain challenges of integration.

For one, a hospital information system should be easily accessible at the point of care. If clinicians must walk to the nursing station to enter data, they will perceive that walk as an interruption of the workflow. As a result, they will not use the system or they will chart the data once the clinical chores have been completed (by that time, they may have forgotten some of the information they intended to chart). A solution to this problem is to provide a computer next to every patient bed, as is the case in LDS hospital, Salt Lake City, Utah. Another impediment to the workflow is having to log on whenever one interacts with the information system. Again, users will either not use the system or (if they must use the system) they will find a way to bypass the problem. For example, one clinician may log onto a computer and other team members may continue to use the system under that particular user name. Clearly, this undermines the purpose of having user identification numbers and passwords. A solution could be to provide biometric scanners next to each computer. Our third example of an impediment to the workflow is an inappropriate human-machine interface. Depending on the clinical setting or the preferences of individual clinicians, the keyboard and the mouse are not always the optimal ways of interacting with a computer. An alternative to typing, is speaking to the computer. Using Philips' SpeechMagic™ speech recognition technology, the Diana Princess of Wales Hospital in Grimsby, UK, could demonstrate a reduction from 17.66 days to 4.56 days in the average time from examination to report authorization.

A prerequisite to integrating a computer application (or a device that generates electronic clinical data) into an existing information system is the seamless exchange of data between the two. A hospital information system that could not obtain data from a laboratory analyzer or a computer tomography scanner would be of limited value, because it could not reconcile all of the patients' data. In an age when computer networks are ubiquitous, it may be hard to understand what the problem is in passing data from one computer to another. The problem is not transferring data, but ensuring that the data are transferred and stored in the correct manner. In other words, even if a computer stores clinical data from another computer, it does not necessarily mean that it stores the data in the correct location. For example, the laboratory results for potassium would become useless if they were stored in the area designated for blood glucose levels.

The key to solving the problem of merging clinical data from disparate sources into one electronic patient record lies in data-interchange standards[40]. Probably, the best-known example of a standard is Health Level 7 (HL7), which regulates the exchange, the management and the integration of health data. Another example is the standard for Digital Imaging and Communications in Medicine (DICOM). Given these standards, would two products from different vendors automatically behave in a 'plug-and-play' fashion? Ideally this should be the case, but in practice the answer is "No." Existing standards are still incomplete and thus vendors interpret certain parts of a standard differently. In future, more gaps of existing standards will be filled, thereby enabling the vision of complete interoperability.

4.   CONCLUSION

In this chapter, we gave an overview of the recent advances and trends in medical information technology. Looking at the development of the medical informatics from the past decades until now, we believe that the field has matured considerably. Medical informatics topics are no longer only of interest to the researchers in the field; government and industry leaders understand the huge potential of information technology in medicine. The next decades will pose many medical challenges such as treating chronic diseases in a continuously aging society or maintaining a high level of health care at lower costs. Without computers we shall not be able to solve the problems of tomorrow.

REFERENCES

1.   L.L. Leape, Error in medicine, *JAMA* **272**(23), 1851-1857 (1994).
2.   Harnessing information technology to improve health care, (July 2005); http://www. hhs.gov/news/press/2004pres/20040427a.html.
3.   National Program for IT in the NHS, (July 2005); www.connectingforhealth.nhs.uk/.
4.   P.C. Tang, C.J. McDonald, Computer-Based Patient-Record Systems, in E.H. Shortliffe, L.E. Perreault (eds.), *Medical Informatics: Computer Applications in Health Care and Biomedicine*, 327-358 (Springer, New York, 2001).
5.   M. Freudenheim, Many Hospitals Resist Computerized Patient Care, *The New York Times*, Issue C:1 (2004).
6.   J.S. Ash, P.N. Gorman, V. Seshadri, W.R. Hersh, Computerized physician order entry in U.S. hospitals: results of a 2002 survey, *J Am Med Inform Assoc* **11**(2), 95-99 (2004).
7.   P. Lawrence, *Workflow handbook 1997*, (John Wiley & Sons, New York, 1997).

8. B.A. Levine, T. Wendler, PACS Systems Integration, in *Handbook of Medical Imaging Vol 3 Display and PACS* edited by Y. Kim, S. Horiii (SPIE Press 2000).

9. M. Fiszman, W.W. Chapman, D. Aronsky, R.S. Evans, P.J. Haug, Automatic detection of acute bacterial pneumonia from chest X-ray reports, *J Am Med Inform Assoc* **7**(6), 593-604 (2000).

10. C. Friedman, P.O. Alderson, J.H. Austin, J.J. Cimino, S.B. Johnson, A general natural-language text processor for clinical radiology, *J Am Med Inform Assoc* **1**(2), 161-174 (1994).

11. G. Hripcsak, C. Friedman, P.O. Alderson, W. DuMouchel, S.B. Johnson, P.D. Clayton, Unlocking clinical data from narrative reports: a study of natural language processing, *Ann Intern Med* **122**(9), 681-688 (1995).

12. F.C. Tsui, J.U. Espino, V.M. Dato, P.H. Gesteland, J. Hutman, M.M. Wagner, Technical description of RODS: a real-time public health surveillance system, *J Am Med Inform Assoc* **10**(5), 399-408 (2003).

13. D.W. Bates, R.S. Evans, H. Murff, P.D. Stetson, L. Pizziferri, G. Hripcsak, Detecting adverse events using information technology, *J Am Med Inform Assoc* **10**(2), 115-128 (2003).

14. G.B. Melton, G. Hripcsak, Automated detection of adverse events using natural language processing of discharge summaries, *J Am Med Inform Assoc* **12**(4), 448-457 (2005).

15. J.C. Prather, D.F. Lobach, L.K. Goodwin, J.W. Hales, M.L. Hage, W.E. Hammond, Medical data mining: knowledge discovery in a clinical data warehouse, *Proc AMIA Annu Fall Symp*, 101-105 (1997).

16. K.J. Cios, G.W. Moore, Uniqueness of medical data mining, *Artif Intell Med* **26**(1-2), 1-24 (2002).

17. A. Steed, D. Alexander, P. Cook, C. Parker, Visualizing diffusion-weighted MRI data using collaborative virtual environment and grid technologies. Paper presented at: *Theory and Practice of Computer Graphics*, Birmingham (2003).

18. caBIG™ web site (July 2005); https://cabig.nci.nih.gov/caBIG/.

19. A. Beuter, L. Glass, M.C. Mackey, M.S. Titcombe, *Nonlinear Dynamics in Physiology and Medicine*, (Springer, New York, 2003).

20. M.C.K. Khoo, *Physiological Control Systems - Analysis, Simulation, and Estimation*, (IEEE Press, New York, 2000).

21. M. Ursino, C.A. Brebbia, G. Pontrelli, E. Magosso, *Proc of the Sixth International Conference on Modelling in Medicine and Biology*, Bologna, (WIT Press 2005).

22. The physiome project, (July27, 2005); http://www.physiome.org/.

23. T. Ferguson, G. Frydman, The first generation of e-patients, *Bmj* **328**(7449), 1148-1149 (2004).

24. G. Eysenbach, T.L. Diepgen, Towards quality management of medical information on the internet: evaluation, labelling, and filtering of information, *Bmj* **317**(7171), 1496-1500 (1998).

25. T.A. Morris, J.R. Guard, S.A. Marine, et al., Approaching equity in consumer health information delivery: NetWellness, *J Am Med Inform Assoc* **4**(1), 6-13 (1997).

26. J.A. Mitchell, J. Fun, A.T. McCray, Design of Genetics Home Reference: a new NLM consumer health resource, *J Am Med Inform Assoc* **11**(6), 439-447 (2004).

27. S. Dickerson, A.M. Reinhart, T.H. Feeley, et al., Patient Internet use for health information at three urban primary care clinics, *J Am Med Inform Assoc* **11**(6), 499-504 (2004).

28. T.R. Eng, A. Maxfield, K. Patrick, M.J. Deering, S.C. Ratzan, D.H. Gustafson, Access to health information and support: a public highway or a private road? *JAMA* **280**(15), 1371-1375 (1998).

29. J. Hsu, J. Huang, J. Kinsman, et al., Use of e-Health services between 1999 and 2002: a growing digital divide, *J Am Med Inform Assoc* **12**(2), 164-171 (2005).

30. A.T. McCray, Promoting health literacy, *J Am Med Inform Assoc* **12**(2), 152-163 (2005).

31. S.C. Porter, Z. Cai, W. Gribbons, D.A. Goldmann, I.S. Kohane, The asthma kiosk: a patient-centered technology for collaborative decision support in the emergency department, *J Am Med Inform Assoc* **11**(6), 458-467 (2004).

32. S.C. Porter, I.S. Kohane, D.A. Goldmann, Parents as partners in obtaining the medication history, *J Am Med Inform Assoc* **12**(3), 299-305 (2005).

33. M.I. Kim, K.B. Johnson, Personal health records: evaluation of functionality and utility, *J Am Med Inform Assoc* **9**(2), 171-180 (2002).

34. A. Hassol, J.M. Walker, D. Kidder, et al., Patient experiences and attitudes about access to a patient electronic health care record and linked web messaging, *J Am Med Inform Assoc* **11**(6), 505-513 (2004).

35. W.J. Winkelman, K.J. Leonard, P.G. Rossos, Patient-perceived usefulness of online electronic medical records: employing grounded theory in the development of information and communication technologies for use by patients living with chronic illness, *J Am Med Inform Assoc* **12**(3), 306-314 (2005).

36. T. Ferguson, Digital doctoring–opportunities and challenges in electronic patient-physician communication, *JAMA* **280**(15), 1361-1362 (1998).

37. K.D. Mandl, I.S. Kohane, A.M. Brandt, Electronic patient-physician communication: problems and promise, *Ann Intern Med* **129**(6), 495-500 (1998).

38. R.H. Friedman, J.E. Stollerman, D.M. Mahoney, L. Rozenblyum, The virtual visit: using telecommunications technology to take care of patients, *J Am Med Inform Assoc* **4**(6), 413-425 (1997).

39. S. Shea, J. Starren, R.S. Weinstock, et al., Columbia University's Informatics for Diabetes Education and Telemedicine (IDEATel) Project: rationale and design, *J Am Med Inform Assoc* **9**(1), 49-62 (2002).

40. C.J. McDonald, The barriers to electronic medical record systems and how to overcome them, *J Am Med Inform Assoc* **4**(3), 213-221 (1997).

Chapter 23

DEVELOPMENTS IN CLINICAL INFORMATION TECHNOLOGY
Integration Opportunities in Electronic Health Records, PACS and Clinical Applications

Kees Smedema, Cor Loef, Bert Verdonck
Philips Medical Systems, Best, The Netherlands

Abstract: After a short introduction into Healthcare-IT three areas where significant developments have taken place will be highlighted: 1) the Electronic Health Record (EHR) as the key component in any health system 2) the PACS which is faced with new challenges for integration with other systems in the hospital to improve workflow efficiency and outcomes and 3) clinical imaging applications where new requirements related to decision support and 3D visualization present new opportunities.

Keywords: Information technology (IT), healthcare-IT (HIT), EHR, picture archiving and communication systems (PACS), clinical applications, image processing

1.   INTRODUCTION

The introduction of IT in Healthcare (HIT) has tremendous opportunities in diverse areas such as improving outcomes, enabling new clinical applications and preventing errors. It also delivers increased efficiency and productivity in healthcare processes, in hospital as well as ambulatory settings. Finally it enables home-care, thus contributing to a more patient-oriented care process.

A typical hospital has between 20 and 100 Healthcare IT applications. There is no agreed structure or nomenclature to distinguish the various systems, and various vendors provide different 'cuts' through the applications. As an example, consider the Philips Xtenity Enterprise System. It populates an Electronic Health Record (EHR) that encompasses all relevant clinical and administrative data related to the patient's episode(s) of

367

G. Spekowius and T. Wendler (Eds.), Advances in Healthcare Technology, 367-384.
© 2006 *Springer. Printed in the Netherlands.*

care. Xtenity Enterprise consists of the following sub-systems (see Figure 23-1):

Core: The Central Data Repository, the Master Patient Index (MPI) and the Reporting System.

Clinical enterprise: Enterprise-wide support for the clinical process; it includes for example Clinical Decision Support (medication, disease management, clinical and financial alternatives), Computerized Physician Order Entry (CPOE), Health Information Management (HIM) and Home Health.

Clinical departmental: A variety of clinical specialties such as pharmacy, laboratory, radiology, oncology and cardiology, and systems for the emergency department and the operating rooms.

Access: Basic patient administrative functions such as Admission Discharge and Transfer (ADT), patient scheduling and registration.

Revenue cycle management: Hospital and physician based billing.

Interoperability and eHealth: Interfaces for external systems such as patient monitoring devices and imaging modalities; also a portal for patients (lab results, medication, health information) and secure access to the EHR for other providers and affiliates.

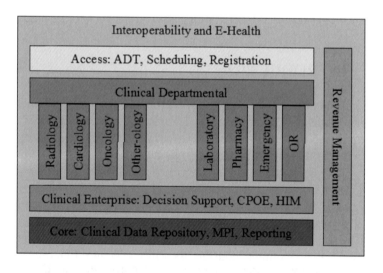

Figure 23-1. Subsystems of a hospital information system.

In this chapter we will concentrate on some of the clinical functionality supported by IT that has seen rapid development over the past years:

EHR is the key component through which health information can be communicated. However its definition is fuzzy and its introduction and use presents many challenges.

Image management and distribution (also called PACS) has always been at the forefront of IT developments in healthcare, and is continuously presented with new challenges.

Imaging applications provide new opportunities in decision support (CAD) and 3D visualization and are moving from stand-alone workstations to applications that are well integrated in the PACS workflow.

2. DEVELOPMENTS IN THE ELECTRONIC HEALTH RECORD

There is a general belief and increasing worldwide evidence that the development of an Electronic Health Record (EHR) and the enabling healthcare IT infrastructure has enormous potential to improve the safety, quality, and efficiency of health care[1].

Direct access to computer-based clinical information, such as laboratory and radiology results, can reduce redundancy in diagnostic procedures and improve quality in decision-making. The availability of complete patient information at the point of care, together with clinical decision support systems such as those for medication order entry, can prevent many errors and injuries caused by medical management rather than by the underlying disease or condition of the patient from occurring. Via a secure healthcare IT infrastructure, patient information can be shared amongst all authorized participants in the health care community. A national healthcare IT infrastructure also has great potential to objectives of national importance, such as improved and informed public health services. A more advanced health information infrastructure is also crucial for various forms of biomedical and health systems research, as well as for educating patients, informal caregivers, and citizens.

2.1 The electronic health record concept

There are many different views of what constitutes an EHR system. Some EHR systems include virtually all patient data, while others are limited to certain types of data. Some EHR systems facilitate decision support such as preventive service reminders, alerts concerning possible drug interactions, clinical guideline-driven prompts, while others do not. Most current EHR systems are healthcare enterprise specific, and only a few provide strong support for communication and interoperability across the health providers in a community. EHR functionalities need to be effective in many different care settings: hospital, ambulatory care, nursing home, care in the community, home health agencies, pharmacies, and dental care.

The primary use of EHR systems is to support the delivery of personal health care services, including care delivery, care management, care support processes, and administrative processes.

There are also important secondary uses, including education, regulation, clinical and health services research, public health and national security, and policy support. The users of EHR systems are both individual users and institutional users. In considering the core functionalities of EHR systems, it is important to recognize these many potential uses:

Health information management. Care providers require relevant information to make sound clinical decisions e.g. medical and nursing diagnoses, a medication list, allergies and drug sensitivities, laboratory test results, radiology reports. Too much information and data may overwhelm or distract the end user, so EHR systems must have well designed interfaces that allow generating relevant selections or cross-sections of this data.

Order entry / order management. The EHR supports the clinical workflow process by computerized physician order entry (CPOE) systems for medication orders, laboratory, microbiology, pathology, radiology, nursing, and supply orders, as well as for ancillary services and consults.

Decision support. Computerized decision support systems support drug prescription and screening for drug interactions, diagnosis and disease treatment and management, detection of adverse events and disease outbreaks, and computer reminders and prompts for preventive practices.

Electronic communication. Support for the effective communication among health care team members and other care partners is critical to the provision of quality health care, especially for those patients with chronic conditions, who characteristically have multiple providers in multiple settings that must coordinate care plans.

Patient support. Functions in this category include patient education to improve control of chronic illnesses in primary care, and self-testing by patients during home tele-monitoring.

Administrative processes. Support for billing and claims management, and reporting tools to support drug recalls and assistance in identifying candidates for chronic disease management programs.

Reporting and population health management. These functions support the institutions with the multiple public and private sector reporting requirements they have for patient safety, quality and outcomes, as well as for public health.

2.2 The IHE initiative's role for the EHR

There is no worldwide EHR standard at present, but there are many efforts underway for many years to define one, or at least a set of compatible ones, most notably in HL7, ISO, and CEN. The current standardization work in HL7 has a focus on the definition of a functional model for the EHR.

Rather than waiting for an all encompassing EHR standard, the IHE initiative[2] (Integrating the Healthcare Enterprise) has embarked, in its IT Infrastructure domain, on a very pragmatic approach to share relevant health information in a cross-enterprise setting. With the introduction of new Integration Profiles addressing these requirements, IHE is well positioned to build regional health networks linking interoperable EHR systems.

The goal is to offer a consistent, standards-based and functional solution for EHR systems. The foundation is formed by the Cross-Enterprise Document Sharing (XDS) Profile. XDS works together with other IHE Integration Profiles for patient identifier management across independent identification domains, and security and privacy measures providing authentication, auditing, and access control. XDS allows information exchange between EHRs in care settings, which together constitute a federated and distributed longitudinal EHR. It is not based on any broad EHR information model (because that does not exist yet), but follows the document paradigm by registration of clinical documents using well-established standards in a document registry. A minimum set of relevant meta-data elements, such as a Patient Identifier, has been defined to identify the documents for registration in the registry and later retrieval from the document repositories.

A particular clinical care community will define the document content that can be shared and the standards it is based on. For example, in the Radiology domain an XDS for Imaging Information Profile has been created, which allows for the exchange of DICOM medical images and diagnostic reports. Another example is the Patient Care Coordination domain, in which a Content Profile for the Medical Discharge Summary using an HL7 Clinical Document Architecture (CDA) document has been created. By starting with a secure document-sharing infrastructure, regional health information networks have a platform available that allows the further extensions with clinical content using more specialized coded terminology.

2.3 EHR deployment challenges

In addition to technical challenges, there are many policies, financial and organizational challenges that must be addressed to facilitate the adoption and deployment of HER systems.

Challenge: Required national scope and approach. The adoption and introduction of a nation-wide EHR needs a clear, broadly motivating and communicated vision and practical adoption strategy. Achieving the buy-in of the public as health care consumer, including health plan beneficiaries, patients, and family members is also essential for success.

Many countries in the world are currently engaged in a national approach for HIT and the EHR. In the USA the position of the National Coordinator for Health Information Technology was created, charged with the development, maintenance, and oversight of a strategic plan for nationwide adoption of health information technology.

Also the EU prepares the introduction of an EHR through its eHealth program, and many countries, e.g. England, Netherlands, Denmark, Italy, have started HIT and EHR introduction programs.

Challenge: Investments needed. Considerable investment in hardware, software, and the broadband networking capacity for EHR is required to realize its potential benefits.

Challenge: Introduction of financial incentives. A major complicating factor for adoption of the EHR in the healthcare sector is that the stakeholder incentives must be aligned across the stakeholders to foster EHR adoption. There are many stakeholders, and the investment cost need to be taken by one stakeholder, while the return on investment benefits another stakeholder. To achieve widespread implementation, some external funding or incentive programs will be necessary.

Challenge: Standards adoption. At present, almost all EHRs are based on proprietary information models within EHR systems, with little or no interoperability between EHR systems and little or no ability to share EHR information beyond the immediate boundary of a single healthcare organization. What is lacking is semantic interoperability, the ability for information shared by systems to be understood at the level of formally defined domain concepts, so that information is computer processable by the receiving system.

Semantic interoperability is necessary for automatic computer processing to underpin the real value-added EHR clinical applications such as intelligent decision support and care planning. In order to achieve this, a definition is needed of a standardized set of domain-specific clinical templates using standardized terminologies, in a collaborative effort between healthcare professionals, the industry, and standard development organization. The active involvement of the healthcare professionals is essential in this process. The IHE initiative is a good example of such a collaborative effort, which should be supported by the government. The government should promote the adoption of well-founded HIT standards.

Challenge: Workflow and ease of use of the EHR. The main purpose of an EHR is to support the collaborative service provision by institutions or individual healthcare providers. The collaborative service provision only works if the information is easily available in an appropriate format for the tasks at hand. Even though EHR information is available, it will only be used if accessing the information is very simple and intuitive, and is perfectly suited for the specific tasks in the workflow. Because the workflow and clinical work practice has a tendency to be slightly different in each healthcare organization and setting, there is a need to assist healthcare organizations to reengineer business processes using HIT. And HIT products should be adaptable to these varying workflows.

Challenge: Extra effort to enter information. Entering information is extra work for the clinician. The benefits and value come only when also other patient information is available, relevant for the clinical case, and entered by a distant co-worker. This is a typical global benefit, which does not exist initially when the participation level is still low.

3. DEVELOPMENTS IN PACS AND ITS INTEGRATION IN THE HEALTHCARE ENTERPRISE

Vendors selling PACS systems and hospitals installing PACS systems nowadays have different challenges than in the past. The innovative hospitals (early adopters) could cope with unexpected situations during the introduction. They discovered the challenges of workflow integration between modalities, HIS, RIS and PACS and they worked with the vendors to solve interoperability problems in a customized fashion. Together with the vendors, the IHE program (Integrating the Healthcare Enterprise) was conceived[2]. The hospitals that decide now on a PACS have quite different expectations and they want to see immediate benefits in efficiency and quality. There are many new developments in the healthcare enterprise, which present new challenges for the PACS vendor as well as for the hospital.

Table 23-1 lists some of the major issues for the introduction of PACS, in the past, and now. This list is not getting smaller as continuously new issues are coming up. Note that many key-issues of the past have been solved in a specific context, but re-appear later, for example speed of image-communication as a result of new multi-slice CT scanners.

Table 23-1. Key issues of PACS introduction.

Time	Issues
6 years ago	Cost-benefit questions.
	Technology not quite available (bandwidth, access speed to 1st image, storage capacity, display resolution, processor speed).
3 years ago	Workflow integration (with imaging modalities, RIS, HIS).
	Integration with speech recognition systems.
	Hardware obsolescence and refresh.
	Distribution of images outside of Radiology
	Other business models: Application Service Provider (ASP), Pay-per-exam.
Now	New issues in workflow integration: Master Patient Index, imaging applications, hospital mergers.
	Management of all images, including visible light, cardiology.
	New paradigms for reporting.
	Security and privacy, single log-on.
	New developments in modalities: data explosion (CT, MR), not only images but also other data (measurements, CAD), reports.
	Information integration: EHR, access to other clinical information.

3.1   Challenges in workflow integration

For most cases the workflow integration between modalities, HIS, RIS and PACS is very well defined by the IHE (Integrating the Healthcare Enterprise) program[2]. One of the first profiles defined by the IHE was the so-called Scheduled Workflow profile for radiology. It is based on the existing standards of DICOM and HL7, and it restricts the many options in implementing these standards in such a way that the information exchange between the different systems should be 'plug and play'. The scheduled workflow profile also takes care of emergency patients but it does not yet address all the variations that may exist.

Requirements for sub-specialty radiology workflow. The IHE Scheduled Workflow profile is not (yet) sufficient for workflow in specific situations. Nuclear Medicine for example has made a special profile for its images. But also for Mammography, Radiation Oncology, Surgery and the Operating Room there are new workflow requirements and IHE has initiated activities in these areas. Note that, although IHE started in Radiology, it has extended to other disciplines as well. This makes it possible to couple image workflow to workflow related to other diagnostic information, e.g. for Cardiology where images, ECGs, reports, measurements and Electro-Physiological data are involved.

Additional images through post-processing. More and more clinical applications are executed on PACS workstations, rather than, or, in addition to, modality workstations. These post-processing applications often produce new images after the exam was finished at the modality and these new images must be archived on the PACS. However, these images were never ordered through the RIS. Because it should be possible to find all images through querying the RIS, special measures have to be taken to make RIS and PACS information consistent.

Personal display protocols. Personal display protocols provide the possibility to customize the screen(s) depending on the preferences of the radiologists. For example screen layout for new and prior images in stack- or tile-view can be predefined. This is an important productivity feature. To implement this the PACS needs DICOM header information such as type of exam, body part, etc. to launch the appropriate display protocol. If, however, the modality-base does not provide all DICOM information, it takes considerable effort to implement the right display protocols at the time of installation.

The 'time-to-first-image' on the PACS viewing station maybe dependent on the personal display protocol if it forces a certain image order, which is different from the order in which the modality sends the images. The PACS is usually capable of re-ordering images, but that may increase the time-to-first-image. It is much better that the modality is able to customize the order of sending, because in that case an optimal speed can be found. Note that the order in which images are sent by the modality is not specified in any standard.

Other workflow complexities. Many of these workflow issues (and we have not been exhaustive) are rather complex. With the early PACS adopters, there was sufficient knowledge available to appreciate the complexity and understand that the solution was unique to a particular hospital. If, however, PACS is viewed as a commodity, which can be introduced with minimal support in any hospital, the complexities will not be understood and the customer can easily become dissatisfied. That is why a basic knowledge in this area for the hospital staff is essential. This knowledge will also help the hospital to do the right purchases in the future in order to prevent the continuous burden of making and supporting hospital-specific solutions.

3.2   The challenge to manage all images

A PACS should support the management of all images, not only the radiology images. This is easily said, but not easily done. Only archiving of images is not sufficient. We need to support the workflow in the hospital. This is well understood in the radiology department, where IHE has specified the relevant profiles. It is also reasonably well understood for

Cardiology, where IHE has just agreed on workflow profiles for the handling of cath and echo images and for ECGs.

However in other areas we often have no available 'standard' infrastructure for ordering, scheduling and reporting (pathology, endoscopy, dental, radiotherapy, ophthalmology). If we want a system to manage all images we have to make sure that the PACS database is able to manage all these images despite the fact that their meta-data (patient, study and exam information) are produced by different information systems. At present this requires proprietary solutions until appropriate IHE profiles are developed for all these situations.

3.3   Challenges in reporting

Medical images are being acquired in order to answer a clinical question and to report this answer. The report is directly used in the clinical workflow, while in most cases the images are just archived for later reference. The report can consist of a wide variety of information[3,4]: Unstructured text (often in radiology), measurements, diagnostic codes, CAD results, etc. In the integration of the PACS in the healthcare enterprise, reporting is still a very big challenge[5].

Different reporting systems. Reporting is often done in different departmental systems. In radiology it is usually the RIS that keeps the reports. There is a trend to combine the RIS and the PACS in one information system. Other clinical disciplines have often their own 'vertically' (i.e. it is a system supporting only one clinical discipline) integrated system to manage reports, numerical data and images. For example a Cardiac Ultrasound Image Management System will probably not only manage cardiac studies of different modalities, but it will also manage diagnostic findings and measurements. Hence it is not an option to simply extend the radiology PACS systems to allow archiving of non-radiology images, because other clinical disciplines have their own ways to handle images and other data in one integrated image and report management system. Unless the radiology PACS will also take care of reporting and measurements, the integrated management of all image types will not be feasible.

HL7 or DICOM? In most hospitals the HIS manages the clinical reports. HL7 is used for access and communication of these reports. Traditionally the radiology department has always been separate with archiving reports in the RIS, for various good reasons. HL7 is also used to access reports in the RIS. In order to take care of non-image results in radiology, DICOM has defined so-called structured report (SR) objects. We are now confronted with 'cultural' differences between the traditional reports in a HIS or RIS with

HL7 as a standard communication protocol, and the structured reports as defined in DICOM, meant for data associated with images. Probably DICOM SR will be used as a communication protocol whenever the non-image information is directly transmitted from the modality or the modality workstation, because modalities typically do not support HL7. Whether this information is kept in DICOM SR format when managed in other information system remains to be seen. Also HL7 has now defined a way to define structure in information through the Component Document Architecture (CDA).

3.4 Challenges in security and privacy

Requirements for security and privacy have to be solved at the enterprise level. We cannot isolate the PACS from the rest of the healthcare enterprise.

This means that the PACS should be able to implement the enterprise rules for security and privacy. IHE has specified the so-called Audit Trail and Node Authentication (ATNA) for this. In addition, the PACS will have to log all accesses to its database such that it will always be possible to trace who has accessed which information. More and more there is a requirement for so-called single-login. This means that with one login procedure the user has access to several systems such as the PACS and the RIS, even if they come from different vendors. Based on the CCOW[7] developments, which were taken over by HL7, IHE has introduced a special profile for this: Patient Synchronized Applications, which allows single-login for any number of applications.

3.5 New developments in imaging modalities

New developments in modalities have an impact on the PACS system, and on the way where and how the imaging applications are used in the healthcare enterprise:

The ever-increasing speed of modality acquisition has again opened the debate about what to do with all this information. In Ultrasound we are used to the situation that only clips are stored, because to store everything would not serve any clinical purpose, and it is simply too much information. In other modalities, due to new acquisition techniques, we will get close to the same situation. In any case the data explosion will cause the development of new ways for diagnosis and reporting[3].

Modalities used to produce only images. However also other data are now being sent: Measurements (Ultrasound for example), spectroscopy data (MR) and quantitative data as a result of image analysis (CAD). It was already mentioned that this opens new challenges how to deal with the non-image information: As part of the image (e.g. for spectroscopy in the enhanced MR DICOM object), as a separate DICOM Structured Report (e.g. for Ultrasound measurements and Mammography reports) or as an HL7 message (no examples yet).

Diagnosis is more often based on images from different modalities in such a way that the modalities are already combined in the radiology-room, such as PET-CT, and SPECT-CT. This has changed the workflow in the radiology department, and after some time, when the new procedure has 'settled', new IHE profiles have to be developed for these cases, and PACS systems will have to implement these.

The diagnostic process in modalities is more and more integrated with the therapeutic process, e.g. by allowing surgical interventions at our near the modalities. This will have its effect on the way the images are used, and a PACS system will have to support these developments in the future.

3.6   Images integrated in the electronic health record

For PACS, there are two ways to look at the EHR, as a provider and as a user:

As a provider, the image and report information is part of the EHR. This means that image and report information should be accessible through any EHR system even though it is not physically part of it. This requires that the PACS and/or RIS can be interfaced with a Master Patient Index in order to uniquely identify the patient. IHE has recognized this requirement also and it has defined a profile for the interface to a Master Patient Index (MPI) called Patient Identifier Cross Referencing (PIX).

As a user, it should be possible to access from the PACS workstation not only the radiology images and reports, but also all other relevant information about the patient, e.g. allergies, laboratory results and current medications. Since there is no standard EHR this is not trivial and currently proprietary and hospital specific solutions are required.

4.   INTEGRATING IMAGE PROCESSING APPLICATIONS INTO PACS

Image acquisition devices typically include post-processing applications to enhance images in order to best represent the clinical problem of interest. Dedicated processing workstations were developed to off-load acquisition consoles from the more time-consuming image analysis tasks, and to create a work spot for the reporting radiologist. However, since PACS workstations also give access to prior images and data from other imaging modalities, they are the ultimate reporting work spot.

Due to the fast adoption of technological advances in image acquisition systems, and due to the swift increase in computer memory and computing power advanced image analysis software packages are now regularly made available on PACS workstations. This may dramatically increase the flexibility of PACS work spots, avoiding users to hop around various systems in a department in order to get a task done. But the trend is bound to a number of constraints.

4.1 Advanced viewing and image processing on PACS

4.1.1 PACS workstation evolution: From 2D to 3D

The original PACS workstation was designed for viewing X-ray radiographs on a dedicated, high-end workstation with high-resolution grayscale displays. These systems were optimized for 2D images with large amounts of pixels per image but typically few images per exam and per patient.

This traditional PACS workstation is transforming now into a more flexible work spot, running on off-the-shelve hardware and supporting medium-resolution color displays. It adds specific viewing features for other modality images such as Computed Tomography (CT), Magnetic Resonance (MR), Ultrasound (US) or Nuclear Medicine (NM): stacks of 2D images with less pixels per image but large amounts of images per exam and per patient. And finally, it becomes feasible to run advanced image processing and image analysis applications on the same systems.

Initially images were tiled on screen, similar to how images were laid out on film. However, browsing through image stacks with a cine tool, automatically or under user control, is the exclusive advantage of a computer when compared to film.

With the huge increase of images generated by multi-slice CT and parallel MR new viewing tools are needed, e.g. allowing tiled layout with skipping of slices, combining consecutive slices with a maximum or average operation ('slice thickening'), interactive MPR tools to allow direct coronal or sagittal viewing, etc.

Finally, when the 2D image stacks are compiled into volumetric or three-dimensional (3D) data, direct projection viewing becomes feasible. Techniques such as maximum intensity projection, surface and volume rendering, initiated from default presets, with interactive manipulation of view settings give direct access to the 3D nature of this medical data.

The 3D visualizations may be used as reference or roadmap images when they give an intuitive overview of the anatomy of interest, or to assist in problem solving when they give good spatial insight in complex three-dimensional structures. They always need links to the original slice data before coming to conclusive diagnosis. Examples are shown in Figures 23-2 and 23-3.

Although the exact impact and value of 3D visualization on the diagnostic viewing process remains to be determined, the trend towards using more direct 3D viewing is set.

4.1.2   Advanced and clinical applications

Combinations of 2D and 3D viewers and image processing tools are often bundled into 'advanced applications'. These rich toolsets are required and need optimization for each imaging modality.

Dedicated image processing applications are developed to support answering specific clinical questions. These 'clinical applications' are designed by combining specific viewing functions, by tuning of advanced toolsets, adding specific image processing algorithms and dedicated reporting tools.

Traditionally these advanced and clinical applications have been developed on separate, advanced, image-processing workstations. However, making such applications available on PACS workstations opens new possibilities because of the availability of prior images and reports, and the integration with other IT systems such as radiology or hospital information systems, or electronic health records.

4.1.3   Increase efficiency

PACS is geared to efficiency: reducing waiting times for patients, improving quality and throughput of radiographers and radiologist, and reducing overall costs. Only then the investments in these systems pay off with satisfied patients and profitable hospitals. Workstation performance and functionality is a key factor in obtaining this efficiency. Bringing the right tools, to the right people, at the right time, at the right place is necessary to guarantee the optimal workflow through a radiology department, and beyond. Bringing advanced and clinical applications to the people that need them, in the working environment they are most accustomed to, avoids them to hop around multiple systems and disturb multiple people before completing a specific task. Therefore we believe that integrating a complete set of advanced and clinical applications onto the same workstation is an unavoidable requirement for today's PACS.

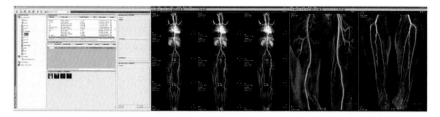

Figure 23-2. Total body MR Angiography. Rich viewing format on 3 monitors, with an information window on the left, and on the right maximum intensity projection images that are automatically sorted.

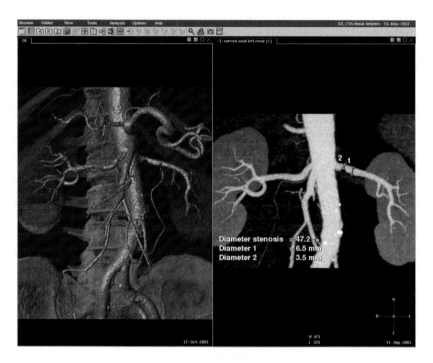

Figure 23-3. CT Angiography showing renal stenosis. Combined view with maximum intensity projection and volume rendering.

4.2 Constraints

4.2.1 Computer hardware

Advanced SW tools that process large amounts of (image) data typically require more performing hardware configurations. Computer and network hardware need to be tailored for the transfer of large amounts of image data, and the SW applications need to be optimized for performance, while some applications may need color, e.g. for native visualization of color Doppler US or for 3D color visualizations.

4.2.2   Application design

Clinical SW applications require specific user training to ensure proper interpretation of results and to avoid potentially dangerous misuse. When such applications are proliferated throughout the radiology department, or beyond, usage may need to be restricted to the intended and trained users.

On the other hand, it may be very worthwhile to provide certain applications to more users, e.g. to let the orthopedic specialist manipulate 3D views of a complex bone fracture. This may imply however that such applications, typically developed for an experienced radiologist, need to be adapted and optimized to different users.

PACS workstations are designed to optimally support the workflow of a radiology department. Worklists and process status are continuously tracked and adapted to ensure an efficient flow of patients, images and reports through the department and the hospital. Adding image processing and analysis steps into this workflow needs to be explicitly supported in order to avoid congestion and confusion in the system.

Finally, the design of the user interface of the application needs to be sufficiently consistent with the user interface of the native PACS workstation, especially when these applications are made by different software vendors. If not, conflicting user interface concepts may totally confuse the user, and result in an unusable system. This is particularly important for mouse usage, screen layout, button icons and terminology.

De-facto standards as imposed by Microsoft[6] for example can cater for a more unified general user experience of modern applications. Medical terminology standards may also help to avoid confusion. But so far there is no standardization of medical image processing specifics, let alone of a medical image processing user interface.

4.2.3   Interoperability

Although strong consolidation takes place between the vendors of imaging modalities and PACS, compiling a complete set of applications from a single SW vendor is often impossible.

Bringing 3rd party applications to a PACS is only possible when that party and the PACS supplier agree to adapt and integrate their SW applications, or when that party implements an open and published application programming interface for that PACS vendor. Difficulties also exist in optimizing performance and computer memory usage between applications from different vendors. Industry standards for this task are still immature, although DICOM defines rich image information models for most imaging modalities now, and CCOW standardizes methods for visual integration of healthcare applications (CCOW stands for the Clinical Context Object Workgroup)[7].

Clinical applications typically need more descriptive image attributes then are needed for simple image viewing. Although the DICOM standard is currently very mature and in wide-spread use, still quite some interoperability problems exist when processing data from one system on another system.

The reporting results of clinical applications need to be viewable and storable in the PACS, and therefore the application need to integrate with the normal report flow of the PACS.

5. CONCLUSION

With respect to the EHR we experience momentum in many countries toward implementation of a national or regional EHR. The IHE initiative is supportive to these EHR adoption strategies with the creation of a large number of clearly defined Integration Profiles for departments inside the healthcare enterprise, but also for the cross-enterprise regional health information networks. However, many challenges still need to be addressed: technical standards adoption, clinical knowledge encoding standards, overcome differences in working practice, collaboration along the clinical pathway, alignment of financial incentives, legal issues, and last but not least the patient's privacy.

The PACS system has evolved to an efficient environment for radiology departments. However, hospitals and vendors are continuously challenged to adapt their PACS to the changing environment in the healthcare enterprise to enable more efficient workflow, better quality diagnosis, and a better integration into the EHR-based systems of the near future.

PACS workstations become capable of running clinical and advanced software applications. This may dramatically increase the flexibility of PACS work spots, avoiding users to hop around various systems in a department in order to get a task done. However, a long list of practical constraints needs to be tackled before the efficiency promises can be made true.

REFERENCES

1. *Crossing the Quality Chasm: A New Health System for the 21ˢᵗ Century*, (National Academy Press, Washington, D.C., 2001).
2. Integrating the healthcare enterprise, IHE; www.ihe.net/index.cfm.
3. D.L. Weiss, *SCAR University 2004 Course Syllabus*, 49-53, (SCAR University Publications, Vancouver, 2004).
4. C. Loef, R. Truyen, Evidence and Diagnostic Reporting in the IHE Context, *Academic Radiology* **12**(5), 620-625 (2005).
5. K. Smedema, Opportunities and Challenges in PACS, *Medicamundi* **46**(2), 2-7, (2002).
6. Microsoft Windows User Experience: Official Guidelines for User Interface Developers and Designers, ISBN 0-7356-0566-1, (Microsoft Press, 2004).
7. CCOW; www.hl7.org/special/Committees/ccow_sigvi.htm and www.ccow-info.com.

Chapter 24

COMPUTER AIDED DETECTION & QUANTIFICATION

Concepts and Results with Respect to Pulmonary Nodules in High Resolution CT Data

Rafael Wiemker[1], Patrik Rogalla[2], Dag Wormanns[3], Thomas Bülow[1], Roland Opfer[1], Ahmet Ekin[1], Thomas Blaffert[1], Ori Hay[4], Ekta Dharaiya[5], Roel Truyen[6], Joost Peters[6], Eike Hein[2], Valentina Romano[2], Florian Beyer[3]

[1]*Philips Research, Hamburg, Germany;* [2]*Charité Hospital, Humboldt University, Berlin, Germany;* [3]*University Hospital Münster, Germany;* [4]*Philips Medical Systems, Haifa, Israel;* [5]*Philips Medical Systems, Cleveland, OH, USA;* [6]*Philips Medical Systems Medical, Best, The Netherlands*

Abstract: With the superb spatial resolution of modern multi-slice CT scanners and their ability to complete a high resolution thoracic scan within one breath hold, software algorithms for computer aided detection (CAD) of pulmonary nodules are now reaching high sensitivity levels at moderate false positive rates. Pilot studies indicate that CAD software modules can serve as a powerful tool for diagnostic quality assurance. Equally important are tools for fast and accurate automatic three-dimensional volume measurement of detected nodules. Computer aided diagnosis (CADx) tools such as automated three-dimensional quantification of contrast enhancement in dynamic CT help to exclude benign nodules and reduce biopsies.

Keywords: Computer aided diagnosis, lung cancer screening, differential diagnosis, pulmonary nodules, quantitative contrast enhanced CT, ultra-low-dose CT

1.   INTRODUCTION

Computer aided detection and automatic marking of lesions and anomalies in medical image data is a software technology that has gained rising interest in the last years. In principle, it is applicable to all kinds of

385

G. Spekowius and T. Wendler (Eds.), Advances in Healthcare Technology, 385-401.
© 2006 *Springer. Printed in the Netherlands.*

medical images (2D, 3D, and higher dimensional) and signals (1 dimensional) from all kinds of scanners (e.g. CT, MR, US, PET, SPECT, ECG) and for all kinds of organs (lung, colon, kidneys, liver, brain, vascular system, etc). In this chapter we want to concentrate on concepts related to pulmonary nodules and their manifestation on CT, for the medical reason that lung cancer is the cancer with the highest mortality, and the technical reason that, after X-ray mammography, CT is currently seen as the modality with the next highest potential for CAD software.

Two main areas have to be distinguished where computer assistance can be used. The *computer aided detection* (CAD) of pulmonary nodules as such, be they malignant or benign, calcified, solid or sub-solid. The results of CAD are markers that draw the attention of the reader to locations of suspicious anomalies (Figure 24-1). The second area is *computer aided quantification (CAQ)* or even more ambitious *computer aided diagnosis* (CADx) of a detected nodule, and aims at the differential diagnosis between malignant and benign pulmonary nodules. Only a fraction of the pulmonary nodules are malignant carcinomas from lung cancer or metastases from cancers in other organs. It is well known that the fraction of nodules which are actually malignant decreases when smaller and smaller nodules are considered[1,2] as they become detectable by the still increasing resolution of multi-slice CT scanners[3].

As software technologies, computer aided detection and diagnosis aim for three main objectives:

- **Diagnostic quality assurance:** By detecting and marking suspicious lesions, CAD can help avoid potential nodules from being overlooked by the radiologist.
- **To increase therapy success by early detection of cancer:** By down-staging the typical stage when a cancer is diagnosed; it is hoped that detection at an earlier stage increases the survival rates.
- **Reduction of biopsies:** By computation of growth rates and doubling times of lesions between follow-up examinations, for non-invasively differential diagnosis to avoid the risks associated with invasive procedures like needle-biopsies or resection surgeries.

Within the context of CAD and CADx for pulmonary nodules, a number of separate technical tasks can assist the reading radiologist. In this chapter we want to address several concepts and discuss the underlying principles, problems and preliminary results:

- Enhanced viewing for optimal visual detection of lung nodules
- Automated detection and prompting of nodules

- Automated three-dimensional volumetry and follow-up matching of nodules for growth-rate computation
- Contrast-uptake measurement with dynamic CT to differentiate benign and malignant lung nodules.

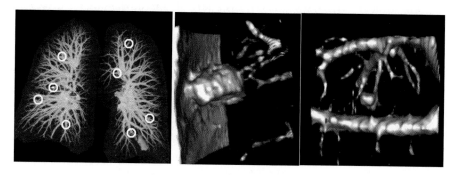

Figure 24-1. CAD markings of lung nodules (left), and renderings of nodules attached to the lung wall (middle) and to pulmonary vessels (middle, right).

1.1   Lung cancer

Cancer of the lung and bronchus is the second most common cancer type. However, due to its aggressiveness, lung cancer is the number one cause of all cancer-related deaths, with more than 150 000 deaths in the USA each year[4].

Pulmonary nodules are among the most common focal pulmonary lesions. The presence or absence of pulmonary nodules is of great importance in the differential diagnosis of lung diseases[5,6]. Therefore the detection and diagnosis of pulmonary nodules in CT data sets of the thorax is a standard procedure in radiological practice. Pulmonary nodules are often benign, or may be metastases from various cancer types, but they may also be an indication for primary lung cancer.

The early detection of lung nodules is crucial, both for close observation or biopsy to differentiate between benign or malignant nodules, and for timely therapy. Among the most common methods to detect pulmonary nodules are chest X-ray and CT. Fiber optic bronchoscopy is also used but has limited value for finding nodules other than those directly attached to the larger airways. CT offers better contrast than chest X-ray between nodule and background with no overlapping structures, and several studies have shown that CT can detect smaller, earlier stage nodules with a higher sensitivity than chest X-ray[7].

In the last years CT technology has undergone a major evolution with the introduction of multi-slice technology. With multi-slice CT, a full lung, thin-slice (<1 mm) scan can be done within a single breath-hold. It is hoped that with the high-resolution CT data available from multi-slice CT scanners cancerous nodules can be recognized while still small and in an early stage of lung cancer. Many researchers assume that this down-staging effect by early detection of lung cancer will ultimately improve the survival rate[1,2].

Moreover, it is hoped that lung cancer screening of high-risk patient groups may significantly increase the rate of lung cancer cases that are diagnosed before the cancer has metastasized. These propositions will be investigated during a large-scale randomized 9-year trial conducted by the US National Cancer Institute (NCI): The National Lung Screening Trial (NLST)[8] has enrolled enroll nearly 50,000 current or former smokers at a total of 30 clinical sites throughout the USA. Similar trials are underway in the Netherlands (NELSON, 24,000 people), the United Kingdom (LUCAS, 40,000 people), and France (DEPISCAN, 21,000 people)[9].

1.2   Differential diagnosis of pulmonary nodules

Once one or several pulmonary nodules have been detected in a patient, the likelihood of malignancy has to be determined. A number of different clinical approaches are aimed at differential diagnosis: biopsy, observation of possible growth by follow-up examinations[10], appraisal of morphological features (such as spiculated or smooth margins), measurement of contrast enhancement in a dynamic CT series[11], use of additional modalities such as positron emission tomography (PET), etc. For all these clinical approaches, software modules for *computer aided quantification* can be used, not only to speed up the workflow, but also to make the necessary measurements themselves more accurate, less prone to error, and more repeatable. Going beyond pure quantification, *computer aided diagnosis* software (CADx) can then estimate likelihood for malignancy versus benignity.

From the various needs for quantification of lung nodules in CT, the volume measurement (volumetry) of a detected nodule is the most immediate (for reporting) and the most basic (for detection of possible growth in a follow-up examination).

2.   COMPUTER ENHANCED VISUALIZATION FOR OPTIMAL VISUAL DETECTION

Lung nodules can be detected particularly well by CT, since they show good contrast in the lung parenchyma and – in contrast to projection X-ray –

cannot be hidden by ribs or other overlying structures. Although in principle detectable in CT, a non-negligible fraction of small nodules may be overlooked by the radiologist, particularly if they are located centrally and hidden in a maze of vessels of similar size (Figure 24-2). This may be even more of an issue, as modern multi-slice scanners can produce up to 800 slices for a thoracic CT exam with sub-millimeter slice thickness. All the small vessels have to be checked for their 3D-connectivity in order to rule-out the presence of possible nodules.

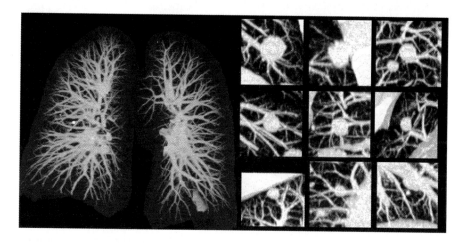

Figure 24-2. Left: Maximum intensity projection (MIP) of the lung segmented out of a high-resolution CT data set. Right: Examples of nodules of varying size (2–20 mm diameter), hidden in the maze of vessels.

For the human observer, a major difficulty in visual detection of lung nodule lies in the fact that in axial slice images the lung nodules can easily be confused with the cross sections of pulmonary vessels. Displaying maximum intensity projections (MIPs) of the lung region is of limited use since nodules will be occluded in the maze of the pulmonary vessels due to their similar Hounsfield (HU) values.

We propose a visualization technique[12] which removes the disturbing vessel structures from the MIP and thus provides a clear view of the lung nodules. The structures that obscure the view are all the structures outside the lungs (the chest wall including bones, the heart, etc.) on the one hand and the pulmonary vessels on the other hand. Consequently, an automatic segmentation of the lungs is performed in order to exclude all exterior structures from the display. Secondly, the pulmonary vessel tree is automatically extracted and then suppressed.

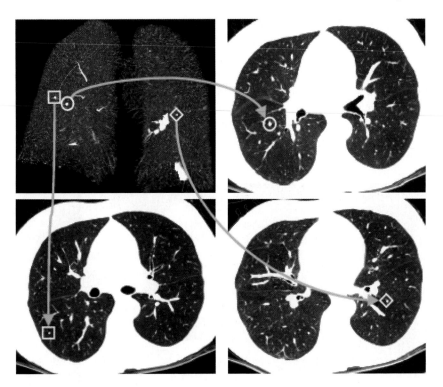

Figure 24-3. Upper left: A coronal MIP of the lung with suppressed vessel tree (compare Figure 24-2). A mouse click on one of the nodules which stand out prominently in the display transfers to the corresponding axial slice.

The principal technical challenge is a careful segmentation of the vessel tree, such that no vascularized nodules that are connected to the vessel tree are erroneously suppressed.

Figure 24-3 shows the method applied to CT datasets acquired with a Philips Brilliance 40-slice scanner (in-plane resolution 0.7 mm, reconstruction interval 0.45 mm, slice thickness 0.9 mm). In the maximum intensity projection (MIP) of the extracted lung after suppression of the segmented vessel tree, lung nodules down to absorption values of about -600 HU are clearly visible. The effect is most striking in interactive mode, where the user can change the viewing direction. It can also be noticed that some vessel segments have been missed by the extraction step. Also some chest wall tissue is still visible. Nevertheless, most overlying tissue is excluded from the MIP and lung nodules become clearly visible at a single glance.

The enhanced visualization scheme suggested here appears promising to reduce the number of false negatives (missed nodules) in visual lung nodule detection.

3.   COMPUTER AIDED DETECTION

In contrast to optimal visualization as described in the last section, the concept of computer aided detection (CAD) means that a visual prompt like an arrow or an ring is drawn at distinct locations of the displayed image in order to call the attention of the reading physician to potential anomalies.

Computer assistance for detecting lung nodules in CT data sets is a straightforward concept and has been suggested and investigated as early as 1989[13,14,15]. The underlying idea is not that the diagnosis is delegated to a machine, but rather that a machine algorithm acts as a support to the radiologist and points out locations of suspicious objects, so that the overall sensitivity (detection rate) is raised. This could be important particularly in screening situations with a massive reviewing load of CT studies, to detect single so far unknown nodules, but also as a significant workflow improvement in oncology therapy follow-up situations, where a multitude of already known nodules have to be assessed for monitoring therapy success.

The principal problem of CAD is that inevitably false markers (so called false positives, pointing to structures which are either not nodules or medically irrelevant) come with the true positive marks. The aim then is to develop software algorithms that hold the false positive rate per patient data set as low as possible while retaining a high sensitivity (detection rate)[16].

The CAD algorithm we have suggested[17] works on pure geometric reasoning. It assumes that any blob-like solid structure (which may also be on one side attached to a plane-like structure, the lung wall) may be a candidate for a pulmonary nodule, if all connecting vessels are significantly smaller in diameter than the central blob-like structure.

A pilot study of a lung nodule CAD system was conducted on images from the radiology department at the Charité university hospital Berlin. The images were acquired in the years 2000–2001 by a 4-slice scanner over the entire thorax at 1 mm slice thickness, 120 kV and 100 mAs.

The automated detection showed a sensitivity of 84% (detection rate including nodules of all sizes). If the minimum nodule size for detection was set to 2 mm, the sensitivity was 95% with 4.4 false positives per patient. For nodules greater than 4 mm, the sensitivity was 96% with 0.5 false positives per patient.

However, we would not necessarily expect such a high detection rate at an equally low false positive rate in all clinical settings. Exams may be taken with low-dose or ultra-low dose imaging protocols. Patient compliance with regard to breath hold and lying still may be poor. Also the delineations and regularity of the nodule population in question may vary considerably.

3.1   CAD performance comparison

In the medical context, the term true positive often refers to a detected nodule that has turned out to be truly malignant. In the context of CAD, a marker is considered as a true positive marker even it points at a benign or calcified nodule; false positive markings are then those which do not point at nodules at all (but at scars, bronchial wall thickenings, motion artifacts, vessel bifurcations, etc). The outcome of computer aided detection is not a yes/no decision for a given image, but rather markings at certain locations; therefore the term 'true negative' is not defined and a normalized specificity cannot be given. Instead, the performance of CAD is usually given as sensitivity (detection rate) and false positive rate (false positive markings per CT study).

Experience with clinical studies has shown that the measured detection rates achieved by CAD systems as well as by radiologists themselves clearly depend on the number of co-reading radiologists: the more co-readers participate, the more suspicious lesions will inevitably be found, and thus the individual sensitivity of each participating radiologist and CAD system will decrease. But even though the absolute sensitivity figures have to be appreciated with care, all clinical studies have agreed in that a significant number of nodules have been detected by the additional CAD software alone, while being overlooked by all co-reading radiologists[18]. Therefore, CAD can be seen as a strong quality assurance tool.

Up to now it is hard to compare the performance of the different CAD algorithms, as they have all been tested in different settings, on different patient data sets, and acquired with different scanners and imaging protocols.

In order to allow a more objective comparison of CAD performance, the US National Cancer Institute has formed a consortium to build up a lung image database with consensus based diagnostic findings, which could then be used to validate and improve computer aided detection software[19].

3.2   CAD performance on ultra-low-dose CT

For lung cancer screening with CT, i.e. for asymptomatic patients, the feasibility of low-dose or even ultra-low-dose CT exams is of particular interest. Therefore we have tested CAD algorithms on ultra-low-dose scans of the Charité University Hospital Berlin, which were recorded with the very low tube current setting of 5-9 mA. It was possible to directly compare the CAD performance to the standard dose images that were acquired of each patient in the same exam session. The double CT examination of the patient was possible because the ultra-low-dose data was reconstructed from the raw data of the scout scan (which was performed with a rotating CT gantry), so that the patient was not exposed to more ionizing radiation than usual.

A pilot study was conducted on 18 patient data sets, for which both standard and ultra-low-dose scans were available. Double reading of two experienced thoracic radiologists revealed a total of 44 lung nodules.

For any CAD algorithm, the trade-off between false positives and detection rate leads to a range of possible operating points. A performance comparison that is independent of a specific operating point can be made by virtue of an FROC curve (free response receiver operating characteristic)[16]. The performance of our CAD algorithm for nodules with a diameter ≥ 2.5 mm is shown in Figure 24-4. The CAD algorithm was applied without any change to both standard-dose and ultra-low-dose images. At one operating point on standard dose images, a sensitivity of 90% was achieved at a rate of 10 mean false positives per patient, a sensitivity of 80% was achieved at a rate of 5 mean false positives per patient. For the ultra-low-dose data the CAD software achieved 83% sensitivity at a rate of 10 mean false positives per patient, and a sensitivity of 76% at a rate of 5 mean false positives per patient.

Appraisal of the two FROC curves indicates that the CAD shows only a slight performance decrease on ultra-low-dose CT images, but seems generally feasible. This is particularly interesting with respect to lung cancer screening of asymptomatic patients.

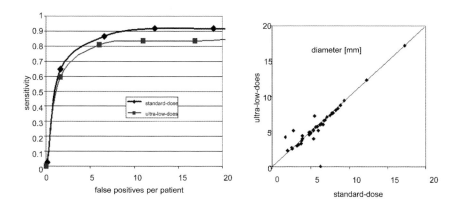

Figure 24-4. Left: FROC curves describing the performance trade-off between detection rate and false positive rate for standard-dose and ultra-low-dose CT (lower curve), for nodules larger than 2.5 mm diameter. Right: Correlation between computer measured volume-equivalent nodule diameter in standard-dose and ultra-low-dose CT (correlation 0.92).

4.   COMPUTER AIDED VOLUMETRY OF PULMONARY NODULES

Nodule volumetry is important for the detection of possible growth between follow-up examinations and computation of growth rates (volume doubling times) for small indeterminate nodules to evaluate the likelihood of malignancy. It is also important in oncology for monitoring the success of cancer therapy. Follow-up of small lung nodules becomes even more important with the increasing number of small nodules detected in thin-slice CT data.

Computer-aided three-dimensional volumetry promises a better sensitivity than manually guided diameter-measurements in a single image slice, since an actual doubling of the nodule volume means a diameter increase of a factor of only $^3\sqrt{2}$ or 26%, which for small nodules might easily be overlooked in the measurement error range.

The main technical challenge for automatic three-dimensional segmentation of nodules is that the image processing algorithm must be able to separate the nodule from the lung wall or attached vessels in a consistent way. The automated segmentation should also yield consistent results when the nodule is imaged with different CT slice thickness settings[20, 21].

For validation of automatic volumetry, we have conducted comparisons of manual measurements between two radiologists, and between manual versus automated volume segmentation. The correlation between the manual measurements by two radiologists was 0.987. There was also a strong correlation between automated and manual segmentation with the correlation coefficient equal to 0.972 and 0.986 for the two radiologists respectively. So the agreement between manual and computer aided volumetry proved to be equally good as the agreement between the two human readers. The automated measurements required minimal user interaction with average volume estimation time per nodule of about a second. Slicewise manual measurements on the other hand took an average of five minutes per nodule[22].

4.1   Nodule volumetry with ultra-low-dose CT

It is an important question whether computer aided nodule volumetry is also feasible on ultra-low-dose CT data, despite its higher image noise. Therefore we have compared the nodule volumetry results for patients scanned twice with standard-dose and ultra-low-dose CT (data material as described in section 3.2). The computer-estimated volume-equivalent diameters show good correlation between ultra-low-dose and standard-dose (see Figure 24-4, correlation coefficient of 0.92), so that both protocols could be used for follow-up monitoring.

4.2 Follow-up registration and matching of nodules

Evaluating the potential growth or shrinkage of pulmonary nodules between a former CT exam and a current follow-up exam is a routine task in radiology practice, not only for diagnosis of detected nodules, but also for monitoring the response to oncological therapy. The typical manual matching procedure is quite time consuming; the user has to separately scroll through the slice stacks of the two studies and locate each nodule and then locate the same nodule in the follow-up study, perform the volumetry and copy down the results. In contrast, the computer assisted matching indicates the corresponding nodule location in the other dataset when the user points to the nodule in either one of the datasets (see Figure 24-5). Moreover, a list of matching pairs is automatically compiled for all nodules found in the two datasets (detected both manually and/or by CAD).

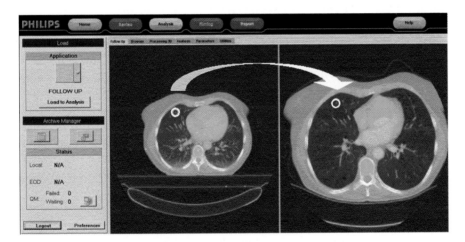

Figure 24-5. Automated matching of a nodule between follow-up exams reconstructed with different imaging protocol parameters (field-of-view).

To perform such a statistical growth analysis with measurement and matching in a manual fashion is of course possible, but might simply not be undertaken for all cases in the clinical practice with high caseload pressure. Therefore, the computer aided follow-up matching may be more than a convenience tool but indeed contribute to diagnostic quality assurance.

The automatic nodule matching approach described by Blaffert[23] starts out by segmenting the lungs out of the overall thoracic CT data volume of the current and former study. The two lung volume images are geometrically registered (aligned) using an affine coordinate transformation until optimal cross-correlation is reached. Using highly optimized image processing methods, the optimal alignment of the two lung volumes can be reached in typically 5 seconds.

In general, an affine coordinate transformation is not expected to always suffice for the alignment of the same lung between a former and current CT study, since the possibly different respiratory state and patient pose on the CT table may necessitate the use of elastic registration. Current state-of-the-art elastic image registration algorithms are still too time consuming, but are expected to reach the performance required for clinical real time applications soon.

5.   CONTRAST UPTAKE MEASUREMENT FOR DIFFERENTIAL DIAGNOSIS

Differential diagnosis of incidentally found pulmonary nodules is a very common clinical problem. The widespread use of multislice CT scanners has led to an increase of incidentally detected small nodules. Possible options to differentiate benign and malignant nodules are follow-up with growth assessment, biopsy, surgical resection, analysis of the nodule morphology on high resolution CT images, contrast enhanced dynamic CT, and PET/CT examinations. However, CT-guided or bronchoscopic biopsy of small nodules is difficult to perform, and surgical resection is a very invasive procedure (in relation to the highly probably benign nature of small nodules). Thus, non-invasive tests for reliable distinction between benign and malignant nodules are highly desirable. Analysis of nodule morphology alone is currently not known to be sufficiently reliable, and PET/CT shows a lack of sensitivity for detection of malignancy in small nodules[24].

Swensen et al.[11] have suggested that due to angiogenesis every malignant pulmonary nodule visible at CT should exhibit enhancement after intravenous injection of contrast media. Inversely, lack of enhancement should virtually exclude malignancy. Even though the sensitivity of this quantitative contrast-enhanced CT (QECT) is high (above 90%), the specificity of dynamic CT is known to be moderate (below 50%). However, despite its known moderate specificity, dynamic CT serves to effectively reduce the number of necessary biopsies, since all non-enhancing nodules do not require work-up.

Quantitative contrast-enhanced CT (QECT) requires precise density measurement in pulmonary nodules at CT for reliable detection of enhancement, which is suspicious for malignancy. The mean Hounsfield value of the nodule in question is measured in a native scan and in e.g. four subsequent CT scans 1, 2, 3, and 4 minutes after administration of contrast agent. However, the measurement of the mean Hounsfield value is not without pitfalls. The estimated mean Hounsfield number of a nodule may easily vary in an interval of ±100 HU (depending on the selected volume of interest or segmentation of the nodule, Figure 24-5), which is 10 times higher than the expected enhancement, which we want to quantify. Here, computer aided quantification can be a valuable tool for diagnostic quality assurance.

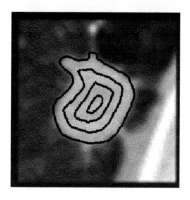 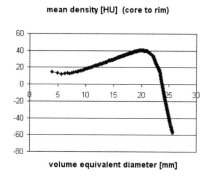

Figure 24-6. Computer aided three-dimensional measurement of the mean Hounsfield value from nodule core to boundary, showing the functional dependence of the estimated mean Hounsfield value and the estimated volume of a nodule.

In contrast to an average enhancement number from an arbitrary volume of interest, we suggest a radially resolved enhancement curve[25] which is capable to convey more detailed information, and more reliable comparison between pre- and post-contrast scans, e.g. for partial enhancement such as rim enhancement. This measurement and visualization method promises to be a valuable tool for differential diagnosis between malignant and benign lesions.

Figure 24-6 shows a malignant lesion (carcinoma), which was auto-matically segmented in 3D. Lung wall and attached vessels were cut-off. Successively large Volumes of Interest (VOI) are defined from the center of the segmented region moving outward. The Hounsfield values within each of the growing volumes of interest are averaged to yield a mean Hounsfield value. Then the distance to the boundary is gradually lowered, and more and more voxels are continuously added to the VOI, leading to a gradual inflation of the VOI towards the segmentation boundary until it completely fills the segmented nodule. For each VOI a cumulative mean Hounsfield value is computed from all voxels aggregated so far, yielding a continuous mean-Hounsfield-curve (Figure 24-7), which can be plotted as a function of volume-equivalent diameter.

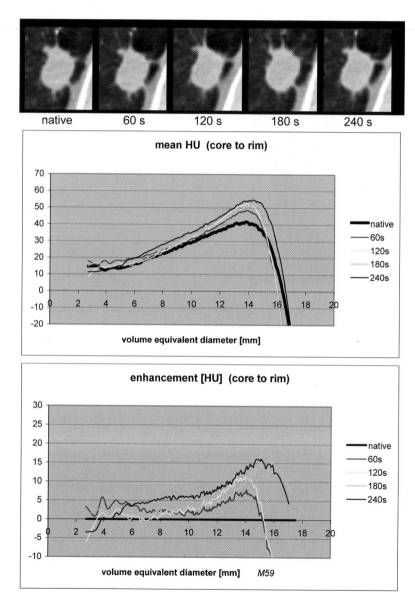

Figure 24-7. Example of radially resolved mean-Hounsfield and contrast-uptake curves for a malignant nodule exhibiting rim enhancement.

The resulting enhancement curves convey information to the reading physician whether there is significant enhancement present, and whether it is present more in the core or towards the rim of the nodule. Moreover, the ensemble of mean-Hounsfield-curves gives a good indication whether the measurements are stable (parallel course of the curves), or if the measurement is possibly unreliable due to problems of segmentation, misalignment (registration), cardiac motion artifacts, or incomparable respiratory state of the different series of the dynamic CT dataset.

6.   OTHER AREAS OF INVESTIGATION

Going beyond detection and quantification of pulmonary nodules, *computer aided diagnosis* software (CADx) may be able to estimate a likelihood for malignancy versus benignity, by comparing the measured values in a multidimensional feature space to known benign and malignant example populations[26]. It may also be helpful to automatically retrieve similar cases with known diagnosis from a database and display them together with their findings to the radiologist[27].

Other CAD applications concerning thoracic CT imaging are the detection and quantification of pulmonary emboli[28], emphysema, airway diseases[29], and parenchymal infiltrations. Most of the tasks described in this chapter can in a similar fashion be applied to polyps in the colon, which may develop into colonic cancer[30].

7.   CONCLUSION

With the advent of multi-slice CT scanners and the possibility to acquire sub-millimeter slice data over the whole thorax within a single breath-hold, software algorithms for computer aided detection and quantification start to reach a level of sensitivity and specificity which can make significant contributions to diagnostic quality assurance, and can provide radiology departments with the increased safety of a 'second reader' at low cost.

For computed tomography, the currently most advanced clinical CAD applications are related to lung as well as to colon cancer. The CAD applications provide automated and reproducible computer aided detection and three-dimensional volumetry of lesions, which is important for diagnostic quality assurance, acceleration of clinical workflow, and reduction of biopsies.

With ever refining spatial, dynamic, and temporal resolution of medical imaging scanners, more applications of computer aided detection and quantification are currently emerging.

REFERENCES

1. C.I. Henschke, D.I. McCauley, D.F. Yankelevitz, D.P. Naidich, G. McGuinness, O.S. Miettinen, D.M. Libby, M.W. Pasmantier, J. Koizumi, N.K. Altorki, J.P. Smith, Early Lung Cancer Action Project: overall design and findings from baseline screening, *Lancet* **354**(9173), 99-105 (1999).

2. S. Diederich, D. Wormanns, M. Semik, M. Thomas, H. Lenzen, N. Roos, W. Heindel, Screening for early lung cancer with low-dose spiral CT: prevalence in 817 asymptomatic smokers, *Radiology* **222**(3), 773-781 (2002).

3. F. Fischbach, F. Knollmann, V. Griesshaber, T. Freund, E. Akkol, R. Felix, Detection of pulmonary nodules by multislice computed tomography: improved detection rate with reduced slice thickness, *European Radiology* **13**(10), 2378-2383 (2003).

4. United States National Cancer Institute; http://www.cancer.gov/statistics.

5. M. Prokop, M. Galanski, *Spiral and Multislice Computed Tomography of the Body,* (Thieme Medical Publishers, Stuttgart, 2003).

6. W.R. Webb, N.L. Müller, D.P. Naidich, *High Resolution CT of the Lung*, second edition, (Lippincott-Raven Publishers, Philadelphia, 1996).

7. P.B. Bach, M.J. Kelley, R.C. Tate, D.C. McCrory, Screening for Lung Cancer: A Review of the Current Literatur, *Chest* **123**, 72S-82S (2003).

8. National Lung Cancer Screening Trial, United States National Cancer Institute; http://www.cancer.gov/nlst.

9. S. Diederich, D. Wormanns, W. Heindel, Lung Cancer Screening with Low-Dose CT, *European Journal of Radiology* **45**(1), 2-7 (2003).

10. D. Wormanns, S. Diederich, Characterization of small pulmonary nodules by CT, *European Radiology* **14**(8), 1380-1391 (2004).

11. S.J. Swensen, R.W. Viggiano, D.E. Midthun, N.L. Muller, A. Sherrick, K. Yamashita, D.P. Naidich, E.F. Patz, T.E. Hartman, J.R. Muhm, A.L. Weaver, Lung nodule enhancement at CT: a multicenter study, *Radiology* **214**, 73-80 (2000).

12. T. Bülow, R. Wiemker, C. Lorenz, S. Renisch, T. Blaffert, A Method for Lung Nodule Visualization from Multi-slice CT data, *Proc Computer Assisted Radiology and Surgery CARS 2005,* 1127-1131 (2005).

13. F. Preteux, N. Merlet, P. Grenier, M. Mouellhi, Algorithms for automated evaluation of pulmonary lesions by high resolution CT via image analysis, *RSNA*, 416 (1989).

14. F. Preteux, A Non-Stationary Markovian Modeling for the Lung Nodule Detection in CT, *Proc Computer Assisted Radiology CARS 91*, 199-204 (1991).

15. M. Giger, K. Bae, H. MacMahon, Computerized Detection of Pulmonary Nodules in Computed Tomography Images, *Investigative Radiology* **29**(4), 459-465 (1994).

16. P.C. Bunch, J.F. Hamilton, G.K. Sanderson, A.H. Simmons, A free response approach to the measurement and characterization of radiographic observer performance, *Proc SPIE 1977*, **127**, 124-135 (1977).

17. R. Wiemker, P. Rogalla, A. Zwartkruis, T. Blaffert, Computer Aided Lung Nodule Detection on High Resolution CT Data, *Proc SPIE Medical Imaging 2002*, **4684**, 677-688 (2002).

18. C.L. Novak, J. Qian, L. Fan, D. Naidich, J.P. Ko, A.N. Rubinowitz, Inter-observer variations on interpretation of multislice CT lung-cancer screening studies and the implications for computer-aided diagnosis, *Proc SPIE Medical Imaging Conference 2002*, **4680**, 68-79 (2002).

19. S.G. Armato, G. McLennan, M.F. McNitt-Gray, C.R. Meyer, D. Yankelevitz, D.R. Aberle, C.I. Henschke, E.A. Hoffman, E.A. Kazerooni, H. MacMahon, A.P. Reeves, B.Y. Croft, L.P. Clarke, Lung image database consortium: developing a resource for the medical imaging research community, *Radiology* **232**(3), 739-748 (2004).

20. R. Wiemker, P. Rogalla, T. Blaffert, D. Sifri, O. Hay, E. Shah, R. Truyen, T. Fleiter, Aspects of computer-aided detection and volumetry of pulmonary nodules using multislice CT, *British Journal of Radiology* **78**, S46-S56 (2005).

21. R. Wiemker, P. Rogalla, E. Hein, T. Blaffert, P. Rösch, Computer Aided Segmentation of Pulmonary Nodules: Automated Vasculature Cutoff in Thick- and Thinslice CT, *Proc Computer Assisted Radiology and Surgery CARS 2003*, 965-790 (2003).

22. O. Hay, D. Sifri, Y. Srinivas, R. Wiemker, Evaluation of Automatic Volumetric Segmentation of Lung Nodules in Standard and Low Dose CT Scans, *RSNA* (2003).

23. T. Blaffert, R. Wiemker, Comparison of different follow-up lung registration methods with and without segmentation, *Proc SPIE Medical Imaging 2004*, **5370**, 1701-1708 (2004).

24. M.K. Gould, C.C. Maclean, W.G. Kuschner, C.E. Rydzak, D.K. Owens, Accuracy of Positron Emission Tomography for Diagnosis of Pulmonary Nodules and Mass Lesions, *Journal of the American Medical Society* **285**(7), 914-924 (2001).

25. R. Wiemker, D. Wormanns, F. Beyer, T. Blaffert, T. Bülow, Improved sensitivity of dynamic CT with a new visualization method for radial distribution of lung nodule enhancement, *Proc SPIE Medical Imaging Conference 2005*, **5746**, 486-497 (2005).

26. F. Li, M. Aoyama, J. Shiraishi, H. Abe, Q. Li, K. Suzuki, R. Engelmann, S. Sone, H. Macmahon, K. Doi, Radiologists' performance for differentiating benign from malignant lung nodules on high-resolution CT using computer-estimated likelihood of malignancy, *American Journal of Roentgenology* **183**(5), 1209-1215 (2004).

27. A.M. Aisen, L.S. Broderick, H. Winer-Muram, C.E. Brodley, A.C. Kak, C. Pavlopoulou, J. Dy, C.R. Shyu, A. Marchiori, Automated Automated Storage and Retrieval of Thin-Section CT Images to Assist Diagnosis: System Description and Preliminary Assessment, *Radiology* **228**, 265-270 (2003).

28. M.J. Quist, H. Bouma, C. van Kuijk, O.M. van Delden, F.A. Gerritsen, Computer-Aided Detection of Pulmonary Embolism on Multi-Detector CT, *RSNA* (2004).

29. R. Wiemker, T. Blaffert, T. Bülow, S. Renisch, C. Lorenz, Automated assessment of bronchial lumen, wall thickness and bronchoarterial diameter ratio of the tracheobronchial tree using high-resolution CT, *Proc Computer Assisted Radiology and Surgery CARS 2004*, 967-972 (2004).

30. F.M. Vos, R.E. van Gelder, I.W.O. Serlie, J. Florie, C.Y. Nio, A.S. Glas, F.H. Post, R. Truyen, F.A. Gerritsen, J. Stoker, Three-dimensional display modes for CT colonography: conventional 3D virtual colonoscopy versus unfolded cube projection, *Radiology* **228**, 878-885 (2003).

Chapter 25

MEDICAL DECISION SUPPORT SYSTEMS
The Wide Realm of Possibilities

William P. Lord[1] and Dale C. Wiggins[2]
[1]Philips Research, Briarcliff Manor, NY, USA; [2]Philips Medical Systems, Andover, MA, USA

Abstract: Need and know-how have come together to start in earnest the era of medical decision support systems. Reducing medical errors while saving costs, and discovering new medical knowledge while reducing information overload are among the conflicting needs addressed. Decision support systems span the realms of home health care to enterprise-wide systems to medical research laboratories. Limited use of electronic patient records, incomplete standards, and difficulties in encoding all aspects of the patient encounter are examples of hurdles to overcome. In the short-term we will see more intelligent alerts, earlier indicators of critical conditions discovered by data mining, and context aware displays. In the long-term we hope to see a highly integrated continuum of care with guardian angel and coaching applications helping us not only in illness, but also with our health and wellness.

Keywords: Decision support systems, medical error reduction, electronic patient record, data mining, knowledge representation

1.   INTRODUCTION

Science fiction would have us believe that the manifestation of medical decision support systems requires autonomous robots or holograms that can completely replace humans. Though far more mundane than those of science fiction, medical decision support systems have existed for decades with many now in common use, and saving lives. Today's technologies coupled with the driving forces of standardization efforts, consumer and corporate advocacy, governmental initiatives, and sociological changes in the acceptance of computers in medicine are all escalating the use of more advanced decision support systems. These systems will help answer the cry for reducing medical errors, reducing medical costs, detecting diseases earlier, and achieving preventive medicine.

G. Spekowius and T. Wendler (Eds.), Advances in Healthcare Technology, 403-419.

But what are these existing systems, and what might they be in 5 years, in 10 years? In this chapter you will be introduced to the wide scope of medical decision support applications and the driving forces behind them. We will paint our vision of the future paired with the hurdles in front of us and the technologies to get us there.

Broadly speaking decision support systems are any systems that help in the decision making process. Key in this definition is the word *help*. These systems do not necessarily make decisions, but more times than not just *help* in the decision making process. Accomplishing this can be done in numerous ways as will be demonstrated through examples in the following sections. Similarly, a key word missing in the above definition is *electronic*, or *computer*. There are many non-computer-based decision support systems (i.e., reference books like the *Physicians' Desk Refernce*[1], using colleagues for second opinions). However, we will restrict ourselves to computer-based decision support systems in this chapter.

Our focus in this chapter will be on medical decision support systems outside the domains of medical imaging and bioinformatics, as these have their own dedicated chapters. Core to this chapter will be Clinical Decision Support Systems (CDSS), applications used in a clinical setting by medical professionals to help them make decisions. However, clinical decision support systems alone would be too limiting, so we also include applications for non-professionals, systems used outside of formal clinical environments, and systems to enhance health care research.

2.   DRIVERS

Many drivers are indirectly responsible for the increasing prevalence of and the push for decision support systems, but perhaps the biggest influence has come from two IOM books: *To Err is Human*[2], and *Crossing the Quality Chasm*[3]. Almost single handedly these books have raised the awareness of the number of lives lost per year due to medical errors: 96,000 per year in the United States alone. Far more are injured or suffer an adverse experience due to medical errors. Reducing medical errors has become the number one driver in healthcare today. Unfortunately, the number two driver is close behind and can be seen as conflicting: reducing medical costs. Other drivers that indirectly help promote the use of decision support systems are improving the quality of life, advancing medical science, combating the shortages of physicians and nurses, and making the use of medical knowledge and technology more widespread and timely. As we drill down into these drivers we see directly the influencing factors behind the growing interest in decision support.

2.1 Data overload

Advancing medical technologies are giving us access to more data about patients than ever before. Just as in imaging, where we produce more images than doctors can look at, patient-monitoring equipment provides innumerable real-time physiological data as more parameters can be monitored, and newly developed tests mean more lab values to sort through. All this in a world where information technology allows us to store unlimited amounts of data indefinitely. Meanwhile there is a real or perceived need to run more tests for fear of lawsuits. Data availability does not necessarily lead to better outcomes though, especially when coupled with the need to reduce costs, which can mean less staff available, less training among staff members, or just less time to spend per patient.

Data need to be turned into information. Data are not information unless they are necessary for the current medical decision and are understandable in the time available for the decision. Decision support systems can help with visualization. In imaging this could mean producing a fly through of 4-D data sets or highlighting suspicious areas. For monitoring data this could mean showing trends instead of raw data, and highlighting values outside of expected results.

2.2 High complexity

Devices can be too complex to operate, processes can be too complex to follow, not to mention how complex diagnosing and therapy planning have become with all the new medical knowledge and therapy options. Coupled with complexity is the need for more and better training of users. With the push to reduce costs, systems that allow users with less training to do their job to the level of highly trained individuals will be highly sought after. One solution to help reduce training time is for vendors to have a common interface look, feel, and functionality across their product lines as Philips has done with Vequion. Decision support technologies can also play a role by automating complex workflows, and helping navigate through complex diagnostic and therapeutic decision trees.

2.3 Ubiquitous availability

Where someone lives, works, and vacations can have a direct influence on the quality of medical care they receive. Rural communities as well as impoverished communities often lack world-class medical facilities. Telemedicine offers a partial solution, but can actually increase the number of medical personnel needed per patient case, as you need both local and remote staff. Decision support systems that help bring the expertise directly to locations without experts in a certain area can do so without putting undue burden on the experts. Such systems can be made available to serve people at all levels of the healthcare delivery chain, including radiologists working outside their subspecialty, primary care physicians working with rare conditions, technicians setting up for non-standard imaging exams, and even potential patients in deciding if they need to see a healthcare professional and which one.

3.   DEFINITION BY EXAMPLES

The primary goals of clinical decision support systems are focused on assistance with diagnosis and patient safety. In diagnosis, clinical information is used to enhance decisions. Clinical decision support systems vary greatly in their complexity, function and application. Initially these systems differed from clinical practice guidelines and critical pathways in that they required the input of patient-specific clinical variables and as a result provided patient-specific recommendations. Paper-based guidelines and pathways, in contrast, provide more general suggestions for care and treatment. However, electronic clinical guidelines and electronic critical pathways as part of the clinical decision support system can combine general suggestions with patient-specific clinical information, as will be shown among the examples below.

3.1   Help making difficult decisions

You've just received a patient in the Emergency Department (ED) who is exhibiting signs of hemiparesis and aphasia. You suspect stroke. If this patient has had an ischemic stroke and the onset was within the past three hours, thrombolitics may lead to improvement and even a full recovery. However, if this patient has suffered a hemorrhagic stroke, the same treatment may cause death. What do you do?

Although stated simply in the scenario above the decision is not just a critical one, but also difficult because of the number of factors that must be weighed. Knowledge exists to make the best decision for/with the patient, but today in the United States there are a paucity of hospitals with this knowledge[4]. Decision support systems that lead the ED staff through the recommended battery of questions and tests could make the positive outcomes obtained in certified/designated stroke centers more wide spread[5].

3.2   Help making simple yet repetitive decisions

Performing simple arithmetic calculations and looking up values in tables are certainly skills that nurses and doctors have, but over time errors will be made. Computers on the other hand will perform the same all the time. As a patient do you want a nurse responsible for 10 patients calculating a medication dose based on your body weight in kilograms after obtaining your weight in pounds? How about a first year resident after being woken up at 2:30 in the morning?

Among the most common forms of decision support systems are drug-dosing calculators. These computer-based programs calculate appropriate doses of medications after clinicians input key data.

Physiologic calculations are also provided in advanced bedside monitors and information systems. These calculations utilize existing information and proven formulas to eliminate errors and save valuable clinician time.

The potential exists for more advanced automation via closed loop and/or clinician-directed closed loop systems. These systems would monitor the patient's variance from a target and apply or ask for therapy to bring the patient back. Glucose levels could be an early target for these types of systems. Specific examples of closed loop therapy have already been applied. For example, Kouchoukos and Sheppard[6] built a computer-based system in 1967 that was used in the observation and treatment of patients following cardiac surgical procedures. The system performed automatic control of blood infusion and vasodilating agents by closed loop feedback control techniques. Excessive blood loss was detected via hourly evaluation of chest tube drainage patterns following surgery. The infusion rate of pharmacologic agents was calculated according to a specified dosage. According to literature, the use of the system contributed to the reduction of patient time spent in the unit to 24 hours or less for the majority of the patients.

3.3   Help reducing time, errors, and variance of practice

For years clerical staff have set up radiologists' workspaces for reading films. Current and previous films are pre-fetched and arranged on rotating light boxes, alternators, to speed up the process by which they read films. Everything the radiologists will need to make decisions about the films is within their reach and in the order they will need it. On the other hand, clinical decisions by doctors in the various intensive care units, for example, require looking through many pages of a paper-based

*medical record or screens of a an electronic medical record. Why can't
the efficiency afforded radiologists be more widespread?*

Clinical guidelines, critical pathways, bundles, standing orders, and other
varieties of recommendations are all knowledge sources for what to do in
various situations[7]. If a computer system can use these in the way a clerical
staff uses knowledge of how radiologists practice, then given the decision an
intensivist in the Medical ICU has to make next about a patient, the
computer system should be able to anticipate the information required to
make the decision. If so, the system can then pre-fetch and arrange the
information in such a way as to help speed up the decision making process.
As time is related to cost, money can be saved.

Additionally, because all the recommended information required to make
a decision is pre-fetched and displayed in an easy-to-view manner, errors of
omission will be reduced. Likewise, such a system can be set up so that all
staff using the system will be making their decision starting from the same
set of information, thereby reducing the variance in practice among staff
members.

3.4   Help in combining imaging and non-imaging information for diagnoses

*A 53-years old marketing executive just had a state-of-the-art thoracic CT
scan. She was a heavy smoker for 20 years, but quit 8 years ago. The
radiologist is looking at her CT scan on a workstation accompanied by
a CAD (Computer-Aided Detection) system, which can help identify
suspicious lesions. Several of the lung nodules have a diameter of 1 mm.
Can the radiologist determine that these nodules are malignant or benign
without ordering a biopsy or repeating a CT scan in half a year?*

Diagnosis is one of the most difficult tasks clinicians face everyday, it
carries with it many serious implications, such as prognosis, treatment options,
and often life or death. Early stage cancer diagnosis in asymptomatic
patients is an especially a challenging task even for experienced physicians.
About 1.4 million new cancer cases (excluding basal and squamous cell skin
cancer) are expected to be diagnosed in the USA alone in 2005 and cancer is
the second leading cause of the death in the USA[8].

Early detection and diagnosis of suspicious lesions allow for earlier
intervention, which lead to better prognosis for the patients. While recent
advances in imaging modalities (e.g. 128-slice CT scanners), molecular
imaging, and genomics make possible the diagnosis of cancer at an earlier

stage than ever before; it also creates a huge amount of data (images, lab reports, findings) that have to be interpreted by radiologists and/or oncologists. Computer Aided Diagnosis (CADx) can facilitate fast and accurate diagnosis and can increase workflow[9]. However, it is important to emphasize, that these system should provide only a second opinion to the clinicians, which they can use to help form a diagnosis or improve their confidence.

While some CAD systems that help to localize abnormalities (e.g. tumors) have already received FDA approvals and started to be 'must-haves' with imaging equipment (e.g. CAD for breast cancer), CADx systems are still mostly in research and development stages. CADx systems, more so than CAD systems, require state-of-the-art thin slice CT scans to perform well. Multiple 3D characterizations of lesions are derived from thin slice CT scans by the CADx systems. This information combined with patient information (e.g. age, sex, family history, cancer history, etc.), findings from molecular imaging, and findings from molecular diagnostics may all be used to build CADx systems that clinicians will use and trust. Desired output of CADx systems include a likelihood estimate of malignancy, or pointers to similar cases with known diagnoses[10].

3.5 Help in staying aware of critical changes

The alarm from the ECG monitor for the patient in MICU room 3 has just gone off for the sixth time in only two hours into your shift. Mr. James has been particularly restless today, and in the previous five times the alarm was caused by artifacts generated by his excessive movement. When the alarm goes off for the sixth time you happen to be on the phone with another patient's cardiologist, one that you have been trying to get a hold of for the past 45 minutes. Do you finish your conversation with the cardiologist or go check out the alarm?

Studies have shown that upwards of 96% of patient monitoring alarms are not significant[11]. Recent studies have shown that utilizing multiple hemo-dynamic signals can be an effective way to screen out many of these false alarms[12]. These so called intelligent alarms can positively impact patient safety and improve the overall clinical workflow.

An example of advanced alarming is an Advanced Event Surveillance (AES) application[13]. This application provides a way for clinicians to correlate parameter information in a way that it is easier to interpret changes in a patient's condition. AES allows the clinician to combine their choice of parameters and set a deviation threshold, combined with delay times. For example: Heart rate 10% change in 60 seconds *or* 6 bpm for 60 seconds.

The resultant type of notification can be selected depending on the severity of condition.

In clinical practice AES can be used by clinicians to enter protocol requirements. An example of this is sepsis. All four physiologic parameters (HR, RR, BP and temperature) recommended by current practice guidelines are routinely available in critical care monitoring. The laboratory parameters of CO_2, WBC and serum lactate that are also part of early identification can be measured easily, quickly and with minimal expense. When used together, this information may provide early recognition of sepsis.

3.6   Help reducing the education and experience required

When seventy-two year old Emily Madison had called into the living room five minutes ago to tell her seventy-six year old husband, Andrew, that dinner was ready, all she heard back was a muffled groan. She just assumed that it was because his beloved Yankees were losing again, and yelled back "just Tivo it and come eat." Now, when she walks in she finds him slumped in his chair and unresponsive. What can she do?

Perhaps the poster child for how decision support can put advanced capabilities into the hands of untrained or minimally trained people is the Automated External Defibrillator (AED) such as the Philips HeartStart Home Defibrillator[14]. AEDs for home use are now available in the United States on-line and in stores without a prescription. Although some training is recommended, most people can operate the HeartStart Home Defibrillator without previous training. From the time the unit is opened, very simple pictures and voice prompts lead the user through each step of its use. Decisions that 15 years ago had to be made by highly trained physicians, nurses, and paramedics, are now made by the AED. The current day user does not have to differentiate between atrial fibrillation and ventricular fibrillation, ventricular tachycardia and asystole, or even know what 200 watts/second is. All this knowledge is built into the AED.

3.7   Help in knowledge discovery

Thousands of patient cases from various ICU facilities at multiple hospitals have been collected into one database. Contained within this database are all the reasons for admissions, monitored data (ECG, SpO2, arterial blood pressure, etc.), medication administrations, lab results, nurses' notes, final outcomes, and more. In this wealth of data, is there new knowledge to be discovered?

Data mining, the analysis of data sets for the purpose of discovering new knowledge, helps in that the knowledge discovered can be used in making subsequent clinical decisions. An example of this is work from Philips Research that uses data mining of large ICU/CCU data sets to help determine the proper parameters for a predictive index of patient instability[15]. Figure 5-1 shows a subset of the types of data that new knowledge will hopefully be drawn from. Methods currently exist for predicting mortality at the time of hospital admission; however, they are not adequate predictors of patient deterioration during the course of stay.

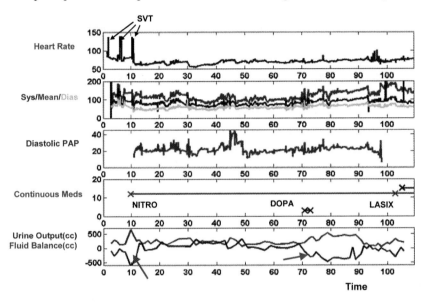

Figure 25-1. Sample of some ICU parameters used in data mining for knowledge discovery.

Two common pathways for a patient's condition to deteriorate in the ICU are single-organ system failure (SOSF) and multi-organ system failure (MOSF). SOSF and MOSF have multiple causes, but all frequently indicate that the patient's condition is worsening, which usually results in a poor outcome. Early identification of SOSF or MOSF by identifying the initial signs of patient deterioration could lead to earlier interventions and in turn, better outcomes. But what are these signs? This is where data mining comes in.

Working with a large database of ICU/CCU patient cases collected from a consortium of Boston area hospitals, universities, and companies, Philips Research performed data mining on the database to discover similarities among patient cases where the patients ended up having SOSF or MOSF. Key to this whole process is that the outcomes of the patients were known.

After applicable verification resulting early indicators can be set up as part of an existing real-time patient monitoring system.

4.   TECHNOLOGIES

Implementing the capabilities described above in the scenarios requires multiple technologies, which can be grouped into two main categories: knowledge discovery, and knowledge representation and interpretation. Far too many technologies exist to cover in this chapter, however we present the goals behind using a class of decision support technology along with a brief mention of some of the algorithms themselves.

4.1   Knowledge discovery from data (KDD)

Knowledge discovery from data, also known as data mining, attempts to find potentially useful relations from data sets, with the goal that discovered knowledge can eventually be used to help predict some medical event. Discovered relationships may or may not be easily understood by humans. Acceptance of new knowledge discovered by some of the various methods discussed below is greater and quicker when the causality between the signs discovered and outcomes observed is easily explained. In other words, there is an explainable mapping from patients' phenotypes to their outcomes. Technologies involved in knowledge discovery for data mining include some combination of databases, statistical analysis, modeling techniques and machine learning. Data mining can be further categorized into algorithm types and specific algorithms as shown in Figure 5-2. The three most common algorithm types are:

Classification and regression: Classification is learning a function that maps (classifies) a data item into one of several pre-defined classes, for example mapping a patient's signs and symptoms onto a specific disease. Regression is learning a function that maps a data item to a real-valued prediction variable, for example determining the predictive value of an antigen from a blood test (like PSA) to the probability of having a disease (prostate cancer).

Clustering: Clustering breaks a set of data records into groups of similar content in such a way that the groups are as dissimilar as possible. Clustering is helpful when the user does not know the nature or structure of the data, and is looking to gain insight into the distribution of the data. It is often used as a pre-processing step for classification algorithms.

Dependency modeling: Dependency modeling attempts to find significant dependencies among variables. A simple example would be, if

82% of the time a patient has a specific blood test come back high, a specific test from urinalysis comes back low. The goal is to find much more complex dependencies than the example, like patient acuity indices.

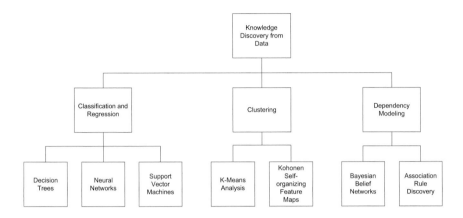

Figure 25-2. Various data mining technologies and representative algorithms.

4.2 Knowledge representation and interpretation

Knowledge representation is about encoding knowledge in an information system in such a way that it can be used later by decision support applications. This goes far beyond storing and retrieving information in/from a database or a data structure in that there is a need for algorithms to interpret the information; it must be understandable to both humans and machines.

Beyond the question of how do you best represent knowledge, is the question of what knowledge do you want to represent, and what do you want to be able to do with it. Four such areas alluded to in Section 3 are:

Differential diagnoses. Determining which of two or more diseases with similar signs and symptoms is currently afflicting the patient is a process that can be aided by algorithms. The type of algorithm to use is dependent on the knowledge known about the patient and the possible diseases. If the causal logic to go from signs and symptoms to diagnosis has been well articulated as a set of rules, then a case-based reasoning system could be the best approach. When the sensitivities and specificities of various tests used to diagnose are well known then a Bayesian Network could offer the best results. When many previous cases with known outcomes are available to learn from, a neural net approach may offer the best results.

Most existing work for CADx follows the same methodology as supervised learning: starting with a collection of data with ground truth, a classifier is trained with the data using a set of features (computed e.g. from diagnostic images) that are believed to have enough discriminant power to distinguish between malignant and benign lesions. Challenges include extracting the features that can discriminate between categories, finding the most relevant features from a feature pool, combining heterogeneous information (e.g. image-based features with patient data), and finding similarity metrics for example-based approaches.

Clinical guidelines. Clinical guidelines along with critical pathways recommend procedural steps and options for next steps based on a patient's condition. Adherence to these guidelines and pathways is generally seen as a way to have more consistent treatment of patients among practitioners and to reduce medical errors. Executable clinical guidelines attempt to follow the course of a patient's care for the purpose of being able to alert users to an action they are about to take that is not the recommended one, advise on what step is next, and to anticipate the care provider's needs for information, order sets, and resources.

Workflow. Closely related to executable clinical guidelines is workflow automation. Whereas clinical guidelines focus on the clinical needs of the patient, workflow focuses on the interaction among care providers, management, and patients. Workflow automation systems allow designers and users to specify actions to automatically take place upon the completion of various tasks. For example, if we look at a patient who has just shown up for an outpatient diagnostic cardiac catheterization, they will first check in at the reception desk. After the receptionist completes this task, notification of the patient's arrival should automatically be sent to the nurse charged with this patient. The nurse may be automatically presented with a task list that specifies steps to take with the patient, like getting a release form signed, drawing blood, obtaining vitals, etc. Any one of these actions, or all of them together may trigger notification of other people that will be involved with the patient to start certain tasks, and so on.

Modeling. Modeling can be used in various ways. One way, not mentioned above, is to help with a differential diagnosis. With a model of a physiological system, patient parameters can be entered into the model to help determine the root cause of why specific parameters are abnormal, like low cardiac output or hypotension. Another use of a physiological model can be to ask 'what if' scenarios. Again the patient's parameters are input to the model, but now we ask "what will happen to this patient if we give him a vasodilator?" or "what will happen to this patient if we reduce the oxygen percentage on her ventilator to 28%?"

5.   IMPEDIMENTS

Medical decision support systems have been around since the 1960's, but the vision from the 60's of what these systems would be doing here in the 21st century is not[16]. Why is this? The following sections present some of the bigger contributing causes.

5.1   Electronic patient record

Access to clinical data in electronic form is essential for creating computer-based decision support systems. Unfortunately this is not the norm. Less than 20% of hospitals are completely digital[17]. Although this situation is a currently a major impediment for decision support systems that require integration of data from all aspects of a patient's care, there are still plenty of opportunities for decision support systems that run on standalone systems or minimally integrated systems, like departmental information systems, lab systems, image review workstations, treatment planning systems, order entry systems, and monitoring systems.

5.2   Standards

Standards like DICOM and HL7 have made great progress in providing standards for many aspects of data capture, storage, and exchange[18,19]. Other standards exist for specialty areas. But even if standards existed for all aspects of clinical care, impediments would still exist:

- Legacy systems may not support standards or the current versions of standards.
- Not all vendors provide solutions that support standards.
- There are multiple standards, sometimes overlapping.
- Standards are continually evolving making today's state-of-the-art systems, tomorrow's legacy systems.
- The granularity of data supported by standards is often too course grained for the requirements of decision support systems. This issue is closely related to the coding of data.

5.3   Coding

Coding is the translation and classification of data, typically from a human readable form to a form that can be processed by a computer. Many coding schemes exist; many overlap, and there are even coding systems that convert from one coding scheme to another. Coding systems suffer from all the impediments of standards, plus more. At first glance it may seem that coding systems excel at coding quantified data like heart rate, blood pressure, ejection fraction, etc., but upon further inspection there are still difficulties. Taking ejection fraction as an example, coding the numbers is easy, but we may need to know by which method was the ejection fraction established (ultrasound, MR, or in a hemodynamic lab), and who or what performed the segmentation? This information may not matter for a specific patient's care, but may matter for a data mining application evaluating the predictive capabilities of ejection fraction as an indicator for a specific condition. Beyond the capabilities of the coding system itself are the difficulties of automating the coding process. Perhaps the most difficult task for automated coding systems is the coding of free text. Without extremely advanced natural language processing capabilities any automated coding system will fail to differentiate the clinical significance of the following two patients' chief complaints: "I get chest pains when I take my dog out for a walk," and "I sometimes get chest pain watching TV."

5.4   Human computer interaction

Like most computer applications, the application's human computer interaction can make or break its acceptance. Many early-day decision support systems failed because of their user interfaces, even though they produced clinically correct and relevant results. Some of the most successful systems of today work almost completely behind the scenes, only becoming apparent upon alert situations. Some of the key issues in designing the human computer interaction of decision support systems are:

- Little to no training should be required to use the system. Designers need to keep in mind that many potential users of a system will not have time to receive training on your (and every other) system in the department. Many nurses work on a per diem basis or are 'floaters' filling in where needed. These people may end up working in a different department each day of the week. Likewise, doctors on rotations, doctors on call, and doctors with practice privileges in multiple hospitals face a similar situation.
- A system must strike the proper balance of being helpful without being annoying. An analogy from the computer world for many is their acceptance of the automatic spell checker with the red underlining of misspelled words, versus their loathing of the 'paperclip guy.'
- A system should improve or fit in as much as possible with normal workflow. A system that requires extra work and/or extra time to use, even if it improves clinical outcomes, will likely be rejected

5.5 Social acceptance

Beyond acceptance of the human computer interface discussed above are other acceptance issues. Key among these is trust. Healthcare professionals will not use decision support systems they don't trust. Trust may come from a number of sources:

- Knowledge of how a systems works, for example knowing and agreeing with the rules a rule-based system uses. (Note that neural network solutions don't meet this requirement and have met reluctance because of it).
- Evidence from clinical trials.
- Positive experience from using the system (the system appears to have both high sensitivity and specificity).
- Recommendations from colleagues and/or professional organizations.

5.6 Costs

Like all other purchases in a professional health care setting, there must be a positive Return on Investment (ROI). With decision support systems the anticipated ROI will be indirect. It is unlikely there will be decision support systems whose use can be directly charged for. A notable exception to this is that the use of certain computer aided detection systems for screening is reimbursable when used as second readers. The return will come from when time saved, errors reduced, training requirements eased, and staffing levels reduced get translated into money.

6. VISION OF THE FUTURE

Our vision of the future for decision support systems is tightly coupled with our vision of the future for electronic patient records. We envision a day when the so-called 'lust to dust' electronic patient records are a reality. Not only would these electronic records store data for the duration of one's life, but they would cover all aspects of your life that contribute to your health and well-being, providing true continuity of care.

Such an electronic patient record capability enables countless decision support possibilities. With proper access to large populations of complete electronic patient records by the medical research community, knowledge discovery through data mining could produce new knowledge at a never-before seen pace. Among the knowledge to be discovered would be early indicators of diseases and conditions. And if genomic data is part of the electronic patient record, personalized medicine will become the norm.

With the electronic patient record being a longitudinal record, guardian angel software could regularly look over the record for early indicators, be they single events, combinations of values, or trends over time. The electronic patient record need not stop with being just a keeper of medical records. Together with new sensors embedded in our everyday clothing and workout clothes, it could also obtain health and wellness data, and fitness data. This further enables applications playing the role of a diet advisor or a fitness coach.

Overall we see decision support adding to the already overwhelming amount of medical knowledge, but still making it easier to practice medicine. Saving time. Saving money. Saving lives. Sense and simplicity.

ACKNOWLEDGEMENTS

The authors of this chapter would like to thank Lilla Boroczky and Larry Eshelman for their contributions to various sections of this chapter. Additionally, we would like to thank Colleen Ennett, Xinxin Zhu, and Larry Eshelman for reviewing earlier versions of this chapter.

REFERENCES

1. *Physicians' Desk Reference*, 59ᵗʰ Edition, (Thomson PDR, 2005).
2. J. Corrigan, L. Kohn, et al., *To Err is Human: Building a Safer Health System*, (National Academy Press, Washington DC, 2000).
3. Institute of Medicine, *Crossing the Quality Chasm: A New Health System for the 21ˢᵗ Century*, (National Academy Press, Washington DC, 2001).
4. Stroke Center Designation and Its Impact on the Practice of Emergency Medicine (2005); http://www.ferne.org/Lectures/aaem_lajolla_0205/bunney_strokecenter_aaem_lajolla_0205.htm.
5. M. Alberts, et al., Recommendations for the Establishment of Primary Stroke Centers, *JAMA* **283**(23), 3102-3109 (2000).
6. L. Sheppard, N. Kouchoukos, M. Kurtis, et al., Automated treatment of critically ill patients following operation, *Ann Surg* **168**, 596-604 (1968).
7. M. Peleg, et al., Comparing Computer-interpretable Guideline Models: A Case-study Approach, *JAMIA* **10**(1), 52-68 (2003).
8. *Cancer Facts and Figures 2005*, (American Cancer Society, Atlanta, 2005).
9. K. Doi, Current status and future potential of computer-aided diagnosis in medical imaging, *The British Journal of Radiology* **78**, S3-S19 (2005).
10. J. Roehrig, The Manufacturer's perspective, *The British Journal of Radiology* **78**, S42-S45 (2005).

11. R. Schoenberg, D. Sands, C. Safran, Making ICU Alarms Meaningful: a comparison of traditional vs. trend-based algorithms, *Proc AMIA Symp*, 379-83 (1999).
12. W. Ali, L. Eshelman, M. Saeed, Identifying Artifacts in Arterial Blood Pressure Using Morphogram Variability, *Computers in Cardiology conference*, 697-700 (2004).
13. Philips Medical Systems, Patient Monitoring – IntelliVue MP40 and MP50 (2005); http://www.medical.philips.com/main/products/patient_monitoring/products.
14. Philips Medical Systems, HeartStart(2005); http://www.heartstarthome.com/content/.
15. G. Moody, R. Mark, A Database to Support Development and Evaluation of Intelligent Intensive Care Monitoring, *Computers in Cardiology* **23**, 657-660 (1996).
16. M. Musen, Y. Shahar, E. Shortliffe, *Medical Informatics: Computer Applications in Health Care and Biomedicine*, edited by E. Shortliffe, et al., 573-609, (Springer, New York, 2001).
17. D. Brailer, E. Terasawa, Use and Adoption of Computer-based Patient Records (2003); http://www.chcf.org/documents/ihealth/UseAdoptionComputerizedPatientRecords.pdf.
18. DICOM – Digital Imaging and Communications in Medicine (2005); http://medical.nema.org/NEMA.
19. Health Level Seven, Inc., Health Level 7 (2005); http://www.hl7.org/.

Chapter 26

BIOINFORMATICS
Overview and Research Opportunities

J. David Schaffer[1], Nevenka Dimitrova[1], Michael Q. Zhang[2]
[1]Philips Research, Briarcliff Manor, NY, USA; [2]Cold Spring Harbor Laboratory, Cold Spring Harbor, NY, USA

Abstract: We present a survey of bioinformatics, first focusing on preclinical research applications where much progress has been made in the last two decades or so. Then we examine clinical applications where there is much excitement about the potential, such as, clinical genotyping, early diagnosis, prognostic disease models, personalized medicine and wellness monitoring. The selection of topics largely reflects our optimism that this potential will begin to be realized in the near future.

Keywords: Sequence analysis, molecular medicine, systems biology, clinical genotyping, early diagnosis, prognostic disease models, personalized medicine, health wellness monitoring

1.   INTRODUCTION

One of the key enabling technologies participating in the genomic medicine revolution has been bioinformatics, or the development of powerful algorithms enabling us to cope with the flood of new molecular information from living systems. It has been argued that the development of the fast sequence matching algorithm BLAST (Basic Local Alignment Search Tool) by Altschul et al.[23] in 1990 was a principle contributor to the rapid advance in molecular biology. Today it is probably the single most used bioinformatic algorithm in the world. Yet, to date, the exciting impacts have been primarily on the basic science, i.e. preclinical. Still there is great optimism that clinical impacts of molecular medicine are to be expected soon, and bioinformatics advances will continue to play a pivotal role. The

G. Spekowius and T. Wendler (Eds.), Advances in Healthcare Technology, 421-438.

spectrum of bioinformatics research and applications is extremely broad, so
we decided to focus on a few topics with potential for clinical impact.

2.   SELECTED PRECLINICAL BIOINFORMATICS TOPICS

2.1   Data collection and dissemination

Bioinformatics is driven by the outpouring of massive genomics data.
The best place to find updated online resources is the two special issues
published annually by Nucleic Acid Research: the January issue is on
databases and the July issue is on Web servers of online analysis tools. The
Bioinformatics Links Directory[1,38] is a good entry point with curated links to
most such molecular resources, tools and databases. The exponential growth
of the sequenced DNAs in the GenBank (Figure 26-1) NCBI[2] repository
nucleotide database is the best testimony of ongoing genomic revolution.
Together with EBI[3] and DDBJ[4], they are the 3 major information databases
in the world, they exchange their sequence data on a daily base to ensure
that the basic sequence information stored in their 'primary databases' are
equivalent. PDB[5] is the biggest repository for 3D bio-macromolecule structure
data.

In addition to basic sequence information there are web resources for the
ever-changing gene nomenclature, HUGO Gene Symbol Database[6], GO[10]
and GeneCards[11], metabolic network information, KEGG[7], and for promoters
and transcription factors, EPD[8] and TRANSFAC[9] respectively.

2.2   Sequence analyses

There are many algorithms in sequence analyses. They may be grouped
by DNA, RNA and protein or single, double, multiple sequence analyses.
Here we only give some typical and yet important examples in each
category.

2.2.1   Comparing sequences

Pairwise comparison and similarity searches: Starting with a molecular sequence, one of the first questions everyone would ask is 'is it similar
or related to a known sequence?' The basic tool is similarity comparison/
alignment; it has three components: a similarity (or distance) measure which
gives a score to a pair of aligned sequences, an objective function to be

optimized and an algorithm to obtain optimal alignment. A scoring matrix provides a numerical value (penalty) to apply to each mutation, be it a deletion, insertion, or substitution. In addition, protein sequence mismatches must account for the similarities/differences of each possible amino acid pair (PAM and BLOSUM matrices). Needleman-Wunsch[54] global alignment algorithm (searching for best alignment of the two entire sequences from the beginnings to ends) and Smith-Waterman[67] local alignment (searching for best subsequence alignment) are best known rigorous (most sensitive) algorithms based on dynamic programming. Since rigorous search is costly, faster approximate algorithms are most often used (e.g. FASTA[58], BLAST[23], BLAT[47]).

Multi- sequence alignment and phylogenetic trees: Aligning multiple sequences is of interest to explore what nucleic acid or protein sequences are most preserved by evolution, thus suggesting critical functions, and may be used to infer the evolutionary distances among species. The optimal alignment of a set of sequences may not contain the optimal pair-wise alignments. ClustalW[73] is the most commonly used program. It uses a progressive method (hierarchical clustering by pairwise alignments) and weights each sequence to reduce redundancy. The recently developed Tcoffee[61] is similar to ClustalW, but it compares segments across the entire sequence set. It can combine sequences and structures, evaluate alignment or integrate several different alignments. Although ClustalW can be used to build phylogenetic trees, Phylip[36] and PAUP[71] are much more accurate, powerful and versatile.

2.2.2 Analyzing DNA sequences

Finding protein coding genes: In bacterial DNA, each protein is encoded by a contiguous fragment called an open reading frame (ORF, beginning with a start codon and ending with a stop codon). In eukaryotes, especially in vertebrates, the coding region is split into several fragments called exons, and the intervening fragments are called introns. Finding eukaryotic protein coding genes is essentially to predict the exon-intron structures. Almost every possible statistical pattern recognition and machine learning algorithms has been applied to this difficult problem (see Zhang[79] for review).

Identification of promoters and transcription factor binding site (TFBS) motifs: In order to study gene regulation and have a better interpretation of microarray expression data, promoter prediction and TFBSs discovery have become important. A number of machine learning approaches that find differences between sets of known promoter and non-promoter sequences have been applied, for example quadratic discriminative analysis

(FirstEF[31]) artificial neural networks (DPF[25], relevance vector machine) and Monte Carlo sampling (Eponine[34]). Because of a lack of protein coding signatures, current promoter predictions are much less reliable than protein coding region predictions, except for CpG island genes (see Bajic et al. 2004[26] for recent review).

Once regulatory regions, such as promoters, are obtained, finding TFBS motifs within these regions may proceed either by enumeration or by alignment to find the enriched motifs (see Tompa et al.[74] for a recent assessment).

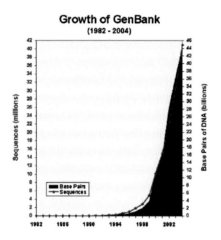

Figure 26-1. Growth of GenBank.

2.3   Microarray analysis

Microarrays typically contain thousands of 'spots' each holding many copies of a different probe molecule (see Figure 26-2). Molecules that were taken from a sample of interest (say tumor cells) and are capable of

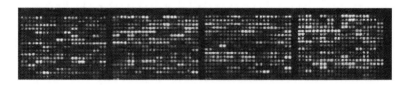

Figure 26-2. A typical microarray.

hybridizing to the probe molecules (cDNA or RNA) are marked with a fluorescent marker and 'washed over' the microarray. Hence, their relative abundance in the sample can be inferred from the luminescence of the spot. Since abundance is relative, a control sample with a contrasting fluorophore is invariably used. By choosing the set of probes, one can assemble a microarray to measure a variety of genetic patterns. The uses of microarrays have expanded from gene-expression profiling (which genes are over/under-expressed in the sample relative to the control) and now include comparing whole genomes (e.g. normal vs. tumor), identifying alternate RNA transcripts, locating genes that have been methylated (turned off by having had methyl groups attached), detecting protein modifications and interactions, and many forms of genotyping. New types of microarrays are still appearing.

2.3.1 Expression microarray analysis

Expression microarrays are used to measure mRNA abundance for large number of genes. The low-level computational tasks[27], such as experimental design and pre-processing (image analysis and normalization), are aimed to reduce uncontrollable sample variations, which may depend on specific types of microarrays. Many data analysis packages can be found from the open source Bioconductor software repository[40].

Normalization: Normalization, critical step for data preprocessing, removes unwanted variances from data by exploiting and enforcing known or assumed invariance of the data[49]. Common approaches include: 1) rescaling by median of all or 'housekeeping' genes or by spike RNA controls, 2) explicit one parameter (log-) or two parameter (asinh-) transformation, 3) local regression smoothing (LOESS), and 4) quantile normalization.

Exploratory analysis: Since the number of genes (measurements) generally far exceeds the number of observations (cases), substantial variable reduction (e.g. low-varying genes filtering) is usually done before any machine learning or statistical algorithms are applied. Exploratory analysis aims to find patterns in the data, common methods include Clustering (genes, cases, or both), Principle Component Analysis (PCA) and Multi-Dimensional Scaling (MDS). Bayesian Networks (BN) have also been used to describe interactions between genes[39].

Identifying differentially expressed genes (DEGs): The most common task of microarray studies is to identify genes that are differentially regulated across different classes of samples; examples are: finding the genes affected by a treatment, or finding marker genes that discriminate cancer from normal tissues. Statistical tests include t-test and permutation test for two groups and

ANOVA/F-test for multi-groups. To correct for multiple testing, often q-value[70] for specifying the smallest False Positive Rate (FPR) is used instead of the conventional p-values. There are also several emerging nonparametric approaches, such as the Empirical Bayes (EB), the Significance Analysis of Microarray (SAM) method and the Mixture Model Method (MMM), seem even more powerful (see e.g. Pan[57] for performance comparison). This is an active research area, a plethora of well-established and new methods are being applied, and a consensus best practice has yet to emerge.

2.3.2   Genomic microarray analysis

Most of the human genome does not express protein ($\approx$98%), so the gene expression microarrays of the previous section, necessarily examine a small fraction of it; hence, the interest in approaches capable of providing a genome-wide view. The major application of genomic microarrays is for localization of DNA binding proteins or for detecting DNA copy number changes, although genomic tiling arrays have also been used to detect novel RNA transcripts[28].

Identification of protein binding sites in chromatin DNA: ChIP-chip is the most popular method for localization of chromatin DNA binding proteins in vivo[43,63]. Combining microarray data (either expression or local-ization data) with promoter analysis for TFBS motif identification is becoming a powerful extension to methods described in section 2.1.2. If positive and negative gene sets extracted from microarray data are available, then motif-discovery turns into a classification problem: identify motifs that best discriminate the two gene sets. If continuous scores are available, then the problem turns into a regression problem: identify motifs that best correlate with these scores. Such analyses are very useful in Gene Regulatory Network (GRN) and Cis Regulatory Modules (CRM) studies[68,44].

Identification of amplification and deletions in the human genome: One of the important applications of genomic arrays in cancer is to detect amplifications (potential oncogene loci) and deletions (potential tumor-suppressor gene loci). ArrayCGH[62] (comparative genomic hybridization) and ROMA[51] (representational oligonucleotide microarray analysis) are two emerging technologies capable of yielding a genome-wide picture of the number of copies of the DNA. The bioinformatics needs include schemes for reducing noise and ways to visualize the enormous amounts of information and focus in on what's of biological significance.

Other types of arrays, such as Alternative Splicing arrays, Protein binding microarray, Protein microarray, Tussie/cell array and microRNA array, etc. are also used. The translation of microarray-based results to clinical applications challenges the technology at all levels. These include robust probe design, uniform sample preparation and increased reproducibility of array measurements as well as advanced data analysis tools (see e.g. Segal et al.[65] for new computational challenges). The recent advances in genomic sciences and array technologies are accelerating the translation of microarrays to clinical applications and will offer enormous potential for improved health care in cancer and a other human diseases.

2.4   Systems biology

Biologists have elucidated the complete gene sequences of several model organisms and provided general understanding of the molecular machinery involved in gene expression. The next logical step is to understand how all the components interact with each other in order to model complex biological systems. It is envisioned that only with this 'systems view' will we improve the accuracy of our diagnostic and therapeutic endeavors.

The field of systems biology emerged at the turn of this century and aims to merge our piecemeal knowledge into comprehensive models of the whole dynamic of these systems. The challenge is daunting; considering the potential of serum proteomics, Weston and Hood[77] warn:

"In addition to the immense repertoire of proteins present, the dynamic range of these proteins is on the order of 10^9, with serum albumin being most abundant (30-50 mg/mL) and low-level proteins such as interleukin-6 present at 0-5 pg/mL)... Identifying proteins at each end of this spectrum in a single experiment is not feasible with current technologies."

"Further complicating the study of the human plasma proteome are temporal and spatial dynamics. The turnover of some proteins is several fold faster than others, and the protein content of the arteries may differ substantially from that of the veins, or the capillary proteome may be specific to its location, etc."

The goal of gene and protein networks research is to quantitatively understand how different genes and their regulating proteins are grouped together in genetic circuits, and how stochastic fluctuations influence gene expression in these complex systems. For example, Thattai and van Oudenaarden[72] focus on the importance of noise in the expression of genes by using both experimental and theoretical approaches. They investigated the bistability that arises from a positive feedback loop in the lactose utilization network of E. Coli. In its simplest form, the network may be modeled as a single positive feedback loop: Lactose uptake induces the synthesis of lactose permease, which in turn promotes the further uptake of lactose. Because of this bistability, the response of a single cell to an external inducer depends on whether the cell had been induced recently, a phenomenon known as hysteresis. The question is how the gene network architecture helps cells remember their history for more than 100 cell generations.

The field is still new, but the reader may find tutorials and pointers to emerging modeling efforts at the web sites of three major systems biology organizations: Europe[12], USA[13] and Japan[14]. In addition, several projects are now ongoing to build models of at least part of the living cell: *The Silicon Cell*[15], *The Virtual Cell*[16], and *E-Cell*[17], and to provide open source tools for this effort[18].

3.   SELECTED CLINICAL BIOINFORMATICS TOPICS

3.1   Clinical genotyping

A dream of long-standing has been the possibility that predisposition to disease and therapy response may be predictable from a person's genome. The well-known link between mutations in the BRCA1/2 genes and breast cancer predisposition[48], and the more recent link between a mutation in the EGFR gene and response to the drug Iressa[56] are just two examples of the results that have encouraged the enthusiasm. The approach proposed is the 'association study' in which the genomes are sequenced from a group of people known to be in a phenotypic group (e.g. prone to disease, responsive to therapy) and those not in this group. The strength of association between a proposed genetic pattern and the phenotypic trait is measured by a simple chi squared type statistic. Operational questions that need to be addressed to advance this paradigm include: how are gene sequences measured, how are candidate genetic patterns selected for testing, what statistical safeguards are needed to minimize false positives and negatives, and how to get the biological validation.

Sequencing an entire genome is both expensive[66] and largely unnecessary. This is because 99.9% of the human genome is common to us all. Hence, interest has focused on Single Nucleotide Polymorphisms (SNPs), or differences of one nucleotide at one locus. Accumulating knowledge of SNPs in the human genome is available from the NCBI (dbSNP[19]) that currently contains over ten million reference SNPs, about half validated. The level of interest may also be gaged by observing that a recent study[45] lists 30 companies with SNP-technology offerings. Hence, there appear to be too many potential genetic variants to make genome-wide association studies practical. Schemes for reducing the numbers of candidates include focusing only on SNPs in protein coding regions and on 'non-synonymous' SNPs (i.e. SNPs that alter the amino acid). Such approaches depend on the common-variant/common-disease (CVCD) hypothesis. Additional help for this paradigm may come as knowledge of which non-synonymous SNPs are most likely to produce deleterious protein alterations and algorithms that exploit this knowledge are being developed. This is referred to as the 'direct' approach[30] and is expected to yield results for single-gene disorders.

An 'indirect' approach involves defining haplotypes. These are sets of SNPs at different loci located in close proximity on the same chromosome; they tend to be inherited as a unit. That is, they exhibit 'linkage disequilibrium' (LD). Hence, the haplotype and not the individual SNPs is proposed as the effective unit of genotype characterization, greatly reducing the combinatorics. Identifying haplotypes poses experimental and bioin-formatic challenges. Some propose family studies, as a way to identify haplotypes related to diseases and their LD, wherein parents and offspring in families with disease prevalence are carefully studied. In contrast, population studies involve collecting genotypes from a suitable sample from, say different ethnic groups, and applying pattern discovery algorithms to locate suitable haplotypes. The HapMap project[20] is an international collaborative project to collect data on about 270 individuals in five populations groups and information on about 600,000 SNPs and make it publicly available. Unsupervised learning algorithms for inferring haplotypes include: The Clark algorithm[29] that begins with one or more homozygous individuals (or heterozygous at at most one locus – a problem for some datasets) and builds its initial haplotype set. It then adds the heterozygous individuals and extends the set as needed only to cover them (a parsimony criterion). Some genotypes may be left unassigned to haplotypes in some datasets. Expectation Minimization (EM) algorithms (e.g. Escoffier et al.[35]) make an initial guess at haplotype frequencies and iteratively converge (with reasonable probability) so all genotypes are assigned. EM algorithms can be computationally challenged by large datasets. Bayesian approaches have been reported to perform better than the previous two classes[69], but all these approaches may fail to exploit some genetic alterations.

Two additional bioinformatics challenges involving haplotypes are the search for haplotype blocks (larger SNP regions that still may satisfy LD criteria[80]) and the location of minimal sets of SNPs that may serve to identify the different genotypes (called tagSNPs). Good haplotype blocks would further reduce the combinatorics of genotype candidates that need to be considered and tagSNPs would reduce the amount of DNA that is needed to genotype new individuals. For a discussion of algorithms for tagSNP identification and the issues related to them (see Crawford and Nickerson[30]).

Clearly, genotype-disease association discovery faces many challenges, substantial population samples and careful matching of controls may be needed as the haplotypes discovered in stratified samples often exhibit substantial differences – genotypes that are meaningful and practical will take work to identify. DNA sequencing measurements are still costly. There appears to be significant opportunities for improved algorithms; for example, complex diseases may resist current approaches calling for more sophisticated pattern discovery methods. Algorithms for the 'static pattern discovery' paradigm discussed in the following section probably apply; genetic algorithms have barely been applied in this domain so far[24].

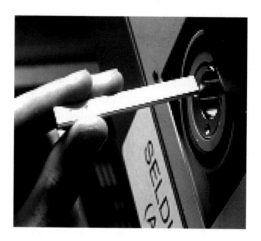

Figure 26-3. A SELDI (surface enhanced laser desorption ionization) chip being inserted into a mass spectrograph.

3.2 Early diagnoses

With the advent of new measurement devices for nucleic acids (e.g. microarrays) and proteins (e.g. mass spectroscopy Figure 26-3), many attempts are being made to discover new diagnostic tests capable of detecting disease much earlier than previously possible[59,76]. The usual protocol involves collecting an array of measurements on a number of patients known to be in one of two (or sometimes more) clinical conditions, say known to be positive or negative for cancer. The bioinformatics challenge is to discover the 'fingerprint' of the disease, the pattern of biomarkers that can be used for diagnosis. Let us call this the static pattern recognition task because the data consist of a single snapshot taken at one instant of time. The methods for DEGs (see section 2.1.3) clearly apply here.

In spite of the promise, this paradigm is fraught with problems and critics have not been shy about pointing them out. Measurement repeatability, normalization of data, the curse of the small clinical samples (not containing enough of the population variability), too many measurements (overfitting risk), poor cross validation (overoptimistic predictions)[53,32]. We take the optimistic position that such difficulties are to be expected with a newly emerging technology and focus on some of the efforts aimed at overcoming each specific challenge.

Probably the most severe challenge is to increase the accuracy of the measurements themselves. While this effort is primarily concerned with the physics and biology of the devices, and recipes for sample preparation (e.g. Saul et al.[64]), there is also a role here for bioinformatics in data normalization. For cDNA microarrays, methods to deal with spatial biases have been recently proposed[78]. For mass spectroscopy, normalization usually at least includes total ion current normalization to correct for differences in overall spectrum intensity. More controversial is within-spectrum normalization[60] wherein the selected measurements are linearly scaled to [0,1] in order to preserve only the relative protein abundances. Another issue with MS data is the choice to do peak identification (requiring specifying a noise cutoff) or binning (merging adjacent intensities to reflect machine precision).

A major bioinformatics issue in this emerging field is how to cope with these datasets that are measurement-rich, but case-poor. One traditional approach to this is to reduce the number of measurements (see section 2.1.3) either by filtering out those that fail to meet some specified criteria of 'signal' (e.g. using a signal to noise cutoff, and/or a cutoff of likelihood that the measurement means are different between the two groups), or by using principle components analysis (PCA). One difficulty with PCA is that results may be difficult to interpret biologically. An alternative approach is sometimes called a 'wrapper' approach in which the space of possible measurement subsets is searched using some form of gradient descent or evolutionary search algorithm, wherein the worth of any proposed subset is evaluated by inducing a classifier and testing its classification accuracy. A risk with the former is the possibility of missing patterns that include measurements that are not strongly discriminating by themselves. The risk with the wrapper approaches is the possibility of discovering patterns that overexploit chance variance in the small samples (overfitting). One method strongly recommended to avoid overfitting is cross-validation. Unfortunately, the scope for cross-validation is severely hampered by the small sample sizes. Michaels et al.[53] have shown how sensitive are the discovered patterns to the specific set of learning cases used. Another issue involves whether or not to use correlated measurements in a classifier. Arguments based upon Vapnik's approach to structured risk minimization[75] dictate the use of the smallest measurement sets that do the job. Another informatics approach to this is an 'ensemble' approach[33] wherein multiple classifiers are derived and the final decision comes from some form of voting scheme (e.g. weighted sum) among them. Another key decision required in a wrapper approach is the choice of classifier. The arguments from risk minimization for using the simplest effective classifier entail assumptions about the homogeneity of the disease classes that in some cases are clearly unsupportable.

In the end, what is an investigator to do? We conjecture that none of the early studies, that have done so much to show the potential and stir excitement, will be shown to have located the best diagnostics. We believe the way forward will be found by a community-wide effort that involves incremental improvements in the measurement devices, careful bioinformatics that lead to new hypotheses about disease mechanisms, and larger studies that include more of the inherent disease variability (and the natural inter-personal variance) and that exploit better screening to reduce the variability that can be controlled.

3.3   Prognostic disease models

The use of modeling in medicine has a long history. Prognostic models have been developed from early 'illness scores' initially devised by experts to try to predict disease outcomes. Later these models used regression methods that required increasing amounts of data. These models may be considered 'static.' Dynamic models have been used in epidemiology for a long time and in the modeling of physiological systems[52] like the cardiovascular[42]. But there is a new opportunity just emerging in this era of molecular medicine: the building of systems biology models (see section 2.1.4) that capture the dynamics of disease at the molecular/cellular level and applying them to medical diagnosis and/or prognosis. In distinction from the 'static pattern recognition' problem mentioned above (see section 2.2.2), this approach is a 'dynamic pattern recognition' task. As such, it requires a series of vectors of measurements taken across the time course of disease.

Without loosing sight of the challenges already mentioned (see section 2.1.4), Weston and Hood[77] also opine that networks have key nodal points where therapy/intervention can effectively be focused. While there are not concrete clinical applications yet, the promise is clear.

3.4   Personalized medicine

The aim of personalized medicine is to find the right therapy for individual patients based on their genotype, environment and lifestyle. A tantalizing example is the Iressa story[56]. It works miraculously for about 10% of the patients with advanced non-small cell lung cancer, those with a mutation of the epidermal growth factor receptor EGFR gene. This dream obviously depends on the maturation of much that has been covered above. In a broad sense, it includes development of genomics-based personalized medicines, predisposition testing (see section 2.2.1), preventive medicine, combination of diagnostics (see section 2.2.2) with therapeutics, and monitoring of therapy. But an additional bioinformatics challenge, not mentioned above will be Clinical Decision Support Systems (CDSS) able to distill the voluminous and complex data into actionable clinical recommendations, whether it is preventive, diagnostic, or therapeutic[41]. CDSS involves linking two types of information: patient-specific and knowledge-based[37]. Personal information related to the patient history is documented in patient records. Some personal medical documents, which are already in use to various extents in different countries, include the personal emergency card, the mother-child record, and the vaccination certificate. A promising source of personal medical information is the data stored in the electronic patient record combined with the genomic information from genotyping and from particular molecular diagnostic tests. Molecular imaging enables visualization of cellular and molecular processes that may be used to infer information about the genomic and proteomic profiles. As a result, the bioinformatic analysis of genomic and proteomic profiles may be valuable to assist the interpretation of images using molecular probes. Molecular diagnostics and molecular imaging can provide the two aspects of the disease: molecular diagnostics can provide the information of the exact mutation of a particular gene and classify the exact type of cancer, while molecular imaging can target the very same type of cells with that particular mutation in order to provide diagnostic information and disease staging.

3.5   Health and wellness monitoring

Current methods in bioinformatics have been used for immediate impact in diseases that are at the top of the killer list: heart disease and cancer. However, these technologies may also enable non-invasive and inexpensive first indicators that a regular person is becoming a patient. Nutritional genomics studies the genome-wide influences of nutrition, with a far-reaching potential in the prevention of nutrition-related disease. Nutrition is not like pharmacology or toxicology, where the drug acts upon a single receptor/target and dose related pathological effects are induced with related strong effects on transcriptomic changes. Our daily food consumption consists of complex mixtures of many possibly bioactive chemical compounds, chronically administered in varying composition, and with a multitude of biological reactions based on our genotype.

The role of bioinformatics in nutrigenomics is multifold: to create nutrigenomic databases, to setup special ontologies in using available resources, setup and track laboratory samples being tested and their results, pattern recognition, classification, and data mining, and simulation of complex interactions between genomes, nutrition, and health disparities[21].

A key objective is the development of tools to identify selective and sensitive multi-parameter (pathway supported) biomarkers of prevention (transcriptomic and metabolic profiles or fingerprints) based on the perturbation of homeostasis[22].

Nutrigenomics research will have a profound impact on our understanding of the relationship between the genotype and the environment. The nutritional supplement and functional food industries will continue robust growth in response to advances in nutritional genomics research and its applications [46,55].

4.   CONCLUSIONS

Today we are in the midst of the genomic medicine revolution. This revolution has been sparked by a plethora of new technologies for measuring, analyzing, understanding and manipulating events at the level of biomolecules both in vitro and in vivo. In this chapter we highlighted bioinformatics methods that are at the heart of genomic medicine.

Among the envisioned benefits of this new era are personalized medicine that enables tailoring of therapy to the patient's own unique disease taking genomic information into account. This starts with a scenario where genotyping is available at birth; the phenotype is matched with the genotype in order to propose best diet and lifestyle for optimum health. In addition, personalized medicine will introduce new diagnostics capable of detecting disease as soon as the molecular events begin and long before symptoms are manifest, and therapies capable of correcting the basic biological malfunctions that are the disease by for instance replacing mutated genes or inserting palliative molecules that can compensate for disrupted cell signaling pathways.

REFERENCES

1. http://bioinformatics.ubc.ca/resources/links_directory/.
2. http://www.ncbi.nlm.nih.gov/.
3. http://www.ebi.ac.uk/.
4. http://www.ddbj.nig.ac.jp/.
5. http://www.rcsb.org/pdb/.
6. http://www.gene.ucl.ac.uk/nomenclature/.
7. http://www.genome.ad.jp/kegg/.
8. http://www.epd.isb-sib.ch/.
9. http://www.gene-regulation.de/.
10. http://www.geneontology.org/.
11. http://bioinfo1.weizmann.ac.il/genecards/index.shtml.
12. http://www.systembiology.net/.
13. http://www.systemsbiology.org/.
14. http://www.systems-biology.org/.
15. http://www.siliconcell.net/.
16. http://www.nrcam.uchc.edu/.
17. http://www.e-cell.org/.
18. https://biospice.org/index.php.
19. http://www.ncbi.nlm.nih.gov/SNP/.
20. http://www.hapmap.org/.
21. http://nutrigenomics.ucdavis.edu/bioinformatics.htm.
22. http://www.nugo.org/wp7.
23. S.F. Altschul, W. Gish, W. Miller, E.W. Myers, D.J. Lipman, Basic local alignment search tool, *J Mol Biol* **215**(3), 403-10 (1990).
24. O. Braaten, O.K. Rodningen, I. Nordal, T.P. Leren, The genetic algorithm applied to haplotype data at the LDL receptor locus, *Comput Methods Programs Biomed* **6**(1), 1-9 (2000).
25. V.B. Bajic, S.H. Seah, A. Chong, G. Zhang, J.L. Koh, V. Brusic, Dragon Promoter Finder: recognition of vertebrate RNA polymerase II promoters, *Bioinformatics* **18**(1), 198-199 (2002).
26. V.B. Bajic, S.L. Tan, Y. Suzuki, S. Sugano, Promoter prediction analysis on the whole human genome. *Nat Biotechnol* **22**(11), 1467-1473 (2004).
27. B.M. Bolstad, F. Collin, K.M. Simpson, R.A. Irizarry, T.P. Speed, Experimental design and low-level analysis of microarray data, *Int Rev Neurobiol* **60**, 25-58 (2004).
28. J. Cheng, P. Kapranov, J. Drenkow, S. Dike, S. Brubaker, S. Patel, J. Long, D. Stern, H. Tammana, G. Helt, V. Sementchenko, A. Piccolboni, S. Bekiranov, D.K. Bailey, M. Ganesh, S. Ghosh, I. Bell, D.S. Gerhard, T.R. Gingeras, Transcriptional maps of 10 human chromosomes at 5-nucleotide resolution, *Science* **308**(5725), 1149-1154 (2005).
29. A.G. Clark, Inference of haplotypes from PCR-amplified samples of diploid populations, *Molecular Biology Evol* **7**, 111-122 (1990).
30. D.C. Crawford, D.A. Nickerson, Definition and Clinical Importance of Haplotypes, *Annual Rviews in Medicine* **56**, 303-320 (2005).
31. R.V. Davuluri, MQ Zhang, Computational identification of promoters and first exons in the human genome, *Nat Genet* **29**(4), 412-417 (2001).
32. E. Diamandis, Proteomic patterns in biological fluids: do they represent the future of cancer diagnostics? *Clin Chem* **49**, 1272-1275 (2003).
33. T.G. Dietterich, Ensemble Methods in machine learning, *Lecture Notes in Computer Science* **1857**, 1-15 (Springer, New York, 2000).

34. T.A. Down, T.J. Hubbard, Computational detection and location of transcription start sites in mammalian genomic DNA, *Genome Re*s **12**(3), 458-461 (2002).

35. L. Excoffier, G. Laval, D. Balding, Gametic phase estimation over large genomicregions using an adaptive window approach, *Human Genomics* **1**, 7-19 (2003).

36. J. Felsenstein, Evolutionary trees from DNA sequences: a maximum likelihood approach, *J Mol Evol* **17**(6), 368-376 (1981).

37. W. Fierz, Challenge of personalized health care: to what extent is medicine already individualized and what are the future trends? *Med Sci Monit* **10**(5), RA111-1123 (2004).

38. J.A. Fox, S.L. Butland, S. McMillan, G. Campbell, B.F. Ouellette, The Bioinformatics Links Directory: a compilation of molecular biology web servers, *Nucleic Acids Res* **1**(33)(Web Server issue), W3-24 (2005).

39. N. Friedman, M. Linial, I. Nachman, D. Pe'er, Using Bayesian networks to analyze expression data, *J Comput Biol* **7**(3-4), 601-620 (2000).

40. R.C. Gentleman, V.J. Carey, D.M. Bates, B. Bolstad, M. Dettling, S. Dudoit, B. Ellis, L. Gautier, Y. Ge, J. Gentry, K. Hornik, T. Hothorn, W. Huber, S. Iacus, R. Irizarry, F. Leisch, C. Li, M. Maechler, A.J. Rossini, G. Sawitzki, C. Smith, G. Smyth, L. Tierney, J.Y. Yang, J. Zhang, Bioconductor: open software development for computational biology and bioinformatics, *Genome Biol* **5**(10), R80 (2004).

41. A.G. Guttmacher, F.S. Collins, Genomic Medicine – A Primer, *New England Journal of Medicine* **19**, 1512-1520 (2002).

42. T. Heldt, Computational Models of Cardiovascular response to Orthostatic Stress, PhD. Thesis, MIT (2004).

43. C.E. Horak, M. Snyder, ChIP-chip: a genomic approach for identifying transcription factor binding sites, *Methods Enzymol* **350**, 469-483 (2002).

44. S. Istrail, E.H. Davidson, Logic functions of the genomic cis-regulatory code, *Proc Natl Acad Sci USA* **102**(14), 4954-4959 (2005).

45. K.K. Jain, *Personalized Medicine: Scientific & Commercial Aspects* (Jain Pharma Biotech, Basel, 2005).

46. *Nutritional Genomics: Discovering the Path to Personalized Nutrition*, edited by J. Kaput, R.L. Rodriguez, ISBN: 0-471-68319-1 (Wiley, 2000).

47. W.J. Kent, BLAT–the BLAST-like alignment tool, *Genome Res* **12**(4), 656-664 (2002).

48. M.C. King, J.H. Marks, J.B. Mandell, Breast and ovarian cancer risks due to inherited mutations in BRCA1 and BRCA2, *Science* **302**(5645), 643-646 (2003).

49. D.P. Kreil, R.R. Russell, There is no silver bullet–a guide to low-level data transforms and normalisation methods for microarray data, *Brief Bioinform* **6**(1), 86-97 (2005).

50. C.E. Lawrence, S.F. Altschul, M.S. Boguski, J.S. Liu, A.F. Neuwald, J.C. Wootton., Detecting subtle sequence signals: a Gibbs sampling strategy for multiple alignment. *Science* **262**(5131), 208-214 (1993).

51. R. Lucito, J. Healy, J. Alexander, A. Reiner, D. Esposito, M. Chi, L. Rodgers, A. Brady, J. Sebat, J. Troge, J.A. West, S. Rostan, K.C. Nguyen, S. Powers, K.Q. Ye, A. Olshen, E. Venkatraman, L. Norton, M. Wigler, Representational oligonucleotide microarray analysis: a high-resolution method to detect genome copy number variation, *Genome Res* **13**(10), 2291-2305 (2003).

52. V.Z. Marmarelis, *Nonlinear Dynamic Modeling of Physiological Systems* (Wiley IEEE Press Series, 2004).

53. S. Michiels, S. Koscielny, C. Hill, Prediction of cancer outcome with microarrays: a multiple random validation strategy, *The Lancet* **365**, 488-492 (2005).

54. S.B. Needleman, C.D. Wunsch, A general method applicable to the search for similarities in the amino acid sequence of two proteins, *J Mol Biol* **48**(3), 443-453 (1970).

55. J.M. Ordovas, L. Parnell, *Nutrigenetics and Nutrigenomics*, ISBN: 0-471-68421-X (Josey Bass Publishers, 2005).
56. J.G. Paez, P.A. Janne, J.C. Lee, S. Tracy, H. Greulich, S. Gabriel, P. Herman, F.J. Kaye, N. Lindeman, T.J. Boggon, K. Naoki, H. Sasaki, Y. Fujii, M.J. Eck, W.R. Sellers, B.E. Johnson, M. Meyerson, EGFR Mutations in Lung Cancer: Correlation with Clinical Response to Gefitinib Therapy, *Science* **304**(5676), 1497-1500 (2004).
57. W. Pan, On the use of permutation in and the performance of a class of nonparametric methods to detect differential gene expression, *Bioinformatics* **19**(11), 1333-1340 (2003).
58. W.R. Pearson, D.J. Lipman, Improved tools for biological sequence comparison, *Proc Natl Acad Sci USA* **85**(8), 2444-2448 (1988).
59. E.F. Petricoin, A.M. Ardekani, B.A. Hitt, P.J. Levine, V.A. Fusaro, S.M. Steinberg, G.B. Mills, C. Simone, D.A. Fishman, E.C. Kohn, L.A. Liotta, Use of proteomic patterns in serum to identify ovarian cancer, *The Lancet* **359**, 572-577 (2002).
60. E.F. Petricoin, L. Liotta, SELDI-TOF-based serum proteomic pattern diagnostics for early detection of cancer, *Current Opinion in Biotechnology* **15**, 24-30 (2004).
61. O. Poirot, E. O'Toole, C. Notredame, Tcoffee@igs: A web server for computing, evaluating and combining multiple sequence alignments, *Nucleic Acids Res* **31**(13), 3503-3506 (2003).
62. D. Pinkel, R. Segraves, D. Sudar, S. Clark, I. Poole, D. Kowbel, C. Collins, W.L. Kuo, C. Chen, Y. Zhai, S.H. Dairkee, B.M. Ljung, J.W. Gray, D.G. Albertson, High resolution analysis of DNA copy number variation using comparative genomic hybridization to microarrays, *Nat Genet* **20**(2), 207-211 (1998).
63. B. Ren, B.D. Dynlacht, Use of chromatin immunoprecipitation assays in genome-wide location analysis of mammalian transcription factors, *Methods Enzymol* **376**, 304-315 (2004).
64. R. Saul, P. Russo, S. Seminara, N. Shea, L. Harvey, G. Whiteley, Development of an Automated, Mass Spec-based Clinical Diagnostic System for the Detection of Ovarian Cancer, *ALAM, San Jose* (2005).
65. E. Segal, N. Friedman, N. Kaminski, A. Regev, D. Koller, From signatures to models: understanding cancer using microarrays, *Nat Genet* **37**(Suppl.), S38-S45 (June 2005).
66. J. Shendure, R.D. Mitra, C. Varma, G.M. Church, Advanced Sequencing Technologies: Methods and Goals, *Nature Genetics* **5**, 335-344 (2004).
67. T.F. Smith, M.S. Waterman, Identification of common molecular subsequences, *J Mol Biol* **147**(1), 195-197 (1981).
68. B. van Steensel, Mapping of genetic and epigenetic regulatory networks using microarrays, *Nat Genet* 37(Suppl.), S18-S24 (2005).
69. M. Stephens, N.J. Smith, P. Donnelly, A new statistical method for haplotype reconstruction from population data, *Am J Human Genetics* **68**, 978–989 (2001).
70. J.D. Storey, R. Tibshirani, Statistical significance for genomewide studies, *Proc Natl Acad Sci USA* **100**(16), 9440-9445 (2003).
71. D.L. Swofford, *PAUP*. Phylogenetic Analysis Using Parsimony (*and Other Methods)* (Sinauer Associates, Sunderland, MA, Version 4.0b10a, 1998).
72. M. Thattai, A. van Oudenaarden, Attenuation of noise in ultrasensitive signaling cascades, *Biophysical Journal* **82**, 2943 (2002).
73. J.D. Thompson, D.G. Higgins, T.J. Gibson, CLUSTAL W: improving the sensitivity of progressive multiple sequence alignment through sequence weighting, position-specific gap penalties and weight matrix choice, *Nucleic Acids Res* **22**(22), 4673-4680 (1994).
74. M. Tompa, N. Li, T.L. Bailey, G.M. Church, B. De Moor, E. Eskin, A.V. Favorov, M.C. Frith, Y. Fu, W.J. Kent, V.J. Makeev, A.A. Mironov, W.S. Noble, G. Pavesi, G. Pesole, M. Regnier, N. Simonis, S. Sinha, G. Thijs, J. van Helden, M. Vandenbogaert, Z. Weng,

C. Workman, C. Ye, Z. Zhu, Assessing computational tools for the discovery of transcription factor binding sites, *Nat Biotechnol* **23**(1), 137-144 (2005).

75. V.N. Vapnik, *The nature of statistical learning theory* (Springer, New York, 1995).

76. L.J. van't Veer, H. Dai, M.J. van de Vijver, Y.D. He, A.A.M. Hart, M. Mao, H.L. Peterse, K. van der Kooy, M.J. Marton, A.T. Witteveen, G.J. Schreiber, R.M. Kerkhoven, C. Roberts, P. S. Linsley, R. Bernards, S.H Friend, Gene expression profiling predicts clinical outcome of breast cancer, *Nature* **415**, 530-536 (2002).

77. A.D. Weston, L. Hood, Systems biology, proteomics, and the future of health care: toward predictive, preventative, and personalized medicine, *J Proteome Res* **3**(2), 179-196 (2004).

78. Y.H. Yang, S. Dudoit, P. Luu, D.M. Lin, V. Peng, J. Ngai, T.P. Speed, Normalization for cDNA microarray data: A robust composite method addressing single and multiple slide systematic variation, *Nucleic Acid Research* **30**(4), e15 (2002).

79. M.Q. Zhang, Computational prediction of eukaryotic protein-coding genes, *Nat Rev Genet* **3**(9), 698-709 (2002).

80. X. Zhu, S. Zhang, D. Kan, R. Cooper, Haplotype Block definition and its application, *Pacific Symposium on Biocomputing* **9**, 152-163 (2004).

PART VI: PERSONAL HEALTHCARE

Chapter 27

PERSPECTIVES IN PERSONAL HEALTHCARE
Towards Patient Centric Care

Thomas Zaengel, Eric Thelen, Jeroen Thijs
Philips Research, Aachen, Germany

Abstract: Future healthcare scenarios will increasingly extend from acute care towards prevention and from institutional points-of-care into personal environments. Individuals will take increasing responsibility for managing their own health. We present and analyze trends towards personal healthcare and describe current approaches as well as future visions for healthcare in the 21st century.

Keywords: Aging population, chronic diseases, risk factors, major diseases, prevention, disease management, remote monitoring, aftercare, rehabilitation, activity

1.   VISION

Future healthcare scenarios will more and more include elements of monitoring and therapy outside institutional points-of-care, i.e. healthcare will continue to extend into personal and private environments both for managing risk factors (primary prevention) as well as chronical conditions (secondary prevention). Personal healthcare will take place in the patient's home and will still accompany the patient by means of mobile solutions when on the move.

With prevention becoming increasingly part of the overall healthcare strategy, everyone will regularly be involved – as a 'consumer', before ever becoming a 'patient'. The responsibility of the individual for his or her health status will continue to grow.

This vision is supported by several major worldwide trends:

- **Increased life expectancy** results from continuous advances in healthcare. Today, we are likely to survive many diseases that still were life threatening before. This not only implies that we will live longer, but also that we will acquire more (often chronic and/or degenerative)

439

G. Spekowius and T. Wendler (Eds.), Advances in Healthcare Technology, 439-462.
© 2006 *Springer. Printed in the Netherlands.*

diseases over time, increasing the overall load on our healthcare systems and requiring new ways of effective long-term disease management.

- The availability of more advanced healthcare options comes at a price. Optimum healthcare continues to become ever more **expensive** with the consequence that **healthcare systems** will have to seek more cost-effective solutions, without compromising the quality-of-care. Lower acuity settings including increasing participation of the individual in managing his or her own health status will become mandatory.
- **More information than ever** on health related matters (e.g. risk factors, symptoms, treatment options and progression expectations) has become available through the modern media, including the Internet. Today, the average person is also much better informed about health issues, leading to pro-active consumer behavior and the development of consumer driven healthcare markets.
- Effective prevention and management of many health problems of today require a **change in lifestyle**. This will have to take place in the individual personal environment at home and away, by conscious adaptation of consumer behavior, supported by proper technologies.

Personal healthcare represents a wide space of opportunities and applications. After looking into some relevant trends and statistic in more detail we will give in the final section of this chapter a first outlook on this opportunity space. The following chapters will then address a number of specific opportunities and technologies in more detail.

2.   TRENDS & STATISTICS

In this section, a number of trends related to personal healthcare are presented together with illustrative data points.

2.1   Aging population

The average age of the population is increasing significantly, not only in the developed countries. Figure 27-1 shows the percentage of the world population aged 60 years and older.

The most prominent reasons for this development are:

- Better working conditions.
- Better nutrition.
- Better health care delivery for a broad population.
- Behavioral/lifestyle changes (e.g. reduction in smoking).

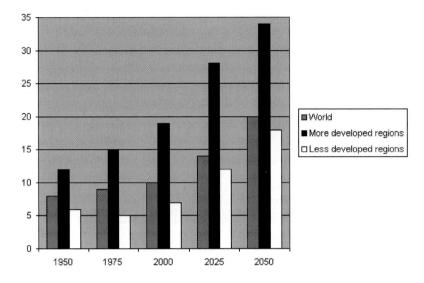

Figure 27-1. Percentage of population aged 60 years and older, between 1950 and 2050[1].

In addition to the increase in life expectancy the decrease of birth rates especially in Europe and Japan increases further the ratio between retired population and working population. In China, this ratio is also expected to increase further due to the introduction of the one-child policy in 1979.

The following facts about the aging population provide a remarkable challenge to the worldwide healthcare systems:

- Population aging is unprecedented in history; the 21st century will witness even more rapid aging than the previous century.
- Population aging is enduring. We will not return to the young populations that our ancestors knew.
- Population aging is pervasive; it is a problem of all world countries, developed as well as non-developed.
- The proportion of older persons is projected to more than double worldwide over the next half century.
- In 2050, up to 33% of the population will be 60+ in developed countries.

In Figure 27-2 the world map shows the development of the percentage of the population aged 60 and older on a per country basis until 2050.

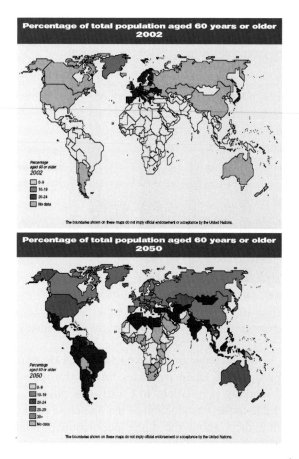

Figure 27-2. Percentage of population aged 60 years and older[2].

2.2   Growth of chronic diseases

As a result of the aging population and the limitations to fundamentally/ completely cure degenerative diseases (but rather turn them into manageable conditions), the world will see an increase of chronic, non-communicable diseases in the coming decades. Chronic diseases are the major cost drivers in the current healthcare system. Therefore cost of and spending on healthcare will substantially increase.

A chronic condition is defined as a health problem that lasts a year or longer, limits what one can do and may require ongoing care. According to the Partnership for Solutions[3], a US based policy research program based at Johns Hopkins University, more than 125 million Americans have at least one chronic condition and 60 million people have multiple conditions. In terms of the American workforce, this translates into a full 40% of employees having at least one chronic health condition. Furthermore, it is projected that by the year 2020, 25% of the American population will be living with multiple chronic conditions, and costs for managing these conditions are estimated to reach $1.07 trillion. The number of people with chronic diseases is expected to increase by more than one percent each year through 2030, as shown in Figure 27-3.

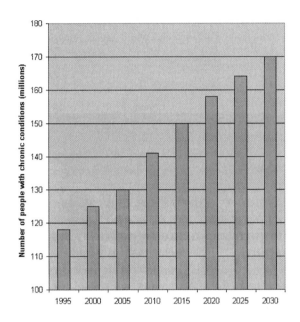

Figure 27-3. Projection of the number of people with chronic conditions in the US[3].

By 2020, over 70 percent of the global burden of disease in developing and newly industrialized countries will be caused by non-communicable diseases, mental health disorders and injuries. Figure 27-4 shows the most prevalent chronic disease is hypertension, followed by arthritis, respiratory diseases and heart diseases.

2.3 Inappropriate lifestyle

The remarkable technology developments of the 20th century have had their inevitable impact on people's lifestyles, especially in the more developed countries.

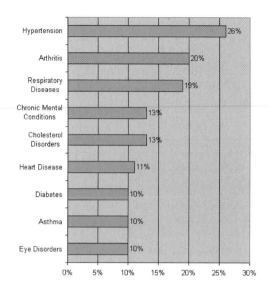

Figure 27-4. Most prevalent chronic diseases in the US[3].

The availability of new means of transportation has reduced our need for moving based on our own abilities. In addition, modern communication and media technologies have motivated an even more sedentary lifestyle. The abundant availability of food – also in many new forms – has altered our nutrition habits. And the ever-increasing pace of our professional lives has raised more attention to the phenomenon of stress. These are just examples.

The evolution of the physiology of our bodies has been unable to follow those developments at the same pace. As a consequence, we are experiencing an increase of 'lifestyle diseases'. Reversing this trend cannot be exclusively realized by managing the resulting diseases – thinking about re-adjusting our lifestyles is required even more importantly. Personal healthcare technologies can support this process.

2.3.1   Physical inactivity

Our current society limits the need for physical activity in our daily lives. However, in order to maintain our health status, our body requires us to make use of our abilities to move. This implies that it is necessary to create additional opportunities for movement, e.g. by means of regular exercising.

In common statistics, the term physical inactivity is used for persons, who report no leisure-time physical activity. A recent World Health Organization (WHO) report recommends at least 30 minutes of regular moderate-intensity physical activity on most days.

The annual estimated cost for diseases associated with physical inactivity (see Table 27-1) in the US in 2000 was $76 billion[4].

Table 27-1. Physical inactivity in the US[4].

	Total prevalence	Total males	Total females
Physical inactivity	38,6%	35,8%	41,0%

Data on levels of physical inactivity across Europe is poor. In general Southern countries have lower levels of physical activity than Northern and Western countries.

In 2002, over 40%[5] of adults in Europe reported no moderate-level physical activity in the past week. Only 15% reported daily moderate-level physical activity, the frequency the WHO suggests is required to reduce the risk for cardiovascular diseases.

2.3.2   Nutrition

Bad nutrition habits have a direct and significant impact on the development of obesity and other important diseases that increase the cardiovascular risk. A high level of cholesterol is widely accepted as an extra risk factor for cardiovascular diseases.

High cholesterol is defined as a total cholesterol level of 200 mg/dl and higher, where levels between 200 mg/dl and 240 mg/dl are considered borderline. A distinction is made between High Density Lipoprotein (HDL, 'Good') and Low Density Lipoprotein (LDL, 'Bad') cholesterol. The higher the level of HDL cholesterol the better, less than 40 mg/dl is considered as a risk factor. For LDL cholesterol levels of 130-159 mg/dl are considered borderline, whereas levels above 160 mg/dl are considered high.

In Europe, cholesterol levels are converted to mmol/l. The threshold for high cholesterol is defined at 6.5 mmol/l.

Roughly half of the U.S. population has an increased level of cholesterol (see Table 27-2), largely caused by bad nutrition habits.

Table 27-2. High cholesterol in USA[4].

	Total population with high cholesterol	LDL cholesterol 130mg/dl or higher	HDL cholesterol less than 40 mg/dl
Prevalence	106,900,000	95,000,000	54,700,000
% of total population	50,7%	45,8%	26,4%

In Europe there are no uniform statistics on LDL and HDL cholesterol levels. Levels vary widely among countries and for men and women. Some examples are listed in Table 27-3.

Generally, Mediterranean countries (Spain, Italy, Greece) have a lower prevalence of high cholesterol.

Table 27-3. Population with high cholesterol in Europe[5].

	Prevalence of levels 6,5 mmol/l and above in men	Prevalence of levels 6,5 mmol/l and above in women
Germany	36%	37%
Northern Sweden	45%	35%
UK-Scotland	35%	36%
Italy	28%	26%

2.3.3   Stress

Stress response describes the condition caused by a person's reaction to physical, chemical, emotional or environmental factors. Stress can refer to physical effort and mental tension. Precise ways of measuring the levels of emotional or psychological stress are not available. Most people feel stress, but they feel it in different amounts and react to it in different ways.

More and more evidence suggests a relationship between the risk of cardiovascular disease and environmental and psychosocial factors. These factors include job strain, social isolation and personality traits. How stress contributes to heart disease risk is at this time subject to further research.

There are not many statistics about stress, as objective measures for diagnosing do not exist.

A number of surveys have however been conducted. A survey by Roper Starch Worldwide[6] states that globally, 23% of women executives and professionals and 19% of their male peers, say they feel 'super-stressed'.

According to the National Institute for Occupational Safety and Health, $300 billion, or $7,500 per employee, is spent annually in the U.S. on stress-related compensation claims, reduced productivity, absenteeism, health insurance costs, direct medical expenses (nearly 50% higher for workers who report stress), and employee turnover[7].

2.3.4   Smoking

Smoking is usually defined as cigarette use during the preceding month. This definition includes the complete range of smokers from irregular to heavy smoking. Smoking is a major risk factor for cardiovascular diseases and for cancer. In the U.S., more than 20% of the population (almost 50 million citizens) smoke[4]. Prevalence is shown in Table 27-4.

In European statistics, smoking is often defined as regular daily smoking. The average smoking prevalence in Europe is 30%[5]. The strongest deviations are found in the former Yugoslavia (48%), Albania (39%), Greece (38%) and Germany (37%). Lower prevalence is found in Sweden (18%), Portugal (21%), Romania (21%) and Iceland (22%). The numbers date from 1999 to 2002.

Table 27-4. Prevalence of smoking in the US[4].

	Total	Male	Female
Prevalence	48,500,000	26,300,000	21,200,000
Percentage of total population	22,5%	25,2%	20,0%

2.4 Relevant diseases

In this section, we discuss the major disease types in the context of personal healthcare scenarios.

2.4.1 Obesity

Obesity is defined by using the Body Mass Index (BMI). This is calculated as

$$BMI = \frac{weight}{(height)^2}$$

In the definition of obesity a difference has to be made between obesity and overweight. Persons with a BMI between 25 and 30 are considered to be overweight, whereas a person with a BMI greater than 30 is defined to be obese.

Table 27-5 lists the NIH (National Institute of Health) classification of obesity and, combined with waist circumference, the associated disease risk for type 2 diabetes, hypertension and cardiovascular diseases.

Table 27-5. Obesity risk factors[4].

Classification of obesity	BMI	Obesity Class	Disease risk, waist circumference men <102 cm Women <88 cm	Disease risk, waist circumference men >102cm Women >88 cm
Underweight	<18.5			
Normal	18.5-24.9			
Overweight	25.0-29.9		Increased	High
Obesity	30.0-34.9	I	High	Very High
Obesity	35.0-39.9	II	Very High	Very High
Extreme Obesity	>40	III	Extremely High	Extremely High

In Table 27-6 the prevalence of obesity and overweight for the United States is depicted. Figure 27-5 shows the percentage of overweight and obese people in the US.

Table 27-6. Prevalence of overweight and obesity in the US (data from 2002)[4].

	Overweight and obesity in adults (BMI>25)	Obesity in adults (BMI>30)
Prevalence	134,750,000	63,120,000
Percentage of total population	65.1%	30%

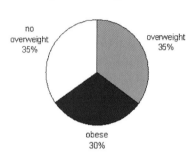

Figure 27-5. Prevalence of obesity and overweight in the US[4].

In Europe, the latest statistics date from the beginning of the 90's[5]. These show that overweight rates in Europe are overall around 50% of the population. Obesity has a prevalence of 15-20% of the population.

2.4.2   Diabetes

Diabetes mellitus is a chronic disease caused by inherited and/or acquired deficiency in production of insulin by the pancreas, or by the ineffectiveness of the insulin produced. Such a deficiency results in increased concentrations of glucose in the blood, which in turn damages many of the body's systems, in particular the blood vessels and nerves. If diabetes is acquired due to obesity or bad nutrition habits, it falls into the category of 'lifestyle diseases' as described above.

More than 194 million people have diabetes worldwide[8] and the number may well double by the year 2025. Much of the increase will occur in the developed countries. In the U.S., the following numbers are known about diabetes prevalence:

Table 27-7. Diabetes prevalence in the US[4].

	Diagnosed diabetes	Undiagnosed diabetes
Prevalence	13,900,000	5,900,000
Percentage of total population	6,7%	2,8%

The values in Table 27-8 accumulate diagnosed and undiagnosed (estimated) diabetes prevalence.

Table 27-8. Diabetes prevalence in Europe[5].

	Undiagnosed and diagnosed diabetes
Prevalence	48,378,000
Percentage of total population	7,8%

In 2002 the direct and indirect cost of diabetes in the US was $132 billion[4]. Diabetes has a broad background and is segmented in a number of types and complications that can occur. An analysis of the needs of diabetics shows the three most important unmet needs of diabetics being painless glucose monitoring, decision support and lifestyle support. New technological solutions in these fields have the potential to fulfill these unmet needs. This will make meaningful contributions by reducing the daily burdens of diabetes management, reducing long-term complications and generally improving the quality of life for diabetics. Chapter 31 discusses diabetes and the management of this disease in more detail.

2.4.3   Hypertension

Hypertension or high blood pressure is defined by the American Heart Association (AHA) as a systolic blood pressure of 140 mm Hg or higher or a diastolic blood pressure of 90 mm Hg or higher. There is a definition for pre-hypertension, which is defined as a systolic pressure of 120-139 mm Hg or a diastolic pressure of 80-89 mm Hg.

Studies have recently shown that for adults aged 40-69 years, each 20 mm Hg increase in systolic blood pressure or 10 mm Hg increase in diastolic blood pressure doubles the risk of death from coronary heart disease.

Nearly 1 in 3 adults has hypertension in the US (see Table 27-9). It is more prevalent in men than in women. The estimated direct and indirect cost of hypertension in 2005 is estimated to be $59.7 billion.

Table 27-9. Prevalence of hypertension in the US[4].

	Total	Male	Female
Prevalence	65,000,000	29,400,000	35,600,000
Percentage of total population	32,3%	31,5%	32,8%

The only reliable data on the prevalence of hypertension in Europe was collected between 1989 and 1997. In these studies hypertension is defined as having a systolic blood pressure over 160 mm Hg. It varies widely from 2% in the south of France and Spain to 17% in former Eastern Germany and

21% in the north of Finland. Since different definitions of hypertension are used, these figures are not comparable to the figures from the US.

Figure 27-6 shows the results of a study conducted in 6 European countries and the US[9] in 2003 on the prevalence of hypertension in major European countries and the US:

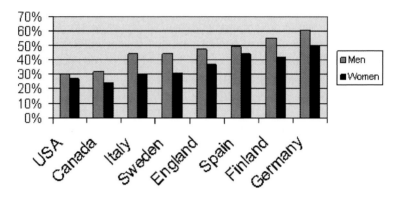

Figure 27-6. Prevalence of Hypertension, ages 35-64yr, USA and Europe compared[9].

This study also used the 140/90 threshold and can therefore be compared to the US figures. According to this study, hypertension is generally higher in European countries, compared to the US.

2.4.4   Asthma

Worldwide between 150 and 300 Million people suffer from asthma[10] and the number is rising. In Western Europe, the number has doubled in the last 10 years. The international patterns of asthma prevalence are not explained by the current knowledge of the physical backgrounds of asthma. Research into these backgrounds and the efficacy of primary and secondary intervention strategies represent key priority areas in the field of asthma research. The rate of asthma increases as communities adopt western lifestyles and become urbanized. With the projected increase in the proportion of the world's population that is urban from 45% to 59% in 2025, there is likely to be a marked increase in the number of asthmatics worldwide over the next two decades. It is estimated that there may be an additional 100 million persons with asthma by 2025.

The map in Figure 27-7 shows the world prevalence of asthma.

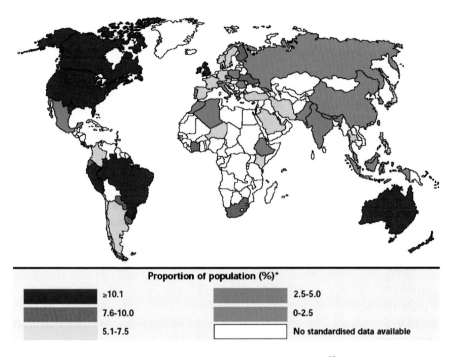

Proportion of population (%)*

≥10.1	2.5-5.0
7.6-10.0	0-2.5
5.1-7.5	No standardised data available

Figure 27-7. Worldwide prevalence of asthma[10].

The economic cost of asthma is considerable both in terms of direct medical costs (such as hospital admissions and cost of pharmaceuticals) and indirect medical costs (such as time lost from work and premature death). In the US, asthma had an economic impact of $14 billion in 2002.

It is estimated that asthma accounts for about 1 in every 250 deaths worldwide. Many of the deaths are preventable, since they often result from suboptimal long-term medical care and delay in obtaining help during the final attack. Annually 180,000 deaths are caused by this condition.

The lack of symptom-based rather than disease-based approaches to the management of respiratory diseases including asthma is one of the major barriers to reduce the burden of asthma. It is therefore needed to develop and promote cost-effective management approaches, which have been proven to reduce morbidity and mortality, and to ensure that optimal treatment is available to as many asthma patients as possible worldwide.

2.4.5 Sleep disorders

A sleep disorder is defined as any difficulties related to sleeping, including:

- Difficulty falling or staying asleep.
- Falling asleep at inappropriate times.
- Excessive total sleep time or abnormal behaviors associated with sleep.

Physicians and sleep specialists typically categorize sleep disorders into four main categories specified by the International Classification of Sleep Disorders[11]. These include:

- Dyssomnias: These are disturbances in the amount, timing, or quality of sleep resulting in excessive daytime sleepiness or insomnia.
- Parasomnias: These are disorders of partial arousal or disorders that interfere with sleep stage transitions, e.g. abnormal events occurring during sleep.
- Medical/psychiatric disorders.
- Proposed sleep disorders: Proposed sleep disorders encompass sleep problems for which there is not enough information available to positively establish them as distinct disorders.

Sleep disorders range from the bothersome to the serious. Insomnia (problems falling or staying asleep) affects 15% of the population. Furthermore, 30% of people will experience short-term insomnia at some point in their lives. The most common types of sleep disorders are discussed in the following.

Sleep apnea: A breathing problem during sleep that creates a sleep disorder. Sleep apnea occurs when a person's breathing is interrupted during sleep. Three types of sleep apnea are obstructive sleep apnea, central sleep apnea and mixed sleep apnea. In obstructive sleep apnea there is an obstruction in the airway. In central sleep apnea the brain signal that instructs the body to breathe is delayed. In mixed sleep apnea, both types are present. Sleep apnea and snoring are a related and common disorder that can lead to serious health problems such as high blood pressure, heart disease, stroke, and may cause a significantly greater mortality risk if untreated. Snoring can be irritating, but can also be a sign of sleep apnea, a more serious disorder where one actually stops breathing during sleep. Sleep apnea affects up to 20% of middle-aged men and 10% of all age groups.

Restless legs syndrome and periodic limb movement during sleep: A neurological disorder characterized by uncomfortable, tingly or creeping sensations in your legs, which create an uncontrollable urge to keep them moving. Restless legs and periodic limb movements are very common, affecting between 15% and 50% of the population, increasing with age. These conditions may lead to difficulty falling asleep or sleepiness due to disrupted sleep.

Narcolepsy: A chronic neurological disorder that impairs the ability of the central nervous system to regulate sleep. Narcolepsy often causes uncontrollable sleep attacks. These may occur while driving, at work or during normal daytime activities. Onset usually occurs during the teenage years and early adulthood.

Parasomnias: Abnormal sleep behaviors are called parasomnias. Two common examples of parasomnias are sleepwalking and bad dreams. Less common parasomnias are nocturnal seizures and REM Sleep Behavior Disorder. Parasomnias are evaluated when there is a suspicion of an underlying medical condition or if the activity is potentially injurious to the patient or others.

2.4.6 Cancer

Cancer is a group of diseases characterized by uncontrolled growth and spread of abnormal cells. If the spread is not controlled, it can result in death. Cancer is caused by both external factors (tobacco, chemicals, radiation, infectious organisms etc.) and internal factors (inherited mutations, hormones etc.). These causal factors may act together or in sequence to initiate or promote carcinogenesis. Cancer is treated by surgery, radiation, chemotherapy, hormones and immunotherapy.

An estimated 9.8 million Americans have a history of Cancer[12] (2001). Worldwide 11 million new cases of cancer are reported every year. In the US, these are about 1.4 million, in Europe 2.7 million. Table 27-10 shows leading sites for new cases of cancer are found to be in the US.

Table 27-10. Leading sites for new cases of cancer in the US[12].

Men	Women
Prostate 33%	Breast 32%
Lung and Bronchus 13%	Lung and Bronchus 13%
Colon and Rectum 10%	Colon and Rectum 11%

Cancer in lung & bronchus is the leading cause of death related to cancer. Worldwide around 7 million people die of cancer yearly. In 2005, 570,000 people in the US are expected to die of cancer, meaning more than 1,500 people per day. This makes it the second leading cause of death in the US, exceeded only by heart disease. Overall costs for cancer in the US were estimated at $189.8 billion in 2004.

2.4.7 Cardiovascular diseases

In the United States over 70 million people are suffering from one or more types of cardiovascular diseases (CVD)[4]. This corresponds to more than 1 in 3 persons. Almost half of this population is estimated to be age 65 or older. The highest contributors to this number are:

- Coronary heart disease
  (including myocardial infarction and angina pectoris):   18%
- Congestive heart failure: 7%
- Stroke: 7%

The average annual rates of first major cardiovascular events rise from 7 per 1000 men aged 35-44 to 68 per 1000 men aged 85-94. For women, comparable rates occur 10 years later in life.

An estimated 17 million people die of CVD worldwide every year. Cardiovascular diseases accounted for 1 of every 2.6 deaths in the US in 2002. Since 1900, CVD has been the number one killer in the US and Europe. In the US, 1.4 million people die of CVD every year (1 death every 34 seconds). In 2005, estimated direct and indirect costs of CVD (in the U.S.) are $393.5 billion.

2.4.8   Depression

Depression is a common mental disorder that comes with depressed mood, loss of interest or pleasure, feelings of guilt or low self-esteem, disturbed sleep or appetite, low energy, and poor concentration. These problems can become chronic or recurrent and lead to substantial impairments in an individual's ability to take care of his or her everyday responsibilities.

Depression affects about 121 million people worldwide[13]. Fewer than 25% of those affected have access to effective treatment. Depression can be reliably diagnosed in primary care. Antidepressant medications and brief, structured forms of psychotherapy are effective for 60-80% of those affected and can be delivered in primary care. However, fewer than 25% of those affected (in some countries fewer than 10%) receive such treatments. Barriers to effective care include the lack of resources, lack of trained providers, and the social stigma associated with mental disorders including depression.

2.5   Challenges for healthcare systems

The trends described above pose significant challenges to the healthcare systems all over the world. In general, it is acknowledged that a public healthcare system is an important part of the social welfare system of any country. However, with the currently visible developments, an insurance model will eventually no longer be sustainable. With a larger portion of the population achieving a high age and with major diseases becoming rather chronic than lethal, adjustments within the healthcare systems will become necessary. Examples that are already visible in some countries and in some areas of healthcare may include bonus systems for a healthy lifestyle and the increasing responsibility of the individual with respect to private financing of healthcare options.

In this context, technology providers are often asked to enable cost reductions. While this may be possible for certain areas, where the effectiveness of healthcare delivery can still be optimized, it is historically, however, more likely that new healthcare options will even further increase the cost requirements for optimal medical care instead of solving the financing problem.

2.5.1   Global cost structure

Healthcare spending continues to rise at the fastest rate in history. Over 2002, healthcare expenditures increased by 7.7%, four times the inflation in 2003.

In 2003, total healthcare spending in the US was $1.7 trillion[14]. This accounts for about 15% of the Gross Domestic Product (GDP). In 2015, more than 18% of GDP will be spent on healthcare. In the US, the out-of-pocket spending is also rising. In 2003, total out-of-pocket spending was $230 billion, an average of more than $750 per citizen.

Healthcare spending in Europe is shown in Table 27-11.

Table 27-11. Healthcare spending in Europe in 2003[15].

	Healthcare expenditure, % of GDP
Switzerland	10.9%
Germany	10.7%
France	9.5%

Main cost drivers in healthcare are shown in the Figure 27-8 for the US. Main cost drivers are hospital care and physician services. As can be seen from the figure, the cost share for hospital care is continuously going down to eventually 27.9% in 2010. At the same time, the cost share for prescription drugs increases.

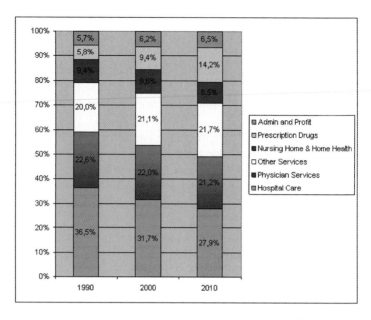

Figure 27-8. Cost structure of healthcare in the US[16].

Healthcare costs are mainly dominated by the costs for chronic conditions[3]. 83% of healthcare spending in the US is spent on chronic diseases. Figure 27-9 shows what share of the offered services people with chronic conditions make use of. People with chronic conditions are the heaviest users of healthcare services and the major costs for the services are accounted to chronic patients.

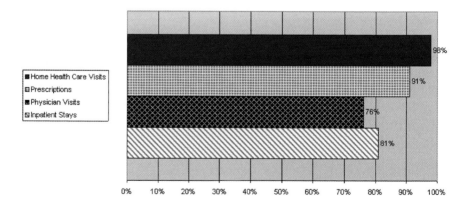

Figure 27-9. Percentage of healthcare services used by chronic patients in the US[3].

3.   APPLICATION SCENARIOS

In this section, we discuss typical personal healthcare application scenarios. We will see that personal healthcare concepts can be applied in all phases of the care cycle (from prevention to rehabilitation) and for various medical conditions.

A common aspect for personal healthcare solutions is that they usually realize a 'closed feedback-loop' between the acquisition of data on the personal health status and the recommended action that should be taken. The following three phases can be distinguished in this context.

Acquisition and pre-processing: Pertinent physiological parameters need to be accurately measured. The measuring methods should be unobtrusive and convenient (e.g. body-worn solutions). For some applications, the availability of continuous readings is beneficial. Due to the special measurement situation, the obtained data will not be directly comparable to data gathered in a clinical environment. While mishandling by the user should be avoided by means of suitable interaction design, movement artifacts and other challenges of the mobile solution need to be dealt with on a signal processing or algorithmic level.

Interpretation: The pre-processed data needs to be automatically interpreted in order to generate higher-level information. For ECG monitoring, e.g., various parameters have to be extracted from the signal in order to enable a proper analysis of the function of the heart.

Feedback & therapy (recommendation): Based on the results of the interpretation step, possibly taking also further higher level information into account from other sources, feedback and therapy will be initiated:

- Either in a closed local loop providing recommendations and/or treatment directly to the patient (by means of home/portable/wearable/implanted equipment).
- Or by invoking professional interaction in an outer loop as needed, which may also be invoked for longer-term surveillance/remote patient management. The hand-over between these two loops is the most critical design parameter of the personal healthcare solution.

The 'feedback loop of personal healthcare' (see Figure 27-10) is closed by monitoring the success of the actions that were triggered by the system response, which implies starting over again with the data acquisition step.

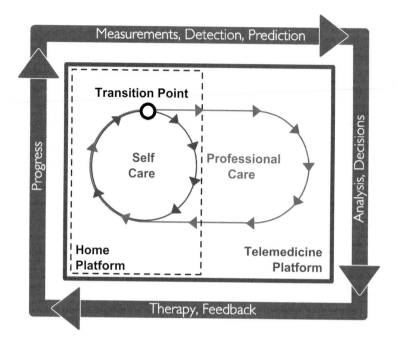

Figure 27-10. The feedback loop of personal healthcare.

3.1   Primary prevention

The individual lifestyle plays the most important role in preventing diseases. The medical community has already developed recommendations on how to effectively prevent diseases, clearly e.g. in the field of cardiovascular diseases. Within the care cycle, the balance continues to shift towards more investments into preventive lifestyles. But although prevention is known to be a very efficient approach to fight diseases, it has not been consistently and successfully implemented so far. We talk about 'primary prevention', if preventive measures are taken prior to a first acute event and the actual outbreak of a disease.

The following personal healthcare application scenarios support primary prevention:

- **Sports & fitness:** Encouraging a more active lifestyle; motivating more frequent and more regular exercise.
- **Weight management:** Supporting active management of weight and avoiding overweight and obesity.
- **Health monitoring:** Allowing regular monitoring of the true health status and enabling to take early action in case of irregularities

- **Elderly care:** Assistance for daily activities in order to avoid negative consequences of age-related problems (e.g. falling).

3.2   Emergency support

The ability to take quick and confident action often determines the difference between life and death in acute medical emergencies. Personal healthcare technology can help to empower people in the environment of the victim to take action. The most prominent example is the Heartstart home defibrillator, which can save the life of a patient in the event of a sudden cardiac arrest. The device is designed to be used by anybody and guides the user through the procedure by means of step-by-step voice instructions. Chapter 29 discusses home defibrillation and the Heartstart product in more detail.

3.3   Early discharge from hospital

An ambition of personal healthcare towards cost-saving for the medical system is to reduce the number of days that patients have to stay in the hospital by enabling a sufficient level of care also in the home environment. The following examples illustrate how personal healthcare scenarios can influence the decision to release patients from hospital earlier than before.

Drug titration: Continuous monitoring of health parameters related to (onset of) drug therapy; adjusting the regular dose to the individually suitable level (today, patients are often kept in the hospital during this drug titration phase).

Relapse detection: Enabling an effective and early detection of relapses with an accuracy that previously would have required observation in hospital.

Depression management: Allowing a close supervision of the disease state for depressive patients, so that acute depressive episodes can be detected sufficiently early in order to take appropriate action, even when the patient is not in the hospital.

3.4   Rehabilitation and restoration

'Rehabilitation' describes the process of recovering from a disease or another event step-by-step by regaining prior strength or potentially learning alternative skills. 'Restoration' means the repair, enhancement or replacement of ability via an intervention or with the help of technology.

Rehabilitation or restoration programs can be run for a large variety of health problems, e.g. related to brain, heart, eyes, ears, skin, muscles or bones. During rehabilitation programs, many patients experience a severe drop in performance after they are released into their home environment. This often occurs due to a lack of guidance and patient awareness and compliance. While most programs still require a significant amount of professional interaction, scenarios that extend into the personal environment can already be envisioned:

- **Stroke rehabilitation:** Making use of the plasticity of the human brain in order to retrain specific (e.g. mechanic or linguistic) abilities after a stroke that has caused neurological deficiencies; extending the rehabilitation exercises from the rehabilitation center into the home environment without loss of quality.
- **Heart rehabilitation:** Running and monitoring a program dedicated to increase the strength of the heart muscle, e.g. after suffering from a severe cardiac event.
- **Eye care:** Providing the most appropriate type of glasses or directly removing the visual deficiency by means of laser surgery
- **Ear care:** Providing optimized hearing aids in order to compensate for a loss in hearing ability with the help of miniaturized acoustic signal processing technology.
- **Skin care:** Treating a variation of skin problems, from strictly medical conditions (e.g. after a burn injury) to mostly beauty related aspects (e.g. avoiding or removing wrinkles).

3.5   Secondary prevention

After a first health-related event (e.g. a heart attack or a stroke), special measures have to be taken, in addition to fighting the root causes, in order to avoid reoccurrence.

Such 'secondary prevention' can usually rely on higher motivation and compliance rates, since the patient now knows exactly what is at stake and that the risk is not negligible.

Personal healthcare application scenarios can support secondary prevention in various ways:

- **Continuous monitoring:** Providing the confidence that everything is alright and under control at any given moment and that a new major health event will be detected immediately; reducing the patient's stress of continuously being afraid.
- **Lifestyle adaptation:** Offering (interactive) guidance after a major e.g. cardiovascular event, e.g. encouraging useful exercising on just the right level, in combination with continuous monitoring.

- **Educational programs:** Reducing the fear of reoccurrence by keeping the patient informed about the disease and raising the awareness e.g. of early symptoms.

3.6 Disease management

After a chronic disease has been diagnosed, two major objectives become an element of everyday-life for the affected patient: Preventing the disease from further progressing and living with the consequences of the disease in its current state. It becomes important to 'manage' the disease.

The person most directly involved in any long-term disease management effort is the patient himself. Self-care, ideally based on well-defined and evidence-based guidelines and supported by easy-to-use tools, always is an important element, supported by interactions with professional caregivers.

This implies that disease management is another important application area for personal healthcare:

- **Heart failure management:** Preventing critical conditions by early detection of decompensation (accumulation of water in the lung due to insufficient heart activity).
- **Diabetes management:** Preventing a worsening of the condition by regular monitoring of blood glucose levels and aiming at adjusting towards a balanced value (diabetes care is discussed in more detail in Chapter 31).
- **Asthma management:** Adjusting the amount of medication to the current need and avoiding strong asthma attacks by early warning.
- **Pain management:** Offering quick and effective relief in situations of recurrent acute pain (e.g. migraine).

Philips has developed a telemedicine platform for disease management applications. Chapter 30 discusses this system (called Motiva) in more detail.

REFERENCES

1. United Nations, *Report on world population aging 1950-2050*, ch2, 11 (United Nations, New York, 2002).
2. United Nations Programme on Ageing, World Population 2002 Wall Chart (September 15, 2005); http://www.un.org/esa/population/publications/ageing/Graph.pdf.
3. Johns Hopkins University, Partnership for solutions, Web factbook: Chronic conditions: Making the case for ongoing care, September 2004 Update (September 15, 2005); http://www.partnershipforsolutions.com/DMS/files/chronicbook2004.pdf.

4. American Heart Association, *Heart Disease and Stroke Statistics – 2005 Update*, (American Heart Association, Dallas, 2004).

5. S. Petersen, V. Peto, M. Rayner, J. Leal, R. Luengo-Fernandez and A. Gray, *2005 European cardiovascular disease statistics* (British Heart Foundation, London, 2005).

6. Roper Starch Reports Worldwide, *Global Consumers 2000 study* (Roper-Starch, New York, 2000).

7. Stress Directions Inc., Website on Stress Statistics (September 15, 2005); http://www.stressdirections. com/corporate/stress_organizations/stress_statistics.html.

8. International Diabetes Federation, *Diabetes Atlas 2nd edition* (International Diabetes Federation, Brussels, 2003).

9. K. Wolf-Maier et al., Hypertension, Prevalence and Blood Pressure Levels in 6 European Countries, Canada and the United States, *JAMA*, **289**, 2363-2369 (2003).

10. M. Masoli et al., Global Initiative on Asthma GINA, *Global Burden of Asthma* (September 15, 2005); http://www.ginasthma.com/download.asp?intId=29.

11. Diagnostic Classification Steering Committee, M.J. Thorpy, Chairman, *ICSD – International classification of sleep disorders: Diagnostic and coding manual* (American Sleep Disorders Association, Rochester, 1990).

12. American Cancer Society, *Cancer Facts and Figures 2005* (American Cancer Society, Atlanta, 2005).

13. World Health Organization, Fact sheet mental and neurological disorders, 2001 (September 15, 2005); http://www.who.int/mediacentre/factsheets/fs265/en/.

14. National Coalition on Health Care, Facts on the cost of healthcare (September 15, 2005); http://www.nchc.org/facts/cost.shtml.

15. OECD, Organization for Economic Co-Operation and Development, *Health at a Glance OECD indicators 2003* (OECD, Paris, 2003).

16. Center for MediCare and MediAid Services, Office of the Actuary, Fact sheets (September 15, 2005); http://www.cms.hhs.gov/charts.

Chapter 28

ON-BODY SENSORS FOR PERSONAL HEALTHCARE
Integration Examples, Implementation Challenges and Emerging Technologies

Olaf Such[1], Jens Muehlsteff[1], Robert Pinter[1], Xavier Aubert[1], Thomas Falck[1], Martin Elixmann[1], Harald Reiter[1], Eric Cohen-Solal[2], Balasundar Raju[2], John Petruzzello[2], Andreas Brauers[1], Jeroen Thijs[1], Claudia Igney[1]
[1]Philips Research, Aachen, Germany; [2]Philips Research, Briarcliff Manor, NY, USA

Abstract: This chapter gives an overview on core technologies that are crucial for the implementation of personal healthcare monitoring devices, with a main focus on cardiovascular applications. The topics covered include dry ECG electrode characterization, activity classification from raw motion data as context information, algorithmic challenges for these applications and wireless network requirements. These elements are integrated into a smart sensor system, of which an example is presented. An ultrasound system for detecting blood flow in resuscitation applications is described, and emerging technologies for Heart Rate detection with unobtrusive ballistocardiography, radar sensors and magnetic impedance cardiography are shown.

Keywords: Sensor principles, vital body signs, smart sensors, on-body electronics, dry electrodes, ECG, radar, impedance cardiography

1.   INTRODUCTION

In this section, we give an illustrative overview over a selection of core technologies that are crucial for the implementation of personal healthcare monitoring devices. Due to the broad nature of this field, the examples given are by no means exhaustive, but can hopefully scratch the surface of this evolving new discipline.

As pointed out in Chapter 27, personal healthcare in our understanding will require in-depth understanding not only of medical needs and requirements, but - possibly even more so - of user acceptance, both from the

G. Spekowius and T. Wendler (Eds.), Advances in Healthcare Technology, 463-488.

perspective of the professional caregiver and from the perspective of the end-user. We usually refer to the latter as 'customer' or 'user', and not as a 'patient'. This stems from our belief that due to the trend towards consumerization in healthcare and a more informed user base, the end user will - directly or indirectly - influence the standard of medical diagnosis and treatment more and more, especially when the potential impact on his or her daily life is high.

Our main focus is on cardiovascular applications and thus most of our sensor work is aimed at cardiography. A key for user acceptance is comfort and ease of use of the monitoring device that must be worn, and therefore the first part of this paper is on dry electrode technology. Due to the badly controllable environment in a personal healthcare setting, motion artifact is a common issue in these applications. We address this by activity monitoring to provide context information and improve the vital body sign interpretation. Classified motion data alone can also give a good insight into the activity profile of the user, which is of high diagnostic interest in itself.

Digital signal processing (DSP) and the algorithmic challenges in personal healthcare is another important issue addressed in this Chapter. Apart from the user demand to be able to interface easily to their personal devices, a typical personal healthcare system will also require a form of data exchange with the established healthcare providers. Thus we also present research on wireless connectivity playing a crucial role in the overall picture of connected healthcare. In the following sections we then give examples how the several technologies can be integrated into consumer friendly devices and solutions. One is the on-body monitoring device for a lay user, the MyHeart Cardio Belt. The other applies Ultrasound Transducers to detect blood flow in resuscitation applications - an excellent example of a 'smart sensor' concept. Finally, we describe a number of emerging sensor technologies that we see as promising due to their specific advantages.

2.   DRY ELECTRODES FOR ECG SENSING

To pick up electrical signals from or to apply electrical currents to a person's body one essential component is to realize an appropriate electrode-skin contact via electrodes. The contact, which primarily consists of a conducting coated material placed on the bare skin, must have sufficient electrical properties and, crucial for personal healthcare applications, should not induce skin irritation during long-term usage. Dry electrode systems are therefore preferred in many long term monitoring scenarios, and they have distinctive features that make them stand out from the classical designs that use special hydro-gels.

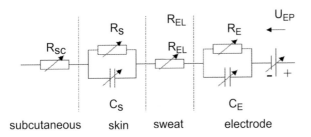

Figure 28-1. Equivalent circuit modeling electrical behavior of skin-electrode contact.

Skin-electrode contacts can be electrically described with a simplified equivalent circuit shown in Figure 28-1. An important contribution to the total impedance is made by the stratum corneum[1] (R_S, C_S), which is the uppermost skin layer and consists of dead cells with sweat glands. It has a thickness of 10...15 μm and the sweat gland distribution inside depends on the skin type as well as the position of the electrode on the body. A conductive bridge from the skin to the electrode is established by an additional electrolyte and/or the sweat produced by the glands. The conversion from ionic to electric current takes place at the electrode surface modeled by a parallel circuit of a capacitor C_E and resistor R_E.

Additionally there are two voltage sources at the skin and electrode summarized by U_{EP}. The electrical characteristics of the electrodes have a strong impact on the system performance and have to be evaluated for a concrete system[2]. Since electrodes interact with the skin, interesting parameters for monitoring purposes are: warm up times, impedance variations[3], equilibrium impedances, noise[4] and motion artifacts on different subjects.

Today in clinical practice medical Ag-AgCl electrodes are commonly used and have very good electrical properties due to low polarization voltages. But since they are normally glued to the skin and require the use of electrode paste, their applicability in personal healthcare applications especially for long-term use is limited.

As mentioned, dry electrodes are a step towards personal healthcare requirements. They normally use only sweat produced by the glands for a conductive bridge from the skin to the electrode. The electrodes need not be glued to the skin, can be easily integrated into clothing and show very good mechanical, biological as well as chemical robustness. Figure 28-2 shows two different examples of electrode technologies for ECG monitoring with functional clothing.

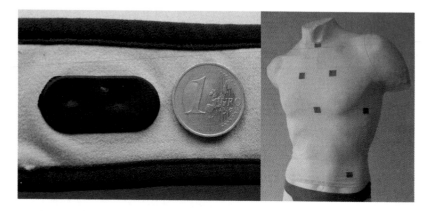

Figure 28-2. Dry electrode made of conductive rubber and integrated into a garment with shielded cable (left), textile electrodes in a garment for unobtrusive sensing of ECG (right), developed in MyHeart (European project IST-2002-507816).

The following paragraph discusses dry electrodes based on conductive rubber[5] and their essential electrical characteristics. Detailed information on the temporal behavior of these dry electrodes can be seen in Figure 28-3, in which the variation of the absolute value of the skin-electrode impedance of four subjects is shown after the rubber electrodes had been placed without any skin preparation. The impedance decreases monotonically over time to an equilibrium value. Subjects 1, 3, 4 have quite different impedances after 5 min. All subjects showed a two-stage process (marked in Figure 28-3), which can be explained by a moisture change in skin during creation of the sweat bridge.

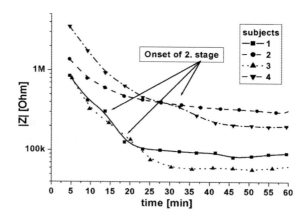

Figure 28-3. Temporal behavior of absolute skin-electrode impedance of 4 subjects; measured at 1Hz, 500nA and same contact pressures[5].

For subject 1 it took about 25 minutes to reach an equilibrium value of (100 ± 20) kΩ whereas for subject 4 the equilibrium was reached after 60 min with (200 ± 30) kΩ. Typical times observed for 10 subjects crossing 1 MΩ have been between 3 min…15 min. Equilibrium values of impedance have been observed in the range of 50 kΩ…350 kΩ probably due to differences in skin properties like skin thickness and sweat composition. The signal trace of subject 2 shows the impact of hairs having the highest impedance value with a more capacitive influence[6,7].

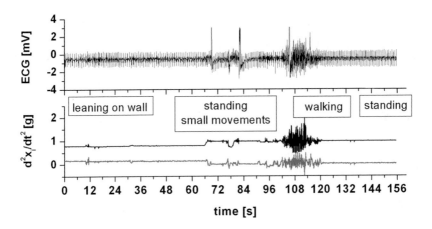

Figure 28-4. Typical ECG-trace (upper diagram) and lateral (grey) and vertical (black) acceleration signals (lower diagram) of a patient wearing the electrodes on the waist; Movement artifact on the ECG signal is apparent.

Typical traces of an ECG gathered by these electrodes, together with 2D-acceleration signals simultaneously measured during a day of normal subject activity are shown in the upper and lower part in Figure 28-4[8]. The electrode positions were at the hip. From 0…26s the patient was leaning against a wall. This is visible in the acceleration signals by the projection of the 1g gravity vector onto both axes. The heart rate was about 73min^{-1}.

In the second state the patient was standing (full projection of 1g on one axis) with small movements. This caused artifacts in the ECG signal in some cases (visible in Figure 28-4). During the third state the patient did a short fast walk in the room. The movements caused strong movements artifacts in the ECG, which makes it impossible to calculate heart rate during this period. In the last phase the patient was again standing at rest and the heart rate was about 112min^{-1}.

As shown, the dry electrodes induce motion artifacts in the ECG signal. Therefore, the overall system performance of such systems is limited and has to be evaluated for each specific application. But these electrodes do offer the opportunity to realize monitoring of vital parameters by sensors placed in a textile 'second skin' in a very comfortable manner with potentially good acceptance by the end-user.

3.   ACTIVITY MONITORING

Based on the Smart Sensor Cardio-Belt design, during which the electrode classification work discussed above was performed, we realized a personal healthcare on-body monitoring system. As mentioned, this includes an acceleration sensor in the system picks up motion along a horizontal (g_x) and a vertical axis (g_y). Apart from using these signals as an indication of corrupt ECG signal, it was evaluated whether this data can be analyzed for activity classification. The activity sensor was located near the spine of the person wearing the system, at waist level, in the person's centre of gravity. Activity data from several subjects undergoing a defined stress test comprising different levels and types of activity were recorded.

The sensor was an integrated MEMS accelerometer [ADXL202, Analog Devices] with a horizontal x and a vertical y axis, a full-scale of +/- 2 g and an analogue voltage output for each of the axes. The sensor signals were sampled at 204.8 Hz with a resolution of 12 bit. The unprocessed data were stored on-body in the system's 64MB flash memory. Upon completion of the exercise all data were downloaded to a PC for the signal processing.

In order to record and evaluate motion data, a stress test course was designed comprising eleven actions that are typical in real life[9]:

(1, 2, 3)	Walking (slow, normal, fast)
(4, 5)	Jogging (slow, fast)
(6, 7, 8)	Walk up a staircase (slow, normal, fast)
(9, 10, 11)	Walk down a staircase (slow, normal, fast)

Motion data of 10 persons were recorded. Four of them completed the stress test course five times in order to improve the quality of the database and to test the repeatability of the measurement. The evaluation approach was based on sorting every two-dimensional acceleration sample into a two-dimensional histogram M_a with elements of pre-defined size $\Delta a_x = \Delta a_y$ and calculating how often every histogram element was hit by one of the acceleration samples.

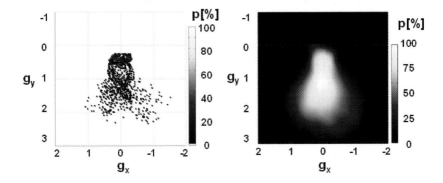

Figure 28-5. Example histograms (left: discrete and right: interpolated), of acceleration events recorded on a person walking fast. The axis g_x and g_y are in acceleration in g, lateral and vertical respectively. The brightness indicates how often the different events occurred (normalized). This pattern was used to classify the activity type.

Figure 28-5 shows an example histogram of acceleration events for a person walking fast. By zero-padding, filtering and averaging a number of these histograms for all abovementioned types of motion, a database containing interpolated acceleration templates was created. For the classification of motion patterns according to these templates a k-nearest neighbor classifier was evaluated on the acquired data using cross-validation.

Table 28-1. Correct classifications in % for one pattern out of four after grouping

Motion pattern	% correct:			
Walking	85	0	5	10
Running	0	100	0	0
Upstairs	5	2	87	6
Downstairs	6	0	2	92
Classified as:	Walking	Running	Upstairs	Downstairs

The best classification result (i.e. the percentage of correctly classified motion patterns) evaluated using the data of all subjects was 53%, while the classification of motion patterns from single persons yielded up to 79.09% of correct classification. Performance on 1 out of 11 types of motion was typically over 60%, and by grouping, this was vastly improved, since only very related motion patterns caused false classifications. If the choice is limited to only four possible classes of motion the overall classification result increases to 91% (see Table 28-1).

These results can then be used to perform context analysis and even enable energy expenditure calculations based essentially on the same input data[10], yielding a much more meaningful diagnostic dataset on otherwise undocumented and uncontrollable user behavior, which is a core issue in most long term personal healthcare monitoring concepts.

4.   ALGORITHMIC CHALLENGES IN PERSONAL HEALTHCARE APPLICATIONS

A sensor application as described requires suitable algorithms to provide meaningful information from the raw and distorted input signal. With the availability of ever growing computational resources, there is also a trend in the medical world to take advantage of still more complex DSP techniques[11]. Their prime role is to provide the experts with more detailed information opening the way to earlier diagnostics and safer treatments. For personal healthcare applications, the trend is similar though the requirements and expectations show distinctive features.

First, as has been shown above, due to the recording conditions occurring in real life and low constraints on the user, biomedical signals captured in home surroundings are prone to artifacts of various types. It is quite common for a given application to observe data samples ranging from 'clean' and stable, to 'noisy' but still interpretable, up to the complete loss of any workable content. The common motion artifacts caused by body movement and/or walking, represent a real challenge for the effective deployment of most body sensors in ambulatory situations.

Second, additional sources of variability are often introduced in the home care environment, as opposed to the controlled conditions prevalent in the clinical world. For instance, within real-life activities, the dynamic range of heart rate and blood pressure is significantly larger than at rest and this puts even more emphasis on robustness issues.

Third, in healthcare practice, it is often necessary to process the acquired signals up to the stage of medically relevant parameters that can be easily interpreted by the user himself. This leads to severe reliability constraints to ensure the required accuracy. To some extent, the algorithms are expected to assess the validity of their results before communicating them.

A last factor concerns the amount of computational resources that might be reasonably spent for healthcare applications. Here too, there is a large scope of possible situations with very distinct requirements, depending on the use model. In any case, to keep technology affordable, software solutions with small footprint and low CPU needs will be definitely favored and there is a strong motivation for miniaturization and clever user interfaces, including wireless connections.

To summarize, healthcare algorithms will have to deal successfully with a number of specific requirements, four of them appearing mostly relevant:

1. The ability to cope with (motion) artifacts.
2. The robustness against multiple sources of variabilities induced by users in real-life conditions.
3. The reliability in terms of stability and accuracy, possibly requiring personalization.
4. The use of limited computational resources.

Keeping in mind that biomedical signals are per se already variable across subjects, it can be inferred that the personal healthcare environment is especially challenging due to the additional sources of variability introduced by the sensors and the uncontrolled recording conditions.

4.1   Example case: Heart rate estimation from chair equipped with a piezofoil

By embedding a piezofoil in the seat of an ordinary chair, it is possible to measure the movements generated by the cardiac contractions. Hence, the heart rate of a sitting person can be estimated in a most discreet fashion. It has to be made clear, however, that the transducer signal exhibits a large variety of patterns, besides being frequently corrupted by motion artifacts, making this a typical challenge for personal healthcare algorithms. Compared to the traditional electro-cardiogram (ECG) 'R peak' detection, the task requires a more elaborate design. In this section, a solution that has been shown to be viable is briefly sketched. The raw incoming signal is pre-processed with standard filtering techniques to enhance the most informative components lying between 1 and 30 Hz. Owing to the relative abundance of data, the current solution rests on a prior segmentation of the signal to locate the intervals exhibiting a clear periodic structure while discarding the other parts, as shown in Figure 28-6.

The algorithm proceeds in three main steps:

1. Segmentation to locate 'artifact-free' intervals.
2. Periodicity detection over the selected segments.
3. Estimation of the local (instantaneous) heart rate period.

The segmentation is obtained with a classifier fed with local signal characteristics such as the envelope amplitude, the gradient intensity and Zero-Crossing-Rates (ZCR). The decision thresholds have been tuned on a small number of representative samples of 'workable' and 'noisy' signals.

The portions of signal tagged as corrupted by motion artifacts are simply ignored. The presence of periodic patterns is sought in the 'artifact-free' intervals based on a modified pulse detector and, after being roughly located,

'RR' intervals are estimated for each pair of successive pulses, using a shifted match measure[12].

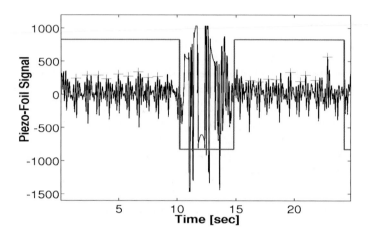

Figure 28-6. Example of a processed piezofoil signal with motion artifacts in [10, 15] sec. It shows the automatic segmentation and the detected pulses marked with a '+'.

The heart rate values are displayed online after appropriate smoothing over a minimal number of consecutive RR estimates, subjected to a variance criterion. The algorithm works almost entirely in the time domain, which insures both the accuracy of the period estimation and the efficiency of the computations based on a small set of arithmetic instructions.

A demonstration system has been set up with a wireless connection sending the digitized signal to a standard PC running the whole algorithm in real-time. Preliminary tests have shown that when the person sitting on the piezofoil chair undergoes standard ECG monitoring simultaneously, both methods achieve almost identical heart rate values, apart from the intervals corrupted by motion artifacts.

5. WIRELESS CONNECTIVITY FOR PERSONAL HEALTHCARE

The absence of wires between sensors as well as low-power operation is of course crucial for acceptance in home care settings. For instance, this enables medical sensors to be hidden in items of clothing or furniture. Advanced low-power wireless technology and intelligent power management systems will ensure that they operate for months or years from tiny batteries.

Philips Research is participating in the Body Area System for Ubiquitous Multimedia Applications (BASUMA) project[13] sponsored by the German Federal Ministry of Economics and Labour (BMWA). The technical outcome of this cooperation will be a body-area network platform for in-home patient monitoring that fits the two core requirements of any home care solution: *Convenience* and *reliability*. This immediately translates into the need for an easy to set up, interference free and low maintenance, hence low power solution, with guaranteed Quality of Service. Containing any number and kind of inter-communicating sensors, these body-area networks monitor vital functions such as heart rate, activity, respiration and others. They will make intelligent decisions about a patient's state of health and pass on relevant data to the patient or to health-care professionals, according to home care protocols advised by the medical specialists.

While body area networking is a new approach, it needs to have industry standards as its basis to ensure technological robustness and smooth interoperability. The platform it is based on should allow the creation of ad hoc networks over short distances, enabling components in the network to find each other very quickly without disturbing the data flow. Though available standards offer a solid technological basis, there is currently no comprehensive solution available that meets the stringent requirements for medical applications. Table 28-2 provides an overview of candidate wireless standards that come into consideration. From this it is obvious that IEEE 802.11b wireless LAN technology is power hungry to such an extent that users would need to replace the batteries already after a few hours of operation. In this respect, the wireless personal area standards Bluetooth and IEEE 802.15.4 are much better suited for battery-powered body sensor networks. However, IEEE 802.15.4 scores over Bluetooth due to its faster and more flexible and scalable networking features, while consuming less energy, processing, and memory resources. In addition IEEE 802.15.4 lays the foundation for ZigBee adding multi-hop networking and an application support layer enabling wireless connectivity of ambient sensors scattered all over the user's home. Therefore as of today, IEEE 802.15.4 turns out to be the standard wireless technology of choice for body sensor networks.

A first version of this wireless body sensor platform called AquisGrain (see Figure 28-7) developed by Philips Research enables wireless patient monitoring of several vital signs. This platform builds on the low-power wireless radio and communication standards IEEE 802.15.4[14] and ZigBee[15] that are about to be widely adopted by industry for monitoring patients from both inside and outside a clinical facility[16]. In addition to the radio and processing hardware, AquisGrain contains the wireless networking protocols and middleware required for ensuring medical grade connectivity, addressing specific requirements in interference mitigation and dynamic channel management. The networking platform concept of the standard can be exploited to let sensors of any kind and any number work together in one body area network.

Table 28-2. Comparison of wireless technologies suitable for wireless healthcare at home.

	IEEE 802.11bWiFi	IEEE 802.15.1Bluetooth	IEEE 802.15.4
Data rate	11Mb/s	1Mb/s	250kb/s (@2,4GHz)
Range	100m	100m	10-30m
Network size	32	8	65,535
Join time	<3s	<10s	<<1s
Real time support	No	No	Reserved time slots
Protocol complexity	Medium	High	Simple
Stack Size	100KB	256KB	5KB (Zigbee 48KB)
Power consumption	400-700mW	200mW	40mW

In a prototype application, this low power AquisGrain system has also been integrated with a mobile cellular phone to allow constant mobile monitoring. The phone collects various vital-sign data from the sensors and is capable of sending it to a care-provider's back-end system over any available data network, such as GPRS, Bluetooth or a WLAN access point.

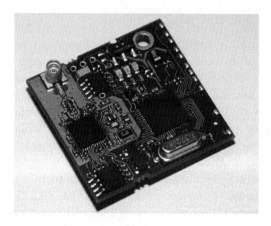

Figure 28-7. IEEE 802.15.4 and ZigBee compliant wireless sensor platform *AquisGrain.*

Together with public research institutions Philips is already working on the next generation of AquisGrain, which will be based on a single chip low-rate ultra-wide band radio IEEE 802.15.3[17], yielding higher bandwidth, which leads to energy savings and prolongs battery life by sending data in a burst mode, providing more robust wireless networking and supporting exact position of sensors and patients.

6. A SMART SENSOR INTEGRATION EXAMPLE

In order to be able to test assumptions on user interaction and to verify medical hypotheses, it is crucial to have access to a platform that enables easy to use and unobtrusive monitoring: A 'Smart Sensor'. We define this as a miniaturized electronic platform that extends the properties of a sensor-only device by providing processing power for algorithms and connectivity directly in the same package. Specifically, a smart sensor combines vital body sign sensors with data acquisition of the sensor signals, the pre-processing (denoising, filtering), and the processing power to analyze the sensor signals and calculate respective results out of the analysis. In addition, such a smart sensor provides connectivity with a wireless link to contact and interact with the outside world. Hence, a Smart Sensor typically consists of all the components discussed above: Multiple transducers, processing hardware, appropriate algorithms, and typically uses some form of connectivity solution.

A good example for this is a smart sensor ECG device (Figure 28-8) to be worn on the body, hence the term 'on-body electronics'. It is used for the purpose of monitoring, diagnosing and giving therapy recommendations for prevention and early diagnosis of cardio vascular diseases in daily life. This system is currently developed in the European Project MyHeart (IST-2002-507816) coordinated by Philips Research.

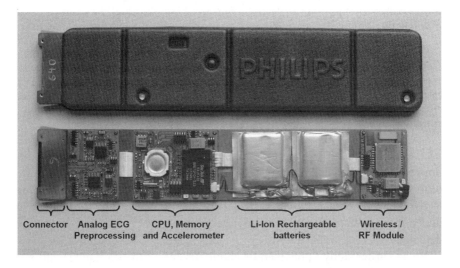

Figure 28-8. Example of a smart sensor device for use in daily life. The packaging is of soft and flexible material and allows comfortable insertion into items of clothing, which enables easy long term monitoring for home care. The modular approach enables configuration with other analog front ends or communication modules to support different requirements easily.

The system measures ECG and activity (motion) continuously (Figure 28-9). The sensor data are processed and analyzed allowing diagnosis of arrhythmia in an unobtrusive and comfortable way outside hospitals. 128 MByte of flash memory are available to store acquired sensor data and calculated results on demand. An important design criterion for such smart sensor devices is ultra-low power consumption, which can be achieved by an optimization of system architecture, system control software and the design of the hardware. A suitable system architecture - allowing minimum data transmission via the wireless link by sending results only instead of raw data, providing simple hand-over protocols and automatically switching the system between sleep, idle and high performance states - can reduce power consumption significantly. The average power consumption finally results in 300μA at 3V supply, around 1mW in total.

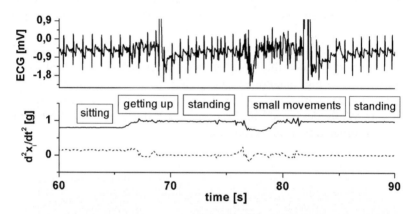

Figure 28-9. ECG and acceleration data collected with a smart sensor system during a motion stress test[8]. It can easily be recognized that the motion during standing up distorts the ECG channel, making an automated diagnosis on this data very challenging. By synchronously observing and classifying the motion or activity, this problem can be alleviated in a smart sensor approach.

Compared to a gel-electrode clinical ECG, the obvious data quality drawbacks of this dry electrode design have to be balanced against the usability advantages of this device concept. Further research has to be done to assess whether it is possible to decorrelate or 'clean up' the data from many of the artifacts by concurrently classifying the activity from the motion detectors.

In an earlier study[5,8], on average about 70% of a full 24h-day (16.8h) was covered by the monitoring system only analyzing the ECG signal. There was no significant difference in the performance of different heart rate detectors.

This value has since been improved due to redesign of the system hardware and form factor, and is typically well above 80%, often reaching 90%.

One major remaining contribution of the signal loss is from short movements during the day (stand up, sit down, short walk, etc.) of the subject, which typically yield to ECG signal loss of about 5...10s at a time. In general there are 10...40 events per hour, which sum up to a signal loss of 1min...8min/h. This means, that during 16 hours of an active day there is an amount of about 10% of bad signal time (2 hours in total) due to short movements that can be masked in a straightforward way. Thus almost 100% of coverage referring to detection of heart rate information can be achieved.

The modular character of the described platform easily allows for the extension of functionality to support additional channels and multiparameter devices, simply by adding and exchanging front-end modules or by linking several systems together in a wireless network as described earlier in this chapter. These systems are in use currently in several patient studies in the MyHeart context and prove robustness and acceptance by users on a daily basis.

7. A NOVEL ULTRASOUND BASED AUTOMATED PULSATILE FLOW DETECTION SYSTEM FOR RESUSCITATION

Sudden cardiac arrest (SCA) is the leading cause of death in developed countries. For SCA patients presenting with ventricular fibrillation (VF) or ventricular tachycardia (VT), early defibrillation applied within a few minutes after cardiac arrest is the only method of successful resuscitation, as has been pointed out in another chapter in this book. Given that a majority of sudden cardiac arrests occur out of the hospital environment, the use of automated external defibrillators (AEDs) in public places by lay responders assumes great importance[18].

Defibrillators currently do not assess the patient's heartbeat or blood circulation and the responder has to manually check for the pulse, a procedure known to be very inaccurate. Several studies have seriously questioned the adequacy of responders to manually assess the pulse[19,20]. Thus, a reliable, noninvasive, automated method to ascertain the presence of blood flow and therefore pulse would be of great benefit in providing care to a sudden cardiac arrest patient before and after defibrillation.

Philips research has assessed an ultrasound Doppler based approach to determine the presence, or absence, of a pulsatile blood flow in the context of resuscitation[21]. In such an application, the objective is to build a completely automated pulse assessment system from acquisition to decision.

Towards this goal, a prototype sensor was built and a new index called *pulsation index* based on a spectral analysis of the Doppler signal, was designed for automated pulse assessment.

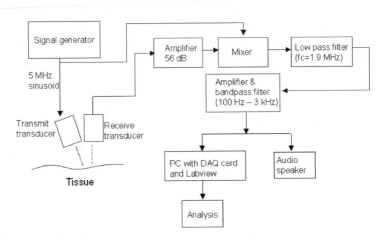

Figure 28-10. Schematic of the experimental CW Doppler setup. The pair of transducers would be placed at the carotid artery location on the neck.

We use a continuous wave (CW) ultrasound Doppler based approach for assessing the pulse of a patient by determining the presence or absence of blood flow in the carotid artery, since the pulse is a direct consequence of the pulsatile blood flow in the artery. The CW Doppler approach was chosen because of the simplified electronics and processing appropriate for the case of unknown carotid artery depth. Figure 28-10 shows a schematic of the CW experimental setup that was designed and built for the experiments.

Experiments were performed to validate and demonstrate the proposed approach. Animals (domestic swines) were used in this study since tissue-mimicking flow phantoms would not capture the complex behavior of the heart after resuscitation. Figure 28-11 represents a typical dataset: Normal heartbeat is present at the start of the experiment and then cardiac arrest (VF) is induced. After about 15 seconds of VF, a defibrillating shock from a defibrillator was applied. The heart then recovered to its normal rhythm. The ultrasound transducers were held on top of the carotid artery location. The ECG and Arterial Blood Pressure (ABP) signals were also continuously monitored to serve as ground truths for the electrical and mechanical activities of the heart.

Collected data were very useful for the development of a new metric, the pulsation index. The idea is to pick a specific Doppler frequency band and analyze the temporal variations within that band of the Doppler power. When a pulsatile flow is present, this quantity would show a periodic behavior that represents the changes from systole to diastole within a cardiac cycle.

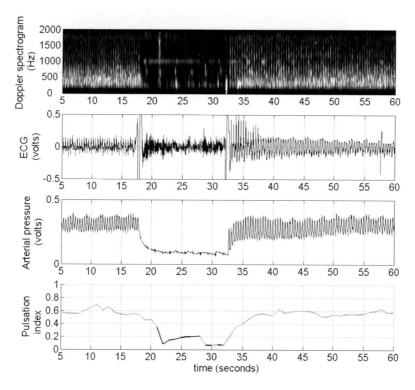

Figure 28-11. Typical dataset showing cardiac arrest and resuscitation. It also shows the proposed pulsation index that non-invasively reflects what is happening and gives an assessment of the pulse state. The shading of the lower trace indicates the frequency band for which the index was the highest. The pulsation index is essentially the same during the VF and PEA periods[21].

Using this fact, it is possible to compute a pulsation index measure that represents a pulsatile behavior of the flow. The Doppler power in several frequency bands is computed as a function of time, followed by the computation of the auto-correlations and power spectra. A peak-searching algorithm then determines the frequency at which the power spectrum is a maximum. The fraction of the total power contained within a narrow band around this frequency is determined. For the case of normal pulsatile flow one would expect that a significant portion of the total power is present in this narrow band whereas it would not be the case when pulsatile flow is absent.

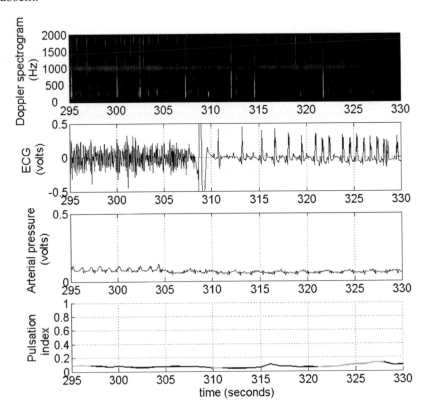

Figure 28-12. Pulsation index for the case of VF and transition to PEA. At about 308 seconds, a defibrillating shock was applied and the ECG returned to normal state, but the ABP did not.

Hence a pulsation index based on this fraction could be used to differentiate the presence or absence of a pulse. We propose the ratio of the power in a narrow band around the peak frequency to that of the total power excluding the second harmonic to be the pulsation index. This quantity is close to zero for no flow (e.g., VF) and close to unity when there is a periodic, pulsatile flow. As shown in Figure 28-11, this new metric is following precisely what is happening during cardiac arrest and resuscitation.

It was also shown on data obtained for a specific condition called pulseless electrical activity (PEA) that the pulsation index was low, showing the absence of a pulse even when the ECG was normal. Thus this index has the potential to robustly indicate the pulse state. An example is given by

Figure 28-12. In this example, there is a return to a normal ECG that is not followed by a return of spontaneous circulation (ROSC), i.e, a beating heart. This work demonstrates the ability of ultrasound-based techniques to bring useful and critical information for applications targeting less-trained users. These applications require the sensing device to be more than a simple acquisition system and must address a more complete functionality set and is thus a typical use case of a 'smart sensor'.

8.   EMERGING SENSOR TECHNOLOGIES

While the technologies mentioned up to here are relatively well accepted in the medical world, we are also investigating solutions with emerging sensors that have found their way only into niches of clinical practice up to today. There are two underlying reasons why they could be more attractive in a personal healthcare surrounding: Firstly, due to convenience requirements, it is often necessary to perform the data acquisition remotely and without body contact, or to hide the measuring function in clothes or furniture. Secondly, some emerging technologies allow measurements that were impossible up to now, and thus the medical world has to be trained to read them. This may lead to the same slow adoption into clinical practice that was needed before pulse oximetry became standard, but could be accelerated by automated smart sensors that can provide a diagnosis directly. We believe that there is a great potential in quite a number of these emerging technologies, and a few examples can be presented in the following:

8.1   Ballistocardiography with piezofoils

Inside the human body there are a number of motion sources due to mechanical movements: The heart (pump movement, heart valve movement), respiration, voice, snoring, flows and congestion. These cause acoustical waves to propagate through the body, making them detectable at the surface passively and non-invasively.

For instance, it is possible to detect the heart movement with so-called *ballistocardiography*[22,23]. This is a technique of measuring the movements of the body imparted by the ballistic forces (recoil and impact) associated with cardiac contraction and ejection of blood and with the deceleration of blood flow through the large blood vessels. These minute movements are translated by a pickup device (e.g. a Piezo sensor) and are then suitably amplified and recorded.

Suitable sensors can be made from materials that have a piezo effect like $BaTiO_3$, Quartz and PVF_2 (polyvenyldifluoride)[24]. Under external pressure the internal stress varies and the material responds with the appearance of measurable voltage. This effect is technically used to measure dynamic variation of pressures and forces. The sensor must be mechanically coupled to the signal source in an appropriate way, but unlike ultrasound probes, in most cases no coupling gel is needed for acoustic audio range sensing.

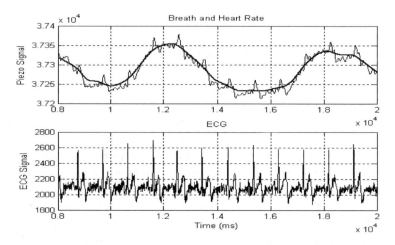

Figure 28-13. Piezo signal (upper diagram) and synchronously measured ECG (lower diagram); the subject was at rest and sat on a Piezo foil placed on the seat cover. The low-pass filtered Piezo signal (thick line) shows the breathing cycle.

The signal of a piezofoil sensor (size 30 cm x 60 cm) with a 44-year-old male sitting on a chair at rest is shown in Figure 28-13. The foil was placed between the subject and the chair.

The foil sensor in the chair detects heart rate as well as respiration quite well when the person is at rest. Respiration can be seen as a variation with frequency components <0.5Hz extracted by a low pass filter (Figure 28-13). An oscillation of about ¾ RR-time, which starts synchronously with the R-peak in the ECG signal, is an indicator of the ballistic heart movements. The signal shape and signal strength depend strongly on the position of the subject on the chair, since the mechanical coupling changes. Small body movements (leg, arm, head turns) by the subject result in a temporary signal loss, as the distortion caused by the movement will be several orders of magnitude higher than the heart rate signal. Automatic exploitation of the measurements thus requires significant effort in the classification of signals and signal processing.

Piezo sensors offer broad opportunities to passively measure the acoustic spectra generated by signal sources in the body. The sensors are simple, potentially very low power, and cheap. Only a single sensor site is required, unlike biopotential recordings always needing multiple sites. Sensors can be integrated into furniture[24,25] and allow for unobtrusive monitoring of breathing and heart rate. Data interpretation of acoustic sound spectra is a growing field and will become an important future method for extracting medically relevant parameters without human interaction.

8.2   Impedance measurements

Essentially, one can also detect the movement of tissue and fluids in the body by the methods known as *Bio-Impedance technologies*. There are two basic methods that can be discussed: Electrical (galvanic contact) and RF and magnetic (non-contact) principles. The electrical systems, delivering the a so-called Impedance Cardiography (ICG) signal, are historically older and more accepted in clinical practice, but all require a low-ohmic connection electrode pair to drive the excitation current into the body, making them only partially attractive for personal healthcare use, where dry electrodes and contactless technologies are preferred for improved convenience. More interesting is the use of remote heart rate sensing by RF Radar and Magnetic Impedance measurements. These sensors can be implemented in a way that they disappear into the daily surroundings of a user, due to the lack of glued electrodes or even any direct body contact. In the following, we present examples of two system approaches: *RF continuous wave Doppler radar* and *Magnetic Impedance measurement*, also termed 'inductive bio-impedance'.

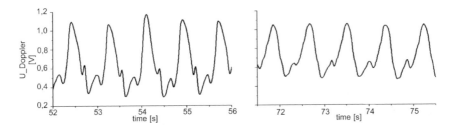

Figure 28-14. Doppler radar signals measured at two different positions. The morphology of the signal is clearly different, which is due to differences in measurement depth and motion of the tissue borders underneath the sensor. The heart rate can be extracted easily from this data that is free of respiratory signal components.

In the following, we describe a Doppler radar sensor based on a on the commercially available microwave motion sensor HFMD24 (Micro Systems Engineering GmbH, Germany). It contains a 2.45 GHz oscillator, transmitter and a receiver in the same housing. The setup has been described elsewhere[26,27] earlier. In Figure 28-14 two measurements at different positions on the thorax are shown. It is apparent that the radar signal depends substantially on the position on the thorax as predicted by the theory[27]. After synchronization of the radar signal and the ICG using the ECG, the ICG can be compared to the radar signal. The time derived radar signal shows good correlation to the ICG (Figure 28-15). Further research will provide insights into the diagnostic value of these morphological characteristics.

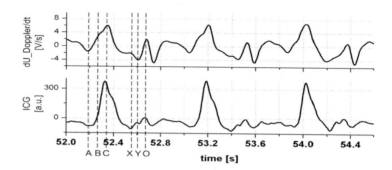

Figure 28-15. The standard characteristic points in the Impedance Cardiograph ICG[26] (A, B, C, X, Y, O) related to phases of the heart cycle also appear in the Doppler radar signal.

Contactless heart rate and heart rate variability measurements are obviously possible with the sensor. However, different measurement positions on the thorax yield substantial differences in the received signal, which requires further investigation. We believe that the simplicity of use could offer significant advantages in the practical assessment of the heart's mechanical activity, compared to the somewhat clumsy use of multiple electrodes in ICG or even imaging modalities. As said earlier, CW Doppler radar is non-contact and can be applied through clothing easily.

Based on similar interaction principles, but different frequency range and transducer techniques, magnetic induction impedance measurement uses the concept of a time varying magnetic field. This induces eddy currents in the conductive tissue, which perturb the field, so a change in the conductivity of the tissue can be detected. The primary field for excitation is about 100 to 100000 times larger than the secondary field induced in the tissue, making this a challenging task[28]. Tarjan and McFee first investigated magnetic induction impedance for biological measurements in 1968[29]. Due to progress in high precision, high frequency electronics with digital waveform synthesizers and lock-in amplifiers, signal quality could be vastly improved since then[28,30].

Typically the measurements are carried out between 100kHz up to 20MHz. In this measurement a frequency of 4MHz was used.

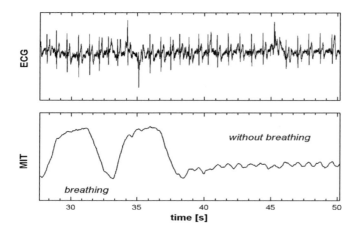

Figure 28-16. Magnetic induction signal measured at 4MHz during a breath hold test. An ECG was used to show synchronicity of the heart activity and the MIT signal.

The system consists of an excitation coil and a measurement coil, which were realized as PCBs. The normal of the excitation coil was directed in the z-direction. The B_x-measurement coil was oriented with its normal in the x-direction. A PC was used to control the lock-in amplifier that is at the heart of this set-up. The imaginary component was used for vital signs detection. To allow a comparison the values from the lock-in amplifier and a synchronous ECG were fed to a measurement box. The coil array was placed underneath a wooden bed and the test person lay on his stomach. To measure vital signs the test person was breathing in intervals. A detailed description can be found in the paper by Igney et al.[30].

The breathing values are typically 10 times larger than signals due to a heartbeat. Figure 28-16 shows measurements at 4MHz with and without breathing. Figure 28-17 shows the same measurement during a phase when the breath was held. By suitable filtering, it is possible to derive the heartbeat signal even while breathing. Respiration signals are easily detected due to their large values compared with heart signals. Filtering allows separating both signals, however, due to the difference in frequency.

The major advantage of both the Radar and the Magnetic Induction Impedance principles lies in the fact that due to their non contact property, they lend themselves easily to integration in textiles and pieces of furniture, making them virtually invisible, and potentially offer 2D imaging capability[31]. Also, unlike ECG, they deliver additional *functional* information about blood movement or respiration otherwise only accessible by Ultrasound, microphones or optical sensors, which all require close skin coupling. Thus, we believe that these concepts will play an important role in practical personal healthcare implementations in the future.

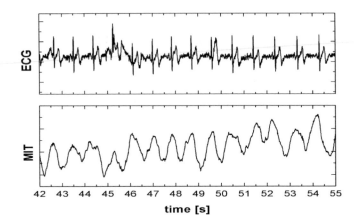

Figure 28-17. The same signal as above, taken from 42 to 55 seconds, when the test person held his breath. A similar signal can be obtained when breathing is filtered with a high pass 4th Butterworth filter with a cut off frequency at 1 Hz.

9.   SUMMARY AND CONCLUSION

Smart body-worn and close-to-body sensors will have a major impact on the realization of personal healthcare systems and solutions. These will allow vital body sign acquisition and thus are at the foundation of any such system. The above sections were chosen to selectively highlight some of the manifold possibilities that have been under research in recent years and include more standard approaches as well as innovative ideas in a more exploratory phase.

Although the goal will always be to have the best possible signal quality, usability, convenience and cost constraints set hard limits to develop against. Hence, as shown, the signal quality will typically be degraded in some form, especially in mobile and ambulatory settings, where motion artifact plays a major role. This insight necessitates the inclusion of detection and classification elements for motion, or activity, in the system, and it is an optimal approach to integrate this into the on-body electronics. This allows robust information extraction in otherwise uncontrolled environments, a key difference to clinical requirements.

The intention of personal healthcare systems is also usually to make a system understandable for a less professional user, compared with clinical equipment. This alone requires intelligence in the sensor in order to make the data interpretation intuitive, while keeping reliability high. At the same time, implementing automatic interpretation on the sensor is also a highly efficient way of compressing data, which has beneficial effects on the required bandwidth in wireless networks. Therefore, intelligent algorithms running on multiple sensor streams are needed for robust operation.

As stated earlier in the introduction, this topic cannot be covered in full breadth and depth in the given format. This chapter is an overview of research that could offer a glimpse of what will be possible in personal sensor systems in the coming years. By combining expertise from transducer or electrode design, alternative methods of gaining pulse or flow information, well-tuned algorithms and packaging and user acceptance knowledge, new sensor systems emerge that will - together with the appropriate system design - allow breakthrough innovations potentially changing the standard of care.

REFERENCES

1. O.G. Martinsen, S. Grimnes, H.P. Schwan, Interface Phenomena and Dielectric Properties of Biological Tissue, *Encyclopedia of Surface and Colloid Science*, (New Decker Encyclopedias, 2002).
2. P. Zipp, H. Ahrens, A model of Bioelectrode Motion Artifact and Reduction of Artifact by Amplifier Input Stage Design, *J Biomed Engng* **1**, 273-276 (1979).
3. T. Yamamoto, Y. Yamamoto, Analysis for the change of skin impedance, *Med Biol Eng Comp* **15**, 219-227 (1977).
4. E. Huigen, A. Peper, C.A. Grimbergen, Investigation into the origin of noise of surface electrodes, *Med Biol Eng Comp* **40**, 332-338 (2002).
5. J. Muehlsteff, O. Such, Dry electrodes for monitoring of vital signs in functional textiles, *26th IEEE EMBS 2004* **26**, 2212-1215 (2004).
6. G.E. Bergey, R.D. Squires, W.C. Sipple, Electrocardiogram Recording with Pasteless Electrodes, *IEEE Transactions on Biomedical Engineering* **18**(3), 206-211 (1971).
7. R.M. David, W.M. Portnoy, Insulated Electrocardiogram Electrodes, *Med Bio Eng* **10**, 742-751 (1972).
8. J. Muehlsteff et al., Wearable Approach for continuous ECG- and Activity Patient Monitoring, *26th IEEE EMBS 2004* **26**, 2184-2187 (2004).
9. A. Schnitzer, O. Such, G. Schmitz, Ein tragbares System für die Bewegungsanalyse zur Unterstützung des kardiologischen Dauermonitoring, *Proc DGBMT 2005: Biomedizin-ische Technik* **49**(2), 252 (2005).
10. G. Plasqui, A.M.C.P. Joosen, A.D. Kester, A.H.C. Goris, K.R. Westerterp, Measuring free-living energy expenditure and physical activity with tri-axial accelerometry, *Obes Res*, in press (2005).
11. Rangaraj M. Rangayyan, Biomedical Signal Analysis, *IEEE Press Series in Biomedical Engineering*, edited by M. Akay (J. Wiley & Sons, 2002).
12. F. Freitag, J. Corbalan, J. Labarta, A Dynamic Periodicity Detector: application to speed up computation, *Proc 15th Int. Parallel & Distributed Processing Symposium (IPDPS-01), San Francisco, April 2001*, 6 (2001).
13. BASUMA project; http://www.basuma.de.
14. IEEE 802.15.4-2003, Standard for Telecommunications and Information Exchange Between Systems - LAN/MAN Specific Requirements - Part 15.4: Wireless Medium

Access Control (MAC) and Physical Layer (PHY); Specifications for Low-Rate Wireless Personal Area Networks (2003).

15. ZigBee Alliance, ZigBee Specification, Document 053474r06, Version 1.0 (2004).

16. B.K. Schuerenberg, PANs Could Pipe Short-Range Data - New wireless network standard could be used to monitor patients from both inside and outside a clinical facility, *Mobile Health Data, July 2005* (2005).

17. IEEE P802.15.3, Draft Standard for Telecommunications and Information Exchange Between Systems - LAN/MAN Specific Requirements - Part 15.3: Wireless Medium Access Control (MAC) and Physical Layer (PHY) Specifications for High-Rate Wireless Personal Area Networks (HR-WPANs), Draft Version D17 (2003).

18. A.P. Hallstrom, J.P. Ornato et al., Public-access defibrillation and survival after out-of-hospital cardiac arrest, *New England Journal of Medicine* **351**, 637-646 (2004).

19. J. Bahr, H. Klingler, W. Panzer, et al., Skills of lay people in checking the carotid pulse, *Resuscitation* **35**(1), 23-26 (1997).

20. B. Eberle, W.F. Dick, T. Schneider, et al., Checking the carotid pulse check: diagnostic accuracy of first responders in patients with and without a pulse, *Resuscitation* **33**(2), 107-116 (1996).

21. B. Raju, E. Cohen-Solal, S. Ayati, A novel Ultrasound based automated pulsatile flow detection method for resuscitation, *IASTED - BioMED conference, Innsbruck, Feb. 2005* (2005).

22. Eblen-Zajjur A simple ballistocardiographic system for a medical cardiovascular physiology course, *Adv Physiol Educ* **27**(1-4), 224-229 (2003).

23. G. Pagnacco, E. Oggero, P.F. O'Reilly, M.J. Warnecke, N. Berme, Design and testing of a 6-component ballistocardiographic bed, *Biomed Sci Instrum* **35**, 57-62 (1999).

24. J. Lekkala, M. Paajanen, EMFi-New electret material for sensors and actuators, *IEEE ISE, Delphi, Greece, 1999*, 743-746 (1999).

25. J. Morgenstern, H. Schettler, M. Wolf, P. Wolf, A contactless cardiorespiratory monitoring system, *J Perinat Med* **19**(1), 164-169 (1991).

26. J.A.J. Thijs, J. Mühlsteff, O. Such, R. Pinter, C.H. Igney, A Comparison of Continuous Wave Doppler Radar to Impedance Cardiography for Analysis of Mechanical Heart Activity, *Proc IEEE EMBC* 2005 (2005).

27. R. Elfring, Master Thesis, Institute of High Frequency Technology, Aachen University of Technology (RWTH Aachen, 2003).

28. S. Watson, A. Morris, R.J. Williams, H. Griffiths, W. Gough, A primary-field compensation scheme for planar array magnetic induction tomography, *Physiol Meas* **25**, 271-279 (2004).

29. P.P. Tarjan and R. McFee, Electrodeless measurements of the effective resistivity of the human torso and head by magnetic induction, *IEEE Trans Biomed Eng* **15**, 266-78 (1968).

30. C.H. Igney, R. Pinter, J. Mühlsteff, A. Brauers, O. Such, Planar magnetic induction impedance measurement system with normal sensor alignment for vital signs detection, *Proc EIT Conference, London,* in press (2005).

31. H. Griffiths, Magnetic Induction Tomography, in: *Electrical Impedance Tomography - Methods, History and Applications*, edited by D.S. Holder (Institute of Physics Publishing, Bristol and Philadelphia, 2005).

Chapter 29

AUTOMATED EXTERNAL DEFIBRILLATORS FOR LAYPERSON USE
Technology to Change the Sudden Cardiac Arrest Treatment Paradigm

Chuck Little, Wendy B. Katzman
Philips Medical Systems, Seattle, WA, USA

Abstract: Sudden cardiac arrest (SCA) is a leading cause of death worldwide. Unlike other epidemics of this magnitude, there exists a definitive and proven therapy for SCA caused by ventricular fibrillation, which is defibrillation. It is estimated that fewer than 5% of people who experience sudden cardiac arrest survive, however, largely because a defibrillator does not arrive in time. Traditionally, defibrillators required extensive training, were large, bulky, maintenance-intensive, and expensive equipment, which limited their widespread deployment. Philips seized the opportunity and has since pioneered numerous technological solutions that have fundamentally changed how sudden cardiac arrest is treated around the world.

Keywords: AED, automated external defibrillator, defibrillator, sudden cardiac arrest, ventricular fibrillation, Heartstream

1. SUDDEN CARDIAC ARREST

Heart disease is a leading cause of death worldwide with no regard for geography, gender, or socio-economic status. It claims nearly 17 million lives each year[1]. In the United States and Europe alone, approximately one million of these deaths are from a specific heart condition called sudden cardiac arrest (SCA)[2,3]. In the U.S., sudden cardiac arrest claims more lives each year than breast cancer[4], prostate cancer[4], AIDS[4], traffic accidents[4], handguns[4], and house fires[5] *combined*.

Different from a heart attack, which is caused by a blockage in an artery, SCA is an electrical malfunction of the heart typically associated with an abnormal heart rhythm known as ventricular fibrillation (VF). Sudden

G. Spekowius and T. Wendler (Eds.), Advances in Healthcare Technology, 489-503.

cardiac arrest usually strikes without warning and the majority of people have no previously recognized symptoms of heart disease[2].

Unlike other epidemics of this magnitude, there exists a definitive and proven therapy for ventricular fibrillation. This therapy is defibrillation - the application of an electric shock to the heart - applied to the patient's chest with a defibrillator. Defibrillation eliminates the ventricular fibrillation and allows a coordinated electrical rhythm and pumping action to resume. For the best chance of survival from SCA caused by VF, a defibrillator should be used within 5 minutes. For every minute that goes by without defibrillation, the chance of survival decreases by 7-10%. After the first few minutes, survival is unlikely. The American Heart Association estimates that fewer than 5% of people who experience sudden cardiac arrest survive largely because a defibrillator does not arrive in time6.

In 1996, the U.S. Food and Drug Administration (FDA) cleared the Heartstream[i] ForeRunner automated external defibrillator (AED), which heralded a new era in the field of defibrillation. The ForeRunner was small, portable, easy-to-use, and less expensive than its emergency room counterparts. Defibrillation therapy was now packaged in a revolutionary way that made it practical to put defibrillators in the hands of non-medically trained responders in order to speed delivery of defibrillation to victims.

Starting with the ForeRunner, a number of pioneering technological solutions have fundamentally changed how sudden cardiac arrest is treated around the world.

2.   HISTORICAL OVERVIEW: HEARTSTREAM AND THE FORERUNNER AED

Heartstream was founded by five individuals in 1992 with the mission of improving survival from sudden cardiac arrest. The vision was to improve access to AEDs by developing and deploying devices that could be used by virtually anyone to help save a life. The team understood from the beginning that survival depended upon early defibrillation and that in order to achieve it, widespread accessibility was mandatory. The goal was to develop a technological solution that would overcome the limitations of previous generations of defibrillators. Namely, the product had to be easy to operate,

---

[i] Heartstream, Inc. was founded in 1992. In 1998, the Hewlett-Packard Company (HP) acquired Heartstream. In 1999, HP created an independent test and measurement company, which included the Heartstream Operation. The new company was called Agilent Technologies. In 2001, Agilent Technologies' medical business was acquired by Philips Medical Systems.

virtually maintenance free, reliable, rugged, small, lightweight, and relatively inexpensive to own.

Initially, the technology would be targeted towards emergency medical responders, such as paramedics and EMTs who were often trained to defibrillate, but who did not usually carry defibrillators as standard equipment. At the time, only 25% of ambulances and only 10-15% of fire companies with emergency "first-response" responsibilities were equipped with portable external defibrillators[7]. From the beginning, however, the Heartstream founders envisioned a day when their AEDs would be used by millions of first responders, which they believed would someday include lay responders in the home as well.

With this vision, a small development team set out to revolutionize the treatment of sudden cardiac arrest.

2.1 Biphasic waveform therapy

For the first 30 years of commercial external defibrillation, monophasic waveforms were used to deliver the "electric medicine" to treat SCA. With such waveforms, current throughout the pulse flows in one direction from one electrode pad through the body to the other electrode pad. To perform defibrillation with this technology, it was generally accepted at the time that between 200 and 360 joules of energy should be delivered. While a monophasic waveform was considered effective and relatively easy to create, it required a significant source of energy. The heavy rechargeable batteries typically used to power the pulse generator were expensive and maintenance intensive[8].

In the late 1980s, the biphasic waveform was introduced to implantable-cardioverter defibrillators (ICDs) in order to reduce the size, weight, and battery requirements of these devices. In a brief time, the biphasic waveform became the standard therapy in nearly all ICDs. With a biphasic waveform, the direction of the current flowing between the electrode pads placed on the patient's chest is reversed part way through the pulse. Importantly, less energy is required to achieve defibrillation efficacy comparable with monophasic waveforms. This means that the defibrillator itself and its energy source can be smaller and lighter[8]. Comparative studies of ICDs in humans demonstrated superior results of biphasic defibrillation over mono-phasic defibrillation[9,10]. Based on these results, scientists at Heartstream hypothesized that implementing a biphasic waveform in an AED could potentially result in smaller, lighter, and less costly AEDs appropriate for use by laypersons.

Heartstream chose to develop a 150 J biphasic waveform to facilitate the design of a portable AED. In addition, the team believed that the lower-energy 150 J biphasic waveform would help minimize dysfunction associated with higher energy shocks. The 150 J low-energy biphasic waveform was developed and validated first in an animal trial, which found that biphasic waveform techniques could be employed to achieve high defibrillation efficacy[11]. A pilot study in humans showed that the low-energy biphasic shocks were as effective as the higher-energy monophasic shocks[12].

Following the pilot study, Heartstream conducted the largest comparative study of defibrillation waveforms that has been performed to date[13]. The study results demonstrated that initial 130 J biphasic waveform shocks defibrillated as well as initial 200 J monophasic waveform shocks traditionally used in standard defibrillators. In a smaller subset of patients, the efficacies of 115 or 130 J initial biphasic shocks were not statistically different from 360 J initial monophasic shocks.

Once commercial shipments of the ForeRunner began in December 1996, researchers were eager to observe the field performance of the SMART Biphasic waveform. Two published studies resulted, which both concluded that the SMART Biphasic waveform was able to terminate long-duration VF at rates above those previously published for monophasic shocks[14,15].

Results of the only multi-center, randomized, controlled trial comparing the SMART Biphasic waveform to various monophasic waveforms in the out-of-hospital setting were published in 2000[16]. This study concluded that the SMART Biphasic waveform defibrillated at higher rates than the monophasic waveforms.

With its introduction in 1996, the ForeRunner became the first commercially available AED to use a low-energy biphasic waveform. Over the next several years, the AED industry embarked on the "energy wars," whereby multiple manufacturers made arguments for sticking with monophasic waveforms. Now virtually every AED on the market offers some variation of a biphasic waveform. Led by Philips, the biphasic waveform became the industry standard.

2.2 Impedance-controlled defibrillation

A defibrillator delivers "electric medicine." For a defibrillation pulse to be effective in terminating ventricular fibrillation, a sufficient "dose" of current must reach the heart. With external defibrillation, the electricity must first travel through skin, muscle, bone, organs, and other tissues. The defibrillator's design and construction must take into account that the electrical resistance, or *impedance*, of the chest varies significantly from person to person. Impedance is influenced by several anatomical and physiological factors and cannot be estimated by looking at a person.

Traditionally, to ensure that defibrillation would be effective on most patients, defibrillators were designed to deliver a high dose of energy such that victims with high chest impedances would receive sufficient current to defibrillate their hearts. This meant that on a relatively frequent basis, victims with low chest impedances potentially received substantially higher amounts of current than was necessary.

The challenge was to design a defibrillator that could effectively measure and compensate for patient impedance in order to deliver the correct dose of current (and energy) on the *first* shock. Rather than delivering a high dose of energy to all victims regardless of need, the ForeRunner was designed to use a special method of instantaneously measuring chest impedance and automatically optimizing the waveform for each victim. This innovative process, called impedance-controlled defibrillation, compensates for patient impedance variations across a wide range of the anticipated patient population. The ForeRunner was designed to measure impedance and dynamically vary the waveform's attributes accordingly on every shock, making it unnecessary to increase the energy on successive shocks. The optimal therapy (or dose) would be delivered starting with the first shock.

As the most well studied external defibrillator waveform, substantial evidence now supports that the low-energy 150 J biphasic waveform performs as well as or, in most studies, far better than the "gold standard" monophasic defibrillation waveform on the first shock without the need to escalate[17,18,19].

2.3 Advanced patient diagnosis and safety

All AEDs analyze ECG information to make therapy recommendations based upon proprietary computational processes that are commonly referred to as algorithms. Algorithm performance is evaluated on two criteria: sensitivity - the ability of an algorithm to correctly detect life-threatening ventricular arrhythmias; and specificity - the ability of the algorithm to correctly discriminate normal rhythms or arrhythmias that should not be shocked. The key is to retain a likelihood of shocking rhythms that need it while reducing the possibility of an accidental or inappropriate delivery of a shock.

Heartstream developed revolutionary detection system known as "SMART Analysis" to allow sophisticated and accurate rhythm interpretation beyond simple rate-based analysis. The system used four key parameters, including rapidity of signal conduction, ECG amplitude, heart rate, and stability of

ECG complexes. No single parameter could lead to a "shock advised." The SMART Analysis system was tested against a database of more than 3,000 ECG rhythms, comprised of a wide variety of rhythms and patient settings. All rhythms were reviewed and classified as shockable and non-shockable by three independent, board-certified cardiologists. With the SMART Analysis system, the ForeRunner could automatically determine if a shock was appropriate, eliminating the need for the user to be trained in electrocardiogram interpretation. Furthermore, ForeRunner was designed to activate the shock button only when a shockable rhythm was identified. Following clearance, a study of the first 100 consecutive uses of the ForeRunner reported that SMART Analysis correctly identified all patients who required a shock (100% sensitivity) and all patients who did not require a shock (100% specificity)[14].

In order for SMART Analysis to work effectively, it requires relatively "clean" ECG signals from the patient. Touching the patient or trying to perform CPR during analysis can induce "artifact," which is an unwanted electrical signal present in the ECG data but unrelated to the electrical characteristics of the heart. Artifact can cause an incorrect analysis and potentially lead to an inappropriate shock/no shock decision. Some types of artifact are controllable, such as touching the pads, moving the patient, radio transmissions, or ground transport. Other types are non-controllable and may be caused by electrical interference, patient seizures, or an implantable pacemaker. SMART Analysis was engineered to "see through" many kinds of non-controllable artifact signals and correctly assess the signal from the heart. It was also designed to detect many other controllable, artifact signals and interrupt the analysis if the ECG was significantly corrupted and direct the user to troubleshoot the problem.

2.4   Ease of maintenance

By incorporating a low-energy, biphasic waveform, the energy storage and delivery challenges were significantly reduced. To power the ForeRunner, the Heartstream team selected a lithium-based battery system. It offered long-life batteries that required essentially no maintenance, were highly reliable, and were a fraction of the size and weight of rechargeable batteries. At the time, lithium batteries were increasingly being used in a range of medical and non-medical applications. A well-known and proven example was cardiac pacemakers. Lithium-based batteries were also widely used in the camera industry as they provided a dense source of energy for flash and motorized film advance photography. Mass production of lithium batteries to support the camera industry alone made them readily available and cost-effective[8].

The lithium battery system, coupled with automated self-testing, made the ForeRunner virtually maintenance free. The need for recharging was eliminated. Once a lithium battery pack was inserted in the ForeRunner, it automatically performed a comprehensive self-test of the battery and the internal circuitry and continued to perform these tests on a daily basis. Periodically, the ForeRunner would perform an internal discharge and verify its calibration. Each battery cartridge was typically capable of maintaining the device in a state of readiness for more than one year (or about 100 shocks). Similar to a fire extinguisher, the ForeRunner had a visual status indicator that could be checked at a glance to ensure it was ready for use[8].

2.5   Intuitive operation

Previously, emergency responders who defibrillated had to remember the protocol, including the number of shocks before pausing for CPR and the energy level for each shock. The goal was to help automate the protocol so that a broad group of users with minimal training could effectively use the product. Furthermore, the user interface had to be intuitive so that the user could move quickly through the steps in order to deliver the first shock if needed. Simplicity seemed like an obvious concept, but the team soon discovered that simplicity is difficult. From the beginning, real-world testing became a key component of the Heartstream industrial design process.

The industrial design team developed several symbols, or icons, to communicate with the user, which were considered a key innovation from a human factors standpoint. These icons were developed and refined through several rounds of design and real-world testing. Once such example was the icon developed to assist with proper pad placement, which is commonly recognized as the most difficult part of using an AED. In an innovative move, the team decided to put pictures of the pad placement on the electrode pads themselves. After testing several versions of the "trodeman" icon, they arrived at the design that is still used today. It took the insight of adding a circle around the pad to be placed that finally helped people understand pad placement.

The team's focus on the importance of industrial design was widely recognized and handsomely rewarded. In 1997, Heartstream received two prestigious Industrial Design Excellence Awards (IDEA) for its break-through in AED technology design. The ForeRunner captured a Gold award, the IDEA's highest honor, in the category of Medical & Scientific Products and a Silver award in the category of Design Exploration. *Popular Science* cited the ForeRunner in its end-of-year "Best of What's New" issue and called it "one of the year's 100 greatest achievements in science and technology." The ForeRunner was a finalist in the Computerworld Smithsonian Awards and received the German Red Dot Award for High Design Excellence. Finally, in Peter S. Cohen's book, *The Technology Leaders: How America's Most Profitable High-Tech Companies Innovate Their Way to Success*, Heartstream was cited as one of America's most innovative technology leaders.

The awards in combination with studies of successful use by non-traditional emergency responders, such as security guards and flight attendants, helped demonstrate ForeRunner's ease of use[20,21]. However, one published study clearly highlighted the ease of use of the ForeRunner and caught the interest of the popular press when it reported that paramedics trained to use the device were only moderately faster at deploying the AED than sixth graders in a simulated response scenario using the ForeRunner without training[22].

2.6 Small, lightweight, and rugged

Early AEDs weighed up to 20 pounds and were as bulky as a portable typewriter. The use of innovative technology and materials resulted in a durable product the size of a hardcover book that weighed just 4 pounds, making it the lightest AED then available. For emergency responders already weighed down by equipment, an AED that fit compactly into an already crowded emergency vehicle and did not add substantially to the load of equipment carried to the emergency site made it a much more attractive tool.

The ForeRunner was designed to withstand a wide variety of adverse conditions commonly encountered in the "real" out-of-hospital emergency world, including water, mud, dust, and severe impact. The solid-state components were housed in a high-impact polycarbonate casing and were extensively tested. The team even went so far as to drive over a ForeRunner with a fire truck. It still worked.

2.7 Launching the ForeRunner AED

On September 12, 1996, Heartstream launched the ForeRunner AED (Figure 29-1). Over the next 48 hours, nearly every major news media outlet in the United States picked up the story reaching over 100 million Americans with the news. Shortly thereafter, American Airlines announced their decision to equip their fleet with ForeRunner AEDs. This unprecedented decision garnered widespread media coverage as well, even finding its way into David Letterman's monologue one night on *The Late Show with David Letterman*. The launch media coverage as well as that surrounding many of the subsequent sales and saves around the country played an important role in raising awareness about sudden cardiac arrest and the need for early defibrillation. Previously, this was a topic not covered by the popular press. This awareness helped fuel the momentum behind the growing AED movement.

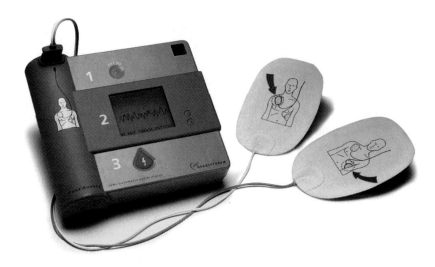

Figure 29-1. The Heartstream ForeRunner AED.

2.8   The true measure of success

With more than 500,000 people passing through Grand Central Terminal each day, the Metro North Railroad/Grand Central Terminal emergency response team felt that since they traveled to emergency situations in the terminal by way of an electric cart, the lightweight, durable ForeRunner AED would be a welcome addition to their first aid procedures. When their ForeRunners arrived on July 2, 1997, that had no idea they would need to use one so soon.

Bob Adams, a 41-year-old lawyer, was healthy, athletic, and had no history of heart disease. On July 3, 1997 he was about to catch the commuter train home from Grand Central when he collapsed. Within four minutes of starting CPR and using their new ForeRunner, the emergency responders had Bob's heart beating normally and he regained consciousness. Bob was taken to a local hospital where he made a full recovery.

Bob, his wife, and his three young children traveled to Heartstream that December for the annual holiday party. "I'm alive today because of two things," Bob told the team, "Technology and the people who came to my aid." Bob's visit started a long tradition that continues today of survivors coming to Heartstream to share their incredible stories. Each story serves to inspire the team and reaffirms their commitment to developing and designing defibrillators as if the life of someone they love depends upon it.

3.   TECHNOLOGY SOLUTIONS FOR THE YOUNGEST PATIENTS

In 2001, a study was published that underscored the need for treatment of infants and children with AEDs[23]. Previously, AEDs, including the ForeRunner, had only been cleared for use on people over the age of 8 or weighing more than 55 pounds. Yet, an estimated 5,000-7,000 children were dying from SCA each year without exhibiting prior symptoms[24].

The team faced several challenges as they set out to develop a solution to treat infants and children. They had to confirm that the FR2's (the next generation of the ForeRunner introduced in 2000) analysis algorithm could effectively analyze pediatric arrhythmias. They had to determine how to reduce the energy delivered to these small patients. Finally, they had to ensure that the infant/child solution was easy to use and did not complicate adult defibrillation.

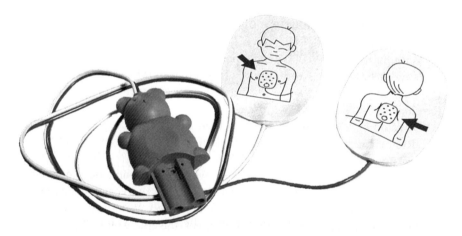

Figure 29-2. Philips infant/child pads.

In May 2001, Philips became the first manufacturer to obtain FDA clearance permitting use of an AED on infants and children under the age of eight (Figure 29-2). The related patent - granted for the process of attenuating defibrillation energy to an appropriate level for pediatric defibrillation - has been placed to the public domain to permit other manufacturers to develop pediatric solutions for their AEDs. To date, four other AED manufacturers have used this technology to develop infant/child pads for their AEDs.

4. BRINGING DEFIBRILLATORS HOME

From the time Heartstream was founded, the team envisioned a day when defibrillators would be as commonplace as fire extinguishers. It had long been recognized that the majority of sudden cardiac arrests happen in the home. Many estimates place the figure near 80%[25]. Given the growing acceptance of AEDs on airplanes, and in airports, workplaces, and communities, the home was the next logical frontier.

The use of defibrillators in the home was much more than a new marketing opportunity. A home defibrillator would represent the first time in the history of medical products that this type of lifesaving therapy would be packaged for broad consumer use. The development of such a product had to be taken seriously and responsibly in order to deliver a device that would truly support broad consumer use.

The technology platform developed for the ForeRunner and FR2, and proven in billions of hours of field service provided the underlying architecture for the home defibrillator, including the low-energy SMART Biphasic waveform, the SMART Analysis system, the artifact detection system, the battery technology, and the automated self-test. These technologies would address the safety and reliability requirements. The ForeRunner had proven easy to operate in the field, but it was primarily used by trained first responders typically with a duty to respond. The team recognized that the key to the home defibrillator would be the human factors as it had to be so easy that virtually anyone could use it in an emergency.

Thousands of hours were spent studying the way people use AEDs to fully understand the next product evolution that had to take place in order to develop the ideal defibrillator for broad consumer use from a human factors standpoint. Once again, the industrial design team employed an iterative design process to develop what would become the Philips HeartStart Home Defibrillator. Iterations of the device were field tested with targeted users in libraries, malls, and senior centers and the results significantly influenced the design process.

4.1 Launching the first home defibrillator

In November 2002, FDA clearance of the Philips HeartStart Home Defibrillator (Figure 29-3) was announced. It was the first new-generation defibrillator specifically designed for the home. Its introduction met with media broad interest, receiving an astounding 500,000,000 media impressions in the first few weeks following launch, including major TV events like *The Tonight Show* by Jay Leno or *Saturday Night Live's Weekend Update*. These mainstream mentions were an important indication that the defibrillator was permeating American culture - a key step towards gaining acceptance of this new technology into people's everyday lives.

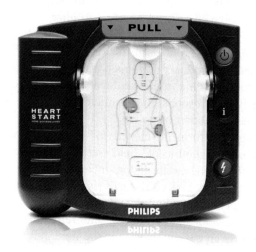

Figure 29-3. The Philips HeartStart Home Defibrillator.

The technological achievements of the Heartstream design team were recognized with numerous design awards including, *BusinessWeek/USA Today* "Best Product of the Year," a *BusinessWeek*/Industrial Design Excellence Award (Gold) 2003, and a Medical Design Excellence Award 2003. In addition, *Popular Science* named HeartStart "Best of What's New".

4.2 Making widespread availability a reality

While the HeartStart Home Defibrillator faced little overt opposition from the medical community, it was not readily embraced. In order to purchase a defibrillator, a consumer had to obtain a prescription from his or her physician. The prescription itself put physicians in an awkward position.

It is virtually impossible for a physician to predict who will suffer a sudden cardiac arrest, when it will occur, and who will be present to use the defibrillator. For whom was the physician writing a prescription?

Philips had begun discussions with the FDA regarding removal of the prescription requirement in 1999. At first, the idea was met with skepticism. Yet, Philips firmly believed that without removal of the prescription requirement, widespread access to defibrillators would be constrained. Such constraints would continue to limit the choice of Americans to be prepared for life-threatening SCA emergencies.

As a result, pursued over-the-counter (OTC) clearance for the HeartStart Home Defibrillator has been pursued. The FDA and Philips worked together for years to understand the requirements of an OTC defibrillator. In order to receive OTC clearance, it had to demonstrated that the device had an established history of safe use and that it could be used safely and for its intended purpose based upon its labeling alone.

In terms of establishing its history of safe use, Philips drew upon the vast field performance data amassed since the introduction of the ForeRunner in 1996. During that time, AEDs had accumulated an impressive and substantial track record. Philips also undertook two studies to demonstrate that the HeartStart Home Defibrillator could be used safely and for its intended purpose based upon its labeling alone.

In September 2004, the FDA cleared the Philips HeartStart Home Defibrillator as the first and only defibrillator available without a prescription. It was an historic moment in the AED movement. This move eliminated one of the most significant barriers to widespread access and was an important step in helping to make the HeartStart Home Defibrillator more easily available to consumers for home use, where the majority of cardiac arrests occur. Again, the news generated broad media coverage, including being named a "Best Product of the Year" by *Fortune* magazine.

With the prescription requirement removed, Philips was able to pursue traditional distribution for the HeartStart Home Defibrillator. The product became available at several leading consumer retailers such as Amazon.com, Drugstore.com, Staples.com, Walgreens.com, CVS.com, and Sam's Club. These new avenues of distribution were an important step forward in making the product more widely accessible and giving both the problem of sudden cardiac arrest and the solution of HeartStart greater visibility.

5.   LOOKING TOWARDS THE FUTURE

The research work done by Philips has played a critical role in helping to make defibrillation an effective therapy. It has led to important changes in defibrillation protocols, the adoption throughout the industry of a more effective waveform, and solutions for the youngest victims. We plan to stay at the forefront of resuscitation research and to continue making contributions that drive the industry.

Philips also plans to maintain its leadership role in developing innovative technology solutions to treat SCA because until every person is within a few minutes of a defibrillator, there will continue to be a need for technology that helps increase accessibility. This will also include developing solutions for patients for whom their event is unwitnessed, defibrillation is delayed, or CPR is required.

We are also looking beyond the treatment of sudden cardiac arrest. As a result of the aging of the post-WWII generation there is an ever-increasing need for technologies that address a range of cardiac-related conditions. One such technology in development leverages our world-renowned expertise in wearable electronics, as described in Chapter 28. Scientists are developing a wearable, wireless monitoring system that can warn patients with underlying health problems, assist clinicians in the diagnosis and monitoring of patients at risk, and automatically alert emergency services in the case of an acute medical event. This technology is designed to disappear into its surroundings from where it can work seamlessly to improve quality of life or personal healthcare.

REFERENCES

1.   World Health Organization, Cardiovascular disease: prevention and control (May 31, 2005); http://www.who.int/dietphysicalactivity/publications/facts/cvd/en/.
2.   American Heart Association, *Heart Disease and Stroke Statistics-2005 Update* (American Heart Association, Dallas, 2004).
3.   S. Sans et al., The burden of cardiovascular diseases mortality in Europe. Task Force of the European Society of Cardiology on Cardiovascular Mortality and Morbidity Statistics in Europe, *Eur Heart J* **18**, 1231-1248 (1997).
4.   National Center for Health Statistics, National Vital Statistics Report. Hyattsville, Maryland, *Public Health Service* **48**(11), (2000).
5.   FEMA/United States Fire Administration, *A Profile of Fire in the United States 1989-1998*, 12th ed. (1999).
6.   American Heart Association, *2002 Heart and Stroke Statistical Update* (American Heart Association, Dallas, 2001).
7.   J.E. Brodey, So many die needlessly: Broken cardiac rescue chain, p. 8 sec. B, *New York Times*, March 30 (1994).
8.   C. Morgan, Advances in AED technology, *JEMS* **22**(1), 12-15 (1997).

9. R.A. Winkle et al., Improved low energy defibrillation efficacy in man with the use of biphasic truncated exponential waveform, *Am Heart J* **117**(1), 122-127 (1997).

10. G.H. Bardy et al., A prospective randomized evaluation of biphasic versus monophasic waveform pulses on defibrillation efficacy in humans, *JACC* **14**(3), 728-733 (1989).

11. B. Gliner et al., Transthoracic defibrillation of swine with monophasic and biphasic waveforms, *Circulation* **92**, 1634-1643 (1995).

12. G.H. Bardy et al., Truncated biphasic pulses for transthoracic defibrillation, *Circulation* **91**, 1768-1774 (1995).

13. G.H. Bardy et al., Multicenter comparison of truncated biphasic shocks and standard damped sine wave monophasic shocks for transthoracic ventricular defibrillation, *Circulation* **94**, 2507-2514 (1996).

14. J. Poole et al., Low-energy impedance-compensating biphasic waveforms terminate ventricular fibrillation at high rates in victims of out-of-hospital cardiac arrest, *J Clin Electrophysiology* **8**, 1373-1385 (1997).

15. B. Gliner et al., Treatment of out-of-hospital cardiac arrest with a low-energy impedance-compensating biphasic waveform automatic external defibrillator, *Biomed Instrum Technol* **32**, 631-644 (1998).

16. T. Schneider et al., Multicenter, randomized, controlled trial of 150-J biphasic shocks compared with 200- to 360-J monophasic shocks in the resuscitation of out-of-hospital cardiac arrest victims, *Circulation* **102**, 1780-1787 (2000).

17. R.D. White et al., Patient outcomes following defibrillation with a low energy biphasic truncated exponential waveform in out-of-hospital cardiac arrest, *Resuscitation* **49**, 9-14 (2001).

18. Capucci et al., Tripling survival from sudden cardiac arrest via early defibrillation without traditional education in cardiopulmonary resuscitation, *Circulation* **106**, 1065-1070 (2002).

19. R.D. White, Early out-of-hospital experience with an impedance-compensating low-energy biphasic waveform automatic external defibrillator, *Journal of Cardiovascular Electrophysiology* **1**, 203-208 (1997).

20. S. Caffrey et al., Public use of automated external defibrillators, *N Engl J Med* **347**, 1242-1247 (2002).

21. R.L. Page et al., Use of automated external defibrillators by a U.S. airline, *N Engl J Med* **343**, 1210-1216 (2000).

22. J.E. Gundry et al., Comparison of naïve sixth grade children with trained professionals in the use of an automated external defibrillator, *Circulation* **100**, 1703-1707 (1999).

23. D. Atkins et al., Resuscitation science of pediatrics, *Ann Emerg Med* **37**, 41- 48 (2001).

24. W. Tang et al., Pediatric fixed energy biphasic waveform defibrillation using a standard AED and special pediatric electrodes, *Supplement to Circulation* **102**(18)II, 437 (2000).

25. P.E. Litwin et al., The location of collapse and its effect on survival from cardiac arrest, *Ann Emerg Med* **16**, 787-791 (1987).

Chapter 30

REMOTE PATIENT MONITORING SOLUTIONS
Towards Remote Patient Management

David Simons[1], Tadashi Egami[2], and Jeff Perry[2]
[1]Philips Research, Eindhoven, The Netherlands; [2]Philips Medical Systems, Milpitas, CA, USA

Abstract: In this chapter, remote patient monitoring is discussed in terms of domain, applications, benefits, barriers, and existing solutions. In addition, remote patient management is introduced as an enabler to further develop new and improved care models. Examples of today's and tomorrow's Philips activities in this domain are included.

Keywords: Telehealthcare, remote monitoring, home telemonitoring, disease management, Motiva

1.   INTRODUCTION

Over the last decade, healthcare delivery has gradually extended from acute institutional care, to outpatient care and home care. Traditional *outpatient care* involves patients receiving care through visits to a hospital, clinic, or doctor's office for diagnosis or treatment without spending the night. Traditional *home care* typically involves periodic home visits by a nurse or other extended healthcare provider, for the purpose of monitoring and expeditiously treating patients with post-operative or chronic conditions. Home care services may require patients to maintain detailed records about their diet and health to support this care.

Advances in communication and information technology have enabled the delivery of healthcare services at a distance, anywhere outside of clinical settings. Such *telehealthcare* services involve both live audiovisual communication and store-and-forward exchange of digital images and medical information between patients and their care providers, at a distance. In our definition, subsets of telehealthcare services include telemedicine, home telecare, and remote patient monitoring.

505

G. Spekowius and T. Wendler (Eds.), Advances in Healthcare Technology, 505-516.
© 2006 Springer. Printed in the Netherlands.

Telemedicine is used to provide consultative and diagnostic medicine to patients at a distance instead of face-to-face, e.g. when patients are very isolated or when specialist services are in very high demand.

Home telecare is the term given to offering remote care of elderly and vulnerable people, providing care and reassurance needed to allow them to remain living in their own homes, via the collection of contextual data and audiovisual communication.

Remote patient monitoring (RPM), a.k.a. *home telemonitoring*, involves the passive collection of physiological and contextual data of patients in their own environment, using medical devices, software, and optionally environment sensors. This data is transmitted to the remote care provider, either in real-time or intermittently, for review and intervention.

Existing RPM solutions, and future extensions to remote patient *management* are the topic of this chapter.

2.   REMOTE PATIENT MONITORING

Deployment of RPM is driven by two principal concerns: to decrease the total cost of caring for patients with conditions that place them at high risk for hospitalization, and to provide efficiency improvements over models that rely on nurses traveling to residences to care for patients.

To date, RPM has been principally deployed in the *disease management* (DM) domain. DM is a systematic process of managing care of patients with specific diseases or conditions (particularly chronic conditions) across the spectrum of outpatient, inpatient, and ancillary services. The benefits of disease management may include: reducing acute episodes, reducing hospitalizations, reducing variations in care, improving health outcomes, and reducing total costs.

Disease management may involve continuous quality improvement or other management paradigms. It may involve a cyclical process of following practice protocols, measuring the resulting outcomes, feeding those results back to clinicians, and revising protocols as appropriate.

The primary application of DM is in chronic diseases. Table 30-1 lists the top 9 most expensive diseases in the US in 2005[1]. It is observed that chronic diseases make up a significant part of the overall cost, and their prevalence is growing. Also, for many of the expensive diseases, obesity is a risk factor.

Table 30-1. Top-9 most expensive diseases (US).

Ranking	Disease	Yearly cost (billions of $)	Nr. of patients (millions)
#1	Heart Conditions[†]	68	20
#2	Trauma	56	36
#3	Cancer[†]	48	11
#4	Mental illness	48	31
#5	Respiratory[†] ailments	45	50
#6	Hypertension[†]	33	37
#7	Arthritis and joint disorders[†]	32	23
#8	Diabetes[†]	28	14
#9	Back problems	23	18

[†] Overweight is a risk factor (1B adults worldwide are overweight)

Compounding this problem, chronic diseases disproportionately afflict the elderly. In the coming years, the so-called 'age wave' (Figure 30-1) will magnify the problem, if no solutions to reducing incidence or costs are found.

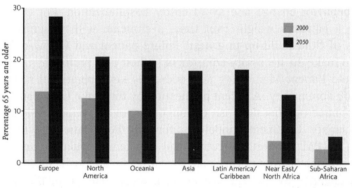

Source: U.S. Bureau of the Census (2000).

Figure 30-1. Proportion of population over 65 by region, 2000 and 2050 (projected).

While all patients with these high-cost conditions would likely benefit from some additional support in the home, remote patient monitoring solutions today are not applied for management of all these diseases. To be effective, the technology must be tailored to the disease-specific care process and made acceptable to the corresponding patient-user group. It must also be provided at a price point that enables the care giving organization to justify investment in the technology. Today, most DM programs mainly use RPM solutions in the management of their cardiac patients (CHF, CAD), diabetes patients, and pulmonary patients (COPD, asthma), starting with the most critical ones.

Of late, RPM is finding new applications in the domain of post-event rehabilitation (e.g. after cardiac surgery), diagnostic monitoring (e.g. of cardiac events), obesity and weight management, and elderly care.

The *benefits* of RPM solutions are broad ranging but can be grouped into economic benefits for the financial risk holders, operational benefits for the providers and quality of life benefits for the patients. A number of studies have already shown dramatic reductions in key cost drivers for the healthcare community through RPM technology leading to positive financial results.

In particular, the TEN-HMS[2] study, sponsored by the European Community, demonstrated a 10% cost saving over pure nurse follow-up, with an ROI of 2.1 when comparing incremental cost savings per patient to additional program fees. In this study of heart failure patients, it was the relative 26% reduction in hospital days per patient that drove the economic savings and increases in quality of life (Figure 30-2). Other studies have shown reduction in costly ER admissions or required home visits by nurses[3]. Monitoring vital signs through RPM solutions with follow-up provides efficient early warning mechanisms for the healthcare community to support patient behavior change and avoid costly hospitalization. For example, by tracking a patient's weight over time, a clinician will recognize pending episodes of fluid build-up in a heart failure patient and follow-up with the patient to make the necessary adjustment to their care protocol.

Remote Patient Monitoring also addresses key operational needs of the healthcare community. A recent publication by the Duke University Medical Center pointed out that there isn't enough time in a day for physicians in the US to satisfy treatment guidelines for all their patients with chronic illnesses[4]. RPM supports effective and efficient population management through automated monitoring and education in line with those evidence-based guidelines for patient management to prevent hospitalizations. Not only is the reach of a disease management organization with a given amount of human resources a bigger patient population, but also the quality of care is enhanced through standardization. This is particularly important given a worldwide shortage of qualified nurses who have typically been the main point of contact with a patient for a disease management service.

Finally, RPM poses significant benefits for the patient in terms of quality of life. Patients have reported feeling more secure with this type of supervision (88% of telemonitoring patients in the TEN-HMS study reported feeling "safer or much safer" while in this type of program.) Patients and caregivers alike appreciate the continued support outside of hospital or physician walls in avoiding hospitalization and exacerbation of their condition. Effective RPM solutions not only increase patient awareness and motivation for healthy behavior but also increase patient confidence in managing their condition.

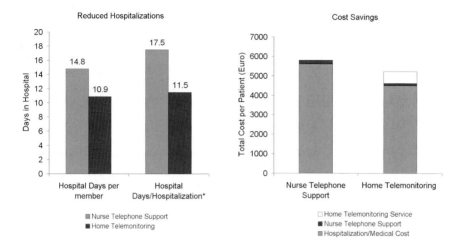

Figure 30-2. Deploying home telemonitoring for heart failure patients reduced both days in hospital (improved quality of life) and total cost of care (see Cleland et al.[2]).

However, a number of *barriers* have prevented broad development and widespread deployment of RPM solutions. These barriers can be segmented into regulatory, financial, cultural and technical categories.

On the regulatory front, a wide variety of organizations and standards may govern the deployment of RPM technologies. In the US, these organizations include the Food and Drug Administration (FDA) and the Federal Communications Commission (FCC). Relevant regulations include the Healthcare Insurance Portability and Accountability Act (HIPAA), promulgated by the Department of Health and Human Services. HIPAA governs the patient health information security and privacy requirements for entities that manage such information.

In Europe, analogues of these organizations and regulations exist on both a European Community level (e.g. the Medical Device Directive) as well as on regional and national levels (e.g. regulations of wireless frequency spaces, privacy and security regulations). As a result, developing solutions that can be deployed on a world-wide basis can be a complex undertaking, realistically accessible only to a few companies who have the resources and domain knowledge to cost-effectively navigate this web of requirements and regulations.

Financial barriers to widespread RPM deployment also exist. First and foremost of these is the absence of well accepted and wide spread reimbursement models to support remote patient care. The traditional health insurance model provides for compensation to health professionals for a wide variety of services provided in hospitals, clinics and doctors' offices. However, these schemes provide little financial compensation for care provided in patient homes or via remote or virtual interactions with patients.

As a result, RPM often suffers from two financial barriers. First is the direct barrier to reimbursement for services rendered. The second, more insidious, barrier is the financial disincentive toward remote management, as effective RPM decreases the need for and revenue from traditional bricks-and-mortar health services.

In turn, this financial disincentive compounds the cultural barrier the traditional healthcare system has to providing continuous remote care. Western healthcare systems have become highly effective at providing acute and emergent care. Corresponding institutions and professional organizations have developed around enhancing these practice models. These institutions in turn may resist or retard the evolution of competitive or non-allied care models.

Finally, some technical barriers exist to cost-effective development and widespread deployment of RPM solutions. In the medical informatics community there is a saying that the wonderful thing about standards is that there are so many of them. Though the healthcare community evidently recognizes the value of interface standardization, the lack any all-powerful standards setting bodies (or comparable de-facto industry standards) has enabled the proliferation of standards, sometimes resulting in several competing standards being developed for the same domain. As a result, creation of plug-and-play devices and services is simply not possible in healthcare today.

Security issues also impact the development of RPM technologies. Policy makers continue to wrestle with setting appropriate expectations, regulations and penalties for the maintenance of healthcare information. Tremendous advances in this area over the last few years have driven changes that make healthcare information more safe and secure than ever before. However, the rapid pace of change, as well as the continued existence of 'legacy' technologies that may not be upgradeable to the latest technical approaches, has proved challenging and expensive for many healthcare technology vendors and customers.

We are convinced that the barriers to RPM can be overcome, and that the benefits will stand out, leading to a wide deployment of RPM.

3. REMOTE PATIENT MONITORING SOLUTIONS

Many solutions for RPM exist today in the market, which is very fragmented. Many players have their own proprietary solutions and individual competencies along the value chain.

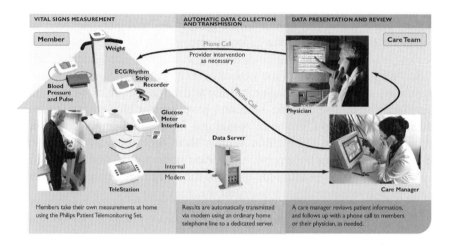

Figure 30-3. Home telemonitoring solution from Philips Telemonitoring Services.

A typical RPM telemonitoring solution consists of the following components (Figure 30-3):

1. **Medical observation devices**, to measure vital signs such as weight, blood pressure, glucose, and ECG rhythm strips. These devices may be stationary, portable, or body-worn, and have wired or low-power wireless connectivity to transmit the measurement to a care station. Today more and more devices appear using Bluetooth radios, though over time this may change to alternative, more suitable radios when they become widely available.

2. One or more **care stations**, either stationary (e.g. PC, dedicated embedded device) or portable (e.g. mobile phone, PDA) that act as an access point and store-and-forward unit for the vital-signs observations. In some cases, if the care station allows for user input, it is also used for gathering subjective input from the patient, via short surveys.

3. **Connectivity** from the patient's homes to a data server at the back-end. Typical RPM solutions are phone-based (POTS) and use dial-up modems to connect intermittently to the data server. Alternative solutions using

cellular networks (e.g. GPRS) and Internet are also being marketed, nowadays.

4. At the back-end **data center** the data for all subscribed patients is being collected and made available for review by nurse care managers. One of the distinguishing features of RPM solutions is the level of specialistic data processing and clinical decision support that is offered to increase the efficiency of the nurse care managers.

5. Typically, the nurse care managers are based in a **call center**, from which they can place a phone call to the patient or corresponding physician, when results fall outside the expected ranges.

So, with today's solutions, objective and subjective patient data are transmitted to the care manager, to allow the most at-risk patients to be prioritized for follow-up. The solutions have proven clinical and financial efficacies[2]. The patient, however, is taking a more passive role – rather than getting the tools and information to help them the positively change their behavior (healthier diet, exercise, medication compliance) and involve them in manage their own health. This is where the extension from remote patient monitoring to remote patient *management* comes into play.

4.   REMOTE PATIENT MANAGEMENT: A NEW PARADIGM IN HEALTH CARE

Management of the chronically ill is still very much driven by the traditional 'bricks and mortar' institutions of the medical community. The majority of those in the generations over 65 rely on their physicians and healthcare network for guidance around daily therapy. Typically, the healthcare community has focused on treating acute conditions and serious exacerbations, not on providing daily support and management. As a result, in this traditional model, patients are largely left to fend for themselves, with the avoidable result that their health status occasionally declines to the point where they must be admitted to a hospital for treatment (Figure 30-4).

The challenge is for the care community to work more creatively and efficiently to drive out these high-cost exacerbations and complications. RPM solutions provide a means to smooth the traditional, reactive care management roller coaster, efficiently detecting when a patient's health status is slipping and enabling the healthcare system to intervene to prevent a high-cost event.

Responsibility and accountability for healthcare costs is increasingly moving toward the consumer. Consumer-driven health and wellness is emerging as an industry, as individuals wish to take more control of all aspects of their health and medical care. Compounding these phenomena, the trend of healthcare systems to push more financial responsibility onto patients is creating incentives for patients to be more savvy consumers of health services. The recent emergence of consumer-directed healthcare plans enables patients who effectively manage their care and risk factors to manage and potentially reduce the direct cost of their healthcare.

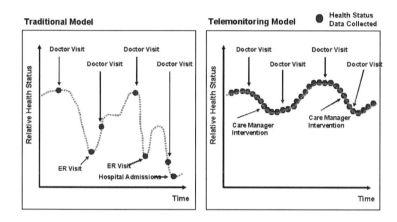

Figure 30-4. Traditional vs. telemonitoring care models.

Technology, in the form of low-cost unobtrusive monitoring devices, pervasive connectivity, and intelligent, personalized applications and services, is poised to play a significant role in this coming transformation. Many of these technology building blocks are crossing over from the consumer and entertainment sectors into healthcare and wellness. For example, Philips' Connected Planet products envision and address a world where consumers can connect and access entertainment, information and services, any place, anytime, anywhere. Philips sees the drivers for Personal Healthcare and Connected Planet technologies being the same – digital convergence, backed by expanding access to a broadband infrastructure and breakthroughs in wireless technologies.

5. MOTIVA – MOVING INTO THE FUTURE

With the Motiva platform[5], Philips is making this convergence vision a reality. Motiva represents a scalable, personalized platform to effectively help healthcare systems manage one of their principal challenges – reducing the total cost of caring for an increasingly elderly population with escalating incidence of chronic illnesses.

The foundation for Motiva is built on half-a-decade of commercial experience supplying telemonitoring solutions, such as the Philips Telemonitoring Services solution (Figure 30-3). Traditional telemonitoring solutions focus on simply collecting patient status information from devices for display and review by care managers. Broad deployment of these solutions has been hindered by both the cost and the complexity of deploying devices into the home. As a result, these monitoring solutions have generally only been deployed for the highest-risk and highest-cost patients, even though studies like TEN-HMS[2] have shown the approach to be cost effective.

The Motiva platform addresses these issues, using technologies that integrate well with normal daily routines and that leverage the cost and scale efficiencies that are common to the consumer electronics domain. For the healthcare system, Motiva enables care providers to more effectively help patients self-manage their conditions. Through an engaging, on-demand multi-media patient interface, delivered over the TV, patients are guided towards healthy behavior, without increasing the demand for costly and scarce live nursing support.

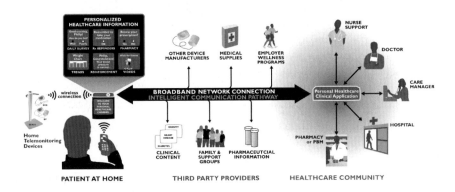

Figure 30-5. Philips Motiva: Leveraging consumer electronics and connectivity to provide secure, reliable health & wellness services to patients at a time and place of their convenience.

Leveraging Philips' understanding of both consumer solutions and the healthcare domain, Motiva combines technologies, form factors and usability models developed for consumer electronics with architectures, security, applications and services designed to meet the needs of healthcare systems. The result is a platform that enables a transformation in how chronic and other complex conditions can be managed – from nurse-and-phone based approaches, to one centered around providing patients with the information, skills and tools they need to effectively manage their conditions themselves (Figure 30-5).

An initial application built on the Motiva platform focuses on supporting the remote management of patients with congestive heart failure (CHF). It comprises a media-rich interactive health channel that is accessible from the patient's own television. This interaction medium works well for the CHF target group of which most patients are older than 55. Also, devices for monitoring weight and blood pressure can be included (Figure 30-6).

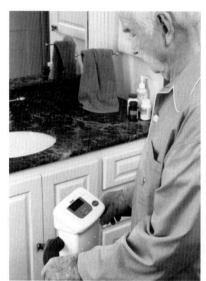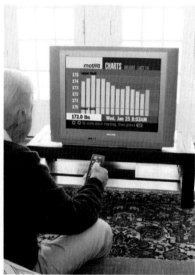

Figure 30-6. Philips Motiva patient self-management components.

At the end of 2004, a usability study of the Motiva system in New Jersey with the Cardiology Associates of the Delaware Valley[5] highlighted strong acceptance by both patients and clinicians. Patients appreciated both the guidance and interactivity that the Motiva solution supports and readily accepted the TV interface.

> "Just as the names suggests, Motiva motivated me to do the right thing... Through personal charts and educational videos sent to me on my TV by my nurse, I learned how to better manage my disease. I weighed myself, took my own blood pressure, answered daily health questions, and the Motiva system tracked how well I was doing. With Motiva, it was easy to learn how improving my lifestyle could help me stay healthier. I'm feeling more in control now."   *- Patient in CADV Study*

At the other end of the care relationship, the clinicians felt that their connection with patients actually improved with the Motiva system, and that they were more aware of the patients' health status.

> "By interacting with patients on a day-to-day basis, we can be more proactive; problems can be detected earlier than they might be otherwise. Chronic cardiac conditions are manageable, but our challenge is to provide patients with the tools and knowledge they need to play a more active role. A patient who is more educated will be more likely to comply with medications, with dietary and fitness recommendations, and in general, to be more involved with their care."
>
> *- Jeffrey H. Kramer, M.D.*
> *Fellow of the American College of Cardiology*
> *Principal investigator for CADV*

The Motiva platform is architected to be extended over time to accommodate applications for other diseases, novel measurement devices (such as unobtrusive, wearable vital sign sensors) and alternative interaction devices (such as web browsers, cell phones, and digital media devices). In addition, the platform is designed to scale toward millions of users and devices, anticipating a future when health and wellness management is a mainstream consumer market.

REFERENCES

1. Forbes on-line article April 14, 2005, The Most Expensive Diseases, based on data from Agency for Healthcare Research and Quality; http://www.forbes.com/science/2005/04 /14/ cx_mh_0414healthcosts.html.
2. J.G.F. Cleland, A. Balk, U. Janssens et al., Noninvasive Home Telemonitoring for Patients With Heart Failure at High Risk of Recurrent Admission and Death (TEN-HMS study), *JACC* **45**(109), 1654-1664 (2005).
3. L.R. Goldberg, et al, Randomized Trial Of A Daily Electronic Home Monitoring System In Patients With Advanced Heart Failure: The Weight Monitoring in Heart Failure (WHARF) Trial, *American Heart Journal* **146**(4), 705-712 (2003).
4. J. Stover, Chronic Disease Management Crippling Primary Care System, DukeMed News, May 31, 2005; http://dukemednews.duke.edu/news/article.php?id=8839.
5. Philips Medical Systems, Motiva; http://www.medical.philips.com/main/products/ telemonitoring/ products/motiva/.

Chapter 31

DIABETIC CARE
Technology Will Improve Diabetics' Quality of Life

Golo von Basum[1], Rufus Driessen[1], Francisco Morales[1], Begonya Otal[2] and Kristiane Schmidt[1]

[1]*Philips Research, Eindhoven, The Netherlands;* [2]*Philips Research, Aachen, Germany*

Abstract: According to the WHO, diabetes is one of the most growing diseases today population-wise[1]. Looking at estimations there will be more than 333 million diabetics by 2025. This justifies efforts to develop new technologies in helping diabetics in their daily life. We briefly describe the background of diabetes, show a potential segmentation of the diabetic population and illustrate their primary needs. Amongst them, we identify the three most important unmet needs, i.e. painless glucose monitoring, decision support, and lifestyle support. We believe that new technological solutions have the potential to fulfill these unmet needs. This will make meaningful contributions by reducing the daily burdens of diabetes management, reducing long-term complications and generally improving the quality of life for diabetics.

Keywords: Diabetes, lifestyle, decision support, non-invasive, diabetes management

1. BACKGROUND ON DIABETES

Diabetes is a metabolic disorder in which the human body either fails to produce or to properly use insulin; a hormone that regulates uptake and transport of glucose. Currently, diabetes affects more than 194 million people worldwide[2]. The number of people suffering from diabetes is rapidly increasing, and is estimated to exceed 333 million by 2025[2]. At least 50% of all people with diabetes are unaware of their condition.

In the long term, diabetes can cause a variety of severe complications, such as blindness, cardiovascular diseases, kidney failure, and lower limb amputations. In most developed countries, diabetes and its complications are already the fourth main cause of death[3].

517

G. Spekowius and T. Wendler (Eds.), Advances in Healthcare Technology, 517-532.

Apart from the enormous physical and emotional burden of the disease and its complications for the individual, diabetes also has a major impact on Healthcare infrastructure and Healthcare expenditures. The American Diabetes Association estimated that in 2002 diabetes cost the US Healthcare System and economy approximately $132 billion[4].

1.1   Types of diabetes

About 5-15% of diabetics are afflicted by what is known as type 1 diabetes[2]. Type 1 diabetes is an autoimmune disease, in which the body's immune system destroys the insulin producing β cells of the pancreas. This results in an inability to produce insulin. Type 1 diabetes tends to occur in people of less than 20 years of age.

The majority of diabetics however suffer from type 2 diabetes, which is usually associated with insulin resistance. In this condition the pancreas cells are able to produce insulin, but the insulin cannot stimulate the uptake of glucose into muscle and adipose cells[5]. Type 2 diabetes is often, but not always, associated with obesity, which in itself can cause insulin resistance. Usually, the condition is diagnosed after the age of 40, and its prevalence increases with age. However, the number of young people and even children with type 2 diabetes is increasing, most likely due to obesity and physical inactivity.

Type 2 diabetes is often preceded by pre-diabetes, an asymptotic condition where blood glucose levels are elevated. Individuals with pre-diabetes are at high risk of progressing to type 2 diabetes, although such progression is not inevitable. Probably over 30% of these individuals will return to normal glucose tolerance over a period of several years[6]. In 2003, worldwide about 314 million people had impaired glucose tolerance (IGT)[2]. Several clinical studies have shown that type 2 diabetes can be prevented or at least delayed by lifestyle changes[7].

Gestational diabetes is defined as IGT that is first detected during pregnancy. About 7% of all pregnancies are affected by gestational diabetes, which is strongly associated with both maternal and fetal complications[8].

1.2   Pathophysiology and complications of diabetes

Without treatment, diabetes results in hyperglycemia, which is a very high level of glucose in the blood (above 10 mmol/l; 180 mg/dl). Even slight hyperglycemia is strongly associated with long-term complications of diabetes[9]. Diabetic people often also suffer from hypoglycemia, which is too low blood glucose levels (below 3 mmol/l; 54 mg/dl). Hypoglycemia is mainly caused by too much insulin and/or too little food intake and can easily be treated by carbohydrate intake. However, if a diabetic person is not able to feel hypoglycemia or if hypoglycemic episodes occur during the night, a life threatening condition could occur.

Insulin stimulates the uptake of glucose into muscle and adipose tissue. In addition, insulin suppresses the release of glucose from the liver and of fatty acids from adipose tissue[10]. The latter explains why most diabetic people also have elevated lipid levels, i.e. cholesterol and triglycerides. Insulin also stimulates nitric oxide (NO) synthase in the vascular endothelium and thus may increase tissue perfusion[11].

Table 31-1 summarizes the long-term complications of diabetes. Microvascular complications are caused by dysfunction of the capillaries and small blood vessels. The main cause for these complications is hyperglycemia. Macrovascular complications are due to alterations in the large blood vessels, for instance arteriosclerosis. Besides hyperglycemia, dyslipidemia (abnormal lipid levels) and hypertension (high blood pressure) are involved in macrovascular complications[5].

Table 31-1. Long-term complications of diabetes.

	Complication	Description
Microvascular	Retinopathy	Damage of eye capillaries, leading cause of blindness.
	Neuropathy	Impairment of nerves, especially in the lower extremities. Loss of sensation, pain (tingling), numbness. Foot ulcers, leading cause for lower limb amputation.
	Nephropathy	Impairment of kidney function. Most common single cause for end-stage renal disease. May require dialysis or kidney transplantation.
Macrovascular	Coronary heart disease	Heart attack, myocardial infarction. Major complication in type 2 diabetes.
	Peripheral arterial disease	Decreased perfusion of lower extremities. Foot ulcers, leading cause for lower limb amputation.
	Cerebrovascular disease	Blockage of blood vessels in the brain. Transient ischemic attacks, stroke.

1.3 Treatment

Until now, there is no cure for diabetes, but optimized treatment can greatly reduce long-term complications. The main target for the treatment of all types of diabetes is glycaemic control, which means bringing the blood glucose levels as close as possible to normal. All type 1 diabetics need to be treated with multiple daily injections of exogenous insulin. The exact amount of insulin that is needed depends on the actual blood glucose level as well as the anticipated intake of carbohydrates (diet) and glucose consumption by the body (muscle activity). The diabetic person must also monitor her blood glucose levels at least three times per day by SMBG (self-monitoring of blood glucose).

For type 2 diabetics, the treatment depends on the severity of β cell failure. A minor fraction of type 2 diabetics requires insulin therapy as described above for type 1. The majority of people with type 2 diabetes use oral agents to lower their glucose levels. Again, the diabetic person has to control the effectiveness of the treatment by performing SMBG. Besides medication, the glucose levels can also be lowered by dietary changes (lowering the carbohydrate intake), weight loss and, most importantly, by physical exercise. During exercise, the uptake and metabolism of glucose is stimulated independently of insulin. In addition, exercise also has been reported to increase insulin sensitivity[5]. For the treatment of pre-diabetes, lifestyle modifications have been shown to be even more effective than treatment with oral agents[7]. For more detailed and in-depth information related to diabetes treatment, refer to the diabetes compendium by Berger[12].

2.   NEEDS OF DIABETICS

2.1   Segmentation of diabetic population

The large population of diabetics consists of many different groups, each with different lifestyles and each dealing with diabetes their own way. We will show seven criteria for a possible segmentation (see Table 31-2) and give examples for specific *needs* and *technologies* in the different groups.

Table 31-2. Segmentation is based on 7 sets of classification criteria.

	Criteria	Range
1	Type of diabetes	Type 1 – type 2 – gestational – pre-diabetes
2	Insulin	Insulin-dependent versus non-insulin-dependent
3	Compliance level	Highly compliant … non-compliant
4	Type of glycaemic management	Self-management … assisted-management
5	Age	Children – adolescents – adults – elderly
6	Diagnosis	Diagnosed versus non-diagnosed
7	Type of chronic complications	Neuropathy, nephropathy, retinopathy, macrovascular

Type of diabetes. The most obvious and commonly used breakdown of the diabetic population is based on the type of the diabetes: type 1, type 2, gestational and pre-diabetes. The segmentation could be extended to those people who are at risk for developing diabetes. A first example for technology related to this criterion is *tight glycaemic control*, which plays an important role in the segments of type 1 diabetes and gestational diabetes. A second example is technology that *supports awareness* of the disease. This is of interest for newly diagnosed diabetics, but is also valid for pre-diabetes and part of the type 2 diabetics. An extension of this technology could be a solution to *support lifestyle*: this can play a role in the total diabetic population.

Insulin. The diabetic population can be divided into insulin-dependent and non-insulin-dependent. All of type 1 diabetics are insulin-dependent, as well as a part of type 2 diabetics. They require insulin therapy to control their blood glucose levels. Technologies for insulin-dependent diabetics could include *decision support* in dosing the right amount of insulin at the right time. Furthermore, a technology is required for *delivering insulin* and other medications into the body. A last example is a *non-invasive* and *quasi-continuous* glucose monitoring technology that would help realizing well-controlled insulin dosing.

Compliance level. The level of compliance in monitoring blood glucose values is a third consideration. While the recommended testing frequency may vary from eight times per day to once a week or even less, in general the actual finger-stick test frequency falls short. The compliance of a diabetic depends mostly on her disease awareness or denial. Also, personal motivation is important when discussing compliance. Although technology may help diabetics to be more motivated, technology by itself is not sufficient. Key technology drivers that will support compliance are *painless and bloodless monitoring*. For non-compliant diabetics, ignorance or denial shows up. Here technology may play a role in *personalizing education* and in *providing meaningful data* that matches the diabetics' compliance level.

Type of glycaemic management. Another way to look at diabetes is to define who is actually performing the day-to-day managing of blood glucose levels. This can either be the diabetic herself (self-management) or somebody else helping the diabetic (assisted-management). In the case of self-management, the user is the diabetic, who needs to integrate monitoring of glucose and administering of medication in daily life. Therefore, *portability* and other *ease-of-use* aspects are important. In the case of assisted glucose management, the user is not the diabetic, but somebody assisting her.

Age. Yet another way to divide the diabetic population is by age: children, adolescents, adults and elderly. Each age-group may require specific technology solutions. An example is that elderly people may require a user interface with *larger displays* and *buttons*.

Diagnosis. Another split of the population is the diagnosed versus the undiagnosed. The undiagnosed is suffering from the same disease as the diabetic but is not aware of it: her blood glucose level will make excursions outside of the normal range. A large part of the type 2 diabetics are undiagnosed. Technology to *screen* and to *identify people* with type 2 diabetes or pre-diabetes will help in reducing its impact.

Type of chronic complications. Finally, chronic complications related to diabetes is another set of classification criteria. A simplified classification is based on macrovascular diseases and microvascular complications. Each of these areas requires specific technologies to avoid, to reduce or to treat the complication. A specific example is technology for *early detection and treatment of foot ulcers*.

This possible segmentation of the diabetic population will help to address the diverse groups of diabetics with individualized technological solutions. Thus, it makes it easier to identify characteristic needs for the separate groups of diabetics.

2.2   Analysis of the diabetics' needs

For undiagnosed people, sometimes a complication of diabetes may give a clue to the presence of the disease. However, these complications are not unavoidable consequences. A healthy, active lifestyle is a lifetime plan. According to that, every diabetic person runs generally through the same basic needs in which lifestyle modifications are essential.

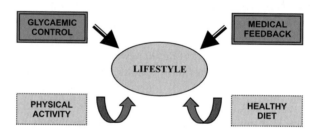

Figure 31-1. Basic diabetic needs, which every diabetic is confronted with.

Figure 31-1 shows the basic needs grouped in four main categories. These four needs, which every diabetic is daily confronted with, are generally described as follows:

Glycaemic control. Tight glycaemic control slows down the onset and progression of diabetes complications. Thus, good diabetes care always begins at home using SMBG. Glycaemic control is the cornerstone for preventing unwanted complications.

Medical feedback. The primary care team plays an important role in diabetes management. Ideally they should be offering step-by-step diabetes self-management education on the one hand, and personalized feedback on the other hand. First of all, they have to pay attention to behavioural changes of all diabetics, such as smoking cessation, adequate nutrition, enough exercise and, above all, right glycaemic control. Moreover, early diagnosis of diabetes is also essential in order to delay or even avoid long-term complications. Last but not least, diabetic people must be reminded of yearly and monthly visits when the time approaches, as a way to increase motivation and compliance.

Physical activity. Physical activity can lower blood glucose, blood pressure, and cholesterol. In addition, regular activity helps insulin to work better and improves blood circulation. Most doctors recommend diabetics to participate in regular aerobic exercise. There is a vital need in increasing motivation for committing to regular exercise and physical activity.

Healthy diet. Food and blood glucose levels are closely correlated. Knowing the food composition – the calories, carbohydrates, protein, and fat – will help in controlling blood glucose levels. Most diabetics will need to make some changes to their eating habits. However, this does not mean that they have to follow a special diet – the diet recommended for people with diabetes is a general healthy diet.

2.3   Key unmet needs

In the following, we will identify those main needs of a diabetic person that will enable her to improve quality of life accordingly to her type of diabetes and personal condition. Within the afore described four groups, the following three key unmet needs are identified:

Painless, blood-free glucose monitoring. Nowadays, diabetics use finger stick meters, which require a fingertip puncture to withdraw a drop of blood. This procedure causes pain and carries risk of infection. It also exposes a diabetic's surroundings to blood and creates an uncomfortable social situation that diabetics strongly avoid. The pain perception during a finger stick test is the major hurdle for frequent testing. Therefore, a painless and if possible non-invasive meter to determine blood glucose values is the most desired tool. Apart from this main feature, accuracy and portability are of fundamental interest. People want reliable blood glucose values, and to measure blood glucose everywhere and whenever it is required. This need is most present in the segments of type 1 and type 2 diabetics, as well as in the gestational diabetics. It also relates to the segment of compliance.

Decision support. Tight glycaemic control increases the risk of hypo-glycaemic events[13]. Diabetics are therefore confronted with the difficulty of keeping their blood glucose values in a very defined regime. Food intake will influence their glucose values, as well as physical activity and of course insulin dosing. Bearing this in mind, every diabetic will find it beneficial not only to measure her current blood glucose level, but also to be able to anticipate its value one or two hours in advance. Easy, comfortable and non-time consuming prediction of blood glucose values is therefore another key unmet need.

Lifestyle support. The basis of managing diabetes nowadays is a change of the lifestyle of the diabetic to prevent long-term complications. These complications are to blame for a reduction in quality of life and in lifetime expectancy. A lifestyle support concept is also a key unmet need and probably the most ambitious to work on, because motivation and educational aspects play the essential role here. Every diabetic requires personalized and continuous coaching in order to manage her disease. Thus, there is on the one hand a need for facilitating relations among diabetics and medical care providers, and on the other hand a need for personal encouragement and responsibility for the own disease.

As portrayed in Figure 31-2, the lifestyle support concept will benefit from the previously identified needs. Generally depicted, the lifestyle support solution will help diabetics to delay or prevent serious complications associated with their disease by providing answers and explanations, as though one had a virtual nurse as a companion.

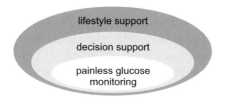

Figure 31-2. The key unmet needs from a diabetic perspective.

The three here presented key unmet needs are a step further in the direction of diabetes management, which will assist every diabetic to keep up with the suggested medical guidelines. These diabetic needs turned into technological solutions will help not only the person in her new way of living, but also the physician to manage the disease.

3.   TECHNOLOGIES AND APPLICATIONS

In this section we describe potential solutions for the afore-mentioned most important unmet needs. These include technologies and applications to address:

- Painless, blood-free monitoring.
- Decision support.
- Lifestyle support.

3.1   Non-invasive glucose monitor

Diabetics from all types need to measure their blood glucose values frequently to ensure tight glycaemic control. From the analysis of the key unmet needs we derived the following three main issues related to glucose monitoring: painless, easy-to-use and sufficiently accurate technology. Such a technology will lead to a much higher acceptance and compliance by the diabetics compared to existing technologies, like finger stick devices. This will help encourage more frequent testing and thus a better control of the diabetes.

Figure 31-3 gives an example how inadequate testing could lead to problems in tracking the correct glucose values. The continuous trace shows the glucose values of a non-diabetic person recorded with a sample interval of five minutes (continuous). This data is taken from literature[14]. We additionally marked points at intervals of two hours. It is obvious that due to this undersampling nearly every excursion of the glucose value is missed. Gough et al. found, that the optimal sampling frequency is in the order of 10 minutes[15].

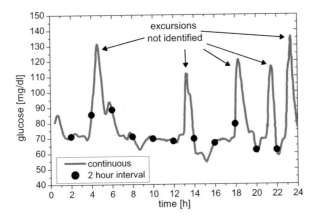

Figure 31-3. Example of undersampling[14].

In the analysis of potential solutions, we will focus on truly non-invasive technologies to ensure the aspect of painless monitoring and avoiding the risk of infection or contamination. This means that these technologies should not require any analyte extracted from the body (e.g. blood or interstitial fluid). Such techniques have been investigated extensively for many years. Khalil[16] has given an excellent overview of the recent developments in the area of non-invasive glucose measurement techniques. The most extensive investigated approaches are optical techniques, which make use of the specific absorption spectrum of glucose. The wavelength regions vary from near infrared (NIR, 800 – 2000 nm) up to the mid infrared (MIR, 2000 – 10000 nm). The optical techniques include diffuse back-reflectance spectroscopy, Raman spectroscopy, attenuated total reflectance (ATR) spectroscopy, optical coherence tomography (OCT), and photoacoustic spectroscopy. All of them assume to be able to measure directly the effect of glucose on the spectrum. Besides these, non-optical methods also have been reported, like *in vivo* electrical impedance measurements.

A common challenge for many non-invasive techniques relates to the measurement volume, where glucose is mainly present in interstitial fluid and capillary blood. When comparing these glucose values with values obtained directly from venous blood, they often show a lag time due to metabolism, vasoconstriction and perfusion. But recent research shows promising results to address this lag time issue[17]. Another difficulty arises from substances present in human skin, which may hamper a correct glucose determination. These factors add up to the challenge of sufficient accuracy and specificity.

Although none of the current non-invasive technologies, which are reported in literature, is able to solve all of these problems, major steps towards sufficient accuracy and specificity have been made[16]. Moreover, we believe that in near future, the problems related to truly non-invasive glucose measurements will be overcome.

3.2   Decision support technology

The second identified unmet need mainly addresses the issue of appropriate glycaemic control. This includes prediction of future glucose values, giving advice for food intake, alerting in case of hypoglycaemia, and advising insulin dosing. Decision support technology should give advice or recommendation to help regulate the blood glucose values on a short-term time scale (e.g. hours).

For any technology addressing this need, it is crucial to develop suitable algorithms helping to predict future glucose values. As for the painless, non-invasive glucose meter, work has been done in this area by different academic groups[15,18,19,20]. The basic scheme for a decision-supporting algorithm is shown in Figure 31-4.

The most important input parameter for a model to predict future glucose values is the history of measured glucose values. It is obvious that the shorter the measuring interval is, the better the prediction algorithms will perform. Thus, the most suited measuring method to enable a decision tool should be a quasi-continuous technology. Apart from pure measurements of glucose values, a good and simple logging of these values is needed. This will give the diabetic a better insight into her disease, and it will also help the care provider to evaluate and to set up the therapeutic treatment.

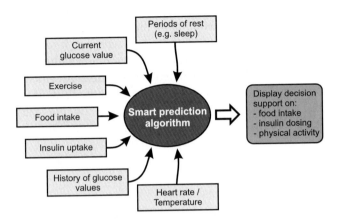

Figure 31-4. Overview of a decision support algorithm.

We mentioned already, that the development of diabetes is strongly affected by the physical condition of the diabetic person, the food intake, and the overall lifestyle situation. All this, of course, has consequences on the short-term change of the blood glucose values. Thus, additional input parameters will improve the prediction model significantly. A tool for decision support should include input for food intake, times and level of exercising, or periods of rest or sleep. Furthermore, other vital body signals like heart rate or temperature will improve the quality of prediction. A major challenge to gather this information is the development of unobtrusive sensors.

A very important point to keep in mind when investigating decision support algorithms, is the unique personal situation of every single diabetic. This requires highly personalized and adaptive tools, which for example take care of the individual metabolism, clinical history, lifestyle situation, or even changes of the diabetes in time. For good predictions, not only past or current actions should be transferred to the algorithm, but also actions planned in the near future. This information could then be considered when calculating glucose and insulin metabolism.

A further feature of decision support should be the advice when to use insulin. Zisser et al.[21] showed that run-to-run control of glucose levels as direct reaction of insulin intake could be used to calculate the personalized best insulin dosing prior to a meal based on the recorded history of the diabetic. The optimal solution would be an intelligent self-learning algorithm, which adapts to the personal situation of the individual diabetic. Apart from concrete actions to change glucose levels, the tool might also give advice on the most suitable measurement intervals, or give an alarm when the next measurement should be taken.

The goal of any new technology enabling decision support should be an easy-to-use and simple application from the diabetics' perspective, relieving them from risks and from the burden of worries. It needs to provide meaningful directives to the diabetic, which are actionable. This will also help to increase the quality of life by enhancing the confidence of a diabetic in taking action related to her condition. Currently there is no good and simple-to-use tool for decision support available on the market, but we believe that algorithms can be developed and implemented in devices for home use.

3.3   Lifestyle support

The life of a person dramatically changes from the moment she is diagnosed with diabetes. This is a very crucial moment in her life because she will be confronted with two major problems:

- You have a chronic, incurable disease that will accompany you for the rest of your life: If you do not change your lifestyle, it will not get better, but it may get worse.
- You have to change your lifestyle in order to keep on living and to avoid potential complications.

This section concentrates on technical options that can improve a diabetic's health during gradual changes in the lifestyle that will match her self-discipline and will empower her, taking away the burden of worries.

Besides the stigma of a chronic disease, the diabetic person has little support dealing with the disease, because almost everything is based on self-treatment. She defines whether to measures glucose levels and when. The calculation of calorie intake is based on her heuristic best guess. The amount of medication is self-dosed, hopefully according to the guidelines given by the general practitioner. She also has to estimate the amount of energy spent during more extenuating physical activity, thus lowering the need of additional amounts of medication. In summary, the disease is always very present in a diabetic's daily life due to the burden of responsibility.

Technology and education of diabetics will enable a change in today's diabetes management. Technology will additionally enable diabetics to start living a more normal life with fewer worries reducing the pressure of responsibility, while maintaining a healthy consciousness of the disease. The former will give people a self-assuring feeling, while the latter is important because diabetics learn to accept the disease rather than denying it. Depending on the level of disease awareness and education, specialized programs can coach diabetics while keeping them motivated to start new phases of treatment and to keep on learning about their disease, and thus inducing more positive changes in the diabetic's lifestyle.

We assume that solutions for lifestyle support must have an integral approach empowering diabetics with autonomy and independence, while keeping them mobile and assuring the right treatment at the right time. We can look at it from two different perspectives: from the diabetic's point of view and from the technological point of view. Furthermore, every perspective can be split in subcategories where the solutions will play a role. We foresee the subcategories as shown in Table 31-3.

Table 31-3. Technology perspectives and subcategories.

Perspective	Subcategory	Definition
Diabetics perspective	Advanced support and coaching	Set of solutions that will support diabetics in their lifestyle changes.
	Healthcare system	General Practitioner, specialists, nurses, hospitals, analysis laboratories.
Technology perspective	Diabetes companion	Portable device that diabetics carry around for lifestyle support.
	Home Health Center	Stationary set of infrastructure based at the diabetic's home that enables data transmission and further diagnostic at home.
	Telemedicine	Support infrastructure that assures that diabetics' data are saved and that proper reporting to the healthcare system occurs at the right time. This might include a two-way communication channel with a Healthcare center, but also a TV set.

Table 31-4 shows the two perspectives with the subcategories, and in addition, some examples of solutions by the technology offerings. These technological solutions will positively influence diabetics' lifestyle and hence their quality of life. We believe that technology and technology trends will make these solutions possible in a foreseeable time horizon. Key technologies that will definitively play an important role are:

- Optical techniques for diagnosis and measurement, but also for treatment
- Self-learning user interfaces that will adapt to diabetics' needs and awareness level
- Miniaturization of electronics for wearable devices and energy management

- Unobtrusive sensors to measure body signals
- Cost-effective biosensors for home use
- Integration of complex systems in meaningful architectures to bring components to an integral system.

Table 31-4. Technological solutions.

		Diabetics' perspective	
		Advanced Support and Coaching	*Healthcare system*
Technology perspective	*Diabetes companion*	• Measures glucose non-invasively • Provides decision support • Reminds that measurement has to be taken • Reminds to take medication • Coaches during exercise • Counts calorie intake • Counts calories consumption	• Downloads data to physician • Keeps track of diabetics' clinical history • Provides ubiquitous information access
	Home Health Center	• Provides decision support • Gives foot care (perfusion, pressure, etc.) • Detects extremity ulcers and decubitus • Measures additional blood analytes to secure compliance • Measures other body quantities	• Informs to contact healthcare provider in case some indicator surpasses a boundary • Broadcasts information to the healthcare provider
	Tele-medicine	• Provides education targeted to a specific diabetic person • Helps to configure • Coaches diabetics to set goals • Helps diabetics to keep motivated	• Physician can change medication / treatment • Education on early screening

Finally, these technological solutions will have to be integrated in the total Healthcare environment to create a diabetic-centered disease management.

4.   CONCLUSIONS

Diabetes is one of the most growing diseases today population-wise. Looking at estimations there will be more than 333 million diabetics by 2025. This justifies efforts to develop new technologies helping people to improve their quality of life. We described a segmentation of the diabetic population, which allows for addressing the diverse groups of diabetics with individualized solutions. For this segmentations seven separate criteria are selected. From the numerous general needs of diabetics, we identified the three most important needs, which could be fulfilled by breakthrough inventions. These technologies include truly non-invasive blood glucose monitors, decision support tools and lifestyle support. All mentioned technologies are currently not available on the market, but we believe that it is possible to overcome most of the current restrictions. This will help the majority of diabetics reduce the burden of their disease, improve their daily living and significantly reduce long-term complications associated with elevated blood glucose values.

ACKNOWLEDGEMENTS

We would like to thank Gerald Lucassen, Rachel Thilwind, Markus Laubscher, Sieglinde Neerken and Dan Barton for their useful comments on the manuscript.

REFERENCES

1. World Health Organization (September 16, 2005); http://www.who.int/dietphysicalactivity/publications/facts/diabetes.
2. International Diabetes Federation, *Diabetes Atlas, Second Edition* (International Diabetes Federation, Brussels, 2003).
3. International Diabetes Federation, *Diabetes and Cardiovascular Disease: Time to Act* (International Diabetes Federation, Brussels, 2001).
4. P. Hogan, T. Dall, P. Nikolov, Economic costs of diabetes in the US in 2002, *Diabetes Care* **26**(3), 917-932 (2003).
5. S.A. Ross, E.A. Gulve, M. Wang, Chemistry and biochemistry of type 2 diabetes, *Chem Rev* **104**(3), 1255-1282 (2004).
6. K.G. Alberti, The clinical implications of impaired glucose tolerance, *Diabet Med* **13**(11), 927-937 (1996).
7. M. Laakso, Prevention of type 2 diabetes, *Curr Mol Med* **5**(3), 365-374 (2005).
8. T.L. Setji, A.J. Brown, M.N. Feinglos, Gestational Diabetes Mellitus, *Clin Diabetes* **23**(1), 17-24 (2005).
9. I.M. Stratton, A.I. Adler, H.A. Neil, D.R. Matthews, S.E. Manley, C.A. Cull, D. Hadden, R.C. Turner, R.R. Holman, Association of glycaemia with macrovascular and microvascular complications of type 2 diabetes (UKPDS 35): prospective observational study, *B M J* **321**(7258), 405-412 (2000).
10. M. Stumvoll, B.J. Goldstein, T.W. van Haeften, Type 2 diabetes: principles of pathogenesis and therapy, *Lancet* **365**(9467), 1333-1346 (2005).
11. K. Shinozaki, K. Ayajiki, A. Kashiwagi, M. Masada, and T. Okamura, Malfunction of vascular control in lifestyle-related diseases: mechanisms underlying endothelial dysfunction in the insulin-resistant state, *J Pharmacol Sci* **96**(4), 401-405 (2004).

12. M. Berger, *Diabetes mellitus* (Urban & Fischer, München, 2000).

13. American Diabetes Association, Implications of the Diabetes Control and Complications Trial, *Diabetes Care* **25**(Supplement 1), 25-27 (2002).

14. Project for Glucose Monitoring and Control (September 16, 2005); http://www.glucosecontrol. ucsd.edu/data.html.

15. D.A. Gough, K. Kreutz-Delgado, T.M. Bremer, Frequency characterization of blood glucose dynamics, *Ann Biomed Eng* **31**(1), 91-97 (2003).

16. O.S. Khalil, Non-invasive glucose measurement technologies: an update from 1999 to the dawn of the new millennium, *Diabetes Technol Ther* **6**(5), 660-697 (2004).

17. P.J. Stout, J.R. Racchini, M.E. Hilgers, A novel approach to mitigating the physiological lag between blood and interstitial fluid glucose measurements, *Diabetes Technol Ther* **6**(5), 635-644 (2004).

18. C.C. Palerm, J.P. Willis, J. Desemone, B.W. Bequette, Hypoglycemia prediction and detection using optimal estimation, *Diabetes Technol Ther* **7**(1), 3-14 (2005).

19. E.J. Knobbe and B. Buckingham, The extended Kalman filter for continuous glucose monitoring, *Diabetes Technol Ther* **7**(1), 15-27 (2005).

20. C. Cobelli, D.M. Bier, and E. Ferrannini, Modeling glucose metabolism in man: theory and practice, *Horm Metab Res Suppl* **24**, 1-10 (1990).

21. H. Zisser, L. Jovanovic, F. Doyle, III, P. Ospina, C. Owens, Run-to-run control of meal-related insulin dosing, *Diabetes Technol Ther* **7**(1), 48-57 (2005).

Index

Philips Research Book Series

1. H.J. Bergveld, W.S. Kruijt and P.H.L. Notten: *Battery Management Systems.* 2002   ISBN 1-4020-0832-5

2. W. Verhaegh, E. Aarts and J. Korst (eds.): *Algorithms in Ambient Intelligence.* 2004   ISBN 1-4020-1757-X

3. P. van der Stok (ed.): *Dynamic and Robust Streaming in and between Connected Consumer-Electronic Devices.* 2005   ISBN 1-4020-3453-9

4. E. Meinders, A.V. Mijritskii, L. van Pieterson and M. Wuttig: *Phase-Change Optical Recording Media.* 2006   ISBN 1-4020-4216-7

5. S. Mukherjee, E. Aarts, R. Roovers, F. Widdershoven and M. Ouwerkerk (eds.): *AmIware.* Hardware Technology Drivers of Ambient Intelligence. 2006
          ISBN 1-4020-4197-7

6. G. Spekowius and T. Wendler (eds.): *Advances in Healthcare Technology.* Shaping the Future of Medical Care. 2006   ISBN 1-4020-4383-X

springer.com